Community and Population Health

Eighth Edition

Lawrence W. Green, B.S., M.P.H., Dr. P.H

Professor and Head
Division of Preventive Medicine and Health Promotion
Department of Health Care and Epidemiology;
Director, Institute of Health Promotion Research
University of British Columbia
Vancouver, British Columbia

Judith M. Ottoson, B.S.N., M.P.H., Ed.D.

Associate Professor
Department of Educational Studies
Faculty of Education
University of British Columbia
Vancouver, British Columbia

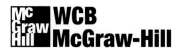
WCB
McGraw-Hill

Boston   Burr Ridge, IL   Dubuque, IA   Madison, WI   New York   San Francisco   St. Louis
Bangkok   Bogotá   Caracas   Lisbon   Madrid
Mexico City   Milan   New Delhi   Seoul   Singapore   Sydney   Taipei   Toronto

WCB/McGraw-Hill

A Division of The **McGraw·Hill** *Companies*

Vice president and editorial director: *Kevin T. Kane*
Publisher: *Edward E. Bartell*
Executive editor: *Vicki Malinee*
Developmental editor: *Sarah Reed*
Marketing manager: *Pamela S. Cooper*
Senior project manager: *Peggy J. Selle*
Production supervisor: *Mary E. Haas*
Coordinator of freelance design: *Michelle D. Whitaker*
Photo research coordinator: *Lori Hancock*
Compositor: *Shepherd, Inc.*
Typeface: *10/12 Times Roman*
Printer: *R. R. Donnelley & Sons Company/Crawfordsville, IN*

Freelance cover designer: *Mary Nowakowski, Cunningham & Welch Design Group, Inc.*
Cover illustration: © *Boris Lyubner; Stock Illustration Source*

Library of Congress Cataloging-in-Publication Data

Green, Lawrence W.
    [Community health]
    Community and population health / Lawrence W. Green, Judith M.
Ottoson. — 8th ed.
        p.   cm.
    Previous eds. published under the title: Community health.
    Includes bibliographical references and index.
    ISBN 0–8151–2542–9
    1. Public health.   2. Public health—United States.   I. Ottoson,
Judith M.   II. Title.
    RA425.G73   1999   98–15984
    362.1—dc21   CIP

www.mhhe.com

Coming together is a beginning,
Staying together is progress,
Working together is success,
Laughing together makes it all worthwhile

Contents in Brief

Contents

Part Five
Health Organization, Resources, and Services 551

Preface

Community health has evolved at the intersection of many disciplines and sectors working locally or regionally. Their common purpose has been to blend the influences of public health, school health, occupational health, social and recreational services, mass media, housing, transportation, self-care, and mutual aid in the service of whole populations. The growing scope and magnitude of influences on local populations from outside the local community has forced the recognition of the limits of community health as it has been conceived and practiced in the past. We have attempted to address some of these limitations in this new edition of our book.

This eighth edition retains its essential features as a general textbook for undergraduate and introductory graduate courses in community health or public health. The change in title to include the term *population health* is mostly an acknowledgment that much of what had been called community health was increasingly the work of multiple disciplines, local organizations, and agencies with populations that do not constitute communities in the traditional sense of geographically cohesive jurisdictions. Two other departures of this edition from previous editions are its inclusion of more international comparisons and its inclusion of World Wide Web sites as resources for further pursuit of the topics and issues introduced here. These three changes are not coincidental. The expansion of the Internet and the proliferation of Web sites have signaled the growing awareness and recognition of the interconnectedness and interdependence of human populations everywhere.

Adding *Population Health* to the Title

We define population health in the glossary as "The status of a category of people with respect to their well-being and the determinants of that status." The growing recognition of categories of people who do not constitute communities, either in the geographical sense or in the organizational sense, rendered "community health" alone in the title inadequate. We continue to believe that the community is the ideal center of gravity between highly centralized planning and control of health at national, state, or provincial levels and totally decentralized control and consequent responsibility heaped on families and individuals. In the new global economies, however, communities alone no longer have the power or concentration of resources to control or look after all the needs of their residents or constituents.

Population health has emerged as an expression of the common concerns of community health and public health with the determinants of the health status of whole populations. The population groupings or the organizations addressing their health, increasingly, may not share common territory, except the earth itself. Public health has tended to emphasize governmental responsibility at all levels for the protection of the health of populations. Community health has tended to emphasize the joint responsibility of governmental health agencies and other organizations and sectors for local collaborative action to achieve improvements in health. It was easier in the past to equate local with community, but community has taken on other meanings, and local health action has become increasingly regional and dependent on broader social determinants of health.

Recent Developments

Since 1993 when our seventh edition went to press, momentous historical developments have buffeted a rapidly changing landscape for community and population health. The Liberal Party formed a new government in Canada under Jean Chrétien in a wave of dissatisfaction with the economy and strong public sentiment to preserve the health care system that had been criticized in the American health care reform debates. In 1994, the 103rd Congress of the United States and the governments of Canada and Mexico approved the North American Free Trade Agreement. This has made the North American countries increasingly interdependent. In the same year and the years since, the U.S. Congress has failed to pass health care reform proposals that would have brought U.S. and Canadian health systems into greater alignment. We have attempted to reflect these changes by giving greater attention to the comparisons of U.S. and Canadian experiences.

Soon after the seventh edition was published in 1994, the U.S. Congress also passed a major crime bill with a ban on assault weapons, inspired in part by the differences in firearm-related deaths and injuries between the United States and Canada. Congress also passed that year the Brady law, requiring a waiting period for handgun purchases; the Family and Medical Leave Act; an abortion clinic access bill; and a national service program to encourage young people in community service. Besides health care reform, Congress also failed to pass proposed campaign finance and lobby reform, Congressional reorganization, welfare reform, and the Superfund overhaul, all of which were debated in the Congressional elections of that year, and held out as possibilities in the seventh edition of this book.

When the 104th Congress convened in January 1995, President Clinton was in his third year and a new Republican majority controlled the House and Senate. They presented an ambitious legislative program of downsizing federal budgets in their "Contract with America." Budget deadlocks between Congress and the White House resulted in two partial shutdowns of the U.S. government in 1995 and 1996. In one of its most significant actions for population health, Congress repealed the national highway speed limits. In 1995, Canada passed its own extensions of gun control and struggled with a national scandal over tainted blood supplies.

In 1996, the 104th Congress would have dealt further blows to community and population health if the President had not exercised effective vetoes. One was an abortion bill that would have banned an abortion method known as late-term or partial-birth abortion. Congress did pass and the President signed laws reforming welfare and health insurance. Landmark welfare legislation authorized states to establish their own welfare programs using block grants from the federal government. It required most adult recipients to find work within two years, established a lifetime limit of five years on welfare, restricted benefits to noncitizens, and abolished the Aid to Families with Dependent Children (AFDC) program. In response to the most urgent needs denied by the failure of health care reform, the Health Insurance Portability and Accountability Act (formerly the Kennedy-Katzenbaum bill) provided continued coverage for workers who changed jobs and prevented insurance companies from withholding insurance from people with preexisting medical conditions. Finally, Congress passed the Safe Drinking Water amendments requiring municipalities to report on levels of contaminants and establishing a federal fund to upgrade water systems.

On a global scale, the population health story of the year in 1996 was the report of the British government commission on its problem with Mad Cow Disease in its cattle industry. This sent shock waves through the international food industries (rippling still into 1998 with the legal battle between the U.S. cattle industry and TV host Oprah Winfrey). It spooked consumers over food safety more than the earlier outbreaks of salmonella in hamburgers and unpasteurized juices in North America. At the same time, North Americans found encouraging statistical trends reported in the mid-decade review of progress toward the *Healthy People 2000* objectives in the United States and population health reviews in Canada. These showed that crime rates were coming steadily down, teenage pregnancy rates had begun to drop, the number of Americans living below the poverty line dropped, and some 1.4 million Americans moved off food stamps since participation in the program peaked at nearly 28 million people in 1994. On the other side of the ledger, the United States and Canada noted a rise in teenage drug use after more than a decade of steady declines. The number of managed care enrollees tripled from 1993 to 1995. Mortality from heart disease and stroke continued their declines, but these masked an ominous development of an obesity epidemic and the leveling off of the declines in smoking rates.

The population health story of the year in 1997 was the crumbling of the tobacco industry's stonewall against admitting fault in tobacco-related deaths. As the federal-industry negotiations to protect the industry against lawsuits unraveled, the states marched on in their legal initiatives to recover health costs from tobacco manufacturers. In 1994, Mississippi filed the first of these lawsuits to recover smoking-related Medicaid costs. In 1995, in other states, Blue Cross and Blue Shield also filed suits. Whistle blowers within tobacco companies revealed industry attempts to target adolescents and to conceal research on nicotine addiction. In 1996, the Liggett Group broke with other tobacco companies, agreeing to settle its share of the Mississippi suit. In 1997, the tobacco industry settled with forty states for $368.5 billion and changes to the way the industry advertises and does business, in exchange for protection from future suits in these states. Tobacco stocks rose on Wall Street on news of these settlements, but the blanket protection sought with the federal negotiations was not signed by the president. In 1998, British Columbia announced the appointment of a legal team to undertake the first Canadian provincial initiative to file suit against the industry under its Tobacco Damages Recovery Act.

Crossing the Millennium

As we review recent developments, this book also provides a historical look at the advances and changes in community health and the challenges remaining for the twenty-first century. While safe water exists in much of the developed world, it is still threatened at times such as the great floods of 1996 and the ice storms and El Niño floods of 1998 when parts of the United States and Canada were once again boiling water to assure its safety. While some of the infectious diseases that killed populations in this last millennium are long conquered, new threats exist such as HIV/AIDS and "superbugs" resistant to antibiotics. We also carry into the new millennium the consequences of past lifestyle and environmental choices, such as smoking and pollution. While political and moral debates continue over issues such as abortion, new ethical dimensions are pressed with the arrival of Dolly the cloned sheep. Will human cloning follow? These are just some of the debates and issues addressed in this revised edition. While some of these challenges call for new strategies based on research and technological approaches, others bring us back to educational and public health basics. The past is prolog.

Features

Readability   We continually work to make this book comprehensive and reader friendly. We have shortened average sentence length in each chapter and defined more terms in the glossary.

Pedagogy   We have added "Issues and Controversies" boxes to engage the reader more actively in the content and to provoke critical thinking. WebLinks are provided at the end of each chapter listing several Internet addresses that can provide additional resources for some of the information discussed in the chapter. A number of informational boxes appear within each chapter to provide added detail on some of the material mentioned in the text.

Illustrations, Photos, and Tables We have replaced almost all of the figures and charts, photographs and tables with new illustrations or data. This has the advantage of giving the new edition a more contemporary and fresh look, and bringing the data up to date. It also means, however, that many of our favorite illustrations and some memorable ones that readers liked will have been sacrificed on the cutting room floor. We encourage instructors to refer back to the previous editions for classroom use of copies of those illustrations that they found most helpful.

Global Impact Our comparison of U.S. and Canadian systems, and contrasts with other systems, are intended to help understand options, as both the United States and Canada face health care reform and health care renewal proposals. In the emerging global economy, no country can afford to be isolated in its view of systems accounting for more than 10 percent of their Gross National Product, as the health care systems do in the United States and Canada. These two countries have the highest expenditures as a percentage of their GNP of any of the western countries. This is more significant when one considers the greater military proportion of budgets these two countries must bear as part of their international peacekeeping and policing responsibilities.

Format As in past editions, the book is divided into five major sections: foundations, health through the life span, promoting community health, environmental health protection, and health resources and services.

Chapter Format One or two paragraphs at the beginning of each section provide organization and continuity. Each chapter begins with a set of objectives, includes updated information, uses case studies and contemporary issues to provoke discussions, and ends with a chapter summary, questions for review, annotated readings, and an updated bibliography.

Glossary and Appendices A glossary defines important terms identified in boldface type when they first appear in the text. Three appendices supplement the content by summarizing areas of community health specialization, common job titles, and graduate degree programs for public and community health accredited by the Council on Education for Public Health.

Supplements The accompanying *Instructor's Manual and Test Bank* have been overhauled thanks to the work of our coauthor Dr. Robert Cadman. New questions have been added to the test bank and all answers confirmed against the text. The Manual's practicality is enhanced by the following: chapter overviews; additional objectives; student assignments; late-breaking headlines; additional resources including web sites; easy test questions; and transparency masters of important illustrations, diagrams, tables, and charts. These transparencies were chosen to help the instructor explain difficult concepts and to illustrate key points.

A computerized test bank is also available to qualified adopters in IBM and Macintosh formats. This allows the instructor to select, edit, delete, or add questions and construct and print tests and answer keys.

Updated Web Site The authors will be maintaining a web site at *http://www.ihpr.ubc.ca* to provide updates and new information related to the contents of the eighth edition of *Community and Population Health*. Students will be able to get late-breaking information on the topics of each chapter.

Acknowledgments

To the students and instructors whose classrooms tested the previous editions, we express sincere thanks again. We also thank the following reviewers whose contributions are reflected in this revision:

Debbie Godfrey-Brown, University of Rhode Island
C. James Frankish, University of British Columbia

Dawn Larson, Mankato State University
Mary Beth Love, San Francisco State University
David Sleet, U.S. Centers for Disease Control and Prevention
Mary Beth Tighe, The Ohio State University

We thank the graduate students, postdoctoral fellows, visiting scholars, faculty associates, and staff, especially Mary Sun, at the University of British Columbia Institute of Health Promotion Research. The Department of Health Care and Epidemiology in the Faculty of Medicine and the Department of Educational Studies in the UBC Faculty of Education also have proved hospitable homes to study health from a community perspective. The importance of engaging populations in their own health and that of their communities reveals itself in the coming chapters. We have had the opportunity to interact with many of the disciplines, professions, and organizations in communities across the United States and Canada that seek to develop their community health resources and programs. Conducting workshops and seminars on these topics over the last few years in Australia, Indonesia, Israel, Italy, Japan, Kuwait, the United Arab Emirates, and Spain have added to our international understanding of community and population health. We are especially indebted to Rob Sanson-Fisher and Newcastle University in Australia and the Azienda Unita Sanitaria Locale of Reggio Emilia in Northern Italy for providing sabbatical opportunities to study community and population health in contexts outside North America.

Among the sponsors of research we have drawn upon in this edition, we are indebted to the Social Sciences and Humanities Research Council, the National Health Research Development Program, the National Cancer Institute of Canada, the Center for Substance Abuse Prevention, and the Royal Society of Canada.

Finally, thanks to family and friends who have promoted our health along the way. We are grateful to Cliff, Harry, and Helga for the strong foundations they gave and to Betty for the foundation she still provides. We hope to have honored those foundations in this book and with Beth and Doug, Jenny and Cesar, and the joyous arrival of curly-headed Madeleine, the next generation. A special thanks to Sophe who has patiently waited through the many months it has taken to finish this book. At long last, Sophe, it is time for a long walk.

LAWRENCE W. GREEN
JUDITH M. OTTOSON

PART ONE
FOUNDATIONS

This journey into community and population health begins with a look at our past and at the foundations on which the structure of community health rests. The foundations are set among our historical roots—not just the happenings of the past but the ideas from primitive to modern that linger in our collective psyche. The essence of the primitive ideas is expressed by St. Augustine, speaking to us from the beginning of the Dark Ages. He said, "All diseases are to be ascribed to demons." The *scientific* foundations of community health, resting sometimes tenuously among these historical roots, address the determinants of health between two of the four components of the health field: *human biology* and *environment*. These are represented in community health by human ecology, demography, and epidemiology. The other two components of the health field are *lifestyle* and *health care organization*. These are represented in community health by the social and behavioral sciences, including political science, economics, and health education.

Chapter *1*

Through the Centuries

*P*rogress might have been all right once, but it's gone on too long.

—Ogden Nash

*Y*ou must be the change you wish to see in the world.

—Mahatma Gandhi

Objectives

When you finish this chapter, you should be able to:

- Distinguish between community health and other forms of population health
- Identify the three essential strategies of community and population health (health promotion, health protection, and health services)

- Describe examples of how the strategies have been reflected in the customs, beliefs, codes, laws, and programs of the major historical eras

Since its founding in 1948, the World Health Organization (**WHO**) has defined **health** as a state of complete physical, mental, and social well-being, not the mere absence of disease or infirmity. Social **well-being** entails the history that has caused a particular population or community to accept some conditions that another community would define as unacceptable. Community health reflects the philosophy, religion, economics, form of government, education, science, aspirations, and folklore of any period. The history of community health chronicles the advances and declines of societies and human conditions. People also define what they consider advances and declines, acceptable and unacceptable conditions. As expressed by

Sir Godfrey Vickers, "The history of public health might well be written as a record of successive redefinings of the unacceptable."

Consider your own community's history over the past few years, with population and industrial growth or decline, with economic improvements or recessions. The headlines related to health in your local newspapers might include issues of abortion, legalization of drugs, increased speed limits, gun control, the aging population, air bags, computer linkage of medical and vital registration records, and smoke-free restaurants. Such controversies reflect community responses to trends in health and technology. They reflect attempts to shape the history of health and community development. Some people regard the reforms signaled by these issues as social advances. Other people see them as infringements of their individual rights or freedoms.

Social collapses in Zaire, Rwanda, and the former Yugoslavia illustrate how civilization depends on the quality and distribution of health in the general population. Population health in turn depends on human advancement and community development in various spheres, not just in the health or medical sector. Cast in historical context, community and population health are the cumulative results of lifestyles and the environment. They are also a barometer of cultural and social conditions that have shaped lifestyles and the environment.

WHAT ARE COMMUNITY AND POPULATION HEALTH?

These characterizations of community or population health might make them seem only the passive consequence of history. Community and population health promotion also represent dynamic human enterprises that shape history. People devote their careers and organizations devote their missions to the promotion or protection of community or population health. Some do so through their influence in other sectors, causing change in transportation, commerce, conservation, welfare, agriculture, housing, law enforcement, recreation, and education, all of which influence health.

Community health refers to the health status of a community and to the organized responsibilities of public health, school health, transportation safety, and other tax-supported functions, with voluntary and private actions, to promote and protect the health of local populations identified as communities. Some populations cannot meet the criteria of a community or do not identify as a community. Chapter 2 will define "community" more fully. **Population health** refers to the health status and the conditions (not necessarily organized) influencing the health of a category of people (for example, women, adolescents, prisoners) whether the people define themselves as a community or not. A population could be a segment of

a community, or a category of people in the several communities of a region. The fundamental distinction between population and community is the degree of organization and identity. Populations may have little or no organization and identity as a group or locality. Communities are one type of population who do have organized arrangements and mutual identity with each other or with their common circumstances.

Community health and *population health* as descriptive terms, with the action terms *promotion, protection,* and *services,* produce six combinations. These combined terms, community health promotion, population health promotion, community health protection, population health protection, community health services, and population health services, identify the targets or channels (community or population) and the strategies for improving or protecting health. These emphasize the collaborative efforts of various public and private sectors in relation to the health of communities or populations. **Community health promotion** seeks to activate *local* organizations and groups or individuals to cause changes in behavior (lifestyle, selfcare, mutual aid, participation in community or political action) or in rules or policies that influence health. These include public health practice; school health practice; the professional practices of medical, dental, nursing, and allied health personnel; and the personal health practices of individuals and families. Community health promotion lies in the areas in which these spheres overlap, as shown in figure 1-1. Additional spheres of action overlap with these and contribute to community health, but usually as a by-product of their primary purposes. Such additional spheres include the worksite, in which employee health promotion, safety, and screening programs address adult health much as school health programs do for children. In addition, the recreational system and the legal system contribute to community health promotion in performing their primary functions. The coordination and integration of these spheres of action make up the practice of community health promotion.

. . . .
Figure 1-1

Overlapping spheres of health action. This book concentrates on the shaded areas in which sectors collaborate to achieve community health and the ways in which the other spheres contribute to population health.

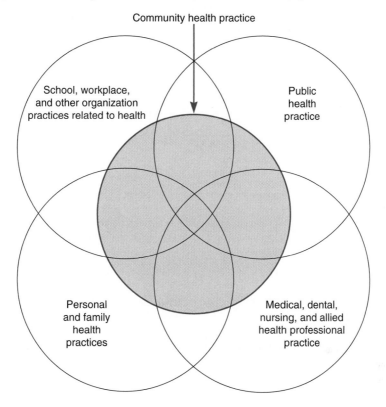

Community health practice

School, workplace, and other organization practices related to health

Public health practice

Personal and family health practices

Medical, dental, nursing, and allied health professional practice

Population health promotion differs from community health promotion only in the scope of the people whose health it might address. The people constituting a population might be residing in multiple communities, states, provinces, or even nations. This might call for health promotion or advocacy efforts at the regional, state, provincial, national, or international levels. The people constituting a population could live within a single community, but might be a defined segment of that community that does not identify itself as a community or subcommunity. A demographic segment might include, for example, all adult males, all women over fifty, all blue-collar workers, or all people living in public housing. These categories do not necessarily lead people to identify themselves as a community. Similarly, the segmentation of the population might be epidemiological, based on disease or risk categories such as all people with diabetes or all people with poor eating habits.

Community health protection is described in part 4 of this book and **community health services** in part 5. These differ from community health promotion in the nature or timing of the actions. Protection and services imply implementing laws, rules, or policies previously passed in the community as a result of health promotion or legislative effort. The work to be done after promotion and passage of the policy, law, or rule is **enforcement** or implementation. This might include

· · · · · · · · · · · · · · · · · · ·

Figure 1-2

Relationships between the strategies in health services, health protection and health promotion, the processes of change they seek to set into motion, the three modifiable determinants of health they can influence, and the ultimate health and social benefits they are expected to yield. (Adapted from Green LW: Prevention and health education in clinical, school, and community settings. In Wallace RB, editor: *Public health and preventive medicine,* ed. 14, Norwalk, CN, 1998, Appleton and Lange.)

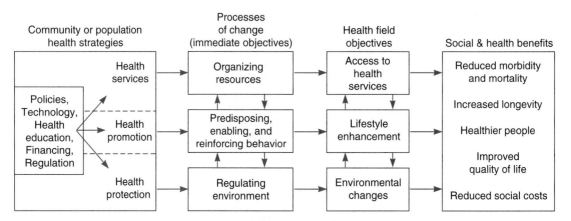

the building of a new water treatment plant, enforcement of highway speed limits and drunk-driving laws, and fines for selling cigarettes to minors. It could include closing of restaurants that violate food handling codes, withdrawal of building permits from contractors who fail to meet housing codes in their construction, or confiscation of firearms carried illegally. Figure 1-2 shows how the population health strategies of promotion, protection, and services relate to each other and the health of populations, whether in communities or in broader regions.

Health promotion, as described in part 3 of this book, is any combination of educational and social supports for people taking greater control of and improving their health. If it is *community* health promotion, the people live in and identify with a geographically defined area, and they use community as a vehicle for change. Health promotion uses educational supports to motivate, enable, and reinforce the actions of high-risk individuals, families, or groups; decision makers; or whole communities through the mass media, schools, industry, and other organizations. *Social* supports

may take the form of economic, political, legal, and organizational changes designed to support actions conducive to health. These actions may include those of the people whose health is in question and the actions of community decision makers, professionals, peers, teachers, employers, parents, and others who may influence health.

Organized community effort defines community health. Some things the individual can do entirely alone, but many health benefits they can attain only through collective action or united community effort. Community health promotion seeks to make the fruits of health science available to all local residents. Population health often requires appeal to higher levels of governmental or social action because the population at risk lives in multiple communities. The population whose health is in question may live dispersed among neighborhoods of a single community or work in various industries. Communities usually attempt to address such dispersion through health promotion, health protection or health services with a **coalition** of multiple organizations within the community.

HISTORY OF COMMUNITY AND POPULATION HEALTH

Other than carvings and drawings, such as the murals on cave walls in Spain recording physical deformities around 25,000 B.C., the earliest records of community health practices were those of the Chinese, Egyptians, and Babylonians.

Chinese Health Practices

The Yellow River region of China, one of the world's most ancient cultural centers, gave birth to Chinese history and health practices. Ancient inscriptions on tortoise shells, and later evidence in books and historic relics, indicate that people dug wells for drinking as early as the Xia and Shang dynasties (twenty-first to eleventh centuries B.C.). Ruins of the Yin dynasty reveal ditches around houses for draining rain water. The Zhou dynasty of the eleventh to seventh century B.C. yields documents mentioning methods of protecting drinking water, killing rats, and preventing rabies. By the second century B.C., Qin dynasty (221 to 207 B.C.) communities had sewers, water spray carts, and latrines.

Accompanying these early environmental health references in Chinese history, many writings from 770 B.C. to the present mention personal hygiene, lifestyle, and preventive medical practices. Confucius (541–479 B.C.) said in the *Anelects: Xiang Dang,* "Putrid fish . . . food with unusual colors . . . food with odd tastes . . . food not well cooked is not to be eaten." Similar wisdom from other sages advised Chinese people to eat, sleep, drink, and work in moderation and with regularity rather than with excess. The Chinese made their tea with boiling water as early as the Tang dynasty (A.D. 618 to 907), protecting themselves from infectious intestinal diseases.

Confucian thought had widespread influence, especially on the rest of Asia. Chinese explorers and traders opened routes to the West and carried herbal medicines and diagnostic and preventive concepts. These included feeling the pulse and acupuncture.

The Sayings of Confucius on Lifestyle and the Pulse

The Master said, "There are three things against which a gentleman should be on his guard. In youth, before his pulse has settled down, he is on his guard against lust. Having reached his prime, when his pulse has become strong, he is on his guard against strife. Having reached old age, when his pulse declines, he is on his guard against avarice."

How did Confucius know about variations of the pulse with age in the fifth century B.C. when the concept of feeling the pulse did not appear in western medical books until the seventeenth century A.D.? How did he use the concept to relate his advice on life cycle, lifestyle, and self-discipline?

Egyptian and Babylonian Health Practices

Excavations in the Nile region, another river cradle of civilization, reveal that the Egyptians had community systems for collecting rain water and for disposing of sewage. Herodotus, in the fifth century B.C., described the hygienic customs of the Egyptians, emphasizing personal cleanliness, frequent baths, simple dress and the use of earth closets for human wastes.

Hammurabi, a great monarch of Babylon who lived around 1900 B.C., formulated a set of laws. Called the Code of Hammurabi, they governed the conduct of physicians and prescribed healthful practices.

Although highly spiritual and astrological in their interpretations of cause and effect, the Egyptians applied knowledge with practicality for the community's protection. They attributed alcoholic intoxication, for example, to the spirits inhabiting the fruit used to make the drink. They regarded the consequences of using alcohol as beneficial in moderation but socially troublesome in excess. One of the oldest temperance tracts, advocating moderation, written in Egypt about 1000 B.C., had text translated as follows: "Don't drink yourself helpless in the beer garden. You speak, and you don't know what you are saying. If you fall down and break your limbs, no one will help you. And your drinking companions will get up and say 'Away with this drunkard.' "

Similar sentiments appeared later in Chinese, Greek, Roman, Indian, and Japanese writings, and in the Old and New Testaments, tolerating alcohol but denouncing excessive drinking and drunkenness.

Hebrew Mosaic Law

The Mosaic law or code of early Hebrew society extended Egyptian ideas of promoting community health through the regulation of human conduct. Human behavior is fundamental in population and individual health. With the Hebrews, a weekly day of rest was a health measure and a religious measure. The Mosaic code channeled family relations and sexual conduct to the interests of community health. Their crude concepts of the spread of disease nevertheless served to support their efforts at prevention. The first practice of preventive medicine was the segregation of lepers, as recorded in Leviticus. Recognition that eating pork sometimes resulted in illness led the Hebrews to regard pork as unclean and later to forbid it in the Jewish diet.

The Mosaic law or code provided for some of the essential elements of modern community health. These included (1) personal and community responsibility for health, (2) maternal health, (3) control of communicable diseases, (4) fumigation, (5) decontamination of buildings, (6) protection of water supplies, (7) disposal of wastes, (8) protection of food, and (9) sanitation of campsites. The Jews lacked fundamental knowledge of the nature of infectious disease spread. Hebrew society nevertheless mobilized community forces against conditions associated with health problems.

The Physical Ideals of Greece

The Classic Greek era extended over the years 460 to 136 B.C. The Greeks excelled in games and gymnastics directed toward their ideal of physical strength, endurance, dexterity, and grace. Harmonious development of all faculties was the guiding philosophy. They supplemented exercise with measures in personal cleanliness. Hippocrates wrote of the relationship of diet to health around 400 B.C. The Classic Period emphasized the individual, as reflected in the Hippocratic Oath. As a consequence, the Greeks of that era gave little attention to environmental protection (see box on page 9). Hippocrates, nevertheless, wrote a definitive treatise on environment and health with his *Airs, Waters, and Places.*

The Greeks did not borrow health practices from other nations. The Hindus of ancient India had practiced surgery for at least a century, but there is no evidence that the Greeks used the Hindu methods of surgery, despite Alexander's conquests on the Indian subcontinent (figure 1-3).

The Roman Empire

The fall of Corinth in 146 B.C. led to a migration of the health knowledge and practices of the Greeks to Rome where the rising Roman Empire welcomed them. In the philosophy of the Romans, however, the state, not the individual, was of primary importance. To the Romans, the individual existed merely to serve the state. With this extreme emphasis on the importance of the state, the influence of Greek hygiene soon faded.

The Romans applied their advanced military, administrative, and engineering sciences in their many community health projects. The registration of citizens and slaves and the taking of a periodic census served to help in planning community health measures, although their primary purpose was mercenary. The Romans innovated modern health protection measures such as regulation of building construction, the prevention of sewage in the streets, and the destruction of decaying goods and buildings. Building regulations provided for ventilation and central heating. Town planning served sanitation through the construction of paved streets with gutters. Street cleaning and repair were standard procedures in the interest of sanitation, although modern health officials regard such measures as serving esthetic more than health objectives. The Romans undertook drainage networks to carry off rain and other water, removal of garbage and rubbish, and public baths as community health measures.

Figure 1-3

Contemporary health problems portrayed in historical perspective tend to idealize the accomplishments and the health of Ancient Greek civilization, but wars took a greater toll than today, and lives were short, even without cigarettes. (Courtesy Office on Smoking and Health, Centers for Disease Control, U.S. Public Health Service.)

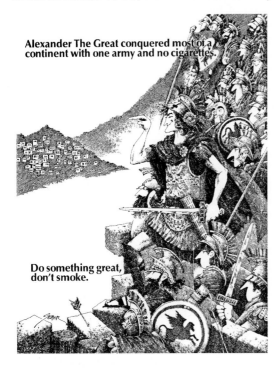

Alexander The Great conquered most of a continent with one army and no cigarettes.

Do something great, don't smoke.

Atmospheric Pollution Began in Ancient Greece and Rome

The Greek and Roman civilizations began the mass production of silver coins more than 2,000 years ago, spewing lead from their smelter emissions into the atmosphere. Recent evidence of pollution reaching the remote Arctic region has been dated in ice samples in the Greenland ice core to these oldest sources of hemispheric pollution. Samples from 500 B.C. to 300 A.D. contained lead in concentrations four times that found in the pre-lead production period. These amounted to 15% of the quantity of lead fallout caused by the modern use of lead additives in gasoline, now outlawed in North America.

Could the Greek or Roman governments have known of the damage they might do to the health of their citizens with lead smeltering? How does a point source of pollution such as a manufacturing plant differ from a diffuse source such as automobile exhausts from the standpoint of environmental protection?

Roman officials had sufficient understanding of health to provide a protected water supply for their cities. Rome brought water from great distances by way of aqueducts, some of which are still incorporated into the water system of Rome. Some of the city sewer systems built during the earliest period still provide drains that serve as part of the current sewer system of Rome. This ability of the Romans to design and construct public water and sewer systems enabled Rome to grow to 800,000 people during the reign of Julius Caesar. The Greek dependence on family wells and private refuse disposal limited the size to which their cities could grow. Corinth at the pinnacle of its greatness had a population of only 35,000.

Most historians attribute the downfall of the Western empire to social degeneration. The term **Byzantine,** which refers to the Eastern Roman Empire, connotes bureaucracy, luxury, and sloth. Even in this atmosphere, Galen (A.D. 130 to 201) did some experimentation relating to health, but his dogmatism limited the value of his work. In contrast to Galen's attempt at least to understand disease was Saint Augustine's (A.D. 354 to 430) foreshadowing of the Dark Ages: "All diseases are to be ascribed to demons."

Dark Ages

The Dark Ages generally refers to the early centuries (A.D. 476 to 1000) of the medieval period of history. Western civilization was in a chaotic, almost formless, state. The only existing science fostered by the state was but a trifle. The emphasis of the time was on the spiritual aspects of life because the clergy were the only educated class. Rejection of the body and glorification of the spirit became the accepted pattern of behavior. The

Church considered it immoral to see one's naked body. People seldom bathed, and they wore dirty garments. The use of perfumes appears to have stemmed from the attempt to conceal body and other unpleasant odors about the person. The more one could neglect and abuse one's body, the more esteemed one was. A legendary example of body neglect is that of Saint Stylites, who sat on top of a pole for sixteen years to expose his body to the abuse of the elements. It was as though health itself had been defined as unacceptable. The poor diets of the time resulted in the use of spices to overcome the bad odor and the foul taste of the food. Masking the symptoms rather than removing the cause of the problems has always retarded the development of community health.

During the sixth and seventh centuries, Islam rose to prominence. After the death of Mohammed, a series of pilgrimages to Mecca began. A cholera epidemic followed each pilgrimage. All through history migrations have been a vehicle for the spread of disease.

Leprosy spread from Egypt to Asia Minor and then to Europe. Most nations decreed lepers "civilly dead," stripping them of their civil rights. They required lepers to wear identifying clothing and to warn of their presence by a bell or a horn. This isolation, however, together with the early death of lepers, almost eliminated leprosy in Europe.

Medieval Pandemics

The later medieval period, from A.D. 1000 to about 1453, is of special interest because of the severe **pandemics** of the time and the attempts to deal with the spread of disease. (*Pandemics* are widespread epidemics, usually affecting more than one country; **epidemics** are outbreaks of a disease that has spread through a population.) Between the years 1096 and 1248, the six great crusades to the Holy Land were of health significance. Providing crusaders fit for the long journey required attention to building the best possible level of health. While the approach was similar to that of the ancient Greeks in building physical prowess, the general result was to improve well-being in only one segment of the population. However, in their journeys the crusaders picked up cholera and spread it; their death rate from it was high.

In 1348 bubonic plague, or the **Black Death,** carved a devastating path from Asia to Africa, the Crimea, Turkey, Greece, Italy, and up through Europe. From 1348 to 1350, 20 percent of the population of Europe died from some combination of bubonic plague and pulmonary anthrax. The deaths in several of the large cities in Europe illustrate the devastation of the pandemic: Paris, 50,000; Seine, 70,000; Marseilles, 16,000 in one month; Vienna, 1,200 daily. The Italian writer Boccaccio reported Florence forgot pity and humanity in its 1348 outbreak of plague. Families deserted their sick. In England 2 million died, representing approximately half the population of the country. London had 100,000 deaths. Over a number of years London's deaths exceeded its births. Had it not been for the influx of people from the rural areas, London's population would have declined steadily. Estimates that approximately 25 million people died of the Black Death in Europe attest to the virulence of the bubonic plague.

Control Measures   The public attributed pandemics variously to storms, comets, famines, drought, crop failures, insects, and poisoning of wells by the Jews. Discerning officials of various communities recognized the possible relationship of crowding, poor sanitation, and migrations to the outbreak and spread of disease. Some communities took steps to establish control measures. In 1377 the city of Rogusa ruled that travelers from plague areas should stop at designated places and remain there free of disease for two months before being allowed to enter the city. Technically, this is the first official **quarantine** method on record. In 1383 Marseilles passed the first quarantine law and erected the first official quarantine station. In Venice the government appointed three guardians of public health and in 1374 denied entry to the city of infected or suspected travelers, ships, or freight. In 1403 Venice imposed a quarantine of forty days on anyone suspected of having the disease.

ISSUES AND CONTROVERSIES
Epidemics in Historical Perspective

Epidemics and pandemics of dreaded diseases have always aroused irrational fears and prejudices. Victims of disease will be ostracized by society, shunned by some members of the medical community, abandoned by some family and friends. Religious fundamentalists will attribute the victims' suffering to God's wrath and just punishment for perversion and sin. As early as 4000 B.C. in Egypt, leprosy evoked the same response; as did the Antonine plague (probably measles) in classical Rome; syphilis and bubonic plague in medieval Europe; cholera and tuberculosis in eighteenth and nineteenth century Europe and North America; and influenza, polio, and Legionnaire's disease in twentieth century North America.

With each epidemic, hysteria develops as a second epidemic. People first deny the reality of the disease, then they search for scapegoats, and then they rush to magical and commercially exploitative cures and protectors. Finally, they isolate the victims and suspected carriers of the disease until society becomes sufficiently educated about the modes of transmission of the disease to treat the victims with greater understanding and compassion.

Epidemics also influence the course of history. Bubonic plague contributed to the collapse of the European economic system, including the bonds of feudalism. Syphilis ushered in dramatic changes in puritanical lifestyles of the Victorian era.

When it first began to be reported in 1981, HIV/AIDS, still without a name, was thought not to be contagious (denial), then dubbed a gay disease, later a Haitian disease, and still later an intravenous drug user's disease (scapegoating). Eventually people began turning to commercial and religious sources for help or protection (exploitation) when the medical profession offered little comfort. They treated victims as "untouchables," barred children from school, and undertakers shunned the bodies of dead AIDS victims (social isolation). How will HIV/AIDS influence modern history? How can communities ensure greater compassion for the carriers of the HIV virus and the victims of AIDS?

Measures to control the spread of disease were not highly effective. The need was for a scientific understanding of the cause and nature of disease and its spread. Scholars of the time who turned to the scientific approach to pestilence suffered public persecution. As a consequence of such resistance, there was little progress in the understanding of disease control or health promotion.

Renaissance

The **Renaissance** represented a revival of learning that germinated in Italy, stimulated by the fall of Constantinople in 1453. For many historians the Renaissance, as the term applies to western and northern Europe, encompasses the period from A.D. 1453 to 1600.

From the standpoint of community health, the Renaissance was particularly important because of

its movement away from **scholasticism** and toward realism. An age of individual scientific endeavor, it ushered in a spirit of inquiry that would lead to the understanding of the cause and nature of infectious disease. The fifteenth and sixteenth centuries produced such distinguished figures as Copernicus, da Vinci, Vesalius, Galileo, and Gilbert. By the middle of the sixteenth century, scholars had differentiated influenza, smallpox, tuberculosis, bubonic plague, leprosy, impetigo, scabies, erysipelas, anthrax, and trachoma. They viewed diphtheria and scarlet fever as one disease but differentiated them from all other diseases.

Fracastoro (1478–1553), a physician of Verona, theorized in 1546 that microorganisms caused disease. He also recognized that sexual relations transmitted syphilis. Learning advanced, but increasing social concentration, expanding trade,

Occupational Health in History

Grinders in the sixteenth century inhaled the silica dust from their grinding and contracted silicosis, or "grinder's disease" as it was known then. Silicosis is common today among U.S. sandblasters in shipbuilding and other industries. For more than thirty years, the United States failed to follow the lead of Great Britain in banning the use of silica in sandblasting operations.

What progress does the law in Great Britain represent for community health? What is the process of the diffusion or spread of problems and progress from one country to another?

and movement of populations tended to spread disease. Knowledge of communicable disease control lagged behind disease spread, and great plagues still harassed Europe.

Colonial Period

As Europeans colonized the rest of the world from 1600 to 1800, community health in North America, Australia, Africa, Asia, and South America responded to health problems in Europe and the contributions that European scholars made to health.

Community Health in Europe   Between 1600 and 1665 Europe suffered three severe pandemics of bubonic plague. The plight of London indicates the severity of the outbreaks. In 1603 a sixth of London's population died of the plague. In 1625 another sixth of the population and in 1665 one out of five of London's residents died from the same disease.

This era produced Descartes (1596–1650), Voltaire (1694–1778), and Boyle (1627–1691). Boyle, an Englishman, recognized the need to analyze the spoiling of food "to give a fair account of certain diseases (fevers as well as others) which will perhaps be never properly understood without an insight into the doctrine of fermentation." William Harvey (1578–1657) fairly accurately described the circulation of human blood. In 1661 Captain John Graunt completed the first study on

vital statistics. In 1658 Thomas Sydenham of England made a differential diagnosis of scarlet fever, malaria, dysentery, and cholera. Some historians contended that most of Sydenham's discoveries were accidental, but chance favors the disciplined mind. Sydenham's methods showed the way for a science of epidemiology.

Athanasius Kircher (1602–1680) examined the blood of plague victims using a microscope with a magnification of thirty-three diameters. This opened a new method of study. In 1676 a Dutch draper and city hall janitor, Anton van Leeuwenhoek (1632–1723), using a microscope with a magnification of 200 diameters, succeeded in seeing bacteria in scrapings from his teeth. He found he could kill them with vinegar, but he never connected this with disease or **asepsis.**

In 1693 an astronomer, Edmund Halley (1656–1742), compiled the Breslau Table of births and funerals, which represented a contribution to the growth of vital statistics. In 1762 M. A. Plenciz, a physician of Vienna, studied scarlet fever and other infectious diseases and concluded that each infectious disease was caused by a specific kind of thing. While he did not identify "thing" factually, his theory predated the discoveries of Louis Pasteur and Robert Koch by a century.

Edward Jenner (1749–1823), a British physician and son of a Gloucestershire minister, scientifically demonstrated the effectiveness of smallpox vaccination. In 1796, using matter from pustules on the arm of a milkmaid who had contracted cowpox, Dr. Jenner vaccinated a young boy. Six weeks later he inoculated the boy with smallpox virus and demonstrated that the boy was immune to smallpox. Dr. Jenner showed scientifically that inoculation with cowpox virus can produce immunity to the smallpox virus. He derived his idea of inoculating with cowpox vaccine to prevent smallpox from the practice of English peasants of allowing themselves to contract cowpox in the knowledge that they would then be safe from smallpox. Some form of smallpox vaccination had been practiced in Turkey before Dr. Jenner's time, but he usually gets credit for the first scientific vaccination.

Health in the Colonies   Only during epidemics did the British, French, Dutch, and Spanish take community health action in their colonies. Their measures consisted of isolation and quarantine. Sanitation consisted of community tidiness or general housecleaning. Social and political action was directed mostly to matters of independence, trade, and land claims (figure 1-4).

Ironically, smallpox, measles, typhus, and scarlet fever aided the European settlers of the Americas. Introduced to the East Coast by the Cabot and Gosnold expeditions, smallpox eliminated 50 percent to 90 percent of the Indians. This enabled the new settlers to colonize with little or no opposition. Smallpox took its toll among the whites as well, however, obliterating some of the early settlements. Some notable pandemics were those of the Massachusetts Bay colonies in 1633, New Netherlands (New York) in 1663, and Boston in 1752. Of Boston's 1752 population of 15,684, only 174 completely escaped the smallpox pandemic. During the life of George Washington, 90 percent of the people who attained the age of twenty-one had had smallpox, and 25 percent of those infected by smallpox died. Consider these statistics against the total eradication of smallpox from the earth declared in 1979.

Yellow fever became a bigger scourge than plague or smallpox during the eighteenth and nineteenth centuries. In 1793 Philadelphia had the greatest single epidemic in America. Of a population of about 37,000, more than 23,000 had the disease and over 4,000 of these died. A citizen's committee appointed to deal with the problem drew up the following set of regulations:

1. Avoid contact with a case.
2. Placard all infected houses.
3. Clean and air the sickroom.
4. Provide hospital accommodations for the poor.
5. Keep streets and wharves clean.
6. Encourage general hygienic measures such as quick private burials, avoidance of fatigue of mind and body, avoidance of intemperance, and adaptation of clothing to the weather.

....

Figure 1-4

Colonial North America had taken up the use of tobacco, but it was a negligible health problem compared with the infectious and communicable diseases that took most smokers' lives before heart disease, cancer, or lung disease could claim them. (Courtesy Office on Smoking and Health, Centers for Disease Control, U.S. Public Health Service.)

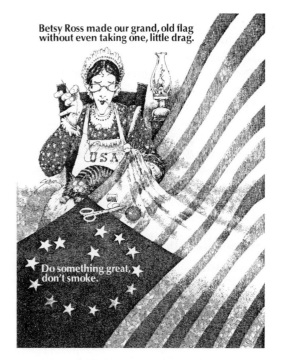

People used vinegar and camphor on handkerchiefs to prevent infection. They burned gunpowder in the streets to combat the disease. Simple and perhaps ineffective as these measures may have been, they represented a sincere attempt of communities to combat the disease based on the fragmentary knowledge people had of yellow fever. Frosty nights on October 17 and 18 ended the epidemic. Citizens of Philadelphia did not understand the "miracle," but we know that the frost killed the **Aedes aegypti** mosquito, the temporary host or vector for yellow fever. We owe a debt to Dr. Benjamin Rush for a magnificent report of the Philadelphia epidemic published in 1815.

Health science advanced in the colonial period mostly during the eighteenth century. Governments and communities addressed issues of occupational hygiene and the safety and well-being of workers. They tackled infant hygiene without any scientific basis but as a humane attempt to give better care to children. They dealt with mental hygiene with methods limited to sympathetic protection and care of the severely mentally ill. Between the years 1692 and 1708 Boston, Salem, and Jamestown passed laws dealing with nuisances and offensive trades.

The superstitions expressed in witchcraft and other practices of the time indicate that the colonial period was hardly one in which to expect any great advances in health science. In America during George Washington's time the average duration of life was about twenty-nine years. Measured by today's standards, the people who wrote the American Declaration of Independence and drew up the U.S. Constitution were extremely young. Few of them were over the age of forty.

Early Nineteenth Century

Between 1800 and 1850 North America experienced rapid industrial expansion. As remarkable as this expansion was, public health activities could not keep up, and many **outbreaks** and epidemics occurred. The rapid growth of cities outstripped other developments. Community and population health could hardly flourish under such conditions.

Community Health Promotion in England

The first half of the nineteenth century saw public health officially recognized in 1837 with community sanitation legislation in England. This indication of an awakening interest in community health led to the appointment of a Factory Commission to study the health conditions of the laboring population of the nation. The Commission laid particular emphasis on the study of child employment conditions. Edwin Chadwick, a civilian who had a special interest in social problems, wrote the Commission's 1842 "Report on the Inquiry into the

Table 1-1
Mean Age of Death and Infant Death Rates, England, 1842

	Mean age of death		Infant deaths per 1000 births
Class	London	England	(England)
Gentry, professional persons, and their families	44	35	100
Tradesmen, shopkeepers, and their families	23	22	167
Wage classes, artisans, laborers, and their families	22	15	250

Based on Chadwick. See Richardson BW: *The health of nations: a review of the works of Edwin Chadwick,* vol 2, London, 1887, Longmans Green.

Sanitary Condition of the Laboring Population of Great Britain." Chadwick's colorful descriptions of the deplorable conditions of the time had more than just a popular appeal. They aroused the determination of well-meaning people to improve the conditions of the laboring class, particularly the child employment conditions. Chadwick's report pointed out that half the children of the working classes died before their fifth birthday. The length of life data reported by Chadwick clearly indicated that inequities in living standards between the gentry and working classes produced inescapably powerful determinants of health and longevity (table 1-1).

Some of England's outstanding literary figures of the time paid the price of such appalling health conditions. Shelley died at the age of 30, Keats at 25, Byron at 36, Robert Burns at 37, Charlotte Bronte at 39, Emily Bronte at 30, and Anne Bronte at 29. On the continent, Chopin died at 40, Mendelssohn at 38, and Schubert at 31.

John Simon was appointed first medical health officer of London in 1848. England was not ready for the reforms that Chadwick's report pointed

Milestones of Colonial North America

1000 Leif Ericsson and other Vikings visit Labrador and Newfoundland

1492 Christopher Columbus claims the "New World" for Spain; he observes the natives, and later his sailors, chewing dried leaves or inhaling their smoke through pipes called "toboca," noting, "it is not within their power to refrain from indulging in the habit."

1497 John Cabot claims Cape Breton Island for England

1541 First French settlement in Americas

1625 Jesuits arrive in Quebec to begin missionary work among the Indians; in New Amsterdam (now New York), the first building law on record in North America governed the types and locations of roof coverings to prevent fire transmission from chimney sparks

1633 Smallpox pandemic of the Massachusetts Bay colonies

1634 First public park, Boston Commons, "plyce for a trayning field and for the feeding of cattell"

1639 Massachusetts colony passed the first act requiring the registration of each birth and death

1640 The Huron nation reduced by half from European diseases

1667 Canada's first census counts 3,215 nonnative inhabitants in 668 families

1746 Massachusetts Bay colonies passed regulations to prevent the pollution of Boston Harbor

1754 Beginning of French and Indian War in America; first phase of struggle between France and Britain in North America

1763 France cedes its North American possessions to Britain by the Treaty of Paris

1776 American Revolutionary War begins for independence from Britain

1780 First local Board of Health, Petersberg, Virginia

1783 American Revolutionary War ends; border between Canada and the United States accepted from Atlantic to Lake of the Woods

1793 Philadelphia epidemic of yellow fever, largest in North America

1797 State boards of health were established in New York and Massachusetts in response to yellow fever outbreaks

1799 First Board of Health, Boston, with Paul Revere as its first president

1812 The United States declares war on Britain, invades Canada from Detroit

1814 Treaty of Ghent ends the War of 1812

1818 The 49th Parallel accepted as U.S.-Canada border from Lake of the Woods to Rocky Mountains

1849 Border extended to Pacific; gold rush in California

1850 Shattuck's report on the health conditions of Massachusetts set standards for several generations and marks beginning of modern era of public health

1857 First quarantine convention met in Philadelphia

1869 First state health department organized, Massachusetts

1870 Louis Riel leads the Metis Indians in resisting Canadian authority in Canada's northwest

1872 American Public Health Association founded

1882 Ontario Board of Health established in Canada's largest province with the motto, "Let not the people perish for lack of knowledge"

1885 Metis defeated in same year as last spike of transcontinental railway is driven in British Columbia

1897 Gold rush in Klondike, stretching European influence and diseases into Eskimo and Inuit populations of last frontiers (Alaska and Yukon), in same year as first Boston Marathon

out, for Simon's general board of health lasted but four years. Nevertheless, Chadwick's report stands as a landmark in the history of population health.

Wars During the early nineteenth century wars were rampant on the American and European con-

tinents. Direct loss of life was less than the losses from epidemics or the destructive potential of modern wars. The death rate among those in battle, however, especially among those wounded, was high. Ironically, these wars contributed to medical and community health advances. In 1815,

during the Napoleonic wars, Delpech first understood the cause of the infection of wounds. Many
of the hundreds of casualties in the hospitals developed gangrene. Delpech noticed the patterns of
gangrene development with dressings on the
wounds. He theorized, fifty years before Lister developed **antiseptic** methods, that "animal-like
matter jumps from one object to another."

In the midnineteenth century the Crimean War
led to such high casualties that nursing had to in-
vent the method of **triage.** Triage sorted the injuries of battleground victims into three categories
of severity and urgency to avoid losing valuable
time and resources on those who could wait or on
those who were certain to die. The method of
triage still persists in emergency room and community disaster procedures.

Health Developments in North America
Not until the close of the first half of the nineteenth century was there a significant North
American development in community health promotion. Lemuel Shattuck (1793–1859) drew up a
health report that was to serve as a guide in the
field of health for the next century. Shattuck was
successively a teacher, historian, sociologist, statistician, and state legislator. Like Chadwick, he
was a not a health professional, but he had an intense and intelligent interest in sanitation. As appointed chair of a legislative committee to study
sanitation and health problems in the Commonwealth of Massachusetts, he wrote its report. Published in 1850, the report revealed Shattuck's insight and foresight. It charted health pathways for
many generations. Many of its provisions remain
to be fully attained. This remarkable document reveals its contemporary relevance in its various
recommendations:

1. Establish state and local boards of health.
2. Collect and analyze vital statistics.
3. Exchange health information.
4. Initiate sanitation programs for towns and
   buildings.
5. Maintain a system of sanitary inspections.

6. Study the health of schoolchildren.
7. Conduct research on tuberculosis.
8. Study and supervise health conditions of
   immigrants.
9. Supervise mental disease.
10. Control alcoholism.
11. Control food adulteration.
12. Control exposure to nostrums.
13. Control smoke nuisances.
14. Construct model tenements.
15. Construct standard public bathing and wash
    houses.
16. Preach health from the pulpit.
17. Teach the science of sanitation in medical
    schools.
18. Introduce prevention as a phase of all medical
    practice.
19. Sponsor routine health examinations.

The wisdom of Shattuck's report stands as a
valued guidepost in the history of public health.
Perhaps because he had less of a flair for writing
that Chadwick, and he used fewer vivid descriptions of appalling conditions, the report produced
no results until 1869. Then Massachusetts established its first state board of health with lay and
health professional membership. The Shattuck report served as the guide for the board in its early
years of activity.

Modern Era of Health
Shattuck's report signaled the modern era of
health, dated from 1850 to the present. An organized, disciplined attack on environmental problems of disease transmission followed from recognizing the importance of a united public approach
to health protection. Health services and health
promotion were to come later.

We can divide the modern era of health into
five phases. The first phase (1850–1880) was the
miasma phase; the second phase (1880–1910), the
bacteriology phase or health protection era; the
third phase (1910–1960), the *health resources* or
health services phase; and the fourth phase
(1960–1975), the *social engineering* phase. The

fifth phase began in the mid 1970s with the *health promotion* period. This phase, called the "second epidemiological revolution," addresses the behavior and lifestyles of individuals, communities, and societies. These are recognized as the major causes of illness, disability, and death. These social and behavioral determinants became the targets for the promotion of community and population health.

Miasma Phase (1850–1880)   The term *miasma* means noxious air or vapor. During the **miasma phase,** communities based their approach to health protection on the misconception that noxious odors caused disease (figure 1-5). For example, people thought gases associated with putrefaction caused diphtheria. Though scientifically unsound, this assumption led to many of the environmental reforms that resulted in some of the greatest health improvements in history. Observations as early as Hippocrates that people who ventured about at dusk often contracted malaria perpetuated the common belief into the late nineteenth century that the particular air existing at dusk caused this disease. Dusk, coincidentally, is a time that mosquito feeding is most intense. The term **malaria** means "bad air." This is an illustrious example of the interpretation of mere coincidence as a cause-and-effect relationship.

Communities directed their disease control efforts largely toward general cleanliness. Garbage and refuse collection became important to communities. They enforced street cleaning relentlessly. These general cleanliness measures usually missed the specific causes of disease and consequently were of limited value in control of disease.

The topics discussed at the first quarantine convention in Philadelphia in 1857 indicate the interests of the time. They included prevention of typhus, cholera, and yellow fever; port quarantine; stagnant and putrid bilge waters, droppings, or drainage from putrescible matter; and filthy bedding, baggage, and clothing of immigrant passengers where they had been confined.

Figure 1-5

The belief during the miasma phase that foul odors, rather than crowding, caused illness and the spread of disease, led public health officials to break holes in the roofs of plague-infected houses in Bombay. (Halftone after C. D. Weldon, from *Harper's Weekly* 43:552, June 3, 1899; courtesy National Library of Medicine.)

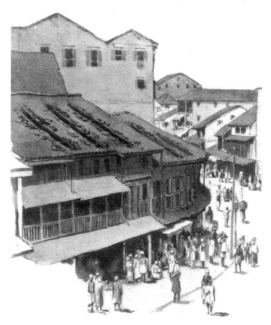

Massachusetts organized the first state health department (the operating arm of the state board of health) in 1869. Dr. Henry Bowdich, the Department's first head, organized the program to address the following six areas:

1. Professional and public education in hygiene
2. Housing
3. Investigation of certain diseases
4. Slaughtering
5. Sale of poisons
6. Conditions of the poor

The American Public Health Association, founded in 1872 at Long Beach, New Jersey, elected Dr. Stephen Smith as its first president. The new association proposed to go beyond the thinking of the quarantine conventions in dealing with sanitation, prevention and transmission of disease, longevity, hospital hygiene, and all other health problems of interest and of concern to the public.

Public health teaching began during this period. An English manual of hygiene edited by E. A. Parkes, professor of military hygiene in the army medical school of England, was published in 1859. The first and subsequent editions were used in the United States. In 1879 A. H. Buck edited his pioneering text, *Hygiene and Public Health*. This volume dealt with environmental sanitation, housing, personal hygiene, child hygiene, school hygiene, industrial hygiene, food sanitation, communicable disease control, disinfection, quarantine, infant mortality, and vital statistics. Dr. J. S. Billings wrote the introduction with foresight regarding the jurisprudence of public health. His concepts, such as the following, reflect the growing influence of medicine in public health:

1. County lines are not natural boundaries and have no relation to causes of disease.
2. Administrative health areas should be large enough and populous enough to require full-time sanitary and executive forces.
3. There should be nonpracticing full-time health officers with medical education.
4. The health officer should have special training for this job.
5. If a municipal board of health is properly constituted so that its relationship to the medical profession is harmonious, it should be charged with the supervision of all medical charities such as hospitals and dispensaries.

The seeds of professional public health preparation were being planted before the next phase of the modern health era was reached.

Bacteriology Phase (1880–1910) Louis Pasteur, Robert Koch, and other bacteriologists who demonstrated that a specific organism causes a specific disease ushered in the bacteriology phase. The knowledge that an organism causes a certain

The Broad Street Pump and John Snow's Epidemiology

As England entered the Crimean War in 1854, a cholera epidemic in the Soho district of London killed more than 500 people in little more than a week. Dr. John Snow, a 41-year-old anesthetist, lived close to the area and began mapping the sources of drinking water of those who died. He traced a cluster to the Broad Street pump. Snow encountered opposition to his suggestion that the pump be closed because the prevailing notion at that time was that bad air caused cholera. He persevered in having the pump handle removed. The outbreak ended soon after that.

This event illustrates two public health principles: First, action often must be taken before conclusive evidence is in hand. Snow constructed epidemiological evidence of the source of the problem, but this was some thirty years before Koch isolated the cholera vibrio, so he could not prove that it was the water and not the air causing the cholera. Second, Snow sought a means to prevent the problem by going to its source rather than merely treating its victims.

In 1992 the Westminister City Council of London unveiled a monument to Dr. Snow: a pump that stands in an open paved area near the site of the original. A plaque tells the story. Nearby, the "John Snow Public House" is frequented by epidemiologists the world over as a place to celebrate their profession and Snow's contribution to their method of research. The pub's management keeps a guest book under the bar for researchers worldwide to sign.

A short distance across the river Thames is the Florence Nightingale Museum, a monument to the pioneer of another health profession. Nightingale's contributions were not only to nursing but also to epidemiology during her service in the Crimean War (1854–1856).

disease made it possible to change from general to specific health protection measures that blocked the routes the causative agents would travel. Even before the specific agents were isolated, the identification of certain vehicles by which they traveled such as water, milk, other foods and insects allowed public health measures to be directed at them (see box on the Broad Street Pump). Laws and health protection programs of this phase sought to protect water supplies, milk, and other foods; eliminate insects; and properly dispose of sewage (figure 1-6). The development of laboratory procedures also advanced the specificity of these measures.

The scientific productivity of the bacteriologists of this period is legendary. The French bacteriologist Louis Pasteur (1822–1895), besides demonstrating that a specific organism causes a specific disease, made other outstanding contributions to **bacteriology.** He discovered the fowl cholera bacillus and developed a method of inoculation against rabies. Robert Koch (1843–1910) discovered the tubercle bacillus and the streptococcus; he also discovered the cholera vibrio, which he demonstrated was transmitted by water, food, and clothing.

During this period Lord Joseph Lister (1827–1912) developed the practical use of phenol (carbolic acid) as an effective antiseptic.

Official public health departments employed bacteriologists, laboratory technicians, sanitation inspectors, sanitary engineers, quarantine officers, and others who specialized in communicable disease control measures. With the extreme emphasis placed on isolation and quarantine during the first two decades of the twentieth century, one might with justification refer to these twenty years as the "tack hammer" period in public health history. To the public, ubiquitous quarantine officers with their hideous placards were the identifying symbol of public health.

Limited as the health protection programs of this period were, they produced a pronounced reduction in deaths in western Europe and in North America.

Health Resources Phase (1910–1960) The first broad-scale assessment of the health status of the people of the United States came with the medical examination of men being inducted into the U.S. armed services during World War I. Even using health standards for induction lower than usual,

....
Figure 1-6
Nineteenth century concerns with food adulteration and inspection were expressed in dramatic novels such as Upton Sinclair's *The Jungle,* and in cartoons such as this depiction of Death handing out contaminated milk to the poor in the street. (Wood engraving after Thomas Nast, *Harper's Weekly* 22:648, Aug. 17, 1878; courtesy National Library of Medicine.)

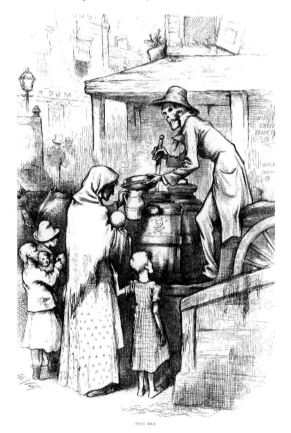

the armed services found it necessary to reject 34 percent of the men examined because of physical and mental disabilities. The nation was appalled to learn that one-third of its youth were unfit for military service. Professional health personnel analyzed the medical examination data on draftees and arrived at a conclusion that was to change the course of public health in the United States.

Milestones of the Bacteriology Phase

1880	Typhoid bacillus discovered Pneumococcus identified Malaria plasmodium discovered
1882	Tubercle bacillus discovered
1883	Rabies treatment successful (Pasteur) Cholera vibrio discovered (Koch)
1884	Diphtheria bacillus identified Federal research laboratory established at Staten Island later named National Institute of Health
1889	Massachusetts Public Health Laboratory and Johns Hopkins Hospital opened with new emphasis on scientific health care
1893	Lawrence, Massachusetts, water treatment plant completed

	Transmission of Texas fever from ticks to cattle demonstrated (Theobald Smith, U.S. Department of Agriculture)
1894	Diphtheria antitoxin successfully demonstrated (Emil von Behring) *Pasteurella pestis*, cause of plague, discovered
1895	Cause of hookworm discovered
1896	African sleeping sickness traced to the tsetse fly
1898	Relation of **Anopheles** mosquito to malaria established (Ronald Ross)
1900	Relation of *Aedes aegypti* mosquito to yellow fever demonstrated (Walter Reed)
1901	Infectious nature of yellow fever established

1902	U.S. Public Health Service established International Sanitary Bureau created First health instruction in schools in New York City
1904	Typhoid fever immunization successful
1905	Spirochete of syphillis identified Grants to Canadian Association for Prevention of Consumption
1906	Pure Food and Drug Act passed Standard methods of water analysis adopted
1908	Chlorination of Jersey City water supply Syphilis successfully treated using arsphenamine *Haemophilus pertussis* identified

Health experts learned from these data that communicable diseases, now controlled quite well, were replaced by other health hazards and problems. Many of the defects reported could have been prevented, and most of the defects could have been corrected. It seemed that public health programs, in their focus on population health protection, had neglected the health of youth as individuals. They concluded that it was necessary to build and maintain the highest possible level of health resources for each individual. Environmental prevention and control of communicable disease was only part of the necessary strategy for community or population health.

State health departments began expanding their programs and directing their efforts toward personal health services and community disease control. This development required administrative reorganization within the state health departments and the inclusion of many new specialties in the health services field.

In 1911 Guilford County, North Carolina, and Yakima County, Washington, organized the first full-time county health departments. The organization of official health departments on a county basis was slow in developing until the second decade of the health resources phase. Then, with financial support from such organizations as the Rockefeller Foundation, the Kellogg Foundation, and the U.S. Public Health Service, county health departments became recognized as important players in the health infrastructure. County health departments with full-time professional personnel gradually displaced city health departments with part-time health officers and nonprofessional personnel. Only a few large cities with full-time professionally prepared personnel still continue to function apart from the 3,102 counties in the United States. Canada, Australia, and some European countries have similar patterns of district or area health agencies.

The largest investments during this era, however, were not in public health services or even in personal preventive health services, but rather in three other expensive resources. These investments included the building of hospitals, the training of professional health personnel, and the development of biomedical knowledge from research. The Hill-Burton Act passed by the U.S. Congress in 1946 provided for the construction of massive facilities for medical care. Medical, nursing, and dental schools proliferated to train the personnel required to staff the new hospitals. Congress also established the National Institutes of Health to generate the research and strengthen the knowledge resource from which scientific medicine and public health could draw new methods, drugs, vaccines, and diagnostic tests.

Voluntary health agencies played an increasingly important role in the promotion of health in the United States, particularly through health education, bringing to public attention the importance of certain health problems. Unfortunately, some of them oversold the importance of relatively rare diseases, causing the public to contribute unnecessary services or resources at the expense of more urgent or pervasive problems. The burden of being solicited for contributions repeatedly by too many voluntary agencies led many communities to establish joint fund-raising through "community chests" and "united campaigns." The voluntary agencies also tended to turn to medical research and medical services, usually at the expense of their public health education function. Thus even private sector resources for community health during this era concentrated in medical rather than health activities.

Social Engineering Phase (1960–1975) By the late 1950s it had become apparent that technical health advances and personal health resources were not equally available to all people. Indeed, large segments of the world and of each community were completely isolated from developments in health. The managing of human resources required that the products of technological developments be made available to every person. The social equity aspects of health gained higher priority in legislation and policy.

Making the advances of health science available to all people posed a pyramid of problems because of the various individuals and groups unable to acquire health knowledge or to obtain health services. The poor—economically, educationally, and socially—often missed the benefits of community health programs. The economic barriers seemed the most urgent. Canada passed sweeping universal coverage provisions for medical care. The United States passed Medicare and Medicaid legislation to put purchasing power in the hands of the elderly, poor and medically indigent to enable them to receive needed health services.

The educational and social isolation of the poor called for outreach to take health resources and services to those who apparently were not receiving the benefits of health programs. The outreach services of public health nurses and indigenous community health workers thus became a mainstay of local health departments.

The U.S. Peace Corps and the Canadian CUSO also attempted to address this need by placing young people with training in health and other professional disciplines into developing countries. The concept was later expanded to include a domestic Peace Corps and all age groups. The Peace Corps continues to recruit from all age and professional groups.

The Civil Rights Act passed by the U.S. Congress in 1964 provided that "no person shall on the ground of race, color or national origin, be excluded from participation in, be denied the benefits of, or be subjected to discrimination under any program or activity receiving Federal financial assistance." The Food Stamp Act in the same year authorized food stamp programs for low-income persons to buy nutritious food for a balanced diet.

The trend in community health programs during the late 1960s was the funneling of federal funds through state and county agencies to provide medical and hospital services for medically deprived groups in the community. Most of the funds went to practicing physicians for professional services rendered to citizens who otherwise would not have had the medical care they needed. County health departments inherited some of the funds for medical services for the poor. This cast an additional burden on county health departments' staffing because the legislation seldom made provisions for additional personnel.

By the late 1960s the redistribution of the resources (health facilities, personnel, and research) developed in earlier decades had achieved greater equity for the poor and the medically indigent. This equalization had occurred in the United States as a result of the "New Frontier" legislation of the Kennedy years and the "War on Poverty" legislation of the Johnson years. European and other countries made even more sweeping social and medical reforms. Citizens in most communities had a growing voice in allocating health resources at the local level. The "maximum feasible participation" provision in most of the U.S. legislative acts required policy and planning bodies for neighborhood health centers and other new entities to include 51 percent lay membership. The 1960s had achieved a closing of much of the gap between high-income and low-income people in their use of medical services.

Increased accessibility of medical care, however, did not universally improve the mortality and morbidity statistics. The differences between the death and disease rates of rich and poor, white and black, urban and rural populations persisted. Indeed, the increasing expenditures on health care (mostly medical care) were not yielding proportionate improvements in the health of nations, populations, or communities. The rapidly escalating costs of medical care were attributed to the expensive medical technology and facilities created by the earlier investments in medical resources. New coverage made these more universally accessible. Health policy in the 1970s, then, devoted much legislation and research to finding ways to contain the costs of medical care and hospital care in this inflationary spiral of supply and demand.

The search for cost-containment strategies in the United States led first to the "health planning" acts of the late 1960s and early 1970s. It then led to "peer review" requirements to encourage medical practitioners to restrain themselves in the use of unnecessary medical procedures. Then it led to new forms of delivery, such as "health maintenance organizations," designed to encourage physicians to keep their patients out of hospitals rather than to admit them unnecessarily. During this period of concentrated tinkering with the *medical* care system, the *health* care system was almost forgotten. State and local health departments lost much of their financial base to medical institutions and much of their political force to health planning agencies. Much of the energy and resources available to them had to be devoted in part to medical care responsibilities.

Health Promotion Phase (1974–Present) By the mid-1970s a renewed interest in disease prevention and health promotion had occurred almost simultaneously in several English-speaking countries. The milestones of this era are marked by a series of influential documents. The United States began the decade with the report of *The President's Committee on Health Education*. The Canadians, however, soon followed with a more comprehensive and influential report by the Minister of National Health and Welfare, *A New Perspective on the Health of Canadians* (Lalonde, 1974). In Great Britain the famous "red book" was issued by the government with the title *Prevention and Health: Everybody's Business, 1976*. The more recent British initiatives in health promotion and disease prevention outline priority objectives for the year 2000 and plans for monitoring progress.

The Americans continued their refocusing with a series of official and still living documents and legislative acts, beginning with the National Health Information and Health Promotion Act of 1976. This Act created the Office of Disease Prevention and Health Promotion, which produced the most influential series of Surgeon General's reports on health promotion and disease prevention,

Milestones of the Social Engineering Phase

1960 U.S. Social Security Amendments authorized grants to states for medical assistance for the aged

1961 Peace Corps and Food Stamp programs established by President Kennedy

1962 Saskatchewan introduces the first Canadian Medicare plan
U.S. Federal Assistance to Migratory Workers Act authorized federal aid for clinics serving migratory agricultural workers and their families

1963 Measles vaccine demonstrated successfully

1964 Civil Rights Act in the United States prohibiting discrimination
Mumps vaccine developed
Canadians get Social Insurance cards
Economic Opportunity Act launches President Johnson's "War on Poverty"
First Surgeon General's Report on Smoking and Health released

1965 Medicare and Medicaid legislation passed as Social Security Amendments

1966 Rubella vaccine trial-tested
Canadian Pension Plan established
Fair Packaging and Labelling Act passed
Model Cities program launched in United States

1967 Medicare and Medicaid begin coverage

1968 U.S. Senate Select Committee on Nutrition and Human Needs established

1969 Rubella vaccine introduced
Canadian abortion law liberalized

1970 National high blood pressure education and screening programs initiated
Family Planning and Population Act signed in United States
Occupational Health and Safety Act signed in United States

1971 White House Conference on Aging held
Sickle Cell Disease Program initiated in United States

President's Committee on Health Education established

1972 Special Supplementary Food Program for Women, Infants, and Children (WIC) initiated in United States

1973 Health Maintenance Organization Assistance Act passed in United States
World Health Assembly, noting widespread dissatisfaction with health service, decides that WHO should collaborate with, not just advise, its Member States in developing national health care systems

1974 Child Abuse Prevention and Treatment Act in the United States
National Institute on Aging established in United States
National Health Planning and Resources Development Act replaced Comprehensive Health Planning and Regional Medical Programs in United States
Safe Drinking Water Act passed in United States

Healthy People (1979) and *Promoting Health, Preventing Disease: Objectives for the Nation* (1980). The current version, *Healthy People 2000* (1991) continues to drive national policy in health promotion and disease prevention. A companion document for communities is *Healthy Communities 2000* (1991).

In the same spirit of shifting policy more toward health promotion, the Australian-Commonwealth Department of Health published *Health Promotion in Australia 1978-79* (Davidson, Chapman, and Hull, 1979) and subsequent reports of the Better Health Commission in the 1980s.

Australian states have been among the most aggressive in the world in attacking tobacco, taxing tobacco to create organizations for health promotion, and restricting advertising. They have taken similarly aggressive, but even more effective action on alcohol and driving and on seat belt use.

The World Health Organization (WHO) spurred the global health promotion movement with its several initiatives under the banner, "Health for All by the Year 2000." In September 1978 representatives of 134 nations met at Alma-Ata in what was still then the USSR, now Russia (figure 1-7). The national representatives pledged

··················

Figure 1-7

In 1978 representatives of 134 nations met at Alma-Ata in the USSR (now Russia) and pledged their support for a worldwide effort to bring about "Health for All by the Year 2000." The approach emphasizes community involvement in setting priorities and goals for population health and primary health care. (WHO photo courtesy World Health Organization.)

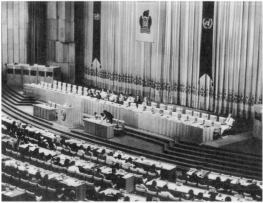

··················

Figure 1-8

In 1986 participants in the First International Conference on Health Promotion from 38 countries met in Ottawa, Canada and hammered out the "Ottawa Charter for Health Promotion." The cover page graphic shown here indicates the six main strategies of the approach advocated for health promotion. (Courtesy World Health Organization, Health Canada.)

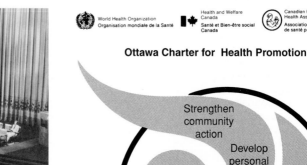

Ottawa Charter for Health Promotion

AN INTERNATIONAL CONFERENCE
ON HEALTH PROMOTION
The move towards a new public health

November 17-21, 1986   Ottawa, Ontario, Canada

their support for a worldwide effort to bring about a new emphasis on primary health care. WHO uses this term to emphasize community participation and more equitable access to basic health services for all than has been achieved by the emphasis on hospitals in the past. In 1986 WHO and the Canadian government co-sponsored the first international conference on health promotion and issued *The Ottawa Charter* (figure 1-8). This document went beyond the Alma-Ata declaration in playing down the importance of the *medical* care system in contributing to *health* care. It emphasized, as had the Lalonde Report in 1974 and the U.S. Surgeon General's Report in 1979, that lifestyle and conditions of living contribute more to health than medical care does. Most countries spend much more on medical and hospital care than on disease prevention and health promotion.

The Ottawa Charter went further than the Lalonde Report and the U.S. Surgeon General's Report in stressing the social and economic aspects of lifestyle. It also emphasized the impor-

tance of community action to enhance opportunities for people to practice healthful lifestyles.

Subsequent Australian, European, and North American health policy documents have attempted to live up to the Ottawa Charter's ideals for health promotion. The Health Promotion Phase was fueled by and retarded by the conservatism of the 1980s and the global recession extending into the early 1990s. National governments sought to reduce federal involvement in states' rights and to

Milestones of the Health Promotion Phase

1974 *A New Perspective on the Health of Canadians* published (Lalonde Report)

1975 National Center for Health Education established in San Francisco

1976 U.S. Health Information and Health Promotion Act signed

1977 WHO announces the eradication of smallpox in Asia and adopts health for all by the year 2000 as target.

1978 National initiatives in childhood immunization, adolescent pregnancy, smoking, and nutrition announced

1979 Australian and U.S. national reports on health promotion released
• Smallpox officially declared eradicated worldwide
• First National Conference on Health Promotion in Occupational Settings sponsored by U.S. Office of Disease Prevention and Health Promotion

1980 Department of Education created, leaving Public Health Service and Health Care Finance Administration in Department of Health and Human Services
• National School Health Evaluation Study sponsored by U.S. Public Health Service documents effectiveness of sustained, comprehensive school health
• First collaborative publication by U.S. Public Health Service and U.S. Department of Agriculture of joint *Dietary Guidelines for Americans*

1981 Public Health Service's *Objectives for the Nation* in disease prevention and health promotion adopted as policy in United States

1982 Block grants to states replace categorical funding of community health programs

1984 New federal reimbursement policies force many community hospitals to close
• U.S. Congress passes laws authorizing new system of labels on cigarettes warning of emphysema, fetal damage, and cancer
• Legislation authorizes federal support for university research centers for disease prevention and health promotion
• European Office of World Health Organization publishes definitions and guiding concepts for health promotion

1985 U.S. Surgeon General's Report on Smoking and Health establishes relationships between smoking and hazardous substances in the workplace

1986 Reports by Australia, Canada, United States, and WHO indicate progress and plans toward objectives in health promotion and health for all
• Ottawa Charter for Health Promotion published by WHO and Canadian Public Health Association following

(continued on next page)

encourage local autonomy and initiative. This has resulted in a relentless decline in federal direct funding to states, provinces, or communities. When viewed in the longer historical perspective, however, this decline began with the earlier social engineering phase. Increasing budget deficits followed the continuous buildup of national investments in local development during the previous health resources phase. Whether communities can rise to the challenges and opportunities to take control of their health in the face of dwindling resources from higher levels of government remains an open question. This book will chronicle some of the principles and examples that have emerged from the past and from recent experiences of communities in controlling their own health.

LESSONS FROM THE PAST, CHALLENGES FOR THE FUTURE

HIV/AIDS, cost containment, and competition preoccupied national health policy and medical care in the 1980s, but they did not displace community interest in health promotion. In the 1990s, new and antibiotic-resistant strains of communicable diseases, managed care, and

Milestones of the Health Promotion Phase (continued)

first International Conference on Health Promotion (figure 1-8)
• Canadian *Achieving Health for All* framework published by Minister of Health
• U.S. Surgeon General's Report on Smoking and Health establishes risks associated with involuntary or passive smoking

1988 First U.S. *Surgeon General's Report on Nutrition and Health*
• Surgeon General's Report on Smoking and Health established nicotine as a highly addictive substance
• National Academy of Science report on *The Future of Public Health* challenged the field of public health to take greater policy development role

1989 International Convention on the Rights of the Child
• U.S. Preventive Services Task Force presents assessment of 169 clinical interventions for health promotion and disease prevention
• U.S. Surgeon General's Report on *Reducing the Health Consequences of Smoking: 25 Years of Progress*

1990 World Summit for Children, New York
• *Healthy People 2000* published by the U.S. Department of Health and Human Services

1991 *Healthy Communities 2000* published by American Public Health Association
• Poliomyelitis elimination in Americas achieved

1992 United Nations Conference on Environment and Development, Rio de Janiero
• The International Conference on Nutrition, Rome
• *Health of the Nation* White Paper published by the Government of Great Britain

1993 World Conference on Human Rights, Vienna

1994 International Conference on Population and Development, Cairo

1995 World Summit for Social Development, Copenhagen
United Nations Fourth World Conference on Women, Beijing
World Health Organization announces it is on track to eradicate polio by the year 2000

1996 Second United Nations Conference on Human Settlements, Istanbul
Pope embraces evolution as "More than just a hypothesis"
First U.S. Surgeon General's Report on *Physical Activity and Health*

1997 States sue the tobacco industry
• Tobacco industry negotiates with U.S. federal government for global settlement
• International Conference on Health Promotion meets for first time in a developing country, Indonesia

---

health care reform became the expressions of the same national concerns. They reminded even the most technologically advanced nations and the most affluent communities that they could not let down their guard against infectious diseases. Nor could they afford to escalate the application of technology without examining the ethical and economic implications for individuals and families. Public health methods of health protection from the nineteenth century continue to have a critical role to play. **Health education** continues to have a voice in the growing recogni-

tion that preventive and community approaches to population health have their greatest potential in health promotion.

One key lesson from the past is that communities sometimes innovate and initiate ideas, methods, strategies, and programs that subsequently become national policy. Indeed, we have seen that most national health-related policies originated in ideas developed in local communities.

Of particular concern with the current emphasis on cost containment and market competition in the health services reform debate is that disadvantaged populations might drop out of sight in the marketing strategies. Of the 34 million Americans left without health insurance at the end of the 1980s, 25 million now have coverage under the 1996 Kennedy-Kassenbaum bill. They now have protection against losing their coverage when they change jobs. The others, mostly unemployed, remain uninsured and their limited income or education makes them unattractive, hard-to-reach markets. The constricted budgets of official health agencies leave them to fend for themselves. Self-care education is only a partial solution. Local health agencies again must pick up the responsibility for outreach to the economically disadvantaged, the socially isolated, the homeless, the immigrant, and other special populations.

Canada has managed to cling to its universal health care system, with some eroding in each province, under the most severe fiscal constraints. A National Forum on Health appointed in 1996 issued draft reports indicating a renewed commitment to the health care system of which Canadians are fiercely proud and protective. The Forum also recommended a focus of attention on the special needs of children, the special problems of employment, the special opportunities of community action, and the special needs for research on population health and determinants of health. We shall examine these determinants of population health and community health in the next chapters.

Migrant workers, mothers, infants, children, adolescents, the chronically ill, and the elderly all need more than health care services. These populations need opportunities at the community level to gain control over the determinants of their health. This effort calls for the enlistment of many community resources, voluntary and official agencies, in many categories of human services besides health.

Creating a favorable environment and favorable living conditions for these people means creating opportunities for self-improvement. This calls for a form of social engineering that was tried in the 1960s in the United States but later was abandoned by the federal government. This approach has been criticized as being paternalistic. To offer people more healthful channels of living and to help them develop the ability to guide their own mode of life, however, is no more paternalistic than to award people state scholarships for a college education. The question for consideration in this book is how this can be done effectively at the community level and when it must depend on higher levels of government or more centralized private sector initiatives.

Modern community health programs cover all citizens of all ages, but of necessity they must give more attention to the people at greatest risk. These usually consist of the least advantaged social, economic, and educational strata. The human ecology involved is apparent. The health of these people affects the dignity, health, and economy of the entire community and reflects the humanity of the community. Abandoned to their own resources, many people would decline in health and consequently in their social condition. Community action for the common good includes protecting and promoting the health of the least advantaged.

These objectives require, increasingly, action outside the clinical and public health settings of the past. The challenges of the future entail more complex lifestyle issues related to risk factors and risk conditions for injury and chronic diseases, which account for the leading causes of death and disability. Community health practice must be centered increasingly in schools, workplaces, recreational settings, and homes. These settings carry the potential to shape the conditions for health protection and the cultures for lifestyles that will promote health.

SUMMARY

This chapter has defined population and community health protection, promotion, and services. It has addressed the historical context of community and population health. Some of the social, cultural, and economic forces that shape history also shape behavior and health simultaneously. To understand and apply these several forces you should draw back from the parochial perspective of your own community to place its health in broader population health perspectives. These include state or provincial, national and international perspectives and trends.

Population and community perspectives on health promotion will gain momentum as more professionals and decision makers recognize the limits of technology. The growing importance of behavioral and social conditions as the key determinants of health will become more apparent as the population ages and quality of life gains greater prominence as a criterion of health.

Heart disease, cancer, stroke, and injuries account for the majority of deaths in Western countries. All of these have as their principal causes one or more behavioral or lifestyle problems. Behavioral and social factors can affect not only the age of onset of these conditions and the reduction in deaths from them, but the severity and limitations of daily activities once they have been diagnosed. The voluntary adoption of behavior conducive to health is the goal of health education. In concert with social and environmental supports for such behavior, health education becomes health promotion. In emphasizing behavior, never lose sight of its historical, social, and environmental origins and constraints. Community and population health promotion and protection address the combination of educational, social, and environmental interventions and in cooperation with clinical health services.

The foregoing historical background can be understood as the repeated redefining of the primary or prevalent causes of illness and death. These have varied from supernatural causes in the primitive and earliest Egyptian through medieval times, to natural causes in the Chinese, Greco-Roman and modern eras, to social causes in the mid-twentieth century, to behavioral and lifestyle causes in the present health promotion period. The behavioral causes of current health problems, however, must be understood and addressed in their historical, cultural, social, economic, and community contexts. Community must be understood in broader population and global contexts.

WEB*Links*

http://www.apha.org
American Public Health Association

http://www.who.org
World Health Organization

http://www.who.dk/policy/ottawa.htm
The Ottawa Charter on Health Promotion

http://www.house.gov/commerce/TobaccoDocs/documents
Congressional collection of previously secret historical files of the tobacco industry.

QUESTIONS FOR REVIEW

1. Why and how does a knowledge of the past in any field of human endeavor benefit those who now work in that field?
2. How has disease altered the course of history?
3. Why should people in the health professions, including those who will work primarily in clinical settings, have a broad knowledge of community health?
4. Why was the Mosaic law or code of special importance to the advancement of the community health movement?
5. How does the political philosophy of a nation affect its health program?
6. What specific lesson in health can the present generation gain from a study of health conditions during the Dark Ages?
7. To what extent did the Renaissance influence the direction of community health?
8. What, in your judgment, was the most important health discovery in Europe during the period of American colonization between 1600 and 1800?
9. How would you evaluate this statement: "Colorful reporting can get more public action than can scientific fact"?
10. How would you evaluate this assertion: "Lowering the death rate among laborers and their families does not improve their lot because it results in a surplus of laborers"?

11. What questionable health practices in the miasma phase of health are still regarded by the general public as important to health?

12. What is the basis for the contention that scientific public health should be dated from 1880?

13. Why did the application of scientific methods have such a profound effect on the death rate in Europe and North America?

14. Why is the postponement of death not sufficient as the objective of a community health program?

15. What is meant by the expression, "Public health is social engineering"?

READINGS

Chesler, E. 1992. *Woman of valor: Margaret Sanger and the birth control movement in America.* New York: Simon & Schuster.

Relentlessly posing the question, Whose body is it?, Margaret Sanger applied her nursing background in the Lower East Side of New York City and opened the first birth-control clinic in the United States in 1916 in Brooklyn. After several weeks the police raided it and jailed Sanger. She went on to lead the birth-control movement through lectures, writing, and international conferences.

Fletcher A. 1996. *Gender, sex and subordination in England 1500–1800.* New Haven: Yale University Press.

During the Shakespearean Tudor and Stuart periods in England, patriarchy and sex roles were sanctioned by the clergy, by royal decree, and by medical models that portrayed males as strong and females as weakened by loss of tears and blood. Family violence and other traditions sanctioned by this culture still persist.

Freeman, M., ed. 1995. *Always Rachel: the letters of Rachel Carson and Dorothy Freeman, 1952–1964,* Boston: Beacon Press.

A biographical look through private letters at the woman whose book, Silent Spring, awakened the world in the early 1960s to the disastrous effects of pesticides and chemical fertilizer on nature and on health.

Kunitz, S. J. 1996. The history of politics of US health care policy for American Indians and Alaskan Natives. *Am J Public Health* 86:1464.

Traces the development of the US federal government's program to provide personal and public health services to indigenous native populations. Chronicles the Indian Health Service and the health status and health care of Indian populations.

Lappe', M. 1994. *Evolutionary medicine.* San Francisco: Sierra Club Books.

Strategies to stop the advance of epidemic drug-resistant bacteria and viruses, tuberculosis, malaria, cancer, and AIDS. Explores the emerging viruses and the linked worlds of evolution and public health.

BIBLIOGRAPHY

Afifi, A. A., and L. Breslow. 1994. The maturing paradigm of public health. *Annu Rev of Public Health* 15:223.

Buck, A. H. 1879. *Hygiene and public health,* Philadelphia: William Wood.

Bullough, B., and G. Rosen. 1992. *Preventive medicine in the United States, 1900–1990: trends and interpretations,* Canton, MA: Science History.

Callahan, D. 1990. *What kind of life: the limits of medical progress.* New York: Simon & Schuster.

Chadwick, E. 1965. *The sanitary condition of the labouring population of Great Britain.* Edinburgh: Edinburgh University Press.

Davidson, L., S. Chapman, and C. Hull. 1979. *Health promotion in Australia 1978–79.* Canberra: Commonwealth of Australia.

DeFries, R. D., ed. 1940. *The development of public health in Canada.* Ottawa: Canadian Public Health Association.

Depew, D. J., and B. H. Weber. 1994. *Darwinism evolving: systems dynamics and the genealogy of natural selection.* Cambridge, MA: MIT Press.

Epp, J. 1986. *Achieving health for all: a framework for health promotion.* Ottawa: Minister of Supply and Services Canada, H 39–102/1986 E.

Elshtain, J. B. 1995. What feminists could learn from Ms. Anthony. *Civilization* 2(6):50.

Flaherty, L. T., M. D. Weist, and B. S. Warner. 1994. School-based mental health services in the United States: history, current models and needs. *Community Mental Health J* 32:341.

Goodman, J. 1993. *Tobacco in history: the cultures of dependence.* New York: Routledge.

Gostin, L. O., P. S. Arno, and A. M. Brandt. 1997. FDA regulation of tobacco advertising and youth smoking: historical, social, and constitutional perspectives. *J Am Med Assoc* 277:410.

Great Britain Expenditures Committee. 1977. *First report from the Expenditures Committee, Session 1976–77, Preventive Medicine.* London: HMSO.

Green, L. W., and M. W. Kreuter. 1990. Health promotion as a public health strategy for the 1990s. *Annu Rev Public Health* 11:319.

Guinta, M. A., and J. P. Allegrante. 1992. The President's Committee on Health Education: a 20-year retrospective on its politics and policy impact. *Am J Public Health* 82:1033.

Health of the nation: white paper. 1992. London: HMSO.

Healthy communities 2000: model standards. 1991. 3d. ed. Washington, DC: American Public Health Association.

Healthy people, the Surgeon General's report on health promotion and disease prevention. 1979. 2 vols. Washington, DC: DHEW (PHS) Pub. No. 79-55071A.

Healthy people 2000: national health promotion and disease prevention objectives. 1991. Boston: Jones and Bartlett Publishing Co.

Henig, R. M. 1993. *A dancing matrix: voyages along the viral frontier.* New York: Knopf; also adapted as Flu pandemic, *New York Times Magazine,* Nov. 29, 1992.

Henig, R. M. 1995. The lessons of syphilis in the age of AIDS. *Civilization* 2(6):36.

Henig, R. M. 1996. *The people's health: a memoir of public health and its evolution at Harvard.* Washington, DC: National Academy Press.

Lalonde, M. 1974. *A new perspective on the health of Canadians: a working document.* Ottawa: Government of Canada.

Lochhead, A. G. 1968. *A history of the Bacteriology Division of the Canada Department of Agriculture, 1923–1955.* Ottawa: Canada Department of Agriculture.

MacDougall, H. 1990. *Activists and advocates: Toronto's health department, 1883–1983.* Toronto and Oxford: Dundurn.

Oppenheimer, G. M. 1996. Prematurity as a public health problem: US policy from the 1920s to the 1960s. *Am J Public Health* 86:870.

Ottawa charter for health promotion. 1986. Ottawa: Canadian Public Health Association.

Preventive medicine USA: a task force report. 1976. New York: Prodist.

Promoting health, preventing disease: objectives for the nation. 1980. Washington, DC: Public Health Service.

Richardson, B. W. 1887. *The health of nations, vol 2, A review of the works of Edwin Chadwick.* London: Longmans Green.

Roberts, J. 1996. British nurses at war 1914–1918: ancillary personnel and the battle for registration. *Nursing Res 45:167.*

Rosner, D., and G. Markowitz. 1991. *Deadly dust: silicosis and the politics of occupational disease in twentieth-century America.* Princeton, NJ: Princeton University Press.

Scherl, D. J., J. Noren, and M. Osterweis, ed. 1992. *Promoting health and preventing disease.* Washington, DC: Association of Academic Health Centers, Health Policy Annual II.

Shattuck, L. 1948. *Report of the Sanitary Commission of Massachusetts, 1850.* Cambridge University Press.

Shattuck, L. 1976. Report to the committee of the City Council appointed to obtain the census of Boston for the year 1845. New York: Arno Press.

Smolan, R., and P. Moffit. 1992. *Medicine's great journey: one hundred years of healing.* Boston: Bulfinch.

Thacker, S. B., R. A. Goodman, and R. C. Dicker. 1990. Training and service in public health practice, 1951–1990: CDC's Epidemic Intelligence Service. *Public Health Rep* 105:599.

Trent, J. W., Jr. 1994. *Inventing the feeble mind: a history of mental retardation in the United States.* Berkeley: University of California Press.

Troyansky, D. 1996. The history of old age in the Western world. *Aging & Society* 16:233.

U.S. Preventive Services Task Force. 1996. *Guide to clinical preventive services: report of the U.S. Preventive Services Task Force. 2nd edition.* Baltimore: Williams & Wilkins.

Vertinsky, P. 1992. Sport and exercise for old women: images of the elderly in the medical and popular literature at the turn of the century. *Int J Hist Sport* 9:83.

Winkelstein Jr., W. 1996. Morton Levin (1904–1995): history in the making. *Am J Epidem* 144:803.

World Health Organization. 1978. *Alma-Ata 1978, Primary health care.* Series, no. 1. Geneva: World Health Organization Health for All.

Chapter *2*

Community Ecology, Organization, and Health

*T*he *major challenge arises . . . from . . . the need to capture community-level change as distinct from population-level change. The latter is adequately reflected in the aggregate scores of individuals, the former most certainly is not.*
—Allen Shiell and Penny Hawe

*S*ense *of community is a feeling that members have of belonging, a feeling that members matter to one another and to the group, and a shared faith that members' needs will be met through their commitment to be together.*
—David W. McMillan

Objectives

When you finish this chapter, you should be able to:

* Identify and describe elements of ecology that apply to community and population health
* Identify the four factors influencing health

* Describe ways in which these factors occur and change in populations and communities
* Distinguish between the natural history of health and the social history of health

---

Population implies many elements. *Community* implies an interdependence of many elements, including people. As one element changes it sets up a chain reaction of adaptations or adjustments in at least some individuals and often in whole populations, organizations, and environments. As described in chapter 1, the history of health reflects the **adaptation** of the human species to its physical and biological environment. Human **ecology** is the study of that relationship as it works in both directions—from human adaptation to the envi-

ronment and from environmental adaptation to human behavior and organization. Centuries of evolution have programmed psychophysical impulses into your inherent responses to the environment. As this chapter will reveal, the environment has changed over the centuries too, partly in response to human behavior. Both have consequences for health.

Besides your genetically endowed drive for survival, you inherit a culture, a society, and a community in which people have organized

31

human resources and technology to ensure survival and enhance quality of life. To understand community health, you need to understand the ecology and organization of communities.

HUMAN ECOLOGY

Society's efforts to organize resources, develop technology, control behavior, and regulate the environment create new problems. Some of these prove harmful to health. The production of nuclear energy, for example, produced a Chernobyl incident. Coal mining strips mountains of protective foliage, causing erosion and flooding. Transporting oil and toxic material by ships, trucks, and trains pollutes the environment when a spill occurs. Computers produce "technostress" and repetitive strain injury. Each of the past methods of meeting society's needs has produced other problems. Social history, then, imposes help and hazard on the natural history of health. The help can be great when organized on a national level, because nations can pool more resources and exercise greater authority than can communities. Yet the hazards are greater when authorities who make highly centralized decisions fail to take into account the special needs and delicate balance of human and other resources at the local community level. For this reason, community health planning and community-based health services are essential to an ecologically sound, culturally sensitive, socially responsive health system. Sustainable development of health depends on sustainable development and conservation of other resources including air, water, soil, trees, and other species of flora and fauna.

The human species has dispersed widely over the planet. Of all forms of life, it possesses the greatest degree of adaptability, being able to adjust to a greater variety of conditions than any other living form. In the Arctic regions or in the tropics, human communities bend nature to their will and solve problems of survival created by environmental conditions. *In solving one problem relating to survival, however, society frequently creates another problem.* Health problems present constant

Table 2-1

Three Dimensions of Ecology

Physical-chemical factors

Climate	Debris
Chemical pollution of water	Soil
Air pollution	Fuel
Radiation	
Noise	

Biological factors

Food production	Poisons and toxic agents
Food conservation	Pathogens
Growth and development	Other parasites
Nutrition	Vectors
Physiological effects	Organic pollution of water

Social, organizational, and behavioral factors

Social structure	Mobility
Communication	Leisure
Consumption	Stress
Learning	Population imbalance
Economics	Culture

challenges. Human beings look for other problems as soon as they have solved one. This search is short because often a new problem is created by the solution to the last.

Communities must plan health programs with this lesson of ecology in mind. Together with the analytical tools of demography and epidemiology in chapter 3, ecological concepts will enable you to assess a community's health problems, trends, and potentials.

Components of Ecology

Human ecology studies the relationships between human beings and their environments. **Society** deals with an environment that is physical, chemical, biological, social, and behavioral (table 2-1). People live in an organic relationship with their environment. They organize themselves as communities in part to alter the environment to their advantage, but there are times when alteration of the environment may work to the disadvantage of specific communities, populations, or individuals.

Adaptation and Sustainable Development

Communities and society modify the course of nature, adapt to nature, and alter conditions to aid in survival. Society even makes it possible for the biologically weak to survive. A common misconception is that this "artificial selection" is **dysgenic** because it enables the "poorest" segments of our species to survive. Biologists reject the notion of artificial selection. It is as much natural selection to use the brain to achieve survival as to use legs and wings.

The human species is neither biologically inferior nor superior to its ancestors of previous centuries. By definition the survivors of any generation were the ones best suited for adaptation and survival in their time. All who survive may be considered fit to survive, even if technology made their survival possible. Civilization recognizes values other than health and biological endowment. Should people with chronic diseases not have the right to live? By making it possible for them to survive, society in return has received the intellectual, artistic, technological, and other benefits that the special gifts of many of these people have made possible. In short, adaptation and survival have become more than biological phenomena; they also have become social and organizational processes.

Conservation is not the hoarding of resources but the wise use and sustainable development of them. Conservation of human resources means the most effective and sustainable use of the environmental factors essential to survival, quality of well-being, and extension of the prime of life. It entails balancing future needs and present requirements. Conservation of human resources gives consideration to climatic conditions; food supply; productive and recreational use of land, fuel, and water; the birthrate; other living forms; and technological development.

Climate and Seasonal Effects on Health

Temperature cycles of the world have had a significant influence not only on the health of the human species but also on the economy and culture of nations. During the glory of Greece and the height of Rome, Europe was in the throes of a cold cycle that provided ideal temperatures for agriculture in the Mediterranean area. Culture flourished in those nations that enjoyed a thriving agriculture, but the nations in northern Europe that had prevailing temperatures too low for growing crops declined culturally and in other respects. During the period of low temperatures, the population of Ireland consisted of sheep, goat, and cattle herders and their families. Vegetable crops were almost nonexistent. Ireland's general culture declined with its economy.

During the Dark Ages, the thermometer swung to the other extreme and reached its peak about A.D. 850. Grapes and other crops usually associated with the Mediterranean area grew abundantly in England. This was when the Vikings were making their explorations of the North American continent and elsewhere. During this hot era, Greece experienced a steady decline as her agriculture and general economy faded. Ireland flourished and probably was the most culturally advanced nation in Europe. A cooling period followed this hot period. Ice that formed in some of the northern nations during the year A.D. 1000 did not begin to melt until the onset of the present upward trend in temperature.

The most recent rising phase of the temperature cycle appears to have begun around 1880, but the rise in temperature was not appreciable until the period beginning in 1930. Since that time there seems to have been a gradual, somewhat irregular, but nonetheless measurable increase in the world's temperature. Glaciers are receding, and objects and forms of life frozen in ice 1,000 years ago are being exposed. How long this upward cycle will continue is unknown, but carbon dioxide is accumulating an atmospheric blanket that holds heat next to the earth, creating a **"greenhouse effect."**

THE HEALTH FIELD CONCEPT

Thousands of things exert some influence on health. The **health field concept** subsumes the thousands of factors under four general categories: human biology, environment, behavior, and health

. . . .

Figure 2-1

Estimated proportions of North American total life years lost before age 75 influenced by each of the four factors in the health field. (Courtesy Centers for Disease Control.)

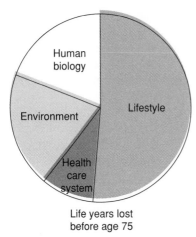

Life years lost
before age 75

care organization. The Canadian and U.S. governments used the health field concept in shifting their national health policies at the beginning of the current health promotion era. Earlier emphasis in health policy was on health care organization and environmental controls of communicable diseases. The new emphases on behavior or lifestyle and on the environment relate to the new leading causes of death and disability: chronic diseases and violent deaths and injuries. The determinants of these sets of leading causes of death and disability are some combination of lifestyle and environmental causes (see figure 2-1).

Human Biology

Human biology encompasses the health outcomes determined by the genetics of the individual, natural growth, and aging. Human biology is a necessary substrate for the remaining three categories, but there is little that individuals or communities can do to alter it except through genetic counseling for the sake of future generations.

Early in the twentieth century only 3 percent of infant deaths were from genetic causes because so many were from environmental causes and infectious diseases. With the greater control of these causes, nearly 33 percent of infant deaths today are attributable to gene-related causes. About 50 percent of spontaneous abortions and 5 percent to 7 percent of stillbirths are caused by chromosomal abnormalities.

Technological advances in screening permit the early detection of many genetic disorders before conception or birth or in newborns. The early diagnosis and treatment or prevention possibilities for many of these problems can guide reproductive decisions and can offer lifelong emotional savings to families and real economic savings to communities and society.

Environment

Environment includes all those factors related to health that are external to the human body. The individual has limited control over some of these. The community may have a larger degree of control. Examples of community control include providing for safe, uncontaminated food, air, water, and drugs; controlling air, water, and noise pollution; disposing garbage and sewage; and preventing spread of communicable diseases. Providing a safe social environment by preventing or controlling injuries and fires, dangerous use of guns, and television programs that glorify and exploit violence are further examples. Urbanization, with resultant crowding and poor housing, is another environmental influence on community health. Isolated rural living also can undermine health under some circumstances.

Swift social change or population growth with disintegration of established community values and their replacement by newer, untested mores may cause alienation and stress. Pursuit of private profit at the cost of common good may result in deterioration of the community environment, health, and quality of life.

Lifestyle and Behavior

Lifestyle, the third category, covers decisions, actions, and living conditions of individuals that affect their health. These include self-imposed risks such as cigarette smoking, overeating, drug misuse, alcoholism, promiscuity, careless driving, unsafe sex, and failure to wear seat belts. The decision to expose oneself to any of these risks, however, may be unconscious or beyond the full control of the individual. Sedentary living without relief from pressure of work or other stressors imposes risks that produce health hazards, but some of these are imposed as much by socioeconomic conditions as by conscious decisions. Lifestyle, therefore, consists of more than personally controlled decisions on daily actions or inactions. It also consists of living conditions.

Health Care Organization

Health care organization, the fourth category in the health field concept, is the one that has received the most attention and money. Its elements are medical practice, nursing, hospitals, nursing homes, dental services, drugs, mental health care, and other community health services. These services use an array of intervention methods, such as bedside nursing and surgery. Application of these usually comes late in the natural history of disease, when patients can expect little in the way of cure but much in the expenditure of effort and cost. Society has developed a dependence on this fourth category while underinvesting in the benefits to be derived from health-related changes in lifestyle and environment.

MODELS OF POPULATION AND COMMUNITY HEALTH

Community health combines the four health field elements of environmental, biomedical, organizational, and behavioral interventions. A clinical procedure might be able to limit its focus to one or two of these elements, but community health practice must keep all four in sight. Community or societal planning and action turn the natural history of individual health into the social history of community or population health.

The **natural history of health** (in a person or population) can be represented by the cycle shown in figure 2-2. Human biology and the environment

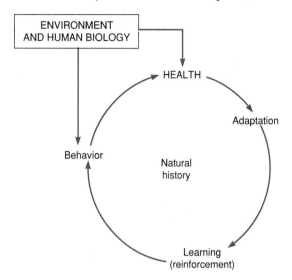

Figure 2-2

The natural history of health before social organization.

combine to influence behavior and health. Behavior, in turn, influences health, and healthy people are better able to adapt to the challenges of life. Some scholars have even defined health as the capability to adapt to life's circumstances.

With rewarding or successful adaptation comes learning the skills and actions that led to the success. This learning reinforces or strengthens those health-promoting or health-protecting behaviors that were most successful. Over a lifetime, people learn many health-promoting and health-protecting behavioral patterns. Over several lifetimes and generations in primitive conditions the healthiest practices tend to survive to be passed on to succeeding generations. All this can occur, however inefficiently, with little or no social organization.

In the process of forming communities, people have imposed another cycle on the natural history of health. They add a social history. They do this by passing information and social influence from parents to children, from neighbor to neighbor, and from elders and other leaders to followers. By this means, behavior becomes more and more organized or "civilized" by

Health Without Social Organization

Consider the "natural" process of health in a pre-historic time when people wandered as nomads without communities. Having little or no organization, they depended on their inherited biological strength and self-protective capacities to contend with the environment. They lived "in harmony" with nature, meaning that they adapted to their genetic endowment and their environment rather than trying to control these factors. Adaptation was made with a minimum of help from other people. Those who survived were the best learners, and their reward (reinforcement) for successful adaptation was survival. In this "natural" state, only three factors directly influenced health—human biology, the environment, and behavior. There was little organization and no health care technology to organize. How has the organization of people into clans, then communities, then governments and nations, influenced the natural history of health?

means of mutual expectations and social influence. Figure 2-3 shows how these socializing influences lead to what sociologists call **"norms"** or "social norms." One generation transmits its norms to the next in the form of culture. Culture, which reflects shared values and purposes sustained over time, shapes the methods and forms of social organizations. Some social organizations, such as churches, include in their mission the control of behavior. Others, such as sanitation and conservation organizations, attempt to control the environment.

Thus the community cycle closes on the **social history of health.** The behavioral and environmental controls exercised by community organizations include behavior related to health and environmental factors related to health. The social history of communities thereby imposes human organization as a fourth influence, for better or for worse, on the natural history of health. Two types of social organization that pertain to community health are consumer health and the organization of health services.

Consumer Health, Market Economics and Equity

The market economist's way of constructing the social cycle in figure 2-3 would be to replace norms with **supply and demand.** A widely practiced or "normative" behavior in relation to goods and services available in the community expresses itself economically as demand. For example, people who shift their purchasing behavior in large numbers from butter to margarine establish a norm and create a demand for more margarine. Demand, in turn, influences supply; if supply is limited, demand influences price. These three economic factors—**demand, supply,** and **price**—produce a social cycle similar to the behavior-norms-values cycle in figure 2-3. Prices equate with cultural values. Prices apply especially well to consumable goods and services. Values apply to consumable goods and to abstract goods such as loyalty, faith, love, and responsibility to care for children and elderly parents.

How does health come into the *Price = Value* equation? Is health a consumable good or an abstract value? If it is a privilege rather than a right, then how much are people willing to pay for health in direct purchase of services? If health is a right, then government must ensure that those who cannot afford the prices attached to health promotion, health protection, and health services still have equal access to them. **Accessibility** and equity in distribution of services and resources requires organization.

Even to people who can afford to pay for health products and services, the community or other level of government has some responsibility to ensure the quality and safety of those products and services. Governments exercise this responsibility through regulations for consumer health protection and standards for public health, hospitals, and other services and resources. Administering and enforcing consumer protection laws requires organization. Also, consumers organize for collective action or advocacy to pass new laws or to educate the public to protect themselves through selective purchasing. These forces put pressure on the

· · · · · · · · · · · · · · · · · ·
F i g u r e   2 - 3

The social history of health has imposed positive and negative influences on health through community organization of behavior, environment, and health care, three of the four elements of the health field.

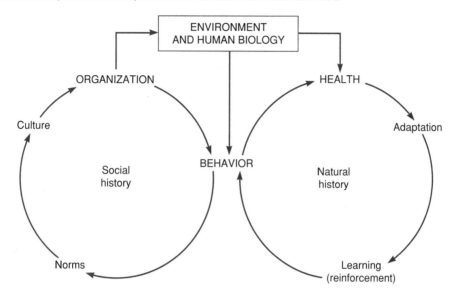

manufacturers, advertisers, and providers of health-related products and services. Companies selling food, toys, and automobiles, for example, feel consumer pressure to give greater attention to the health and safety implications of their practices or lose out in a competitive marketplace.

This "invisible hand" of the marketplace has been particularly invisible in medical care services. The medical profession in the United States, for example, is the only industry legally exempted from most of the economic rules of monopoly. Medicine has also avoided much of the government regulation applied to other social services. Laws restrict other professions from practicing medicine, hence the monopoly. Yet the medical profession enjoys the highest privilege of the professions: self-regulation. Listing of fees is not the custom of medical practitioners. Most medical societies have restrained advertising by physicians. Consumers had little economic information and little encouragement for doctor "shopping." One of the most powerful tools of the consumer in

other marketplaces is shopping for the best prices. Without prior knowledge of fees, patients exert little influence on medicine. New health care reforms, such as managed care competition, are changing the monopoly and self-regulatory aspects of medicine.

Government and health insurance plans further complicate the economic market forces of the medical marketplace by removing the consumer's awareness of the price they are paying for health care services. This "third-party payer" arrangement handles fees for services directly through the insurance company or the government to the medical service providers—hospitals or physicians. This means that the consumer or patient is often unaware of the costs of care, much less financially responsible for their payment. These conditions undermine the potential of competitive economic market forces to control the social history of health. This throws additional responsibilities on society to organize to control the cost and distribution of health resources and services.

····················

Figure 2-4

The place of personal histories and motivation in the development of lifestyle (behavior) and health shows the 1) predisposing factors, 2) enabling factors, and 3) reinforcing factors for behavior, and how these interact with other environmental, social, and individual determinants of community or population health. (Adapted from Green LW, Richard L, Potvin L: Ecological foundations of health promotion. *Amer J Health Promotion* 10:270, 1996.)

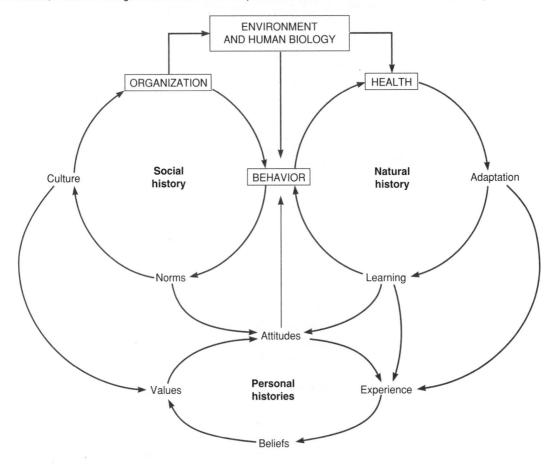

The Individual's Place in Community and Population Health

Ecology focuses attention on the interaction of populations or species and their environments, but the cumulative behavior of individuals is central to the ecological relationship of populations to their environments. A lifetime of individual experience shapes beliefs, values, attitudes, and ultimately behavior, as shown at the bottom of figure 2-4. Beliefs combine with cultural influences to shape

each individual's values. Values are deep-seated, enduring orientations toward social goods and evils, right and wrong, and ethical and unethical behavior. These combine with the perceived norms of behavior to produce in the individual an attitude toward a specific behavior.

Figure 2-4 shows four sources of influence on behavior as a determinant of health. One is the immediate attitude or intention of the individual that *predisposes* him or her to take an action. Organizational and environmental factors combine with innate capacities endowed by human biology to *enable* the individual to take a desired action to promote or protect his or her health. Learning from past experiences *reinforces* the behavior by recalling previous successes and satisfactions associated with a type of behavior. These translate for the individual as anticipated rewards for repeating or generalizing the behavior. How community and population health programs can strengthen the factors that predispose, enable, and reinforce behavior conducive to health will be the subject of chapter 4. Here we will focus on how ecology and organization relate more directly to health. The natural history of health converges with social history and personal histories to influence health through the behavior of individuals and the organization of the environment. The three cycles of figure 2-4 are continuous rather than static. They connect with each other in such a way that everything influences and is influenced by everything else, however indirectly or remotely. This is a central lesson of human ecology.

Tracing the arrows representing causation in figure 2-4, the pivotal factor linking personal and social histories to health is behavior. Personal history can influence health only through behavior. The behavior may be individual action (self-care, lifestyle, or use of health services). It may be collective action (organizing community groups for health, family decisions, neighborhood petition, voter recruitment, or other social process). Collective action results in some change in the organization of health resources or the environment to influence health directly or through behavior.

Organizing Health Services and Technology

Civilized societies recognize the need to provide for the care of their sick, but the demand for and the costs of such care tend to exceed the resources of many communities. When that happens, it compromises the community's greater responsibility to protect the health of all of its citizens. Then its opportunities to promote and protect the health of

Social Ethics in Organized Health Care

Some decisions must be made by the community concerning its own priorities in allocating its resources to social and health services, each with competing interest groups and competing value judgments. Is it more important to spend several million dollars providing for kidney dialysis for a single child who will die without it or to spend half as much for each of two programs to ensure the improved nutrition and immunization of thousands of children in the same community? Few if any of the children would likely die without the nutrition and immunization programs, but hundreds might be healthier, more productive in school, and less likely to contract a disabling or disfiguring disease if the nutrition and immunization programs are maintained.

those who are not sick slip away. Decisions between the best medical care for a few and the best health care for the masses confront those who must allocate community health resources. These decisions become contentious when an aging population with increasing burdens of chronic disease also contains many children and young adults whose needs differ.

Most nations spend over 90 percent of their governmental health budgets on technologically advanced services available only from medical specialists and hospitals. Most Western nations spend less than 5 percent of their health budgets on prevention. The high cost of maintaining the specialized medical services, equipment, and facilities, especially under the market conditions described in the preceding section, has caused the price for medical and nursing care to skyrocket. The inflation of costs in this sector is far beyond the resources of many families and even communities to pay. Medical costs have been soaring at an average increase of 20 percent per year in the United States.

These changing circumstances have caused most families to become reliant on insurance or welfare systems to provide for their medical care. "Catastrophic" care has come to mean anything requiring more than a few days in the hospital. The insurance system, in turn, has had to reorganize its premium structures to cover the outlays for claims made on behalf of the insured by their medical providers. Most families cannot afford these new "health insurance" policies, which are really medical and hospital insurance. They depend increasingly on employer contributions to pay at least a share of the premiums. As a result, labor unions have found more of their progress in collective bargaining taken up by health insurance benefits, leaving less for wages and other benefits. Similarly, employers have found larger percentages of the price on their products being taken up by health insurance benefits to their employees. This means less profit and less investment in growth or modernization and higher prices for most consumer goods.

Many companies have responded to these trends in the competitive private sector by seeking new ways to control the costs of health care. They have supported government efforts to force more competition in the medical care field, while spawning their own versions of self-insurance, managed care organizations, and employee health and fitness programs in the workplace.

Policies to Achieve Greater Equity in Access to Health Resources

As a social experiment in organizing medical care, Great Britain's National Health Service has not entirely solved the ethical and political problems relating to the equitable **allocation** of technology. Canada structured its health care system to address the problems of universal access to affordable care by the average citizen. The federal government in the United States has experimented with a series of adjustments in its policies. These have included policies governing health facility planning; purchasing power for the elderly under Medicare and for the poor under Medicaid; and the market controls on pricing, reimbursements, and competition through managed care. These policies will be the subject of part 4 of this book. We mention them

here to contrast the predominant thrust of national policies to contain costs with the policies addressing the greater determinants of community health in lifestyle and the environment.

Reforming national policies to contain cost in medical care is urgent given that more than 90 percent of the national expenditures for health go into this sector and will increase without reform as populations age. The total contribution to mortality reduction or increased longevity that health care organizations can make is less than 20 percent of the total contribution from all determinants (figure 2-1 p. 34). By this measure, the greatest potential for progress in community and population health clearly lies in programs addressing the environment and lifestyle.

Community health and population health strategies, then, must recognize all four elements of the health field. Communities in democratic societies can exert very little direct control over human biology other than through genetic counseling. This leaves three points for intervention, as shown in figure 1-2, p. 6. Following the terminology adopted in the policies for disease prevention and health promotion in the United States and Canada, the interventions directed at lifestyle are referred to broadly as *health promotion,* those directed at the environment are referred to as *health protection,* those directed at the health care system as *preventive health services.* The three sections of this book following this introductory section are organized around these three broad strategies for community health.

CONCEPT OF COMMUNITY

More than the sum of its populations, a community consists of interdependent social units that transact a common life among the people making up the units. As a social group, functioning with norms of behavior and organization of resources, the community regulates the environment and the behavior of individuals and organizations.

A neighborhood community may exist in a limited territory, but increasingly the functional community consists of a constantly enlarging geographical region. Our concept of community has changed from the limited view that a city in its boundary constitutes a community to a consideration of the interaction of social norms, values, and organizations. We speak of a metropolitan area, implying that the entire area functions as a unified community. In the United States the Metropolitan Statistical Area (MSA) is a county or group of contiguous counties containing at least one city of 50,000 inhabitants or more and a total population of 100,000.

Suburbs and other areas surrounding the legal limits of a city are an integral part of the total community. Erecting hospitals, establishing clinics, and providing other medical services require planning based on estimates of the health needs of the entire population served. By such population-based planning it is possible to organize more efficiently for all people living within the area.

Besides the geographic community, modern communications, the Internet, and rapid transportation have created more widely active and effective communities of interest (such as national advocacy groups). They also produce communities of need (such as minority associations) and communities of solution (such as national voluntary and professional health associations). We will use the term **community,** for most purposes in this book, to refer to a group of inhabitants living in a somewhat localized area under the same general regulations and having common norms, values, and organizations. **Population** refers to any aggregate of individuals, including multiple communities or subcommunities.

Physical Factors

Varying environmental and social influences can identify subcommunities within the community or population. Such subcommunities can consist of towns within counties or ethnic or neighborhood groupings within cities. Therefore in some respects a large metropolitan area can be thought of as a group of villages. Environmental factors to be recognized in assessing community health resources and problems include the physical environment; geography, topography, and climate; neighborhood organization; and industrial conditions.

••••••••••••••••••
Figure 2-5

Water is so critical to the survival, health, and quality of life of a community that women's work in rural areas of some countries consists of many hours each day carrying fresh water from great distances. These women in Nepal carry water urns in baskets from a shared well to their homes. (Photo by N. Willard courtesy World Health Organization.)

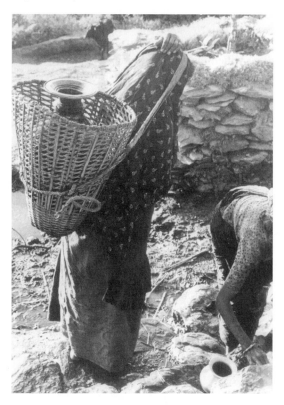

Physical Environment   The physical environment sometimes reflects the community's general health status. This applies to the mental, emotional, and social health of a community and to its physical health. The community that possesses a degree of orderliness, however old or simple its buildings, usually reflects an awareness and a pride in the well-being of its residents. Clean air and water, however, are the most critical environmental factors in health (see figure 2-5 and part 3 of this book).

Geography, Topography, and Climate Geography refers to the surface of the earth. Topography indicates the features of a region or locality. With climate, these two phenomena may cause or contribute to special community health problems. Lowlands, marshy areas, and hot climates give rise to health problems not of concern elsewhere. Such areas contain most of the tropical diseases, but modern air transport can carry them to the cities of temperate regions. Dry, dusty areas may create health conditions differing from those of more humid regions. The minerals of an area, the types of soil, and the functions of the waterways can be significant factors in determining the general health of the local population.

Community Size The traditional notion of a neighborhood was of an area that housed a population for which one elementary school would serve its children. Such a neighborhood ranged in size from 1,000 to 3,000 families. This usually meant an entire population of about 5,000. This is about the size of most census tracts, which form a basic unit of analysis in the U.S. Census counts. Areas deviating from this general pattern are increasingly common, but still can be designated as true neighborhood units. As the birthrate or death rate declines, more people live alone, and more elderly people live without children, the elementary school as a criterion of neighborhood becomes less relevant. As more people relate to friends and coworkers other than their neighbors, the concept of neighborhood itself becomes less compelling as an organizational building block of community (see box).

Many smaller villages and towns tend to lose their younger adults who move away. Disproportionate numbers of the residents of small rural and even nonrural towns are older people. In developing countries the opposite condition arises, with high birthrates in rural areas. With many of their citizens over sixty-five years old, these small communities find themselves faced with low birthrates, high death rates, and the special health problems of the elderly. Many of these communi-

> ### Ecological Building Blocks of Community and Society
>
> In designating 1994 as the International Year of the Family, the United Nations adopted the slogan, "Building the smallest democracy at the heart of society." The UN members thus recognized the family as a building block of a democratic society. How does this building block relate to the neighborhood, the census tract, the suburban area, the city, the county, and the region? Draw concentric circles with the individual in the middle, surrounded by family, friends, neighbors, and other layers of organization to the state or provincial level. Consider what levels of organization need to plan and deliver programs to support or penetrate these concentric circles with information, services, and resources.

ties are unable to keep their hospitals open or to provide the necessary health services for the health needs of their older citizens or children. Some communities are fortunate in being near or part of a large community in which complete health services are available. Health planning agencies are attempting to address the needs of the outlying communities by linking them with urban facilities, resources, and services.

Neighborhood Organization Some of the older, long-established neighborhoods have an amazing unity and rapport. Some of the newer neighborhoods, particularly in the suburban areas, frequently are neighborhoods in area only. Speculative building in the suburbs, combined with a mobile population, tends to produce communities of individuals who are almost transients, with scant allegiance to a common standard for their neighborhood (see figure 2-6). Neighborhoods need time before they feel the influence of schools, churches, and the formation of community groups. Social unity in such neighborhoods is loose. The degree of neighborhood unity, past practices, leadership, and established standards all

• • • • • • • • • • • • • • • • • •
Figure 2-6

This vision of tomorrow's city was displayed by General Motors at the New York World's Fair in 1965. It has come true to a large extent in many metropolitan areas where the automobile has been the reigning mode of transport. Cars fostered suburban sprawl, expanding the areas in which urban workers could live. Abandoning the central city to commercial and industrial use made it less hospitable for residential use. Urban planners now recommend "redensification" of residential settlements in the inner cities. (Photo by General Motors, courtesy World Health Organization.)

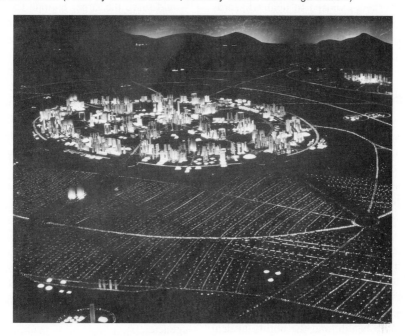

contribute to existing health conditions. More revealing, however, is the nature of the neighborhood unity that exists when a particular health problem or threat arises that the neighbors must deal with on a cooperative basis. A toxic waste problem, a restaurant applying for a liquor license, a school safety hazard, or a store selling cigarettes to minors are examples. Where a long-established neighborhood cohesiveness already exists, the necessary leadership and united support will emerge quickly to initiate a program to solve the health problem summarily. A neighborhood with little cohesiveness will struggle to mobilize the neighborhood's resources. Such a neighborhood may require several years to cope with a health problem that a more cohesive neighborhood will have well in hand in a matter of days. One sees

vivid examples of these variations in the ways different neighborhoods have tackled drug abuse, appeals to city hall for local improvements, and efforts to block developments that present environmental threats or safety hazards.

Industrial Conditions   Health problems arise with particular industrial conditions that either prevail within the community or indirectly affect the community. A "garden city" or a residential community will not have some of the health problems that citizens in a highly industrialized community will encounter. An industry that causes a great deal of noise may create special problems of an emotional and a physical nature. Chemical plants creating noxious odors can affect the social health or quality of life of the community.

A mining community or a logging community living in the shadow of extreme occupational hazards is a community different from one in which industrial injuries are rare. A particular industry will have direct environmental effects on the health of a community. Another will have effects on individual workers exposed to health hazards on the job. If the industry employs a large number of residents, the community tolerates a greater threat or nuisance from its safety hazards or its pollution.

Social and Cultural Factors

A community's character does not lie in the observable physical features of the buildings, industries, size, and topography. Communities distinguish themselves by less visible social and cultural factors. The traditions of the community, its social stratification, its religious influences, its stability or tenure of residence, and other social and cultural processes operate to give the community a distinctive personality. These same factors directly and indirectly influence the health of the community. The cultural and organizational tendencies and capabilities that have evolved over years will affect the recognition of health threats, the promotion of community health, and the ability to deal with health emergencies.

Parochialism, Traditions, and Prejudices

Emerging health problems such as HIV and AIDS, new aspects of old health problems such as drug abuse or tuberculosis, changing health requirements, and new discoveries call for new approaches to health. In some communities long established conventions inhibit attempts to deal with evolving health needs. In some instances these orally transmitted traditions are not readily identifiable but appear as norms of resistance such as, "We have always done it this way," or "Not in our backyard!" Preconceived judgments or values relating to health matters, people having health problems, or public health procedures sometimes present obstacles to health advances in the community. Health biases arising from fear of mental illness, homophobia, or prejudice against people

on welfare, can be as deeply ingrained as a religious bias. Indeed, sometimes they are the same, as with abortion and alcohol.

Another problem of parochial attitudes for community and population health is the resistance of some neighborhoods or communities to reforms that would serve the larger region. Too often people at their neighborhood level resist changes required for the larger good if they see them as requiring some local sacrifice or disadvantage. The slogan, "Think globally and act locally" calls upon individuals and local groups to work cooperatively across regions because many health and environmental threats do not honor jurisdictional boundaries. Among the most contentious issues in urban planning are transportation policies seeking to reduce automobile use in favor of mass transit (see figure 2-6).

Socioeconomic Status (SES)   Individuals, families, and neighborhoods find themselves located in the social stratification of a community or population based on some combination of their income, residence, occupation, or education. The resulting hierarchy of socioeconomic status (SES), graduated into any number of upper, middle, and lower levels, influences lifestyle, which in turn governs environmental exposures, customs, and habits that affect health status. Considerable correlation among income, residence, occupation, and education makes any one of these a reasonable measure of SES. Education (years of school completed) is the most powerful determinant of the four criteria with regard to influence on health-related behavior. Populations of high educational attainment often enjoy the best health status. They respond readily to appeals from health professionals to modify their lifestyles related to smoking cessation, weight control, exercise programs, and immunization. In contrast, populations of a low educational level often suffer the worst health and are more difficult to reach with persuasive health messages. A cultural barrier frequently exists between the efforts of health professionals to educate and the perceptions of people with less education.

Most diseases cut across all strata of society, although they affect the lower strata most.

Prevention and control of communicable diseases by community measures focused on the less privileged groups indirectly protect and thus benefit the entire population. Low-income groups and those of less educational attainment need preventive health services and health promotion activities most, but the entire population will benefit from an overall community health program.

Social Norms Customs and norms imbued with ethical significance can have the force of law. Usually the social norms of a community, such as the norms restraining sexual activity in teenagers, can serve as an asset in the promotion of community health. It is sometimes necessary, however, to change established customs in a community to obtain the necessary gains that modern health procedures can contribute. Tobacco, alcohol, and drug use have become customs or norms in some communities. Reversing the widespread use of such substances is as much a political process as an educational one. Modification of customs in a community usually requires political compromise to reconcile the differing values of different cultural groups. Attempts to eliminate or reverse a custom often generate hostile resistance to a health program. When one generation passes its norms to the next, they become embedded in the culture of the community as values. Effective health programs more often adapt to and accommodate the customs and values of a community than attempt to totally change them.

Religious Influences Communities composed of diverse religious groups living in harmony restrain any particular denomination from dominating the community. The total effect is to enrich community life and to provide a cooperative spirit in which health can flourish. If the community's health leaders seek the support of the many religious groups in the community, they become sensitive to possible conflicts, religious or otherwise, that may undermine a community health program.

Political Factors Among community health strategies that are political, law enforcement is in-

creasingly significant as a factor in modern community health protection and promotion. The caliber of officials a community has and the extent of social-mindedness in its bureaucraisies directly and indirectly affect community health standards. They sometimes need to demonstrate the political will to raise taxes for health services or health promotion. They may need to enforce regulations to control industry for health protection, possibly in the face of strong business or political resistance. Even when official support of community health is inadequate, however, it is often possible through other agencies to promote community health action and to bring political pressure to bear on local government.

Economic Factors The diversity of industry, the fluctuations in the economy, and the extremes of rich and poor are of significance to community health. Different economic conditions mean differences in the amount of money available for food, clothing, housing, and other basic needs. They also mean differences in the amount of money available for health facilities, health services, schools, sanitary facilities, leisure-time activities, and general health promotion programs.

The average family income that a local economy provides directly influences a community's level of health. Vital statistics indicate that people residing in affluent cities live longer than people who reside in low-income cities. The average income, however, may conceal homeless people and others who do not share in the community's wealth. Prosperous communities usually provide more and better medical facilities than impoverished communities, though this is a factor of overrated importance in community or population health.

Growth Rate Population growth sometimes indicates a thriving and healthy community, but growth may cause temporary displacements within a community that may be damaging to health. The community may require additional schools, housing, and services. There may be some disorganization during the time between the occurrence of these new needs and their fulfillment. This is the experience of suburban communities adjacent to large metropolitan areas, especially during periods of heavy immigration and most dramatically with refugee settlements. In such communities the tenure of residence of many of the families is relatively short. Usually the newcomers are young couples with small children. In other communities where families are moving in and out constantly, an unfavorable health situation usually exists. A high number of transient families tends to weaken the stability and social networks that support the health of a community or population.

Organizational Factors

No single local agency or organization has the scope of authority or the necessary resources to encompass all dimensions of a community health strategy. Any community needs a diversity of agencies and individuals to provide services of direct and indirect health significance. Too little coordination or integration of services often leads to duplication and overlapping of functions. Despite the lack of efficient coordination, tax-supported and nontax-supported health services often cooperate and form coalitions to meet specific community health needs.

Official Agencies The official, tax-supported agencies may contribute to the health of a community indirectly, but the majority of their services and programs directly affect individual residents. The most important of these tax-supported agencies is the local or district health department. Other official agencies providing health services include departments of welfare, recreation, transportation, public works, public hospitals, special boards and commissions, public schools, the local housing authority, and the police department.

Voluntary Organizations Health promotion and health services available to communities through voluntary agencies or nontax-supported organizations represent the true spirit of community reflected in the quotations at the beginning of this chapter and in figure 2-7. The giving of donations

Figure 2-7

Voluntary organizations depend on the impulse of people to help others through charitable donations of time, money, materials, or even their own blood and organs. (Courtesy Advertising Council, and Griffin Bacal, Inc.)

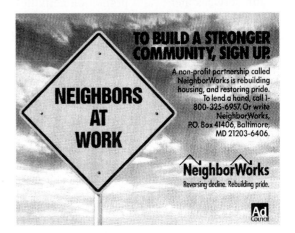

or of blood voluntarily and anonymously to help others less fortunate is an expression of community in its purest form. Civic clubs, church groups, parent-teacher associations, the Red Cross, visiting nurse associations, the United Way, and some community hospitals are examples of nontax-supported services. Special clinical services, and medical care and hospital service plans, may also be available.

National voluntary health organizations may have an indirect effect on the health of any given community and in some instances may play a direct role in the health of individual citizens. These national voluntary health organizations serve several functions, such as educating, conducting demonstrations, supplementing and supporting official health activities, and coordinating community health efforts. Some of these organizations concern themselves with specific diseases. In North America this group includes the American or Canadian Cancer Society, American Heart Association or the Heart and Stroke Foundation of Canada, American or Canadian Lung Associations, and various self-help groups, among others.

Bridging the official and nontax-supported services in many communities are practicing physicians, dentists, nurses, and other health specialists. The organizations that represent them include professional associations such as the local medical society, the dental society, and nursing associations.

TECHNOLOGICAL AND AGRICULTURAL FACTORS

A nation's food supply and its work and leisure patterns influence the health of its people. North America's food and physical activity situations have undergone enormous changes resulting from a convergence of many new technologies applied to farming, work in other spheres, food processing, transportation, and recreational activity. The population living on farms, for example, declined from 31–35 percent of the U.S. and Canadian totals in early decades to less than 3 percent in the 1990s (figure 2-8). During this period the total farm acreage and food production increased, the amount and composition of food consumed changed dramatically, and physical activity slowed to produce a relatively sedentary North American population. We discuss in this chapter some of the global implications of these changes, reserving the more specific health promotion implications for subsequent chapters.

World Hunger and Poverty

Nearly 40 percent of the people in the developing world live in such grinding poverty that they cannot provide themselves with a minimally adequate diet, shelter, education, or health care. Many are unemployed, many more underemployed. This impoverished two-fifths of humanity lack the land to grow its own food. They lack the money to buy it—even in years when local crops are good, world production is high, and storage bins are overflowing. Even doubling food production on present patterns would not materially change the status of the great majority of those who are hungry and malnourished. Eight hundred million people in developing countries are malnourished and more than 8 million deaths of children under five each year are associated with malnutrition.

Inequities as extremes of wealth and poverty persist between and within nations. Three major

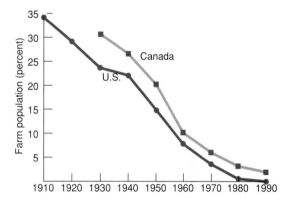

F i g u r e 2 - 8

The farm population, as a percentage of total U.S. and Canadian resident populations, has declined steadily since 1910. (*Sources:* U.S. Bureau of the Census and Statistics Canada.)

national factors give rise to most developing world poverty: inequitable distribution of resources and income, low productivity and slow economic growth, and excessive population increases. As events in Uganda and the former Yugoslavia demonstrate, war and civil disintegration of social order can lead to starvation in even shorter time than the other three conditions combined. Rapid population growth that outstrips economic growth maintains or worsens the cycle of poverty.

The Global Ecology of World Hunger

Solutions to the problem of world hunger can result only from sustainable, equitable, and self-reliant development. The industrialized nations can do their part by providing various forms of development assistance. The effort, however, to ensure equitable development cannot end with economic assistance. Hunger and poverty have ecological roots in political and economic relations among nations. This calls for fundamental changes in global patterns of food production and trade (for example, the General Agreement on Trade and Tariffs of 1993). Such trade agreements can improve the conditions for the developing countries themselves to break the cycle of stagnant agricultural productivity, hunger, poverty, high birthrates, unemployment, and poor health.

Poor nations and poor people depend for their future on the evolution of the international economy as a whole. A number of related factors will govern the general direction of the world economy and the performance of individual communities and developing nations. If the poor nations merely exploit their natural resources as the affluent nations did before them, the improved economic condition will be ecologically unsustainable. It is imperative that policymakers in every nation search for all possible ways to develop sustainable economic growth as the means of overcoming the cycle of hunger, poverty, and poor health.

The rhetoric of the "global economy" sometimes forgets that local community economies have an ecological reality of their own to respect. A community cannot make its decisions about economic development only on the basis of finding a niche in the global economy. It must also consider the sustainability of its own resources, or it risks falling prey to external exploitation and internal depletion of its resources.

Technology

The widespread application of insecticides, weed killers, and fertilizers has reduced the amount of cultivation necessary on farms. Better strains of plants and animals, some through genetic engineering (figure 2-9), and the addition of antibiotics to animal feeds have increased the productivity of farms. Improved methods of food processing, better refrigeration, improved packaging, and better methods of food preservation have reduced food wastes considerably and thus have contributed tangibly to the total food supply.

Such technologies, however, also bear less wholesome results. Chemicals have accumulated in the soil, in the water supply, and in food products. They present new hazards. Environmental health was once concerned primarily with microorganisms. Environmental and occupational health are concerned chiefly with toxic agents of the chemical variety including refrigerants and fossil fuel that escape to the upper atmosphere and threaten the global ozone layer.

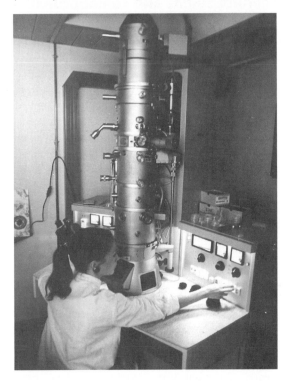

Figure 2-9

The electron microscope made possible some of the genetic studies that have led to the decoding of the gene and the ethical and ecological quandaries that follow. (Courtesy World Health Organization, photo by J Mohr.)

Technology has had as much impact on the behavioral and organizational aspects of the health field as on the environmental aspects. The computer, for example, has revolutionized the ways we handle information and communication. Consequently, it has altered human relationships, creating a newly emerging set of mental, emotional, and social health concerns referred to broadly as technostress and ethical issues concerned with privacy and confidentiality of health information.

Each technological solution to a previous problem brings with it the risk or the reality of new problems it creates. The recognition of this risk cannot hold back the introduction of new technologies,

ISSUES AND CONTROVERSIES
Tampering with Nature?

Gene-splicing is a technology made possible by the electron microscope (figure 2.9) and by the Human Genome Project. It allows scientists to splice a minute bit of genetic material from one organism with another to obtain potentially valuable biological products. At first, great fear gripped the scientific community, then the public, that these techniques could unleash dangerous pathogens through biological warfare or by laboratory accidents. The fears subsided as government health agencies imposed rigorous guidelines for experimentation.

New fears have arisen over the release of commercially engineered organisms and food products for agricultural purposes. The concern is that genetically engineered plants or microbes used in agriculture might harm the ecology if they escaped from their agricultural niche and upset nature's balance. Ecologists point out that the European gypsy moth wreaked havoc in North America because there were no natural predators to keep it in check. Could the same happen with genetically altered agricultural products? Do the new technology's benefits outweigh its risks, assuming that gene splicing should be able to improve the nutritional quality of crops and increase their resistance to pests, disease, and drought? Will gene therapy be allowed to alter the inherited characteristics of newborn children?

---

but does call for an ecological understanding of the radiating impact of each new technology. This understanding can help build societal, community, organizational, and regulatory buffers to protect people from the unintended side effects of a new technology.

QUALITY OF HEALTH

Many people regarded as well still do not have the quality of health that enables them to live as productively, effectively, and enjoyably as they might. They may be free from disabilities and overt symptoms and yet not possess an adequate level of well-being.

Community health seeks not only to minimize disabling defects and disorders, but also to enable the people of the community to do the things they reasonably expect to do with enjoyment and gratification. Not perfect health but a high level of well-being in which an individual finds life productive and stimulating is a realistic goal for residents of every community.

Despite advances in longevity and in communicable disease control during this century, poor health remains prevalent in most communities and many populations. In Western societies most of the serious diseases and disabilities people can control relate to personal habits: drinking, smoking, drug misuse, overeating, poor nutrition, lack of exercise, and careless behavior. Community strategies to support and enable people to change these habits can improve health and the quality of life for individuals and populations.

Not all solutions will be behavioral. Indeed, in the early years of the twenty-first century, as in the first years of the twentieth, the results of basic research, technological development, and environmental modification may offer further control of health problems. Currently, however, knowledge to prevent or to minimize many health problems is not being used to a satisfactory degree.

The challenge, then, is to develop integrated community programs to support better health practices and health protection. Given the ever-increasing social and economic burden of health care costs resulting from negative community conditions and lifestyles, how can governments, community organizations, and individuals work together to improve these conditions?

COMMUNITY ACTION AND INNOVATION

Integrated community programs—as distinct from separate or isolated school health programs, worksite programs, or patient care programs—require a distinct set of concepts, methods, and procedures. How are they different from the numerous applications of the same health programs or interventions used in various organizations within the community? What distinguishes integrated community health programs besides being bigger than their counterparts at the clinical, school, or worksite levels? Are community programs really different from their counterpart interventions in medical and other institutional settings, or do they merely represent the sum of these parts? Besides coordinating the pieces, how do community programs function? Other than reaping the additive effects of small-scale programs, what makes large-scale community programs effective?

These questions are at the heart of a community approach to health. They defy simplistic answers that would merely distinguish community approaches from institutionally-based programs in terms of greater magnitude, scope, or volume. Something more than size holds such community programs together. Their strategies must be more than medical models enlarged; more than pedagogical methods transferred to the media. Their organization must entail more than a step up the bureaucratic ladder from school to district, from neighborhood clinic to city health department or regional hospital.

Levels of Community Intervention and Change

One distinction of integrated community health programs is that change must occur at several levels if the program is to penetrate the whole community (figure 2-10). At the individual level change can be expected to occur among the more affluent citizens without much intervention. For the majority, however, communities must mobilize a more intensive and coordinated effort to be reached and persuade most, especially the poor and socially isolated, to make changes in their behavior or environment. At the organizational level supports for individual change can be mobilized through advocacy, consultation, professional networks, and training of agency leaders and other personnel.

Governmental level local, state, or national tax-supported agencies and legislative bodies can mobilize themselves in support of community programs, or advocacy groups can pressure them to take action. Groups such as Students Against Drunk Driving can demand better enforcement of existing regulations or the passage of more restrictive legislation. Individual health professionals and other citizens also can bring about change in governmental support for community health. They can, for example, give testimony at city council; state, provincial, or national legislative hearings; or at public hearings of government agencies or agencies contemplating revisions of rules, codes, or regulations. Health professionals and local groups also can support governmental action by preparing position papers analyzing the impact of proposed changes. They can present such papers to policy-making bodies, government agencies, and the press. Figure 2-10 suggests other actions and their targets.

This book takes the ecological view that integrated community programs, as compared with the sum of numerous small-scale programs in a community, require a shift in perspective. They require the employment of a set of analytic and programmatic tools distinct from those used with individual patients, students, clients, or customers. The differences between small-scale and community programs reflect the distinctions between clinical and epidemiological methods of analysis. They also reflect differences between psychological and sociological theories; between counseling and mass-media methods of communication; between accounting and economics; and between intra-organizational and inter-organizational levels of planning, management, and intervention.

THE MULTIPLE GOALS AND SECTORS OF COMMUNITY HEALTH

Several countries and many states, provinces, and communities have adopted quantitative goals or objectives in disease prevention and health promotion. The tangibility and the accountability provided by such goals has captured the imagination

....

Figure 2-10

Levels of action for community health intervention suggest roles for various sectors, citizens, and professionals.
(Adapted with permission from Brink SG et al: *Community intervention handbooks for comprehensive health promotion programming,* Atlanta, 1988, Centers for Disease Control.)

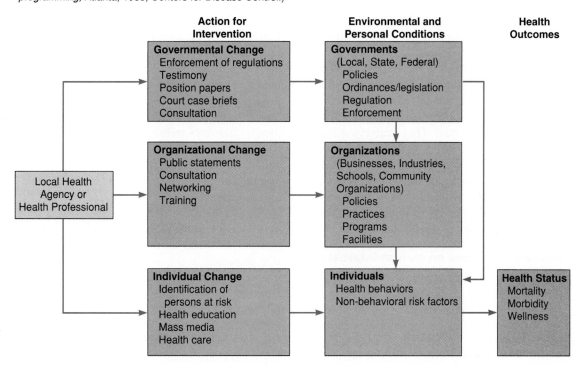

of many health professionals and the commitment of some health organizations. The U.S. Healthy People 2000 objectives, for example, appeared to be gaining momentum in the mid-1990s and programs showed promise of accomplishing many of the objectives by the year 2000. If the enthusiasm and esprit de corps of health professionals and organizations were all that communities needed to accomplish the objectives, the road to health for all by the year 2000 would indeed be smooth.

Health professionals and health agencies alone cannot achieve these broad health goals and objectives. Programs require for their success the active participation of other sectors, other professionals, and other institutions than those primarily identified with health (see figures 1-1 and 2-10). Most of these nonhealth organizations operate at the community level. Schools, workplaces, recre-

ational facilities, social welfare agencies, restaurants, and supermarkets have important roles to play in community health.

Not since the seventeenth century has the medical establishment—or even the public health establishment—been more irrelevant to the task of improving the public's health. They possess the knowledge of what needs to be done, hence the ability to state achievable health objectives. But they are helpless by themselves to achieve most of those objectives. Success depends on reaching people where their daily decisions about the environment and lifestyle are influenced and made. This means reaching them in schools, in workplaces, and in community settings other than medical.

Health organizations and professionals often assume that their own coordinating ability and the compelling nature of health will bring sectors into line. Health professionals indulge such wishful thinking on the mistaken notion that other sectors of human services are all too willing to set their own priorities aside if presented with a health problem or threat. Coordination was easier when epidemics were imminent enough to galvanize concerted community action.

It is remarkable that the disease prevention and health promotion objectives draw any attention at all, considering their remote and sober character. They hardly have the siren appeal of the epidemics and scourges of the past. They scarcely compete even with matters of economics—the dismal science—much less with threats of war and nuclear holocaust. Little wonder then that other sectors and the public at large seem unresponsive when the health sector calls on them to help achieve disease prevention and health promotion objectives.

Building Coalitions on Mutual Interests

Why have nonhealth organizations shown even a glimmer of interest, considering all this? Two reasons seem to account for most of the interest shown by other sectors in community health promotion. One is the perceived demand of the public; the other is the possibility that it could contribute to other goals that they seek.

Coalitions   The mutual interests of many public and private sectors in health issues has led to the development of community coalitions on specific health issues. Coalitions often include representation from recreation, business, media, and welfare sectors and medical and health sectors. Coalitions have their greatest value in bringing multiple agencies together to agree on goals and broad strategy. They sometimes collapse under their own bureaucratic weight when they try to manage programs (see box).

Response to Public Interest   Perceiving a public demand for health promotion, better health protection, or health services, many organizations outside the health field have taken up health-related programs. Commercial interests, in particular, have risen to the challenge of consumer demand.

Many organizations have begun to offer health promotion programs or facilities for their own employees. Some have justified these expenditures on the argument that they gain a competitive edge in attracting and holding the best employees.

How did the consumer demand come about? Can we sustain it or even nurture it to gain even more support from other sectors? Part of the answer to these questions lies in an enlightened public. Continuing health information and education programs will stimulate increased consumer discretion in matters of health. This stimulates commercial and news media to provide more information, some of which strays from fact. This stimulates debate and controversy, further whetting the public's appetite for more health information and education.

The downside to this escalating market of health ideas is the consequent glutting of information and the withering crossfire of health information presented in the media. The "carcinogen of the week" race between the official health agencies, the Food and Drug Administration, and the tobacco and polluting chemical industries makes the legitimate messages of any of them lose credibility and impact. The public pleads for relief from this tumult. The cooperation of public and private organizations in various sectors promises relief for the public caught in this withering crossfire of charges and countercharges. They can do this best through the development of consensus on selected health messages and the dissemination of joint communications such as the Dietary Guidelines for Americans or the Canadian Food Guidelines. The formulation of goals and objectives in disease prevention and health promotion offers such consensus points among community service agencies and commercial organizations that they can present to the public with one voice.

Planning and Implementing Community Programs

Community-wide programs require, above all, more planning and coordination than do small-scale programs. More participants in planning and execution mean more meetings and telephone calls

Caveats on Coalitions

The assumption of many funding agencies in these times of scarce resources and limited budgets is that community health programs need a coalition of local organizations to plan and carry out the program. This assumption is based on the reasonable expectation that the duplication of effort and resources is wasteful and can be avoided through joint planning. The further assumption, however, that after planning such programs jointly, the organizations should remain together in the implementation of the programs, breaks down in many communities. Five caveats on coalitions suggest why:

1. Most organizations will resist giving up resources, credit, visibility, or autonomy at the point of implementing programs.
2. Not everyone insists on being the coordinator, but few wish to be coordinated, resisting the loss of control over their usual ways of doing their work.
3. So much effort and expense goes into maintaining the coalition that little may be left to execute a program.
4. Those who come to the first coalition meeting may be high officials of the several agencies, but to the second meeting they often send their deputies, and they, in turn, send their deputies to the third meeting. By the time the serious coalition work is underway, some of the people attending the coalition meetings have little authority to make decisions on behalf of their respective agencies. Each meeting ends in a stalemate until they can consult with their bosses on actions the coalition would like to take.
5. The reality of implementation, once a good plan is in place, is that it takes flexibility and adaptability in the field. A coalition is an unwieldy instrument for managing the actual implementation of programs.

A solution to this set of caveats could be called The Noah's Arc Principle of Partnering: "Go forth two-by-two." After the coalition has developed agreement on goals, objectives, and a broad strategy, allow the member organizations to pair off in partnerships for implementation. This maximizes the advantages of cooperation while minimizing the disadvantages of trying to manage their activities by an unwieldy coalition.

to achieve consensus, more letters and documents to convey concepts and procedures to more varied actors. The complexities grow exponentially with each organization added to the roster of participants. Coalitions reach a point of efficiency when they can match added organizations into partnership with participating organizations having mutual interests (see box "Caveats on Coalitions").

The number of units (organizations, clinics, schools, persons) reaches a point where newcomers are more likely to be similar to some previous comers. At that point large-scale programs begin to realize an **economy of scale.** This means that for each newcomer the job of planning and coordination gets easier because it is more likely to be repetitious. The cost in time, effort, and resources per unit of production or service goes down as the number of organizations and people reached goes up. Some programs never reach this threshold because their initial planning, production of materials, or coordination fail in the early stages to satisfy early participants and thereby fail to establish the program's reputation and to ensure its **diffusion.**

Diffusion of a new program or practice depends first on satisfying the early adopters and then on timing and placing interventions strategically according to stages in the natural history of the diffusion process. The natural history of the diffusion process across organizations follows a logistic curve similar to that of the diffusion of innovations or ideas in a population as shown in figure 2-11. Theories associated with the diffusion curve describe and explain important features of the diffusion process. One set of features of interest in community health concerns the characteristics and distribution of individuals or organizations according to their relative time of adoption. A second set concerns the forces pushing

....

Figure 2-11

Over time the distribution of people adopting a new idea or innovation tends to follow the normal or bell-shaped curve. Classifying people by standard deviations of their time of adoption from the average time produces categories of adopters who differ also in their response to different communication channels. (From Green LW et al: Diffusion theory extended and applied. In Ward WB, Lewis FM, editors: *Advances in health education and promotion,* vol 3, London, 1991, Jessica Kingsley, pp 91–117.)

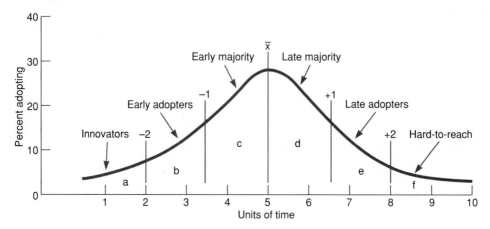

the diffusion process forward and those holding it back at each stage. This same curve describes the diffusion or rate of spread of an infection or epidemic in the community.

The Classification and Distribution of Adopters

Figure 2-11 shows the normal distribution of adoption over time, with the curve divided into standard deviations from the theoretical midpoint of the program or diffusion process. This curve has a vertical axis of percentage of *new* people or organizations adopting an idea or program *at a given point in time.*

A community health program seldom enters at time zero on the adoption curve to stimulate a healthful practice or prevent an unhealthful practice. In free-market economies with extensive communication networks, commercial interests have "skimmed" the innovators and early adopters before government is called upon to take action. The relative deprivation of those who could not avail themselves of privately sponsored programs or services is often the very impetus for government initiative in health. In

the interest of equity, government agencies often undertake large-scale programs in public health when the public redefines previously acceptable circumstances as unacceptable.

When the Food and Drug Administration approves a new drug, vaccine, or medical procedure, for example, it is immediately prescribed to or purchased over the counter by the more affluent segment of the community. Later, the health department may be directed to make the same product available to the poor at reduced cost.

Their late point of entry on the diffusion curve has several implications for community health programs. Certain of these implications distinguish such government or voluntary agency programs from large-scale commercial marketing efforts. Some would like to imagine that all that health agencies need for the success of community health programs is to employ marketing principles and strategies. The implicit criticism that community health agencies have failed where commercial marketing has succeeded is an unfair oversimplification of the task community health faces. A percentage-point gain in the early-adopter phase when commercial interests prevail is much easier to obtain than a percentage-point gain in the late-adopter phase when nonprofit organizations pick up the responsibility to reach the poor or isolated segment of the population.

Innovators and **early adopters** in figure 2-11 typically are more affluent and attuned to the national media. They are cosmopolitans who know the most about health, can afford the most in private purchase of health care products and services, and least need some of the products and services they buy. They are the "upscale" market of Madison Avenue and the social models for the majority. Mass media can suffice in reaching them.

The **middle majority** of people in the diffusion curve (the **early majority** and **late majority** in figure 2-11) attend less to national media and more to local media. They respond less to the media in general than to interpersonal influence. This is why most of the programs in community health put so much emphasis on involving the local media and organizational channels of communication rather than depending on network broadcasts or national publications. This middle majority is the primary target of those public health programs addressing problems for which everybody has lifestyle concerns, such as fitness, stress, nutrition, and injury control programs. These problems and concerns relate to socially and culturally conditioned behaviors embedded in a complex web of lifestyle. This makes organizational and institutional channels essential to the health promotion strategies required to support changes in behavior. The media no longer suffice. To reach people effectively at this stage requires the cooperation of institutions such as schools and of private organizations such as workplaces, clubs, and churches.

The **late adopters** and the "hard-to-reach" in Figure 2-11 are even more likely to be the primary targets of public health campaigns. The people and organizations in these late-adopter categories are typically disadvantaged in economic or status terms. They are socially more isolated or alienated, and they tend to be suspicious of organizations, including government agencies, that purport to help them. Their use of the media is more

exclusively for entertainment, and their membership in organizations or coalitions is sporadic and limited in comparison with that of the earlier adopters. Reaching these people and organizations requires more expensive and labor-intensive forms of community organization, communication, and outreach. Home visits, personal counseling, and small group meetings require more effort and personnel. The payoff is often greater because of this group's high health risk, but the cost per unit of service effectively delivered is necessarily higher.

Communication channels need to adapt their messages to the forces operating variously at successive stages of community programs. Recognizing that many of the forces influencing the diffusion and adoption process are not strictly under the control of individuals, community health promotion programs seek to mobilize organizational, economic, and environmental supports for the changes advocated.

Hypertension control programs and alcoholism detection programs provide examples of organizational strategies that complement communications to the public. These give particular attention to the mobilization of community organizations. They also emphasize the channeling of communications through workplaces and churches where interpersonal influence can complement the formal efforts of the media. In California a media campaign called "Friends Are Good Medicine" appealed to the public to seek out their friends when they felt depressed, bereaved, or under stress. This approach made the reduction of social isolation a means and an end. Encouraging the contact of people with their social support networks served the mental health goals of the program and the diffusion process.

DECENTRALIZATION AND PARTICIPATION

A foundation common to community programs and small-scale programs is the principle of participation. It applies equally to organizations and individuals, to highly educated and illiterate people. Involving people actively in identifying their own needs, setting their own priorities and goals, and planning their own programs of change are helpful processes at the individual, organizational, community, and national levels. The paradox for large-scale programs is that almost by definition they require a degree of centralization of authority and responsibility. Decentralization has occurred most commonly in the implementation of community programs, not in their planning or evaluation. As a result the concept of community participation has a bad reputation in some circles as a form of exploitation, co-optation, or cheap labor for central agencies. Large-scale programs ideally favor localized neighborhood planning, implementation, and evaluation.

Expecting neighborhoods and organizations to implement programs planned elsewhere usually yields only limited local commitment to the goals and methods of the programs. People need to feel at least consulted in assessing their needs and setting priorities, whether the outside "help" comes in the form of finances, technical consultation, or other resources. People are more likely to accept and use those resources if they have participated actively in identifying their own needs and priorities.

An ideal decentralization of community programs is to place the planning and evaluation functions at the local level and the highly specialized resources, including expensive technology and facilities, at the central level. The effective delivery of such programs necessarily depends on central and local organizations. It will occur most effectively with the transfer of some planning and evaluation functions to the local level and with good communication among organizations at each level and between levels (figure 2-12). In these times of growing public discontent with central governments, the opportunities for local control of health planning should be greater. The limitation is the degree to which central organizations pass responsibility to local planning groups without handing off the commensurate authority or resources to implement their programs.

The Community Development Model

Can communities mobilize resources to take control of their own health aspirations if they have depended on central governments to take care of these issues in the past? How can state and national organizations support community health without undermining the initiative and self-reliance that communities need to develop? How can the many sectors collaborate in community health if they each have state, provincial, or national headquarters that direct their priorities? For example, how can the local cancer society and a local company collaborate on a breast cancer program for female employees if both need support and approval from their parent organizations at the regional or corporate level?

A model for community health promotion applying the concepts of decentralized, multisectoral, and participatory planning and implementation is the community development approach. This model has been widely applied with varying success, depending on policy support and effective implementation, in many health promotion initiatives and programs for disease or injury prevention.

Its most influential applications in Australia, Europe, and Canada have been under the "Healthy Cities" and "Healthy Communities" programs. In the United States community development in health has had its most vigorous and sustained push under the PATCH (Planned Approach to Community Health), sponsored by the Centers for Disease Control (figure 2-12).

"Healthy Cities" and "Healthy Communities"

Pilot projects in Toronto and California inspired "Healthy Communities" in Canada and the United States, but the movement has had more formal auspices under the World Health Organization's "Healthy Cities" initiative. The World Health Organization promoted the Healthy Cities movement to encourage city governments to take a broad, multisectoral approach to planning for health promotion. It starts with a broad view of social determinants of health including policies and environmental conditions that influence the health of whole populations. It emphasizes the disparities in health and the need for more equitable distribution of health-related resources from various sectors to close the gaps between subpopulations.

....
Figure 2-12

The Planned Approach to Community Health (PATCH) applies community development principles of participation in planning and multisectoral collaboration with support from central to local levels. At the central levels, "horizontal communication" is encouraged among the organizations that have local counterparts who need to collaborate with their support. (Courtesy Centers for Disease Control and Prevention and the Henry J. Kaiser Family Foundation.)

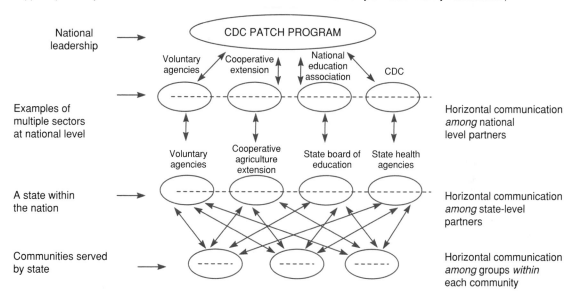

The federal government of Canada briefly supported projects under a Healthy Communities initiative, but following the trends toward decentralization these soon gave way to provincial and local auspices. Use of the term "community" in North America in place of "cities" in Europe reflects the wider range of local auspices for health initiatives in Canada and the United States. In Australia the term for the same program has been "Healthy Towns and Shires," where shires are roughly equivalent to counties in the United States or health regions in Canada.

Planned Approach to Community Health

PATCH first developed in 1983 as a way of reconciling the federal funding requirements that were locked into specific disease categories and the community development principles of local planning for needs communities identify themselves. The designers of PATCH at the U.S. Centers for Disease Control (CDC) based the approach on their own traditions of state and community capac-

ity-building and data-based planning and monitoring of programs. They applied the PRECEDE model of planning and evaluation (described in chapter 4 of this book) and community development principles of local ownership. By 1987, twenty-five PATCH programs had been initiated in twelve states, and by 1998 several hundred were underway across the United States. Dozens more were modeled after this approach in Australia, Canada, Europe, and China.

Similar community development initiatives in health have been sponsored by other U.S. federal agencies and private foundations such as the Henry J. Kaiser Family Foundation, the Robert Wood Johnson Foundation, the Kellogg Foundation, and others. In Canada, similar community development strategies have been sponsored by the Federal-Provincial Heart Health Initiative, tobacco control initiatives, and most of the provincial ministries of health. Table 2-2 provides examples of such projects supported in Canada and the United States.

Table 2-2

Examples of Community Health Projects in the United States and Canada

Community/Aim	Changes made	Measures/Results	Future plans
Anchorage, Alaska Reduce post-neonatal mortality in the native Alaskan community in the Anchorage area	"Nutaqsiivik" (Yupik for "place of renewal") clinic initiated in June, 1994, to focus on patients of known social risk and provide a continuum of services from prenatal period through first year of life.	Days between death increased from an average 34 days to 180 days.	Efforts underway to expand program.
Baton Rouge, Louisiana Reduce injuries and deaths among adolescents due to violence in the Mid City area	Established "A Safe Season" summer program to focus on conflict resolution, personal safety and self-esteem to reduce violent behavior and keep kids in school.	Number of days absent decreased from an average 11.3 days to 5.4 days.	Collaborations with other community groups; piloting teen leadership program.
Camden, New Jersey Improve the health status of women of child-bearing age and their families in the City of Camden	Established team with broad-based community representation. Identified two pilot communities and hired community health facilitators. Projects designed based on ongoing assessment of community need. Establishing local neighborhood "Learning Collaboratives."	Tracking number of primary care visits, women receiving prenatal care, children receiving early immunizations, decreases in ER visits, neonatal infant mortality and very low birth weight babies.	Using HUD and HRET grants to develop a Community Care Network.
Edmonton, Alberta Reduce the incidence of child abuse and neglect in Edmonton	Direct Service Team working on secondary prevention and crisis intervention, as well as a variety of primary prevention activities, to break cycle of abuse.	Will compare three months of child abuse and neglect reports from 1993 and 1995; number of families and children served by DST.	Collaborative is prototype of how services could be offered on province-wide basis; potential merger with another project with similar goals.
Kingsport, Tennessee Reduce preventable injuries to children and adolescents in the Greater Kingsport area resulting from motor vehicle accidents	Improved driver training through introduction of "Drive Smart" curriculum in five high schools; increased public awareness and involvement through public campaign.	Tracking number of students receiving improved training; eventually, number of motor vehicle injuries to children and adolescents. Various indicators of public awareness and involvement.	Implementation of curriculum in seven high schools; expansion of public awareness and involvement.

Location / Aim	Activities	Measures	Future Plans
London, Ontario Reduce injuries due to falls in the elderly in the greater London area	Investigation of reasons for falls in the elderly led to testing variety of interventions, e.g., discharge elderly patients from ER with a walker rather than crutches, weekly exercise programs, curriculum development for bus drivers.	Global measures found not sensitive to project needs. Process measures on specific intervention (number of people attending education sessions, number reporting increase in physical activity).	Team will reconfigure to include key sectors within the community and serve as a catalyst for continuing efforts to reduce falls in the elderly.
Monroe, Louisiana Improve cardiovascular health in the cities of Monroe and West Monroe	Employers offered risk assessment tools to employees, implemented prevention programs, and improved care for heart attack victims in ERs.	Annual evaluation compared to baseline data on number of risk factors identified, heart attack rate, return to work after heart attack and cost. Decreased time from 60 to 27 minutes from presentation with chest pain to thrombolytic therapy.	Sponsoring agency has disbanded. Three efforts continue under their own leadership.
Rochester, New York Improve preventive cardiovascular care in Rochester	Risk assessment tool developed and piloted on hospital patients. Assessment tool used to identify interventions. HMOs have been involved to provide follow-up care.	Tracking reduction in cholesterol level, risk factors. Increase number of people with behavioral change.	Involve private practicing primary care physicians; integrate survey into admissions process, patient education and behavioral changes.
Twin Falls, Idaho Reduce the rate of teen deaths, serious injury and traffic violations due to traffic crashes in Twin Falls	Analysis of DOT data showed lack of skill and poor judgment as major factors in teen crashes. Team developed and tested driver simulator, enrolled 50 teens in pilot education on driving simulator. Data forthcoming.	Developing a community-wide integrated injury surveillance database from police department, ER, hospital and private physician data.	HRET, DOT and other grants will be used to develop a Community Care Network; if effective in preventing teen crashes, simulator will be used in statewide driver training curriculum

Courtesy of the Institute for Healthcare Improvement "Quality Connection."

SUMMARY

Human ecology provides an understanding and appreciation of the interdependence of a human population and its physical and biological setting. This, with an understanding of the social and economic processes of community organization, gives definition to the concept of community. Further understanding from the social and behavioral sciences concerning how people feel about belonging and cooperating gives meaning to the subjective "sense of community." This socially conditioned state of mind makes possible many of the collective efforts and sacrifices of individual pursuits necessary for the promotion and protection of the population's health. Enhancing the health and reducing the social and economic impact of premature death and disability of the entire community are the major goals of community health. Higher morale, greater productivity, and reduction in disease and costs of health care represent the potential benefits of a community health program. This chapter has presented various models to show how these goals and benefits have been accomplished in the past and how they can be achieved in the future.

WEB*Links*

http://www.clsc.org/ciccs/index a.html
Canadian Community Health Centers

http://odphp.osophs.dhhs.gov/pubs/hp2000
Healthy People 2000

http://web.health.gov/healthypeople
Framework for Healthy People 2010

QUESTIONS FOR REVIEW

1. How do individual and community health approaches differ?
2. What constitutes the community in which you live?
3. How do the 4 factors influencing health affect your community?
4. How would you describe the social history of health in the neighborhood in which you live?
5. How can one dramatic incident unite a community in a common health cause?
6. How does diffusion theory inform decisions about community health strategies?
7. How does a particular industry attract a particular type of people with particular health problems?
8. What are some obstacles to and facilitators of community health progress?
9. Is this statement true: "It is impossible to eliminate community customs but not difficult to modify them"?
10. Why should churches have an interest in community health?
11. How does economics enter into community health promotion?
12. Evaluate this statement: "Transient families are community health liabilities."

READINGS

Chesworth, J., ed. 1996. *The ecology of health: issues and alternatives.* Thousand Oaks, CA: Sage Publications, Inc.
Presents discussions of the ethics, issues, and choices linking health and ecology. Environmental issues are debated in relation to public health and cultural contexts.
Herbert, W. 1995. Our identity crisis: in angry times, can we rebuild a true American sense of community? *U.S. News & World Rep,* 6 March.
Assesses the vanishing forms of public discourse, the troubling emergence of meanspritedness, the loss of shared purposes of the early civil rights movement, the decline in voting and other trends reflecting growing tribalism in place of communalism.
Johnson, J. L., L. W. Green, C. J. Frankish, D. R. MacLean, and S. Stachenko. 1996. A dissemination research agenda to strengthen health promotion and disease prevention. *Canadian J Public Health,* 87(Suppl 2):S5.
Reviews the major issues and challenges presented by a series of papers in this compilation of papers on diffusion theory and dissemination research in health promotion and disease prevention.
Karp, R. J., ed. 1993. *Malnourished children in the United States: caught in the cycle of poverty.* New York: Springer Publishing Co.

Examines aspects of malnourishment of children in the United States today, with emphasis on poverty and the cycle it produces in community and population health.

Konrad, E. L. 1996. A multidimensional framework for conceptualizing human services integration initiatives. *New Directions for Evaluation, 69:5.*

A brief history of services integration efforts is presented and a framework is provided that identifies key components of services integration projects and how they may vary by degree of integration.

Richard L., L. Potvin, N. Kishchuk, H. Prlic, and L. W. Green. 1996. Assessment of the integration of the ecological approach in health promotion programs. *Amer J Health Prom, 10:318.*

Proposes a model of the ecological approach in health promotion programs based on systems theory, and assesses forty-four health programs in Canada as to their use of such concepts in their planning.

BIBLIOGRAPHY

Airhihenbuwa, C. O. 1995. *Healthy culture: decolonization of health and education.* Thousand Oaks, CA: Sage Publications, Inc.

Boothroyd, P., L. W. Green, and C. Hertzman, J. Lynan, J. McIntosh, W. Rees, S. Manson-Singer, M Wackernagal, and R, Woollard. 1994. Tools for sustainability: iteration and implementation. In *Ecological public health: from vision to practice,* edited by C. M. Chu and R. Simpson. Nathan, Australia: Griffith University.

Bracht, N., ed. 1990. *Health promotion at the community level.* New York: Sage.

Brink, S. G., D. M. Simons-Morton, G. S. Parcel, and K. M. Tiernan. 1988. Community intervention handbooks for comprehensive health promotion planning. *Fam Community Health* 11:28.

Brownson, R. C., D. M. Koffman, T. E. Novotny, R. G. Hughes, and M. P. Eriksen. 1995. Environmental and policy interventions to control tobacco use and prevent cardiovascular disease. *Health Educ Q* 22:478.

Duhl, L. J. 1996. An ecohistory of health: the role of 'Healthy Cities.' *Amer J Health Prom* 10:258.

Evans, R. G. 1994. Introduction. In *Why are some people healthy and others not?* edited by R. G. Evans, M. L. Barer, and T. R. Marmor. New York: Aldine de Gruyter.

Farquhar, J. W. 1996. The case for dissemination research in health promotion and disease prevention. *Can J Public Health* 87(Suppl. 2):S44.

Frankish, C. J., and L. W. Green. 1994. Organizational and community change as the social scientific basis for disease prevention and health promotion policy. *Advances in Medical Sociology* 4:209.

Green, L. W. 1994. Refocusing health care systems to address both individual care and population health. *Clin Invest Med* 17:133.

Green, L. W., and J. Johnson. 1996. Dissemination and utilization of health promotion and disease prevention knowledge: theory, research and experience. *Can J Public Health* 87(Suppl. 2):S17.

Green, L. W., L. Richard, and L. Potvin. 1996. Ecological foundations of health promotion. *Am J Health Prom* 10:270.

Healthy communities 2000: model standards. 1991. 3d ed. Washington, DC: American Public Health Association.

Hoffman, K. 1994. The strengthening community health program: lessons for community development. In *Health promotion in Canada: provincial, national and international perspectives,* edited by A. Pederson, M. O'Neill, and I. Rootman. Toronto: W. B. Saunders Canada.

Johnson, J. J., L. W. Green, C. J. Frankish, D. MacLean and S. Stachenko. 1996. A dissemination research agenda to strengthen health promotion and disease prevention. *Can J Public Health* 87:S5.

Kay, J. J., and E. Schneider. 1994. Embracing complexity: the challenge of the ecosystem approach. *Alternatives* 20(3):32.

King, L., P. Hawe, and M. Wise. 1996. Dissemination in health promotion in Australia. *Health Prom J Austral* 6(2):4.

McMillan, D. W., and D. M. Chavis. 1986. Sense of community: a definition and theory. *Community Psychol* 14:6.

Macallan, L., and V. Narayan. 1994. Keeping the heart beat in gramplan—a case study in community participation and ownership. *Health Prom Int* 9:13.

MacLean, D. R. 1996. Positioning dissemination in public health policy. *Can J Public Health* 87(Suppl. 2):S40.

MacNeill, J., P. Winsemius, and T. Yakushiji. 1991. *Beyond interdependence: the meshing of the world's economy and the earth's ecology.* London, New York, Toronto: Oxford University Press.

Manson-Singer, S. 1994. The Canadian Healthy Communities project: creating a social movement. In *Health Promotion in Canada: provincial, national and international perspectives,* edited by A. Pederson, M. O'Neill, and I. Rootman. Toronto: W. B. Saunders Canada.

Minkler, M. 1994. Challenges for health promotion in negative consequences, and the common good. *Amer J Health Prom* 8:405.

O'Neill, M. 1989. Community health projects in Quebec: can they participate significantly to promote the health of the population in the years to come? *Health Promotion* 4:189.

Patton, R. D., and W. B. Cissell, ed. 1989. *Community organization: traditional principles and modern applications.* Johnson City, TN: Latchpins.

Robichaud, J. B., and C. Quiviger. 1991. *Active communities.* Ottawa: Canadian Council on Social Development.

Schneider, S. H. 1990. *Global warming.* New York: Random House.

Shiell, A., and P. Hawe. 1996. Health promotion, community development and the tyranny of individualism. *Health Economics* 5:241–247.

Speers, M. A., and T. L. Schmid. 1995. Policy and environmental interventions for the prevention and control of cardiovascular diseases. *Health Educ Q* 22:476.

Stokols, D., J. Allen, and R. L. Bellingham. 1996. The social ecology of health promotion: implications for research and practice. *Amer J Health Prom* 10:247.

Stokols, D., K. R. Pelletier, and J. E. Fielding. 1996. The ecology of work and health: research and policy directions for the promotion of employee health. *Health Educ Q* 23:137.

Stryker, J., and A. R. Jonsen, ed. 1992. *The social impact of AIDS.* Washington, DC: National Academy Press.

Chapter 3

Community and Population Diversity, Demography, and Epidemiology

*T*he primary determinants of disease are mainly economic and social, and therefore its remedies *must also be economic and social.*
—Geoffrey Rose, 1994

I should see the garden far better," said Alice to herself, "if I could get to the top of that hill; *and here's a path that leads straight to it—at least, no . . . how curiously it twists! It's more like a corkscrew than a path!"*
—Lewis Carroll, 1872

Objectives

When you finish this chapter, you should be able to:

- Identify and describe elements of demography that apply to community and population diversity and change
- Compute some basic statistics for an epidemiological analysis

- Distinguish between incidence and prevalence
- Distinguish between life span and life expectancy

Demography reflects population diversity and trends by studying population composition, growth, and movement. Birth, death, and migration data from demography combine with the study of disease transmission and distribution in populations to constitute **epidemiology.**

DEMOGRAPHY

We introduced human ecology, the study of population interactions with physical and biological envi-

ronments, in the last chapter. We extended this to social ecology in examining how these interactions develop as a function of social processes. Demography takes up the study of population trends as measured over time by three sets of data. One consists of vital indexes such as birthrates and death rates. A second consists of measures of population diversity such as ethnic composition, density, rural–urban-suburban residential patterns, and migration. The third consists of socioeconomic indicators such as income, occupation, and educational attainment.

....

Figure 3-1

Seasonal variations in fertility rates (A), whether smoothed by averaging or unadjusted, do not follow the same variations seen in marriage rates (B) because people vary in their fecundity and birth control practices. (*Source:* National Center for Health Statistics, U.S. Department of Health and Human Services, *Monthly Vital Statistics Report,* vol 46, no 6, 1998.)

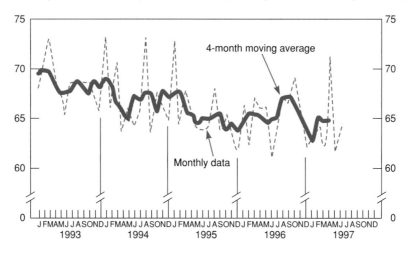

Provisional seasonally adjusted fertility rates per 1,000 women aged 15–44 years: United States, 1993–97

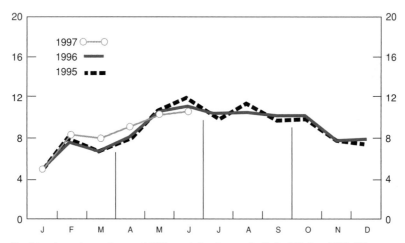

Provisional marriage rates per 1,000 population by month: United States, 1995–97

Seasonal variations in population movement and vital rates result partly from climate and partly from cultural and social conditions affecting employment and traditions associated with seasons and holidays. In North America, for example, the highest death rates tend to occur in the winter months. The holiday season of Christmas and New Year's contribute a large share of the increase through automobile crashes, suicides, and heart attacks. The relatively higher incidence of respiratory conditions and associated deaths in the winter attests to some climatic effect, but not just because of exposure to cold temperatures. Some of it is attributable to being more exposed to the transmission of communicable diseases among people confined indoors. The latter explanation suggests that social norms of adaptation to climatic conditions are important in providing protection and in exposing the individual to additional risks.

The expanding capacity to insulate, heat, and air-condition large indoor spaces brings more people together. Indoor air pollution is becoming as much an issue in community health as outdoor air pollution has been in the past. These expansions of air-tight indoor space have enabled new populations to grow in regions previously considered uninhabitable.

Seasonal adjustments on vital rates are made by averaging monthly rates for several consecutive months, as shown in figure 3-1A. Although North American and European marriage rates follow a predictable pattern of seasonal and monthly variation, fertility rates are much less predictable and less associated with marriage rates than one might expect. The pattern of births is more predictable in some primitive and traditional societies where cultural and social restrictions on birth control are greater. Society imposes positive and negative influences on natural cycles and conditions.

Population Growth

From 1910 to 1997 the world population increased from 1.5 to 5.7 billion (figure 3-2). The rate of increase was such that, if maintained, the population would double in forty years. Mercifully, the world birthrate declined from 34 per 1,000 in 1965 to below 30 per 1,000 in recent years for the first time in recorded demography. This brought the world growth rate closer to that of Western countries such as the United States (figure 3-3). The United Nations predicts that world population will reach 7.6 billion by 2025 and will not stabilize until it reaches the 10 or 11 billion mark projected for the year 2050. Technological, legislative, economic, climatic, and cultural influences on population growth, however, make such long-term predictions highly speculative.

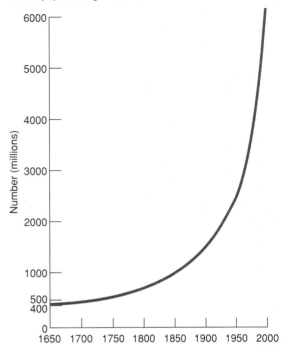

Figure 3-2

World population growth, 1650–2000.

Over 880 million people worldwide are chronically undernourished. Of the 14 million annual deaths of children, malnutrition is a contributing cause in two-thirds of the cases. Where starvation exists, disease flourishes, because the malnourished are more susceptible to infection. Famines cause people to migrate and, by so doing, to spread infectious disease and to redistribute populations as seen in Somalia, Rwanda, and Uganda.

Chapter 2 introduced diffusion theory with a curve that described the growth or spread of an innovation in a population. Exactly the same mathematical principle of growth or spread applies to human population growth and the spread of communicable disease. The essential underpinning of diffusion theory and of demography is the simple mathematical law of nature that defines any spreading or growing process as a logistic function. This means that each new cell, organism, or person

· · · · · · · · · · · · · · · · · · ·

Figure 3-3

Resident population, United States, 1790–1990.

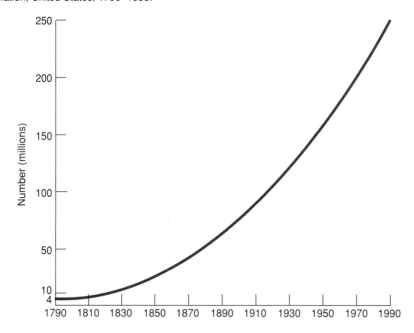

has the possibility, respectively, of dividing, reproducing, or influencing at least one more of its kind. The progression is then geometric: 1 becomes 2, 2 becomes 4, 4 becomes 8, with each generation or unit of time realizing a doubling of the number from the previous generation or unit of time. You can see the shape of this accelerated growth curve by simply plotting the numbers, 1, 2, 4, 8, 16, and 32 on a sheet of graph paper as shown in figure 3-4. This same curve plotted on logarithmic graph paper would take the form of a straight diagonal line, thus the name "logistic function."

The growth curve continues to increase the rate of growth in numbers until it reaches a natural limit. This is where the curve representing the diffusion or epidemic process differs from the reproductive growth curve. All three phenomena have a natural limit on accelerated growth. Thus, the shapes of the curves ultimately are similar, as shown by the broken line forming the S-shaped curve in figure 3-4. However, the causes of the limits differ. Diffusion slows down when the number

of new people available to adopt an innovation no longer exceeds the number of people who have already adopted it. This occurs at the median or halfway point in the existing population. Population growth slows down when the size of the population exceeds the resources available to sustain continued growth. New offspring or their parents starve, cannibalize, or commit suicide, infanticide, or fratricide; or people voluntarily limit their reproduction before their population reaches such limits.

Biotic Potential of a Population

Population changes reflect the **biotic potential** of a population as related to environmental resistance. Environmental resistance results from parasitism, food supply limits, floods, cold, heat, fuel supply, and other factors that may affect life adversely. The biotic potential of the human species is probably a **fecundity** level that would produce a birthrate of 50 per 1,000 per year. The Ukraine attained this rate over a 5-year period and Bengal over a 10-year period. During the 10-year period from 1930 to 1940,

· · · · · · · · · · · · · · · · · · ·

Figure 3-4

The geometric rate of growth or diffusion illustrates how quickly a population can grow or a disease can spread when unchecked. The dotted line reflects the usual S-shaped curve of diffusion, epidemic spread, or reproductive growth when natural limits take hold or when conscious efforts to control the growth or spread are introduced. Consider the implications of the two lines after time 4 for Figures 3-2 and 3-3 assuming the numbers in the y-axis are billions of people.

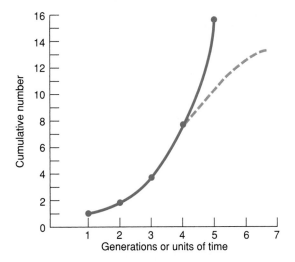

the Warm Springs Indians of Oregon had an average birthrate of 50 per 1,000 per year. Scientific advances in the prevention and correction of human infertility and sterility could raise the present acknowledged maximum human birthrate. Declining family size preferences, however, make it unlikely that most countries, states, provinces, or communities will test the maximum.

Government Policies

A pronatal government policy incorporates inducements and rewards for large families; the reverse is true of antinatal policy. Canadian and U.S. policies have been inconsistent in this regard. The birthrates per 1,000 population and the absolute number of births were falling between 1957 and 1977. A reversal in this trend seemed to correspond with the "prolife" policy. The United States saw more babies born in 1991 than it will see

again until the year 2080 (see chapter 7). This so-called "baby-boomlet" yielded 4.1 million births in 1991, the largest number in 24 years, but still fewer than the 4.3 million births in 1957, the peak year of the postwar baby boom.

The total number of new births minus deaths in a given year make up the **natural increase**. The rate of natural increase is the difference between births per 1,000 population and deaths per 1,000 population. If the United States has a birthrate (figure 3-5) of 16 per 1,000 and a death rate of 8.5 per 1,000, the rate of natural increase is 7.5. When a nation's rate of natural increase begins to approach 2, that nation's population is becoming stable. If deaths exceed births in a population, the population will have a negative rate of natural increase symptomatic of population decline, unless it also receives a large influx of immigrants. Nations with declining birthrates and declining death rates will tend to have high rates of growth in their older populations, as seen in chapter 8.

The addition of 94 million people to the earth each year has its greatest concentrations in the largest populations, China and India, but these countries have achieved remarkable progress in controlling their fertility. China's one-child policy has brought its total fertility rate (average births per woman aged 15–49) to 1.9, well below the U.S. rate of 2.1 (just at replacement level), and Canada's 1.9. By contrast, Nigeria's rate is 6.4. Africa has the world's fastest regional growth rate at 2.9 percent per year, compared with Europe's slowest rate of 0.3 percent per year, and North America's 1.1 percent. Figure 3-6A shows the relative rates of growth produced by total fertility rates in developing and developed regions. Figure 3-6B shows the consequences of these differential rates for the changing distribution of the world's population.

Food Limits and Population

Worldwide, agricultural yields in per capita food production have more than kept pace with population increases. In the 1960s and 1970s food production increased at a faster pace in the developing countries than in the developed countries. The extraordinary increase of 13 percent in the 1980s,

· · · · · · · · · · · · · · · · · · ·

Figure 3-5

Crude birth rates per 1,000 population for successive 12-month periods ending with month indicated, United States, 1992–1997. (*Source:* National Center for Health Statistics, *Monthly Vital Statistics Report,* vol 46, no 6, 1998.)

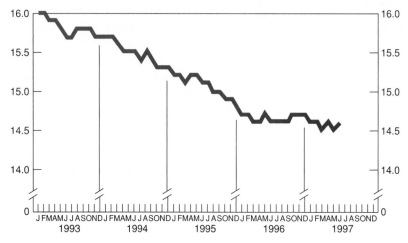

Provisional birth rates per 1,000 population for successive 12-month periods ending with month indicated: United States, 1993–97

· · · · · · · · · · · · · · · · · · ·

Figure 3-6

A) Total fertility rate (average births per woman aged 15–49) estimated for the period 1990–94 for selected regions of the world. B) Consequences of differential growth rates for proportions of the world's population living in the developing and developed regions from 1950–2025.

Total fertility rate

(average births per woman aged 15-49, est. 1990–94) Rate varies widely from region to region.

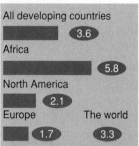

Where people live

The proportions of people living in developed and developing countries are changing rapidly.

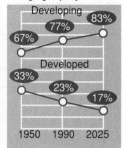

however, was more heavily concentrated in the developed countries as loss of topsoil resulted in widespread declines. Two-thirds of all developing countries witnessed stagnant or reduced agricultural production. Per capita food supplies are becoming smaller where the need is greatest because of much higher population growth rates in the developing countries. In Africa, in particular, food production per capita has declined dramatically in recent years, mainly because of population growth. If present trends continue, substantial portions of the developing world will encounter increasing grain shortages (figure 3-7), followed by hunger and malnutrition as domestic demand outstrips their ability to grow or purchase their own food. **Global warming** and **desertification** will add to the problems, especially in Africa.

The wealth and abundance of food in the developed nations still leave pockets of poor, hungry people within their national borders. Readily identifiable groups with a high incidence of hunger in the United States, for example, are migrant and seasonal farm workers, native Alaskans, American

Figure 3-7

Since 1961, world stocks of rice, wheat, corn, barley, rye, flax, and other edible cereal grains have declined as much as 50 percent, despite increased agricultural yield of the Green Revolution. Without replenishment, the grain reserves from 1995 would have been consumed in the first six weeks of 1996. Supply and demand means that another 90 million mouths to feed in 1997 will drive grain prices up, making the least affluent countries less able to afford to import what they need. (*Sources:* US Department of Agriculture; Canadian Cattlemen's Association; Food and Agricultural Organization.)

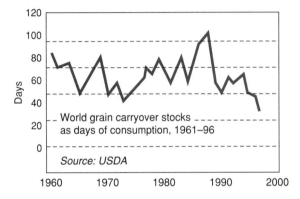

World grain carryover stocks as days of consumption, 1961–96

Source: USDA

The Tragedy of the Commons

Garrett Hardin (1968) revived a scenario first told in 1833 by a mathematical amateur named William Forster Lloyd. It was a rebuttal to the Malthusian doctrine of natural limits on population growth and Adam Smith's notion of "the invisible hand" in economic affairs. Malthus believed that populations would stop growing when resources became too limited to support further growth. Smith believed that individuals pursuing only their own gain would be "led by an invisible hand to promote . . . the public interest." Lloyd created and Hardin popularized the analogy of individual farmers grazing ever-increasing numbers of cows on a common pasture, until each additional cow caused overgrazing to the detriment of all. They applied this analogy to illustrate the tragedy of individual procreation beyond the point of community resources to provide for the sustenance of all. The individual might gain in the short run, but the individual and the community will suffer in the long run.

How might you see the same tragedy in the short-term gratification of industries excessively exploiting natural resources for profit or of indulgent, sedentary, or reckless behavior of individuals? How might these affect the long-term well-being of the community?

Indians, the elderly, and those with incomes below the poverty level. The U.S. Food Stamp, Meals on Wheels, and Women-Infants-Children (WIC) programs have made notable improvements in the nutrition of the poor.

Apart from food limits, the critical problems created by the present population increase and distribution are high prices and inflation, waste disposal, transportation, and fuel supply. These problems challenge economic means, technological creativity, political will, and regional cooperation.

Fuel Limits and Population

The Western world faced a major fuel crisis some 400 years ago when Europe ran out of wood. Since time immemorial wood had provided heat and shelter. The dense forests that covered the continent and the British Isles seemed inexhaustible, and no thought was given to conservation or management. If the population remained relatively sparse and stable, the consequences were not serious. In the sixteenth century, however, prices for firewood and lumber suddenly began to skyrocket with the doubling of population in forty years.

At the same time the mass movement from country to city got under way, creating excessive demands for building material. London grew from 60,000 inhabitants in 1534 to some 530,000 in 1696, making it the largest city in Europe and perhaps in the world. Other pressures contributed to depleting the European forest reserves: the shipbuilding boom in the age of exploration, the soaring production of metal ore mines with their wood-burning smelters, and the rising consumption of wood pulp for paper following the invention of printing.

Eventually coal came to the rescue. A massive shift from wood to coal, along with the discovery of vast new forest reserves in the New World, helped to overcome the crisis. Coal, however, turned out to be much more than a mere substitute; compact and efficient as a fuel, it made possible a whole new technology that led to the industrial revolution. Together with oil, it contributes to many of our worldwide difficulties, including the carbon dioxide added to the atmosphere, producing the "greenhouse effect" discussed in chapter 2.

One lesson of this near-disaster is that there are few final answers. Each solution engenders new problems. Tackling them, however, led society out of the Stone Age—giving hope that the latest oil and nuclear fuel challenges will again be met with some combination of sun, wind, and water sources.

EPIDEMIOLOGY

A companion science to ecology and demography in community health is epidemiology. All three represent perspectives on health that go beyond the individual. Whereas ecology views the individual in the context of environment, demography and epidemiology view the individual in the context of a population. Epidemiology is the science of the causes, frequencies, and distribution of diseases in a population.

Epidemiology differs in two essential respects from the study of medicine. First, epidemiology studies populations or groups rather than individuals; second, in studying whole populations, epidemiology measures health and disease, injury, and disability patterns. Its objective is to find causes (**etiologies**) of disease and patterns of transmission or distribution of disease and injury. Such information enables communities to locate points of intervention before people get sick or injured. In this respect epidemiology is the science of prevention.

Epidemiological methods allow the community health worker to collect, tabulate, analyze, and interpret statistical facts about the occurrence of health problems, risk factors, and deaths in a community. Health professionals trained in clinical sciences sometimes have difficulty standing back from the individual patient to see the larger patterns of disease occurrence in their population of patients, much less in their community. The epidemiological perspective on health enables health workers to specify, describe, and understand such population patterns. From the patterns they can see the common characteristics of those who have a certain problem in contrast to the characteristics of those who do not have the problem. The comparison may reveal the cause or the source of a disease of unknown origin. For example, those who suffered an *E. coli* infection in 1996 had consumed an unpasteurized apple juice product, whereas those without the infection had not. Most of the breakthroughs in medicine, especially preventive medicine, that emerged from the laboratory of an immunologist or a physiologist had their first leads from an epidemiologist or other investigator applying epidemiological methods.

Epidemiology's early preoccupation with epidemics gave it its name. The transmission of communicable diseases in populations, when traced systematically, provided clues to the mode of transmission. Some proved to be airborne, some waterborne, foodborne, or transmitted by an intermediate **host** or vector such as a rat, mosquito, fly, tick, or bird. Such clues enabled community health workers to interrupt the transmission of some diseases through quarantine, pest control, water purification, food protection, immunization, or solid waste disposal (figure 3-8).

The methods of epidemiology have turned from communicable diseases to analyzing chronic diseases; degenerative diseases; and even injuries, addictions, and risk factors such as smoking, hypertension, obesity, and other behavioral patterns. These studies, again, have provided the clues and hypotheses on which advice to the public and further research have been based. The research findings, in turn, lead to strategies for national campaigns against smoking, alcohol and drug misuse, malnutrition, high blood pressure, dental caries, and injuries.

· · · · · · · · · · · · · · · · · ·
Figure 3-8

Animals that harbor diseases transmitted to human beings are referred to in epidemiology as intermediate hosts. Dogs, for example, may harbor rabies. This street scene from New York City in 1879 depicts the shooting of a "mad dog," recognized early in the epidemiological era as a possible source of rabies. (*Source: Harper's Weekly* 23:605, Aug. 2, 1879, after S. D. Erhart sketch. Courtesy National Library of Medicine.)

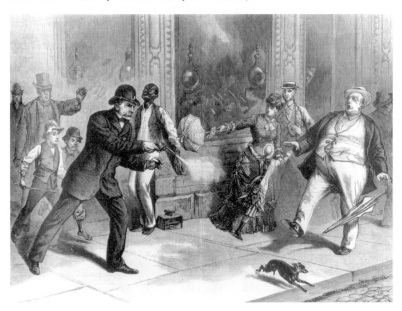

Epidemiological Comparisons

Comparison is the fundamental tool of epidemiological analysis. The frequencies and distribution of diseases are compared by measures of incidence and prevalence. **Incidence** refers to the number of new cases or deaths of the disease or conditions that occur during a given period (week, month, or year). **Prevalence** refers to the number of cases that exist at one time. Thus, incidence measures how rapidly a disease is spreading. As such, it is the most sensitive measure of an outbreak or epidemic of a communicable or acute infectious or toxic agent disease. Prevalence is influenced by incidence and by the duration of the disease or condition, hence its wider use in measuring chronic diseases and disabilities. Figure 3-9 illustrates the incidence of new infections from AIDS by year and the prevalence of AIDS cases for selected countries.

It is difficult to measure the incidence of onset of chronic and degenerative diseases such as AIDS, because they are usually undetected until they reach an acute stage. Incidence rates for morbidity (onset) usually are derived from health department reporting systems that require hospitals, clinics, and even private physicians to report every new case of a communicable or infectious disease they encounter. Prevalence rates usually come from screening and detection programs and special surveys of populations.

To compare the incidence or prevalence of any two groups within a population, or the population of one community with another or with state or national averages, data must be standardized. The all-purpose method of standardization is to construct a **rate** or ratio so that the groups or populations to be compared have a "common denominator." In most comparisons the rate is constructed

· · · · · · · · · · · · · · · · · ·

Figure 3-9

Examples of incidence and prevalence rates can be derived from these two charts on AIDS. A) shows the prevalence of AIDS in selected countries, comparing the number of existing (living) cases per million persons in each country in 1994. The prevalence rate of 380 per million in Canada is the product of the incidence of new cases and the survivorship of those who had AIDS in previous years. B) shows the growing incidence of new cases from 1979 to 1994. (*Sources:* Health Canada: *Quarterly Surveillance Update: AIDS in Canada,* Division of HIV/AIDS Epidemiology, Bureau of Communicable Disease Epidemiology, Laboratory Centre for Disease Control, 1995; and Federal, Provincial and Territorial Advisory Committee on Population Health: *Report on the Health of Canadians, Technical Appendix,* Ottawa, 1996, Health Canada Communications and Consultation Directorate.)

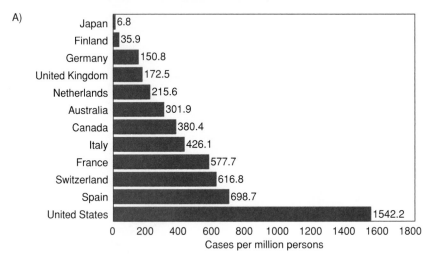

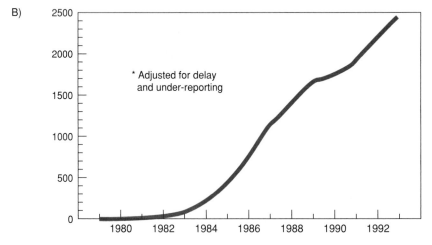

to make a unit of time, usually a year, the common denominator. Thus, the incidence rate is the number of cases per year. This basis for comparison, however, is not adequately standardized unless it is known how large the population was in which the incidence rate occurred. An epidemiological rate, then, is calculated as:

Rate = Number of events per population at risk

Epidemiology makes rates even more comparable by expressing them as events per 100 (percent), or per 1,000 population, or for very rare events, per 10,000 or 100,000 or 1 million population. Figure 3-9A illustrates the prevalence rates of AIDS cases, per one million population in 1994, which permits a comparison among countries or among communities, states, or provinces.

From demography, epidemiology borrows the following formula to calculate **crude death rate:**

Crude death rate =

$$\frac{\text{All deaths during a calendar year}}{\text{Population at midyear}} \times 1,000$$

This rate would be expressed as annual deaths per thousand population.

Age-Specific Rates Mortality varies more by age than by any other demographic variable. Populations and communities also vary widely in their age compositions. Age-specific death rates allow for a comparison between two or more communities or populations with different age distributions. Finding this **age-specific rate** is done simply by dividing the number of deaths within each age group (usually five-year or ten-year groupings) by the midyear population of the corresponding age groups. Then each of these quotients is multiplied by 1,000. This procedure yields a series of rates for comparison, as shown for a North American city in table 3-1.

Several things about such a tabulation of age-specific and race-specific rates should catch your eye. First, you should be surprised that the overall rate for whites is higher than the rate for blacks, even though each of the age-specific rates is lower

Table 3-1

Death Rates per 1000 Population by Age and Race

	White	Black
All ages	15.2	9.8
1 year	13.5	22.6
1–4	0.6	1.0
5–17	0.4	0.5
18–44	1.5	3.6
45–64	10.7	18.8
65+	59.7	61.1

for whites. How can the overall rate for whites be higher than that for blacks if each of the age-specific rates for whites is lower? Herein lies one of the most important lessons of demography and epidemiology. Think about this paradox while we examine a few other features of the tabulation.

The most dramatic differences appear to be between the infant mortality rates and the rates for the 45- to 65-year age group. We will examine infant and childhood mortality in chapter 5, adolescent and adult mortality in chapters 6 and 7, and mortality of the elderly in chapter 8. For now, it is sufficient to note the high rates at the youngest and oldest age ranges, and the greatest differentials between races at the youngest and middle-adulthood age ranges. Once children of either race survive the vulnerable infancy stage, their death rates go down dramatically, then gradually upward from age nine onward. This pattern of age-specific death rates is typical of developed countries, where the communicable diseases of childhood are largely under control. In developing countries, the rates for all ages are higher, but most distinctly higher for the childhood ages.

Relative Risk We can translate the substantial differences between age-specific and race-specific rates as levels of risk. This is precisely what insurance companies do in setting the premiums people have to pay for their policies. Rather than using the simple differences between rates, however, epidemiology expresses relative risk usually as a ratio. The **relative-risk ratio** states the proportionate or multiple risk of death, injury, disease, or disability among those exposed to a risk factor relative to those not exposed.

Relative risk =

$$\frac{\text{Incidence among those exposed}}{\text{Incidence among those not exposed}}$$

The term *incidence* is used. This means that relative risk can apply to any condition for which data are available on the number of cases occurring or discovered over a specified period. With vital statistics such as births and deaths, and with reportable diseases, the period is usually one year. Similar rates apply to pregnancies, automobile crashes, reported symptoms, absenteeism, and other events of community or population health significance. The risk factor can be a demographic characteristic such as age or race, or it can be a behavioral, environmental, or organizational characteristic.

Cause-Specific Rates Data are available from death certificates on the cause of death. Tabulating the causes of death for people in a community, then dividing the total for each cause by the midyear population of the community, yields a series of **cause-specific rates** of mortality. In developed countries the specific mortality rates for heart disease and cancer are much higher than those for communicable diseases. The opposite is true in some developing countries, although this is changing.

Age-Adjusted Rates In examining the question of how the total death rate for whites in Baltimore can be higher than that for blacks when each of the age-specific rates for whites is lower, one must consider the relative risks of death between ages. The population of Baltimore, like that of many cities in the eastern United States, consists disproportionately of older whites and younger blacks. If one multiplies the higher rates for older people by

the larger proportions of whites in those age groups, one gets high numbers of deaths for whites. Then if you add up the products of the multiplications across the entire range, the result will be a higher total for whites than for blacks in the race-specific death rates. This is why comparisons over time (figure 3-10), or between communities or other large, heterogeneous groups, are usually age-adjusted. **Age-adjusted rates** are much like the weighted sum of age-specific rates. The age-adjusted rate uses the proportion (between 0 and 1) of some standard population, such as the national proportion in that age group, to multiply each of the age-specific rates, then sums those products.

Crude Death Rate Versus Age-Adjusted Death Rate Comparing crude death rates over time masks part of the historical trend in declining death rates in developed countries, as seen in figure 3-10. Age-adjusted death rates control for the changing age composition of the population by applying the current age-specific death rates for each age group to a standard population's age distribution. The standard population chosen for the trend analysis shown in figure 3-10 was the population of the United States in 1940. Thus, the crude death rate and the age-adjusted death rate were equivalent for 1940. Why would the age-adjusted rate be so much lower than the crude death rate today than in earlier years? Why is the gap between the two rates still growing in the 1990s?

Crude Death Rate Versus Age-Specific Rates Age-specific death rates are generally higher for older age groups than for younger ones. This means that for any given year the crude death rate, unadjusted for the proportions in each age group that year, will tend to reflect the age-specific rates of the larger age groups. How might this explain the paradox of the Baltimore data? In the early decades of the twentieth century, the younger age groups (under age twenty-five) represented around 50 percent of the total population of the United States, as seen in figure 3-11. As their proportion declined in subsequent decades, the

• • • • • • • • • • • • • • • • • • •

Figure 3-10

The decline in the crude death rate has been less dramatic than the decline in the age-adjusted death rate because the crude rate is based on a population containing more elderly people each year, whereas the age-adjusted rate is based on the standard 1940 U.S. population. (*Source:* National Center for Health Statistics: Annual summary of births, marriages, divorces, and deaths, United States, 1991, *Monthly Vital Statistics Report* 40(13):5, Sept. 30, 1992.)

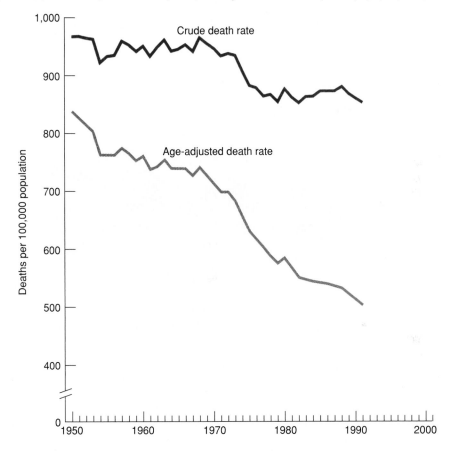

proportion of the older age groups (with higher age specific death rates) increased. This weighting of the population distribution with older and older ages made the crude death rate look as though there was no decrease in mortality during the post-war decades, as reflected in figure 3-10.

Birth Rates   Even the age-adjusted death rate seems to have stalled in its decline during the 1950s and early 1960s, according to the lower slope in figure 3-10. Why would the death rate

have declined faster during World War II than after the war? This phenomenon can be attributed largely to the "baby boom" of the postwar years. It reflects not a slowing of progress in reducing premature death as much as an increased proportion of the population made up of infants and children (see the series of peaks in the middle of figure 3-11). During the same period, the proportion in the oldest age groups with the highest mortality continued to increase. This meant that the three oldest and the youngest age group (under one year) loaded the

· · · · · · · · · · · · · · · · · · · ·

Figure 3-11

Younger age groups are becoming smaller as older age groups grow in their proportion of the total population of most countries. The projected proportions for the U.S. assume constant net immigration of 450,000 persons per year and a slow improvement in life expectancy to 84 years for females and 75 years for males by the year 2050. (Courtesy Metropolitan Life Insurance Co.)

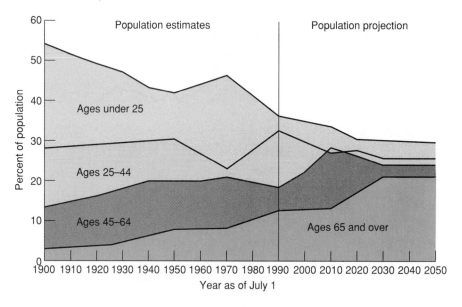

death rates of the 1950s and 1960s with larger numbers of deaths. The dramatic decline in the birth rate in the 1960s allowed the decline in death rates to resume.

These and other rates used by demographers and epidemiologists to compare the fertility, mortality, and health status and trends of populations or communities will be discussed throughout the following chapters.

Host, Agent, and Environment

Concepts underpinning the epidemiological approach to community health include the interaction of host, agent, and environment. The disease host refers to the person in whom the disease resides. The disease agent refers to that which carries or delivers the disease to the person. Epidemiology adds the element of **agent** to the ecological concept of human-environment inter-

action. The development of the germ theory in the late nineteenth century gave rise to the understanding of the role of agents in carrying disease. Communities placed their water supplies under greater control when they realized that water harbored agents of disease.

The epidemiological approach to the host has been to build host resistance to disease and to quarantine the host of a disease so that he or she could not transmit it to others. Community health programs apply the principle of host resistance in mass immunization programs, in maternal and child nutrition programs, and in physical fitness programs. All of these have as part of their function the strengthening of the ability of people to ward off infection, disease, or injury.

Epidemiology views the environment as a means to control the harboring of disease agents in water, air, food, and waste products that might

··················

Figure 3-12

Oswaldo Cruz, an epidemiologist, attained world fame during his lifetime for his victories over vector-borne diseases, especially in Brazil. These were celebrated in newspaper and magazine editorials and cartoons. This caricature from the Parisian journal, *Chanteclair,* appeared in 1911. (*Source:* Photo courtesy World Health Organization, from *Chanteclair,* Paris, 1911.)

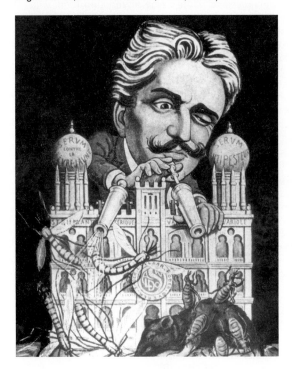

come into contact with people. The control of flies, mosquitoes, rats, and rabid animals (vector control) in the last century reduced yellow fever, malaria, plague, and other pandemic diseases (figure 3-12).

Communities also use epidemiological tools to study the "host resistance" of young children to false advertising, the automobile and alcohol as "agents" of injury, and the social "environment" as a context for shaping healthful lifestyles. These new applications of epidemiological concepts are essential to meet the challenge presented by the

dramatic shift (the "second epidemiological revolution") from communicable diseases to chronic and degenerative diseases and injury.

Epidemics and Pandemics

The term epidemic means "around people" and denotes a condition from a common cause that has affected a large number of people. The term pandemic literally means "all people" and denotes spread of a disease over a considerable area. The term describes a nationwide, continentwide, or worldwide outbreak. An outbreak of a disease may be regarded as an epidemic. The past has seen devastating pandemics of bubonic plague, yellow fever, cholera, smallpox, typhus fever, and syphilis. The 1918–1919 influenza-pneumonia pandemic caused 400,000 deaths in the United States, 10 million deaths in India, and more than 20 million deaths throughout the world. In some developing nations during the 1990s acute infectious disease epidemics such as cholera have occurred. These epidemics usually have centered on a single nation or on a small group of nations. Developing nations are not likely to have devastating pandemics of acute infectious diseases such as occurred in the past, but moderately severe outbreaks will occur for decades. In the more developed nations scientific advances in the field of epidemiology make even a moderate pandemic of an acute infectious disease highly unlikely.

Endemic means "within people" and denotes a condition that persists within geographical areas. Chronic infections still plague vast segments of the population in many nations of the world. Millions of people each year contract malaria, hookworm, ascarids (a roundworm), or leprosy. Asia has 335 million people who harbor the parasitic ascarid. Of the 1 billion people with ascariasis, 20,000 die each year. Each of 335 million Asian people with this parasite will harbor between six and nine adult ascarids. The worms they carry will consume as much food each day as a population of an additional 40,000 people. Indonesia had 15 million cases of yaws before a staff of Indonesians

ISSUES AND CONTROVERSIES
The Tragedy of the Atmosphere

Countries and industries pursuing only their own gain have overloaded the atmosphere with greenhouse gases to the point that everyone is affected by the global warming effects. The countries themselves and the rest of the world will suffer in the long run if the gases cannot be reduced below 1990 levels. The Kyoto conference in December 1997 produced an international treaty that would place greater restrictions on some of the developed countries (including Canada and the United States) than on the developing countries. This leads to opposition to the treaty from the U.S. Congress and some of the Canadian provinces that produce much of the polluting fuels. Congressional opposition has been fueled by advertisements from industries in the United States that portray the treaty as a threat to American economic competitiveness if such large "loopholes" as the exemption of developing countries and Australia give those countries competitive advantage in the global economy. Americans and Canadians as populations also have resisted giving up much of the comfort of their energy-intensive lifestyles in the interest of conserving the environment. The anti-Kyoto treaty advertisements were produced by the same advertising firms who produced the Harry and Louise series that succeeded in killing President Clinton's health care reform initiatives by appealing to the public's worries about not having a choice of their own physicians. How can the global community make progress in safeguarding the environment in the face of resistance from specific countries and the industries and citizens within countries?

---

trained and supplied with penicillin by the United Nations proceeded to wipe out the disease. One injection of penicillin usually cures yaws, so that nearly the entire Indonesian population is free of the disease.

Diphtheria, influenza, measles, meningitis, encephalitis, and other infectious diseases could conceivably break out in pandemic form even in Australia, Europe, and North America. Influenza, for example, reappears in a new form each year around the world. Most regions have controlled these diseases effectively. Smallpox was eradicated worldwide in 1977. Poliomyelitis was eliminated in the Americas as of 1991 and is targeted by the World Health Organization for global eradication by the year 2000 (see box). It is possible, however, that a mutant pathogen of humans may arise with unprecedented virulence. Such an occurrence will challenge society's ability to control the spread of disease, as did the Ebola outbreaks in Africa in 1995. Our ability to solve disease control problems that might arise will depend on rapid application of our knowledge of infection and its control.

Diseases Targeted by the World Health Organization for Eradication or Elimination

1976	Smallpox eradication globally (achieved in Americas in 1970, globally in 1977)
1990	Poliomyelitis elimination in Americas (achieved in 1991)
1991	Dracunculiasis elimination in Pakistan (last endemic area in Asia, achieved 1993)
1995	Dracunculiasis eradication (still endemic in Ghana and Nigeria, though reduced)
	Poliomyelitis elimination in Europe, Western Pacific
	Measles elimination in English-speaking Caribbean
	Neonatal tetanus elimination
2000	Poliomyelitis eradication globally
	Measles elimination in Europe
	Leprosy elimination (defined as <1 case/10,000 population)
2007	Elimination of onchocerciasis in the Americas

LIFE SPAN VERSUS LIFE EXPECTANCY

Life span and life expectancy are distinct phenomena, one biological and the other epidemiological. Life span is the recognized biological limit of life. Considering present knowledge, biologists tend to set the maximum human life span at 120 years. They do not possess reliable data of human beings living beyond this age. The usual report of people living beyond 120 years emanates from primitive areas where unreliable records or no records exist. Biologists suggest that in all probability even the person who lives to age 115 years has shortened his or her life by adverse health practices or circumstances. Scientists recognize that improper dietary practices, infections, excessive fatigue, prolonged exposure, inadequate rest, and other factors may have shortened the life of the person who lives to age 115.

Not all people have a life span of 120 years. Some people probably have a life span considerably below 100 years, as indicated by failure of any member in some lineages to reach the age of sixty years. Life span is an inherited characteristic determined at the time the ovum is fertilized by the sperm. The person can do nothing to extend the inherited span but inadvertently or unwisely does many things to prevent the realization of his or her life span.

Life expectancy, on the other hand, is an epidemiological concept. It refers to the average duration of time that individuals of a given age can expect to live, based on the longevity experience of the population in which they are born. These averages are based on the assumption that the longevity experience of the recent past will prevail in the future. Future developments, however, probably will favor an extension of longevity beyond what past years produced. All averages on expectancy apply to the age group's life expectancy at birth. Individuals within a group will vary, some experiencing an expectancy considerably above the average and some below the average.

Disability-free longevity, or quality life years, has emerged as a replacement for life expectancy to measure more of the quality of life, not just the quantity. This measure quantifies expected degrees of independence and dependence during the average lifetime. It thus serves not only as a better indicator of population health status, but also as a better planning tool to anticipate demands on health care and other services and resources. The United States has not adopted this measure extensively in its statistical reporting. A Canadian child born in 1991 had a total life expectancy of 78, compared with 75.7 for a child born in the United States in the same year (75.8 in 1995). Of the 78 years, the Canadian child could expect 69 years (89 percent of the total life expectancy) to be spent in complete independence from disabling health problems. The balance would be divided between minor dependence (3.2 years), moderate dependence (2.9 years), and heavy dependence (2.2 years). The distributions of these proportions for males and females at birth and at age 65 are shown in figure 3-13.

The United States has computed a related measure of "healthy life years" from life expectancy based on standard life tables coupled with self-reported health status and activity limitation from the National Health Interview Survey. From this analysis, 64 years of life on average (85 percent of the total life expectancy) are estimated to be healthy. Some 11.4 years (15 percent) are estimated to be unhealthy, with limitations of major life activities such as self-care (bathing, grooming, and cooking), recreation, school, and work. The United States appears to be losing ground as health-related quality of life declines despite increases in life expectancy. How much this relates to the subjectivity of self-reported health status and activity limitation, and how much to the actual activity limitations that increase with age in a population with increasing longevity, one can only speculate.

Years of Potential Life Lost, referred to as YPLL, is more widely used in the United States to capture the effects of premature death with greater weight given to deaths at earlier ages. It is a measure, therefore, that is more sensitive to the successes and failures of prevention and health promotion. In the calculation of YPLL before age 75,

· ·

Figure 3-13

Disability-free life years, a measure used in several countries, reflects total life expectancy minus the years of dependency. The shaded areas shown here for Canada reflect dependent proportions of total life expectancy at birth and at age 65. (*Source:* Wilkens R, Chen J, Ng E: The consequences of disease and impairment: trends in disability, dependency and health expectancy from 1986 to 1991. Presentation to the Health Policy Division, Health Canada, April 1995.)

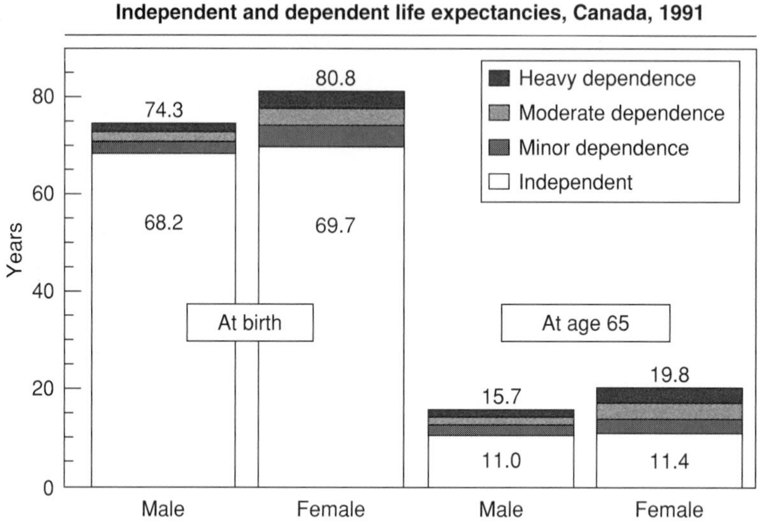

Independent and dependent life expectancies, Canada, 1991

infants who die before their first birthday have lost 74.5 years of life; a person dying at 65 has lost 10 years of potential life. A further elaboration of this measure has been developed, but not yet widely applied, to assess "quality-adjusted life years" or QALYs.

Geographic Differences

Despite the United States' medical, hospital, and other health facilities, along with her favorable economic position, the United States life expectancy does not compare favorably with that in many other industrialized countries. Of 15 countries with the highest life expectancies for males and for which recent comparable data were available, 9 had higher life expectancies at birth for males than the United States. Japan, Iceland, Sweden, and Norway had the longest life expectancies for males. For males in the United States in 1995, life expectancy at birth was estimated at 72.6, for Canada in 1991 it was 74.3. For females the United States longevity in 1995 was 78.9; in Canada in 1991, 80.8.

The people of seven U.S. Midwestern states and the Prairie provinces of Canada consistently have a greater life expectancy than that of the people of most other states and provinces. Iowa, Kansas, Minnesota, Nebraska, North Dakota, Oklahoma, and South Dakota regularly exceed the national life expectancy figures by at least two years and occasionally three years. The national origin of the population, economic means, climate, vocations, living practices, and other factors have been analyzed. None of these by itself consistently distinguishes the population of these states from the population of other states. Two neighboring states, Utah and Nevada, have similar climates and geography but extreme differences of life expectancy, reflecting their differences in lifestyle (75.8 for Utah; 69.3 for Nevada). Most of the geographic differences, then, should be traceable to demographic and cultural or social differences that dictate lifestyle practices and conditions.

The comparison of eight countries that use the disability-free life expectancy at birth measure,

. . . .
Figure 3-14

Disability-free life expectancy at birth in eight OECD countries using this measure show wide geographic variations even within this relatively homogeneous spectrum of economically advanced European and North American countries. How much of this variation is attributable to environment, economics, cultural, social, or organizational factors is unknown. (*Source:* OECD Health Systems: *Facts and Trends,* 1991.)

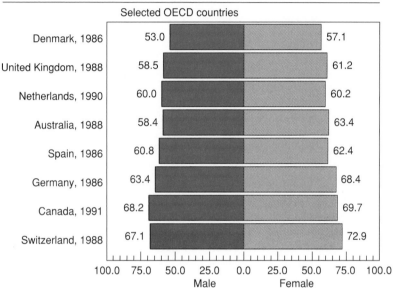

Disability-free life expectancy at birth

Selected OECD countries

	Male	Female
Denmark, 1986	53.0	57.1
United Kingdom, 1988	58.5	61.2
Netherlands, 1990	60.0	60.2
Australia, 1988	58.4	63.4
Spain, 1986	60.8	62.4
Germany, 1986	63.4	68.4
Canada, 1991	68.2	69.7
Switzerland, 1988	67.1	72.9

100.0 75.0 50.0 25.0 0.0 25.0 50.0 75.0 100.0
Male   Female

shown in figure 3-14, reveals widely divergent estimates among the countries sharing highly developed health care systems, similar European cultural heritage, and similar economic affluence. This leaves us, again, to speculate on the possible causes of these differences that might lie in some combination of social differences that dictate lifestyle and conditions of living.

Demographic Differences

In every country, life expectancy and disability-free life expectancy at birth is greater for females than for males. The increased expectation of life at birth continues the general upward trend with the gradual decline in deaths in younger ages. However, the increases are slowing and in the United States black male population actually had a decrease in life expectancy in the 1980s.

Under the mortality conditions prevailing in 1940, a U.S. infant born in that year could expect to live an average of 62.9 years. Between 1940 and 1960, 7 years were added to life expectancy. Only 4 additional years were added between 1965 and 1985. Thus the gain in the earlier 20-year period was greater than the gain during the more recent 20 years.

Females have gained more years than males, especially nonwhite U.S. females, who now have a longer life expectancy than U.S. white males. Although the difference between life expectancy for males and females has increased, the difference between life expectancy for Caucasians and people of all other races in the United States has reduced substantially. In 1950 Caucasians could expect to live about 8 years longer than people of all other races. By 1986 this differential had decreased to 4 years. Since the mid-1980s, however, the black male population in the United States has lost ground.

The greatest gain in life expectancy during the first half of the twentieth century can be attributed to the prevention of deaths in infancy and childhood. Progress has been made in extending the length of life by postponing death in the later age brackets. In 1985 the life expectancy of a person of 40 was nearly 10 years greater than the life expectancy of a person of 40 in the year 1900. Gains in the decade after 1985 were slower.

Risk Factors Determining Life Expectancy

Longevity is a general term that incorporates a vast number of factors significant to individuals interested in estimating their own life expectancy. Fortunately, no one knows precisely when he or she will die. It is possible to establish the approximate probable lifetime by a statistical procedure called health hazard appraisal or health risk appraisal. This questionnaire weighs various characteristics of the individual according to the known population correlation of those characteristics with mortality. This allows individuals to identify with some statistical probability how many years they could add to their lives by changing specific health practices, circumstances, or conditions throughout life. Some factors, however, are not changeable.

Race   At the time of birth, the white male has a life expectancy greater than the nonwhite male, and the white female has an expectancy greater than the nonwhite female. After age 74, however, there is a crossover in the white-nonwhite races for both sexes. Whites enjoy lower mortality rates until age 74, when nonwhite mortality becomes lower and remains so. Nonwhites who have surmounted the economic barriers and environmental hazards to health may represent a hardier group of survivors compared with their white counterparts of similar age. This makes the years of potential life lost before age 65 a more sensitive measure for purposes of detecting differences that may be preventable in earlier years.

Inheritance   Long-lived parents tend to have long-lived offspring. What actually is transmitted is not a single gene for long life. Many genes af-

fect adequate body structure, efficiently functioning organs and systems, resistance to diseases, the ability to recover from injury or disease, the capacity to produce necessary body enzymes, and various other attributes necessary for long life.

Dr. Raymond Pearl, a U.S. biometrist, found that for his subjects ninety years of age or over (longevous group), 46 percent had two long-lived parents, while in the other subjects (control group), only 12 percent had two long-lived parents. The significant difference in the two percentages doubtless represents inherited endowment.

In considering the influence of inheritance on the length of life, one should not overlook that living in a long-lived family usually means certain environmental advantages that could be favorable for longevity. Having both parents living to look after his or her welfare should be an aid to an individual in obtaining his or her highest possible potential, in quality of health and length of life. Certainly gains in the longevity of the general population must be attributed to environmental improvements rather than genetic changes. Inherited longevity still has its advantages in determining one's length of life, but with new knowledge and its applications these advantages are not as great as they were in earlier decades.

Gender   Although the differential between the life expectancy of the female and that of the male declines during the years after birth, she tends to have an advantage all through life. The female appears to inherit a better set of long-wearing qualities. She has less bulky musculature and more flexible soft tissues. She is less prone to heart disorders and arteriosclerosis, thanks partly to hormonal differences. She has lower blood pressure and a higher white cell count, both of which are to her advantage. She engages in less hazardous occupations and less reckless behavior, resulting in injury death rates much lower than those of the male. In the past, she has worked under less daily tension. Even as women increase the intensity and the tension of their lives in vocational pursuits, they seem to possess the means and the social encouragement to give release to their emotions. This is a practice the male could emulate to his benefit.

With emancipation of the female, however, her advantage in longevity may decrease. Adolescent groups contain more female cigarette smokers than male smokers, although females smoke fewer cigarettes and inhale less. Unfortunately, they find it more difficult to stop smoking than do males, and recidivism is higher in females. The habit of cigarette smoking is equated with freedom and social advancement in the advertisements directed at females. Another disadvantageous element is that obesity is more prevalent in females than in males, particularly in the lower socioeconomic groups. As females gain more employment, the differential in mortality may decline.

Education and Occupation   The long-standing recognition of occupation as an element in longevity (see table 1-1 p. 16) incorporates a number of variables. These include the types of individuals who go into various occupations, the hazards and stresses, the economic status, and the educational background of people in these occupations. Longest lived are members of the clergy, lawyers, engineers, teachers, doctors, and farmers, essentially in that order. Next longest lived are business executives, white-collar workers, and skilled manual workers. Shortest lived are the unskilled workers, miners, quarry workers, and granite workers.

Studies indicate that educational attainment correlates consistently with longevity and other measures of health. College graduates have a greater life expectancy than that of the general population. Even noncollege graduates, by the application of sound health principles and the use of available medical and health facilities and services, can extend their life expectancy considerably beyond the average.

Income   Favorable living conditions, associated with adequate income, have a definite influence on longevity. Families with a favorable income are able to avail themselves of medical care, proper nutrition, good housing, and other advantages that make a longer life possible. People living in cities with a high average level of income live longer than those living in cities with a low level of income. The population advantage conferred by high income is no longer operative, however, in very old age groups, that is, those over eighty-five years. After this age, genetic endowment is dominant and socioeconomic status has little influence on further life expectancy in populations.

Marital Status   Married men live longer than single men. Many men in poor health remain single, which partially accounts for the shorter life expectancy of single men. The orderly life of the married man apparently operates to his advantage in preserving his life. Among women, the picture of longevity varies. Up to the age of forty, married women have a greater life expectancy than single women, but thereafter married women and unmarried women have similar life expectancies. Widows survive better than widowers, but this may be the result of gender rather than marital status.

Body Build   An individual inherits a particular type of body that he or she can modify very little through nutrition or other means. Although people of certain body builds live longer than those of other body types, no one is doomed to a short life expectancy merely on the basis of his or her body build. People of average height and weight tend to live longest. As a group, people of very large stature do not live as long as those who are smaller than average. Being extremely underweight during young adulthood has an adverse effect on length of life, whereas those who are somewhat underweight in later years tend to have a favorable life expectancy. Obesity, particularly in the later years of life, has an adverse effect on longevity: people more than 25 percent overweight have a 75 percent higher death rate than those in the average weight category. Obesity is increasing in most countries.

Lifestyle and Habits   Overeating, alcohol and drug misuse, and general excessiveness associated with high-tension living tend to shorten life.

· · · · · · · · · · · · · · · · · · · ·

Figure 3-15

The three leading causes of death for youth account for 61 percent of their deaths in violent injury, whereas for adults 25 and over the three leading causes accounting for 66 percent of their deaths are chronic diseases. The types of community and population programs to prevent premature death must be quite different for these two populations. (*Source:* Centers for Disease Control and Prevention, US Department of Health and Human Services, 1996.)

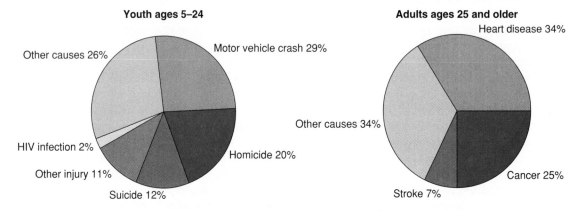

Youth ages 5–24

Other causes 26%
Motor vehicle crash 29%
HIV infection 2%
Other injury 11%
Homicide 20%
Suicide 12%

Adults ages 25 and older

Heart disease 34%
Other causes 34%
Cancer 25%
Stroke 7%

Cigarette smoking and heavy drinking reduce life expectancy. Manual labor, even heavy manual labor, before the age of forty does not appear to affect the length of life, but hard manual labor continued after the age of forty does seem to shorten life expectancy. Generally, people of a temperament that leads to a pattern of moderation in living reap benefits in terms of more years added to their lives. These lifestyle variables, however, are so intertwined with socioeconomic variables that it is difficult to separate them in population analyses.

Blood Pressure Low blood pressure, unless extremely low, favors longevity. The higher the blood pressure, the shorter the life, partially as a result of the relationship of blood pressure to heart and kidney disorders and stroke. Individuals with high blood pressure need not assume they can do nothing to extend their life expectancy. Modern medical treatment and behavioral changes in relation to diet, exercise, and stress management can have a significant effect on reducing blood pressure. Blood pressure, tobacco, diet, and alcohol together account for more than three-fourths of the premature deaths.

COMMUNITY APPLICATIONS

The individual and the community can take effective measures to extend life expectancy, and to improve health, starting with study of the most likely causes of death. More than 76 percent of deaths in any recent year in the United States, Canada, Australia, Japan, Singapore, and most European nations, will have resulted from three causes: cardiovascular diseases, cancer, and injuries. Breaking down these data on the basis of age groups, however, allows a community to be more specific in concentrating attention on the most fruitful points of intervention to prevent premature deaths (figure 3-15). In addition, if the citizens of a community have adequate support in promoting their own quality of health and postponing death, they could extend disability-free life expectancy appreciably in that community. Ten of the twelve leading causes of death are subject to reduction, chiefly through informed individual actions, particularly related to tobacco, diet, and alcohol. Communities can enable individuals to take greater control of informed actions, however, if the communities address the conditions shaping and facilitating or preventing those actions.

A community can contribute to life expectancy through an effective program of health education that gives citizens a knowledge of what they as individuals can do to promote their present health. Health promotion can add support for individuals to control conditions affecting their heart, arteries, kidneys, lungs, and other vital structures. Periodic health-risk appraisals, self-monitoring, and health examinations would give them an assessment of the condition of these vital structures. Such assessments would also warn them against the development of the various chronic disorders of adulthood. People need to adopt a positive health-oriented mode of behavior, emphasizing proper diet and rest, regular exercise, avoidance of tobacco, and moderate use of alcohol. A lifestyle of moderation in a community with value systems, environments and social structures consistent with health can result in healthful living and longevity. A community program of health promotion and health protection should include health education; organizational and environmental changes conducive to healthful living; regulations protecting people from damaging practices by others; and periodic clinical visits for immunizations, tests, or examinations with suitable follow-up. Such a program should yield tangible results in reducing disease and disability. Any community with adequate and accessible health services and facilities is contributing to the quality of life of its citizens.

Research and the diffusion of new knowledge about prevention and control of heart disease, cancer, injury, and other principal causes of death will largely determine the future extension of active and functional life expectancy. A breakthrough in the problem of cancer may have a slight influence on life expectancy. New methods and techniques in heart surgery could increase life expectancy at age fifty by a few months. Reducing automobile-related deaths could have a larger effect on life expectancy. The primary purpose of community health promotion and protection, however, should be to reduce morbidity and improve the quality of life, not merely the addition of years to increasingly disabled lives.

Table 3-2

Health Status Indicators

Indicators of health status	
Mortality	
All causes	Lung cancer
Infant mortality	Breast cancer
Motor vehicle accidents	Cardiovascular diseases
Work-related injuries	Homicides
Suicides	
Morbidity	
Incidence	
Acquired immunodeficiency syndrome	
Measles	
Tuberculosis	
Primary and secondary syphilis	
Indicators of risk	
Low birth weight	
Births to adolescents	
Lack of prenatal care	
Children in poverty	
Poor air quality	

MEASURING PROGRESS

The United States published *Objectives for the Nation* in disease prevention and health promotion in 1981. Since then, *Healthy People 2000* and several editions of model standards for community attainment of the national objectives have inspired other nations, states, provinces, and communities to formulate their community and population health plans with quantified objectives and target dates. In *Healthy People 2000,* the second decade plan for disease prevention and health promotion, the United States laid out 300 specific objectives. A national committee of state and county health officers, together with national organizations, then developed a set of eighteen health status indicators that would be commonly adopted by all states to measure progress toward the objectives for the nation. These are shown in table 3-2.

The *Healthy Communities 2000: Model Standards* document outlines a series of specific objectives for translating national objectives into

Table 3-3

Community Objectives for Monitoring and Surveillance of Health

Focus	Objective*	Indicator
Community health assessment	1. By ____ the community will conduct community health assessments on a periodic basis.	Availability of community health assessment
Health statistical and epidemiological consultation and capacity	2. By ____ the community will have available health statistical and epidemiological consultation and the capacity to: a. Carry out investigations, special studies, and data analyses b. Institute appropriate measures to control conditions of public health significance in the community c. Evaluate the impact of control measures.	A demonstrable system to provide immediate telephone consultation and timely on-site assistance for investigation, control, and evaluation
Quality laboratory services	3. By ____ the community will have access to quality laboratory services necessary for the timely diagnosis/confirmation/identification of diseases, risk factors, and conditions of public health significance.	A demonstrable system of timely access to quality laboratory services.
Identification of underserved populations	4. By ____ the community will be served by an official health agency with capability to conduct surveys in order to identify underserved populations and those demonstrating special needs.	a. Number of surveys conducted b. Availability of survey results
Assessment, monitoring, and evaluation of programs	5. By ____ the health agency will establish a mechanism for the assessment, monitoring, and evaluation of existing programs to measure progress, identify factors that interfere with program effectiveness or efficiency, and determine the need for continuation, refinement, reduction, redirection, or expansion of operations.	Assessment and evaluation mechanisms
Current directory of community programs	6. By ____ the community will have available a current list of community health programs.	List availability
Systematic review of community health services	7. By ____ the community will have a systematic and periodic process to review community health services.	Periodic reports to governing bodies, legislative bodies, elected officials, and the public on current services

Focus	Objective*	Indicator
	8. By ____ health services agencies will establish and maintain a system to review their programs periodically for their sensitivity to individual, family, and community needs, values, experiences, awareness, understanding, language and cultural differences, rights, and dignity.	1. Existence of system to include: a. Policies that provide for public participation in the agency decision-making process b. Documentation of consumer representation on agency boards, councils, committees, commissions, and task forces. c. Written guidelines for and documentation of solicitation of public participation in health care programs d. Existence of consumer education programs e. A stated policy of public access to program information without individual identifiers. 2. Agency personnel composition compared to the community it serves in terms of ethnicity, cultural differences, and principal language spoken in a community a. Existence of a written consumer grievance policy and procedures manual

*In the blank, the community can set a target date for accomplishment of the objective.

achievable community health targets. Each objective or "model standard" provides for the community to set its own reasonable target date for accomplishment of the objective. Each objective also carries one or more indicators of success that can be used to assess progress or attainment of the objective. Examples of objectives and the indicators for monitoring their achievement specific to the epidemiological capacity of the community are shown in table 3-3. Other documents prepared by state and provincial governments, and by other national organizations, guide community groups in similar ways. Some help in applying procedures and measurement tools or indicators in the community's assessment of community needs. Others help community groups measure their progress in meeting those needs.

Future surveillance systems will need to track changes in the public's knowledge of risk factors for particular diseases and conditions, monitor the extent to which people are making changes in their behavior in efforts to reduce their personal or environmental risks, and evaluate their success in maintaining the changes they make. Surveys conducted during the 1980s and 1990s have accumulated a good deal of the necessary baseline data. We will address these questions in the next chapter.

SUMMARY

Promoting and protecting community and population health will have no influence on life span, but can influence life expectancy, especially in the high-risk and poorest sectors of the community. Population health promotion, health protection, and community health services have their greatest potential in directly and indirectly influencing the quality of life that all people of the community will enjoy. We have specific targets toward which to aim our efforts because we know the specific leading causes of death and the population distribution of these risk factors. Programs can be directed into channels leading to likely dividends. Knowing statistically what the causes of disease, disability, and death are most likely to be, the community can concentrate its efforts where they can have the greatest impact on health.

An ecological perspective, supported with demographic and epidemiological methods of analysis, enables the community to understand its health conditions and trends in more comprehensive terms than medical data alone would permit.

WEB*Links*

http://coombs.anu.edu.au/ResFacilities/
DemographyPage.html
Demography and Population Studies

http://www.epibiostat.ucsf.edu/epidem/epidem
.html
The World-Wide Web Virtual Library: Epidemiology

http://www.pitt.edu/HOME/GHNet/GHNet.html
The Global Health Network

http://www.statcan.ca
Statistics Canada (includes information helpful for
audience analysis)

QUESTIONS FOR REVIEW

1. What evidence is there that seasons and climate influence population health?
2. What evidence is there that the advances in health sciences have had a dysgenic effect on human populations?
3. What is meant by the conservation of human resources?
4. For the past forty years the Alaskan glaciers have been shrinking rapidly. What interpretation do you make of this, and what is the significance of the phenomenon?
5. What effect would a constantly rising world temperature have on life expectancy, health, the economy, and the general culture of Canada, Russia, and the Scandinavian and Mediterranean nations?
6. In what type of nation does hunger pose the greatest threat?
7. One county with a rate of natural increase of 16 has a neighboring county with a rate of 4. What differences would you expect to find between the two countries?
8. What has been the effect of the development of DDT on the health and culture of the world?
9. What has been the effect of advances in agricultural technology on the health and culture of the world?
10. Why does Sweden have a greater life expectancy than the United States?
11. What factors probably account for the good disability-free life expectancy of Canadians?
12. Why do females in the United States and Canada live longer than males?
13. Why can a child born in North America expect to live a greater number of years after his or her first birthday anniversary than could have been expected after the day on which he or she was born?
14. How does your community measure up on the objectives in table 3-2?
15. What is the role of economics in life expectancy?

READINGS

Cohen, J. E. 1996. Ten myths of population. *Discover: the world of science* 17(4):42.
  With 5.7 billion people on Earth, and 250 more born every minute, it's critical that we understand the dynamics of human population growth. Yet we cling to a host of half-truths and inventions.

Detels, R., W. W. Holland, J. McEwen, and G. Omen, ed. 1996. *Oxford textbook of public health.* 3d ed. 2 vol. Oxford: Oxford University Press.

This volume of the *Oxford Textbook of Public Health* covers the demographic and epidemiological methods used in the development and analysis of community health information systems, surveys, and demographic data.

Gregg, M. B. 1996. *Field epidemiology.* Oxford & New York: Oxford University Press.

Describes in simple and practical terms the specific tasks and actions needed for successful epidemiologic field investigations. How to conduct surveillance, perform surveys, respond to media, and the legal aspects of field studies.

Hamann, B. 1994. Disease: Identification, prevention and control. St. Louis: Mosby.

Presents information about communicable and chronic diseases and their histories from a nonclinical point of view.

Harkavy, O. 1995. Curbing population growth: an insider's perspective on the population movement. New York and London: Plenum Publishing Corp.

A Ford Foundation program officer for thirty years traces the growth of the modern population control movement from its beginnings in the 1950s, the roles played by the UN and other major organizations, and the role of social sciences, including demography, in understanding the causes and effects of population growth.

Oleske, D. M., ed. 1995. Epidemiology and the delivery of health care services, New York & London: Plenum Publishing Corp.

Shows how epidemiologic principles can be applied to decision-making in health care management and population-based health care.

Stone, D. B., R. Warwick, D. M. Macrina, and J. Pankau. 1996. *Epidemiology.* Madison, WI: Brown & Benchmark.

Introductory text on basic principles and concepts, including host-agent-environment model of epidemiology. Leads student through the steps of investigating a disease outbreak.

BIBLIOGRAPHY

Abernethy, V. D. 1993. *Population politics: the choices that shape our future.* New York & London: Plenum Publishing Corp.

Adams, D. L., ed. 1995. Health issues for women of color: a cultural diversity perspective. Newbury Park, CA: Sage Publications, Inc.

Beaglehole, R., R. Bonita, and T. Kjellstrom. 1993. *Basic epidemiology.* Geneva: World Health Organization.

Bongaarts, J. 1994. Can the growing human population feed itself? *Scientific Amer* 270(3):36.

Clarke, S. C., and B. F. Wilson. 1994. The relative stability of marriages: a cohort approach using vital statistics. *Fam Relations* 43:305.

De Vos, S. M. 1995. *Household composition in Latin America.* New York & London: Plenum.

Evans, R. G., M. L. Barer, and T. R. Marmor, ed. 1994. Why are some people healthy and others not? The determinants of health of populations. New York: Aldine de Gruyter.

Garrett, L. 1993. The coming plague: newly emerging diseases in a world out of balance. New York: Farrar Straus Giroux.

Green, L. W., D. Simons-Morton, and L. Potivin. 1996. Education and life-style determinants of health and disease. In *Oxford textbook of public health.* 3d ed, edited by W. W. Holland, R. Detels, G. Knox, and G. Omen. Oxford: Oxford University Press.

Gruenwald, P. J., A. J. Treno, G. Taff, M. Klitzner. 1996. *Measuring community indicators: a systems approach to drug and alcohol problems.* Newbury Park, CA: Sage Publications, Inc.

Hardin, G. 1968. The tragedy of the commons. *Science* 143: 1243.

Healthy communities 2000: model standards. 1991. 3d ed. Washington, DC: American Public Health Association.

Jenicek, M. 1995. *Epidemiology: the logic of modern medicine.* Ottawa: EpiMed and Canadian Public Health Association.

Kochanek, K. D., J. D. Maurer, and H. M. Rosenberg. 1994. Why did black life expectancy decline from 1984 through 1989 in the United States? *Am J Public Health* 84:938.

Last, J. M., and R. B. Wallace. 1997. *Maxcy-Rosenau-Last public health and preventive medicine.* 14th ed. Norwalk, CT: Appleton & Lange.

Leigh, J. P., and J. F. Fries. 1994. Education, gender, and the compression of morbidity. *Int J Aging Hum Devel* 39:233.

Levy, B. S., and V. W. Sidel, ed. 1996. *War and public health.* Oxford & New York: Oxford University Press.

Lillienfeld, D. E., and P. D. Stolley. 1994. *Foundations of epidemiology.* Oxford & New York: Oxford University Press.

McDowell, I., and C. Newell. 1996. *Measuring health: a guide to rating scales and questionnaires.* Oxford & New York: Oxford University Press.

Molina, C. W., and M. Aguirre-Molina. 1994. *Latino health in the US: a growing challenge.* Washington, DC: American Public Health Association.

Petitti, D. B. 1994. Meta-analysis, decision analysis, and cost-effectiveness analysis. Oxford & New York: Oxford University Press.

Pol, L. G., and R. K. Thomas. 1992. *The demography of health and health care.* New York and London: Plenum.

Population Health Resource Branch. 1995. *Health indicator workbook: a tool for healthy communities.* 2d ed. Victoria, BC: British Columbia Ministry of Health and Ministry Responsible for Seniors.

Population Health Resource Branch. 1995. *Health impact assessment guidelines: a resource for program planning and development.* Victoria, BC: British Columbia Ministry of Health and Ministry Responsible for Seniors.

Van Imhoff, E., A. Kuijsten, P. Hooimeijer, and L. van Wissen, ed. 1995. *Household demography and household modeling.* New York & London: Plenum Publishing Corp.

Wunderlich G. S., ed. 1992. *Toward a national health care survey: a data system for the 21st century.* Washington, DC: National Academy Press.

Chapter 4

Human Behavior, Community and Population Health Education

*H**ealth is the ability to perform certain valued social roles.*

—Talcott Parsons

*H**uman history becomes more and more a race between education and catastrophe.*

—H. G. Wells

Objectives

When you finish this chapter, you should be able to:

- Assess and set behavioral objectives for the factors contributing to a community health or social problem

- Assess and set educational objectives for the factors influencing behavior and lifestyle in the community or population

- Identify principles of, and resources for, educational intervention in community health problems and community development needs

FROM SCIENCE TO APPLICATION

Besides history in chapter 1, we have considered biomedical sciences, ecology, demography, and epidemiology in the previous two chapters. The behavioral and social sciences constitute a fifth scientific foundation in community health. These foundations are interdependent. The relevance of behavior to community health is a matter of how human behavior influences biological, ecological, demographic, and epidemiological processes. As shown in figure 2-3, the behaviors of individuals become the lifestyle norms of populations when practiced by large segments of the community. Norms of fertility and migration behavior accumulate in demographic trends; norms of health behavior show up in social and epidemiological trends.

In the social history of health, normative behavior becomes organized. Organized behavior of a community has a greater impact than individuals on the environment and therefore on the ecology of health. Community organization can work to enhance the environment and to offset or control the destructive effects of human behavior on the environment. Finally, the environment, the social and economic environment in particular, comes full circle to influence behavior and lifestyle.

These interactions give rise to subspecialties among the foundation disciplines. They include scientific fields such as environmental epidemiology, behavioral ecology, behavioral medicine, health psychology, social medicine, medical geography, and social epidemiology. The application and delivery of the scientific products of these subspecialties fall largely to community health workers, especially through health education. **Community or population health education** employs a combination of methods designed to elicit, facilitate, and maintain *voluntary* adaptations of behavior conducive to health. It too has subspecialties in various types of education: patient, school health, population, environmental, sex, nutrition, dental health, mental health, and public health. The broader efforts of community health *promotion,* to be described in the several chapters of part 3, may go beyond voluntary changes in behavior. They may include regulatory and environmental control strategies designed to channel, restrain, or support behavior conducive to health or quality of life for the person, the community, or a population.

HEALTH BEHAVIOR AND LIFESTYLE

Human behavior relates to health in direct and indirect ways. Personal or social behavior has a direct effect on health (arrow *a* in figure 4-1) when it exposes an individual, group, or population to more or less risk of injury, disease, or death. Sometimes the exposure is subtle, as with small but repeated doses of a substance that may become addictive or cumulative in their effect. Drugs and fatty food are examples. At other times behavior may pose an immediate and excessive risk; eating a poisonous or infected food is one example of such behavior. Acute risks to health in food production, distribution, advertising, and consumption have been minimized in the social history of health by the environmental and regulatory controls administered by public health agencies.

Figure 4-1

As applied to the Health Field Concept, behavior or lifestyle has direct (*arrow* **a**) and indirect effects on health through the influence of people's behavior on their personal or community environment or their exposure to environmental hazards (*arrow* **b**) and on the development and use of health services (*arrow* **c**).

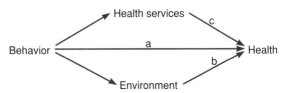

The risks more often accumulate in smaller doses. Chemicals and less lethal or virulent substances (for example, high-fat food) or actions (for example, tanning) have cumulative effects that are nearly imperceptible until they reveal themselves in chronic conditions. These may be obesity, elevated blood pressure or serum cholesterol levels, skin wrinkling, reduced lung function or physical conditioning, drug dependency, lead poisoning, or the diseases themselves (heart disease, cancer, emphysema, atherosclerosis, stroke). Sometimes the first notice of a problem that has been developing for years is sudden death, as with a heart attack or stroke.

Chapter 2 referred to direct behavioral risks and benefits to health as part of the natural cycle of health (see figure 2-2 p. 38). In this cycle, self-protective behavior is a response to prior adaptive experience and environmental influence. The direct ways that behavior influences health, then, involve preventive behavior, health-enhancing behavior, and self-care behavior, including actions to improve or maintain diet and physical fitness.

In the social history of health, behavior has additional *indirect* influence on health through social norms, culture, organization, and environment (see figure 2-3 p. 39). The organizational and environmental routes to health exert additional influences on health, but they, too, relate to behavior. They usually require social action (collective behavior) and planning at a community level.

Figure 2-3 illustrated the relative importance of behavior among the four factors in the health field concept. Besides the direct influence of behavior on health, much of the influence of environment and organization of health services depends on human behavior. Behavior can influence health indirectly through the environment (arrow *b* in figure 4-1) to the degree that people will plan individual or community actions to bring about changes in the environment. Examples of behavioral influences on health through environment include:

• participating in efforts to control toxic waste disposal,
• organizing a lead paint removal program in the neighborhood,
• voting on referenda or for elected officials in support of community water fluoridation,
• advocating drunk-driving laws or other automobile safety provisions,
• writing letters to the editor on food and drug labeling,
• signing a petition on air and water pollution controls, and
• boycotting stores that sell cigarettes to minors.

Behavior can also influence health indirectly through health services (arrow *c* in figure 4-1). This can happen in at least three ways. Individuals, groups, or organizations can

• create and distribute services through action in the legislative and health planning process,
• use available services in a timely and appropriate way, and
• follow the medical or preventive regimens prescribed by their health service providers.

COMMUNITY OR POPULATION HEALTH EDUCATION

Community and population health education seek to elicit, facilitate, and maintain positive health practices in large numbers of people. "Elicit, facilitate, and maintain" refer to the processes of change supported by increasing the understanding, skills, and support people need for voluntary ac-

Figure 4-2

School health education has been a compulsory element in many primary and secondary schools in the past, but many schools now depend on the motivation of teachers in other subject areas and on administrators to achieve comprehensive school health education. (*Source:* PhotoDisc, Inc.)

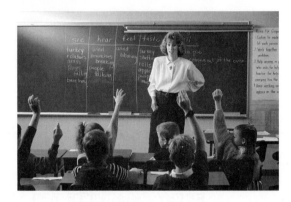

tions conducive to their health. They reflect the efforts of health education to affect factors that predispose, enable, or reinforce behavior related to health. Health education addresses current behavior such as preventive actions, appropriate use of health services, health supervision of children, and adherence to appropriate medical and nutritional regimens. It also must deal with the development in children and youth of a foundation for future health. Within their families and with peers at school, children form predispositions—knowledge, attitudes, and values—that can prevent or promote many of the health problems of later adult life (figure 4-2). Good planning assures that programs combine these various channels of influence appropriately to support voluntary patterns of behavior conducive to health.

Components of Health Education

Community or population health education systematically applies theories and methods from the social and behavioral sciences, epidemiology, ecology, administrative science, and communications. Health education assumes that beneficial

· · · · · · · · · · · · · · · · · ·

Figure 4-3

Mass media health education on smoking has been employed successfully in many countries, states, provinces, and communities to offset some of the influences of mass media advertising by the tobacco industry. (*Source:* Courtesy Department of Training and Health Education, Ministry of Health, Republic of Singapore.)

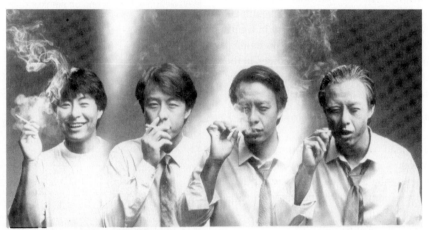

EVERY CIGARETTE YOU SMOKE SHORTENS YOUR LIFE BY 6 MINUTES.

Smoking, far from being 'glamorous', makes you old before your time.
One cigarette cuts 6 minutes off your life.
20 a day for a year cuts one month off your life.
And as for 20 a day for 10 years, well ... you could be headed for an early grave.
There is something you can do.

Stop smoking now before it's too late.

TOWARDS A NATION OF NON-SMOKERS

health behavior will result from a combination of planned, consistent, integrated learning opportunities. This assumption rests on scientific evaluations of health education programs in schools, at worksites, in medical settings, and through the mass media. It also rests on indirect evidence borrowed from experiences outside the fields of health and education. Community development, agricultural extension, social work, marketing, and other enterprises in human services and behavior change have contributed to the understanding of planned change at the community level and in other populations.

Planned experiences to influence voluntary changes in behavior, as distinct from *incidental* learning experiences, link the educational approach to community and population health. We also distinguish health education from other change strategies that may be excessively permissive, legal, or coercive. Behavioral changes resulting from education are by definition voluntary and freely adopted by people, with their knowledge of alternatives and probable consequences. Some behavioral change strategies may have unethical components. Behavior modification techniques, for example, qualify as health education only when people freely request them to achieve a specific behavioral result, such as controlling eating or smoking habits, that they desire. Principles of community health education **planning** call for the participation of consumers, patients, or citizens in the planning process.

Mass media qualify as educational channels for community or population health (figure 4-3) up to the point that commercial or political interests control the media strictly for profit or propaganda. The regulation of advertisers and the media may be necessary as a more coercive, economic, or legal strategy to protect consumers from, for example, deceptive advertising claims concerning the health value of food products. Such was the case when communities took action to restrict the advertising of certain foods and toys on Saturday morning television programs directed at young children. Several countries restrict the advertising of tobacco and alcohol in the mass media. Third World nations took action to restrict the marketing of powdered milk formula for bottle-feeding of babies because it was leading the public to use unsanitary water and bottles in place of breast-feeding.

People may not truly have the resources or support necessary to make independent decisions and to take voluntary actions when some of the determinants of health are factors beyond their control. Whether they were born in a democratic country to affluent and loving parents will set some limits on their ability and will to act independently or to control the determinants of their health.

Such considerations set limits on how much health education alone can achieve health objectives without placing undue responsibility for change on people who are relatively powerless to make such change. This excessive reliance on health education has been referred to as **"victim blaming."** Combining health education with policy and regulatory actions that empower the relatively powerless and restrain the more powerful who might exploit them, overcomes this risk of victim blaming.

Health education will be necessary even when the changes in health risks require regulatory or environmental controls on behavior. For example, health education in a democratic society must precede such controls as drunk driving or seat belt enforcement (figure 4-4) to gain the public understanding and support required to pass legislation. It also helps to gain their cooperation in abiding by the new regulations. Community health promotion, then, is the combination of health education with related organizational, environmental, and economic supports to foster behavior conducive to health. Health promotion will be the subject of chapter 12.

······················

Figure 4-4

The alternative to public health education to achieve some health objectives is legislation and law enforcement. However, these require education of the electorate to pass laws and education of the public to achieve compliance with the laws. Seat belt laws have worked best where the mass media have raised public awareness of police enforcing the laws. (*Source:* U.S. Department of Transportation.)

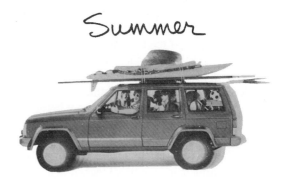

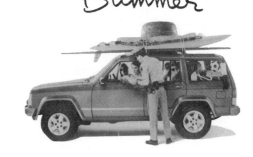

This summer, seatbelt laws are being enforced. So buckle up. Or you might break more than the law. And that would be the biggest bummer of all.

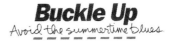

Diagnostic Stage of Educational Planning for Community or Population Health*

A community health or population health plan begins ideally with an analysis of social problems or quality-of-life concerns. It then assesses the incidence, prevalence, and cause of the health problems associated with the social problem in a given population (figure 4-5). The first step, then, is a **social diagnosis** of the *ultimate* community concerns or outcomes (figure 4-5, *bottom*) rather than with immediate input (figure 4-5, *top*). Step 2 is an **epidemiological diagnosis.** Step 3 is a behavioral analysis of the priority health problem to determine specific behaviors causing it. For each behavior implicated in the cause of each health problem, a further analysis of the factors influencing the behavior is needed in step 4 before selecting educational methods. Health education based more on favorite techniques than on systematic analysis of behavior and of the learning problems influencing the behavior will tend to be inefficient if not ineffective. Indeed, the best selection of appropriate behavioral objectives and adequate methods and materials that make up an educational intervention (step 5) depends on the accuracy of the preceding steps in problem diagnosis. Political and legislative decisions often determine some of the priorities and direction of community health programs. Local health planners then develop, from the best epidemiological evidence available, a sound and rational basis for setting the broader objectives of health programs before planning the health education components of the program.

*Footnote: Based on Green, L. W. 1974. Toward cost-benefit evaluations of health education: some concepts, methods, and examples. *Health Educ Q* 2 (Suppl 1):34. The framework described here is referred to as PRECEDE (predisposing, reinforcing, and enabling constructs in educational diagnosis and evaluation). For the latest version of the fuller model combining health education and health promotion, see Green, L. W., and M. W. Kreuter. 1999. *Health promotion planning: an educational and ecological approach.* 3d ed. Mountain View, CA: Mayfield.

Social Diagnosis The ideal starting point in planning would be an assessment of the social concerns of the community or population. Starting with social or quality-of-life concerns rather than health problems ensures that the health planners appreciate the broader context of issues paramount in the community. This step requires an understanding of the subjective concerns and values of the community and objective data on social indicators such as unemployment, housing problems, teenage pregnancy, violence, and poverty.

Consideration of varying community perceptions should take place early in program development. Health programs are not likely to be successful without community support and participation in the planning process.

Epidemiological Diagnosis The social concern or quality-of-life issue in the community or population can be analyzed and redefined as a health problem. This becomes the ultimate target or an overall program goal for a community health or population health program. The sponsoring agency should use the most recent available demographic, vital, and sociocultural statistics to define the characteristics of the subpopulations experiencing the health problem. Planners can review the problem from the perspective of the experience of related agencies with the problem and a review of previously published reports. They can gain perspective on the experience of the community with the health problem by reviewing similar data from other cities, states, or regions. They need to pay particular attention to the rates in subpopulations (age, sex, race, and income groups) within the community or population relative to other communities or in national, state, or provincial rates.

Citizens or lay participants in the planning process at this stage can help identify population subgroups within the community, such as adolescent mothers and preschool youth, who may have special problems and needs. Information on these subpopulations can include geographical distribution; occupational, economic, and educational

· · · · · · · · · · · · · · · · · ·
Figure 4-5

The Precede-Proceed Model for health education planning and evaluation begins at the end of the causal chain (bottom left) with the social diagnosis. Subsequent steps correspond to the causal relationships among factors linking health education to ultimate health and social goals. (*Source:* Adapted from Green LW: Prevention and health education. In Wallace RB, editor: *Public health and preventive medicine,* ed 14, Norwalk, Conn, 1998, Appleton-Century-Crofts.)

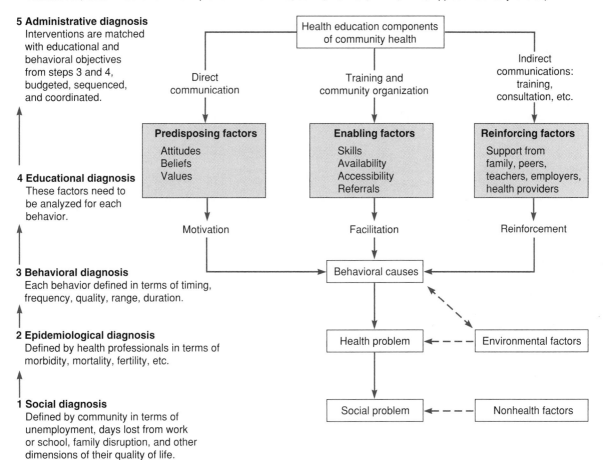

5 Administrative diagnosis
Interventions are matched with educational and behavioral objectives from steps 3 and 4, budgeted, sequenced, and coordinated.

4 Educational diagnosis
These factors need to be analyzed for each behavior.

3 Behavioral diagnosis
Each behavior defined in terms of timing, frequency, quality, range, duration.

2 Epidemiological diagnosis
Defined by health professionals in terms of morbidity, mortality, fertility, etc.

1 Social diagnosis
Defined by community in terms of unemployment, days lost from work or school, family disruption, and other dimensions of their quality of life.

Health education components of community health

Direct communication

Training and community organization

Indirect communications: training, consultation, etc.

Predisposing factors
Attitudes
Beliefs
Values

Enabling factors
Skills
Availability
Accessibility
Referrals

Reinforcing factors
Support from family, peers, teachers, employers, health providers

Motivation

Facilitation

Reinforcement

Behavioral causes

Health problem ← – – – Environmental factors

Social problem ← – – – Nonhealth factors

status; age and sex composition; ethnicity; health indicators, including age-specific morbidity; and service utilization patterns (see box, p. 99).

Behavioral Diagnosis   The definition of the health problem, the program goal, and the high-risk subpopulations should lead to the task of specifying behavioral problems or barriers to the community solution of the health problem (figure 4-6). The following guidelines should be considered in the **behavioral diagnosis:**

• The behaviors presumably contributing to the health problem should be specified as concretely as possible. An inventory of as many possible behavioral causes as one can imagine should be made.

....

Figure 4-6

The U.S. Centers for Disease Control and Prevention provide technical assistance to communities to apply an adaptation of the Precede model, called PATCH (Planned Approach to Community Health). PATCH programs have been developed also in Australia and Canada. (*Source:* Center for Chronic Disease Prevention and Health Promotion, Centers for Disease Control and Prevention, U.S. Department of Health and Human Services.)

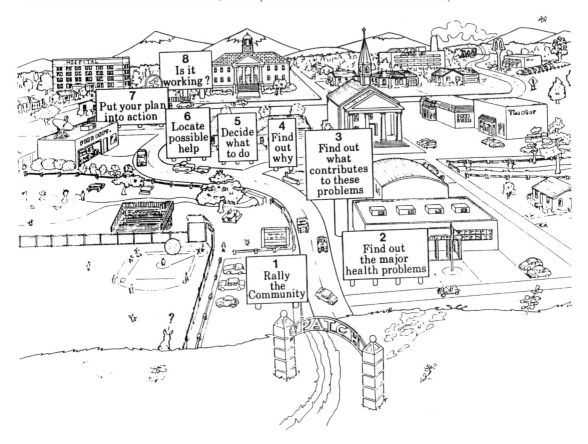

- The nonbehavioral factors (environmental, human biology, and technological factors) contributing to the problem should be identified as determinants for which strategies other than health education must be developed.
- There should be a review of research evidence that the behaviors identified as possible causes are amenable to change through educational interventions and that such change will improve the health problem in question.
- For each health problem, one or more of the relevant dimensions of health behavior should

be identified, as shown in the example in the box titled "Dimensions of Health Behavior."
- An assessment should lead to the selection of specific behaviors that will be the target of the educational interventions. Rarely, if ever, does an agency have the resources necessary to influence all the behaviors contributing to a health problem. An initial selection of some of the behaviors should be made. The selection often must be influenced by policies governing required services of the agency. Priorities might also consider legal and economic factors affecting

Epidemiological Diagnosis Example

Consider an example[*] of health statistics to be reviewed in the epidemiological diagnosis of a community. They include the following rates of maternal and child health in a rural area that is populated mainly by a low-income minority group:

A community maternal death rate of 65.5 per 100,000 births compared to a rate of 18.4 for the state

A community infant death rate of 34.5 per 1,000 compared to a rate of 21.0 for the state

A community fetal death ratio of 24.9 despite an overall decline in the state to 14.6

The health problems that might be identified from these statistics are a high incidence of prematurity, low infant birth weights, a pattern of fetal distress and respiratory distress at delivery, and observed failure of infants to thrive. A visiting nurse service also might report data such as the prevalence of anemia and the incidence of gastrointestinal infections and respiratory diseases.

At this stage difficult decisions must be made to place greater priority on some problems than on others. Patients, consumers, parents, and various health service providers within the community may perceive the problems of mothers and children differently than the sponsoring health agency. The two groups may differ also in ranking the priority of urgency of various health problems. How would you reconcile these competing priorities and perspectives?

[*]Adapted from Green, L. W., S. Deeds, V. L. Wang, R. Windsor, A. Bennet. 1978. Guidelines for health education in maternal and child health. *Int J Health Educ Suppl* 21:1. The maternal and child health examples refer to chapter 5, but the same approach to health education planning can be applied to the problems described in subsequent chapters. A fuller application of the Precede-Proceed Model for community diagnosis and planning is illustrated in chapter 12 in relation to drug misuse. For software demonstrating application of the Precede-Proceed Model to cancer screening and a bibliography of 600 published applications of this model, see Gold, R., L. W. Green, M. W. Kreuter. 1997. EMPOWER, enabling methods of planning and organizing within everyone's reach. Boston: Jones & Bartlett Publishers.

Dimensions of Health Behavior

Behavioral dimension	Example
Time or promptness of the behavior	Prenatal care begins with the first trimester of pregnancy
Frequency of the behavior	Prenatal visits are every sixth week in the second trimester
Quality of the behavior	Foods with low fat content are selected over those high in fat
Range of health behaviors	Prenatal care is obtained, diet control regimen followed, and smoking stopped
Persistence or follow-through with health behavior	All booster shots are obtained following initial immunization or medical care is continued through prenatal, delivery, and postnatal periods

the desired behaviors, agency resources and expertise available, political viability of the educational interventions, the possibility of continued funding, and the probability of quick program success. The reasons for selecting specific behaviors as the priority focus of the educational interventions should be justified.

The two most important objective criteria for selection of priority behavioral targets for health education are (1) the evidence that the behavioral change will make a difference in the reduction of the health problem and (2) the evidence that the behavior is amenable to voluntary change.

Behavioral Diagnosis Example

The behavioral diagnosis identifies factors influencing the health problem and suggests the actions people can take to reduce the problem.

Examples of nonbehavioral factors influencing the previously defined health problems include the following:

Genetic factors

Economic base

Occupation

Environmental isolation

Examples of behavioral remedies of the previously defined health problems include the following:

- Consumption of proper nutritional diet
- Acceptance of medical supervision at each stage from prenatal to postnatal year for mother and child
- Postponement of pregnancy to age 18 and avoidance after medical complications
- Spacing of pregnancies over 24 to 30 months
- Reduction in total number of pregnancies
- Avoidance of physical and emotional stress during pregnancy
- Avoidance of fetal insult (reduction in smoking and in use of alcohol, aspirin, and other drugs)

Educational Diagnosis Example

By assessing the predisposing, enabling, and reinforcing factors influencing the health behaviors in the Behavioral Diagnosis Example box, you can identify the most useful targets on which to concentrate health education. By consulting with the women themselves, you could adapt the health advice to fit the circumstances of these women more appropriately. Examples of the factors identified in an educational diagnosis of maternal and child health follow:

Predisposing factors: Attitude toward pregnancy as a way of fulfilling needs other than reproduction; belief that pregnancy and childbearing are the only acceptable roles for women.

Enabling factors: Scarcity and cost of recommended foods; inaccessibility of emergency care; transportation problems in getting to clinics for prenatal and well-child care; clinic hours that preclude attendance by working women.

Reinforcing factors: Husbands do not support contraceptive behavior; loss of income from inability to work in fields may be an incentive for family planning for some, but exemption from work may reward pregnancy for others; crowded clinic and waiting time does not reward clinic attendance.

How would you use this information?

Educational Diagnosis The behaviors selected can be subjected to further analysis for assessment of their causes. The following sets of factors should be considered as *causes* of each behavior:

- **Predisposing factors:** Knowledge, attitudes, beliefs, and values that motivate people to take appropriate health actions.
- **Enabling factors:** Skills and the accessibility of resources that make it possible for a motivated person to take action.
- **Reinforcing factors:** The attitudes and climate of support from providers of services, families, and community groups that reinforce the health behavior of an individual who is motivated and able to adopt the behavior but who will discontinue the behavior if it is not rewarded.

Planners should consult representatives of the various segments within the agency and community potentially affected by the program. Failure to assess some of these factors and to develop a community health education program addressed to all three sets would seriously limit the impact of the program. Figure 4-5 summarizes the relationships among the factors considered in these procedures.

Administrative Diagnosis Selecting the health education methods for a community health program follows almost automatically from a thorough identification and ranking of predisposing, enabling, and reinforcing factors influencing the health behaviors. Administrative diagnosis then includes the assessment of available resources to support needed methods. The coordination and budgeting of these methods into a timetable that corresponds to the community health program is the next step. Both require constructive participation by staff, other organizations, and area residents. By including other organizations and community members in the planning, one obtains their personal commitment to realizing program success. Most importantly, their participation enables program planners to incorporate the interests, perspectives, and values of various stakeholders into the educational activities of the program. The principle of participation applies usually to representatives of related agencies, institutions, and organizations in the community, to the agency staff who will implement the program activities, and to community residents in the target population.

Organizations in the community may already be channeling funds and efforts into areas related to the proposed educational program. Other resources may have been active in related areas in previous years. It is important to survey these activities and organizations to avoid overlap and to integrate services.

The program plan depends on resources identified through survey information obtained from organizations and agencies at national, state or provincial, and local levels. Some examples of resources include citizens' groups, industry, labor organizations, religious groups, colleges, advertising agencies, drama groups, and pharmacies; local facilities (e.g., libraries, health centers, hospitals, training centers, town halls, gathering places); personnel (e.g., volunteers, agency staff, social workers); communications resources (e.g., numbers of telephones and use of radios, billboards, local television and radio stations, newspapers, newsletters, organization bulletins, Internet and World Wide Web sites); and funding sources available for the educational program through the health service agency itself and related organizations. This identification and assessment of available resources should lead to the further refinement of objectives, strategies, and methods. Advocacy for the reallocation of resources or the changes in policy required to support the program may be necessary at this stage of the planning process.

PLANNING FOR THE DELIVERY OF COMMUNITY HEALTH EDUCATION

The planning steps outlined in this section are not entirely sequential. They begin during the preceding diagnostic stages and continue through the organizational, implementation, and evaluation stages.

Priority Target Populations for Specific Educational Components

A first task of planning the delivery of a program is to identify the people at risk, or those most affected by the health problem. They are the target for and the beneficiaries of most of the educational interventions, and thus constitute the primary target group that the planners should consult. Education must also be directed toward groups not affected by the health problem but in a direct position to influence those who are. These "gatekeepers" and social reinforcers (parents, spouses, teachers, peers, employers, and "opinion leaders") are often an intermediate or additional target population for educational programs.

The primary target group will receive direct communication designed to influence their predisposition to accept the recommended health practices. One intermediate target group for community organization efforts would be directors of other agencies who control resources that would enable or facilitate the health behavior. Another intermediate target group would receive training, consultation, or supervision in reinforcing the recommended health behavior. In relation to the predisposing factors, the planners need to describe the primary target population by their geographical, occupational, economic, educational, age, sex, and ethnicity distributions. The characteristics that provide the basic analysis for the specification of community health programs are also the basis for the development of educational interventions. Planners should consult representative persons from the described population and cooperating agencies in the further development of the educational plans. To develop the enabling factors, planners should identify intermediate target groups including controllers of needed resources for the health behavior. For the reinforcing

ISSUES AND CONTROVERSIES
Education versus Environment

Health education has been displaced in the policy arena by health promotion and more recently population health. These new variations on the health education theme seek to tackle the same problems of social and behavioral determinants of health but they hope to do so by means of environmental changes and socioeconomic changes through policies, organization, and regulation. Health education was seen at some point in the 1970s by policymakers as a method that tended to place all the responsibility for change on the victims of health problems. Still, the policies, regulations, and organizational changes usually depend on a public that is aware, concerned, and informed. An informed electorate to support policy and organizational changes requires health education. Public cooperation with new regulations of their behavior or environment depends on an enlightened public in a democratic society. How do you view the continuum from strategies that depend strictly on bottom-up individual change to strategies that depend strictly on top-down policy and organizational changes that regulate the environment? Under what circumstances are you willing to have government make decisions for you about health matters? Are you willing to have government influence your behavior with respect to diet, smoking in public places, alcohol consumption, physical activity, or immunizations?

factors, they need to work with those who can reinforce the behavior as transmitters of information (see figure 4-7).

Behavioral Objectives

The objectives for behavior change derive from the findings of the behavioral and educational diagnoses. The proper statement of the objectives should lend purpose to the program plan and direction to its implementation. The test of objectives is their ability to communicate expected results. Lucidity and precision in their formulation should accomplish several things. First, these objectives should provide limits to expenditure of time and effort on specific educational interventions. Second, they should identify criteria for measurement of program achievement. Third, they should lead to task analyses for selection, training, and supervision of staff. Finally, these objectives, like others, should provide orientation to cooperating agencies and to the general community.

Time spent on the formulation of objectives in educational planning is especially important because education appears to be more abstract and difficult to define or measure than some of the other activities of community health programs.

Objectives should be expressed as intended outcomes. They may apply to providers and to the organization or system and to the consumers. Each objective should answer the question, *Who* is expected to achieve or become *how much* of *what* by *when, where,* under what *conditions?*

- Who—target groups or individuals expected to change
- How much—the extent of the condition to be obtained
- What—the action, change in behavior, or health practice to be obtained
- When—the time in which the desired condition is to be obtained
- Where—the place in which change will be observed, usually implied within the specification of who.

The desired behaviors (what) should describe what the participants will do or not do as a result of the program that they could not or did not do (as much) before the program. The conditions of the action should be stated in the following way:

- Who—some logical portion (percentage) of the target group

· · · · · · · · · · · · · · · · · ·
Figure 4-7

Health education in villages of Afghanistan requires meeting first with the elders to gain their acceptance and support in approaching others who look up to them. Public health educators plan this step into the assessment of resources for their program. (*Source:* World Health Organization photo.)

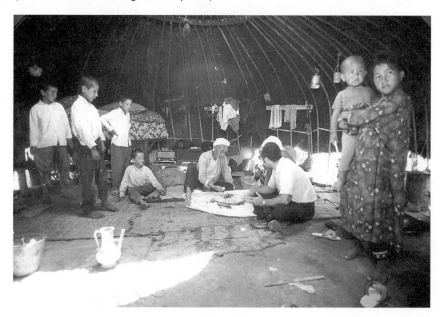

- How much or to what extent— an amount of change that will depend on available resources
- Where—geographical, political, or institutional boundaries derived in part from the original description of the health problem
- When, or how soon, or within what time period— determined by the urgency of the health problem in the community and by the rate of change that can be expected from the amount and type of effort devoted to the program

In most community health or population-based programs, "how much" refers to the number of people or percentage of the population. For individuals "how much" would refer to the level of accomplishment (e.g., monthly prenatal visits). Planners should word their objectives in such a way as to imply their assessment criteria. They should state them in concrete terms with at least an implied, if not stated, scale of measurement that can be used to evaluate progress and achievement of the objective.

Educational and Administrative Objectives

Educational and administrative objectives become the intermediate or subobjectives to the behavioral objectives (figure 4-8). A program must achieve these objectives before it can achieve a change or development in behavior. These intermediate changes emerged from the analysis of the predisposing, enabling, and reinforcing factors in the educational and administrative diagnoses. To avoid a shotgun approach to communications, the planners should consider the knowledge, attitudes, skills, organization, and training required for people to move toward stated objectives. The various types of educational objectives directed at these causes of behavior can be seen at the top of figure 4-8.

Figure 4-8

Types of educational and administrative objectives and their relationship to behavioral objectives and health status objectives of community health programs.

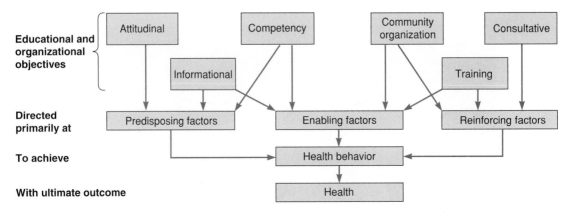

Example of Setting Objectives

The stated program goal for the earlier example (p. 99)—to raise the survival rate of mothers, infants, and children through raising the quality of prenatal care and promoting the optimum growth and development of children—suggests the following health objectives for the community health program:

> To reduce maternal mortality within counties A and B by 10 percent within the first two years and by an additional 15 percent the next three years, continuing until the state average rate is reached

To reduce infant mortality to the state average within 10 years

Behavioral objectives then could take the following form:

In the county, 900 women under 40 who are at risk of problem pregnancy will obtain health checkups the first year of the program

In this group, 80 percent of pregnancies will be detected within the first trimester

Of the pregnant women, 90 percent will obtain monthly prenatal

care for the remainder of their pregnancy

In the first behavioral objective, the following apply:

Who—Women in the county who are under 40 and have selected characteristics (e.g., age, socioeconomic status) associated with high-risk pregnancies

How much—900 women

What—Obtaining health checkups

When—During the first year of the program

Assessment of Barriers and Facilitators to Implementation

Implementing the educational plan requires an assessment of factors that may impede carrying out program activities. At the same time, some characteristics of the community may facilitate program success. The barriers and supports to the program should be assessed.

Barriers to the achievement of educational objectives can assume several forms. Some examples of *social, psychological,* and *cultural* barriers include citizen and staff bias, prejudice, misunderstanding, taboos, unfavorable past experiences, values, norms, social relationships, official disapproval, and rumors. *Communication* obstacles include illiteracy and local vernacular. *Economic*

· · · · · · · · · · · · · · · · · · ·
Figure 4-9

A major barrier to health education and other aspects of population health, especially in rural and remote areas, is the inaccessibility or inconvenience of standing facilities. To overcome this barrier, many health departments have purchased and equipped mobile vans to take services and health education to people where they live or work and to children in schools and recreational areas. (*Source:* Photo by L. Green.)

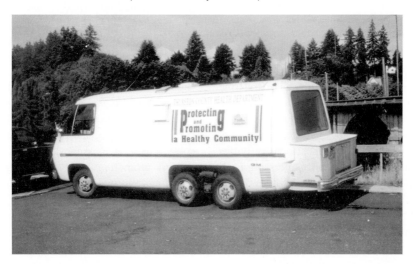

and *physical* barriers include low income and inability to pay for prescribed drugs or the means of transportation to medical services and long distances over difficult terrain to medical or health education facilities (figure 4-9). *Legal* and *administrative* barriers include residence requirements to be eligible for services, legal requirements that the program operate within defined geographical boundaries, and policies or regulations that restrict program implementation.

Facilitators to the achievement of program objectives go beyond the mere absence of barriers. The predispositions of area residents favorable to the implementation of the program may include past and favorable experience with similar programs and high credibility of the program sponsoring agency. Other capabilities facilitating the program might be high education levels of consumers, dynamic and supportive local leaders and organizations, skilled staff with experience, open channels of communication with consumers, and support from other agencies. In addition, some geographical and physical enabling factors may

serve as program assets (e.g., population distribution and density, access to facilities).

The introduction of new or unfamiliar schemes for promoting awareness and health behavior has its greatest opportunity for success when integrated into existing systems of knowledge transfer and influence within the community. Schools, local media, clubs, churches, neighborhoods, and ethnic associations are the most effective channels of communication. Also, planners should identify barriers in additional objectives that indicate how much and when the program will surmount each of the barriers.

THE IMPLEMENTATION STAGE

Implementing the educational components of the community health program follows the development and refinement of the planning operations. At this stage, if involvement of concerned persons has been obtained and detailed written plans are available to staff, volunteers, and cooperating agencies, all will be in agreement over the program's aims and general strategies. One also assumes they are committed to their roles in the educational efforts. To initiate the program will require more specific logistical planning and resource identification; equipment and materials assembly; design of procedures; and training and orientation of staff, volunteers, and cooperating agencies.

Priorities for Implementation

Resources always seem scarce in relation to the great needs in community health. The first line item to be cut when budgets are reduced is often the health education component. To ensure the most economical use of the resources available, priorities among alternative educational activities must be considered. Related to this pressing need for efficiency is the need for effectiveness. This requires the selection of the most effective combination of educational interventions and activities available. The first step is to determine which procedures are feasible, given limited staff, services, money, and time, and then to combine these resources to achieve the best support of program objectives.

To set priorities, obtain opinions and contributions from community members on priorities for educational services. Delineate the areas that will provide the greatest benefits to the most recipients. Phase program activities with a gradual beginning. Limit the number and range of activities, with initial emphasis on areas most amenable to quick and early success and activities requiring minimum staff training. Review the most recent scientific literature on the evaluation of health education methods relevant to the local program to guide these decisions on priorities.

Develop a contingency plan to aid program survival in the event of future reduction of resources. Beyond these general principles, the selection of educational efforts in strategic patterns or combinations depends on the particular circumstances of each site, the particular objectives, and the expectations for sustaining or institutionalizing the program.

Development of Educational Methods and Media

Having set priorities and selected strategies, the program manager can proceed to develop and schedule the use of educational tools, tactics, and methods. Methods, media, and materials can be pretested in the intended audience to determine their acceptability to the particular group and their convenience (time demands, personnel requirements, situational concerns—light, sound). They should also be selected on the basis of their efficiency (fixed costs, continuing costs, space and maintenance requirements, staff and time needs to convey a message), and presumed effectiveness (in communicating messages, arousing attention and interest, promoting interaction, using suitable repetition and message retention techniques, encouraging desired attitudes and adoption of practices).

Interpersonal or two-way communication and demonstration processes provide the most favorable environment for learning, and usually have greater long-term behavioral effects (figure 4-10). One-way communication, such as use of pamphlets, may be appropriate in the early phases of a program or when other methods with more lasting outcomes are not feasible and when the audience is literate. A single educational intervention, however, cannot be relied on to have a significant, lasting impact on an individual's health behavior. Only through repeated educational reinforcement by health staff, aides, community leaders, friends, and family, can health education affect human behavior in the context of today's complex community health problems.

Orientation and Training

Some health workers and allied personnel may be uninformed about methods of health education, while others may feel that educational efforts are too slow, complex, and of dubious efficacy. Training can provide people time to discuss their concerns and develop their competence and confidence. Health education training should be differentiated from technical training related to

....

Figure 4-10

Interpersonal communication with demonstration and opportunities for personal questions to be answered and for participants to practice skills are the ingredients of the most effective health education programs. (*Source:* UNICEF photo by Wolf.)

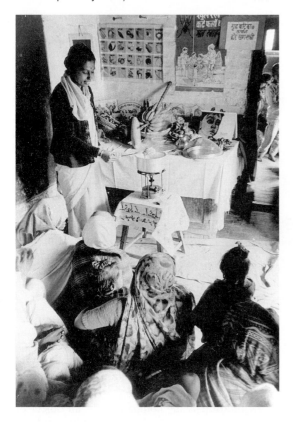

health and medical content. Health education training underscores the attitudinal and behavioral factors essential to long-term health maintenance, the cultural perceptions of the target population, and the necessity of well-planned and properly sustained action. These help achieve the health behavior changes required by the objectives of the community health program.

Staff training may include orientation aimed at sensitizing the staff members to their educational function and to the general objectives of the educa-

tion program. It may also include preparation in recognizing educational opportunities; communication skills; reinforcement techniques, training priorities for those staff members in contact with consumers; and continuing education (figure 4-11).

Volunteers are not free of cost. Proper use of volunteers requires continuous, careful supervision and training. These should be budgeted in the educational plan. A thorough plan for training volunteers might include a content designed to foster their interest in health education and in the program's need for their insight into the attitudes, reactions, and daily lives of the target population. It can also include training in communications skills and teamwork roles and limits of volunteers' responsibility and authority.

Data Collection and Records

Health education planning and evaluation use statistics and financial accounts. These records provide for continuous monitoring of program impact; for supervision, training, and staff development; and for evaluation of program process and outcome. Information collection requiring additional paperwork must always be weighed against other demands for time. Small additions and checklists may be integrated into existing records with little effort and with staff acceptance. For more intensive narrative reporting and recording, special efforts during limited time periods may be acceptable and provide sufficient data without generating staff resistance and unmanageable amounts of paperwork. The educational plan should clearly identify the use and purpose of new forms and records.

Scheduling Implementation

Timing is crucial to the success of the educational plan of action. It requires an analysis of when, where, and who is responsible for implementation. This analysis will provide the starting and completion date required for each activity in relation to the total program. Consideration of the training required, production schedules for material, and staff loads guides the development of timetables.

· · · · · · · · · · · · · · · · · · · ·

Figure 4-11

Intersectoral cooperation includes cooperation among staff in the education sector, the health sector, and the law enforcement sector. Police officers, for example, volunteer time for safety and substance abuse education programs in schools. (*Source:* Lincoln-Lancaster County Health Department, Lincoln, Nebraska.)

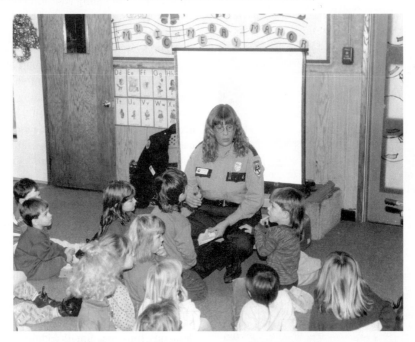

A task analysis and time sequence of activities should integrate the educational implementation with the total program plan. Planners should consider external events when scheduling to avoid conflict with community happenings, school openings, holidays, and related community schedules. The implementing stage is a logical progression from the previous stages of diagnosis, planning, and organizing.

THE EVALUATING STAGES

Good records and documentation, supervisor reports on quality control, and other process evaluation can provide immediate feedback on whether things are working satisfactorily. Peer review among health professionals helps to maintain quality control, but they must base it on standards and documentation of practice. Feedback on patients'

or clients' use and satisfaction should provide data for program adjustment and replanning. Community surveillance will aid in continuous health education planning and evaluation.

Evaluation is the comparison of an object of interest against a standard of acceptability. It is, at the very least, an assessment of the worth of a program, a method, or some other object of interest. It may provide an estimate of the degree to which spent resources result in specified activity and the degree to which performed activities attain goals. The determination of whether the program has met its goals is based on criteria indicated by precise statements of objectives along with subjective impressions and reporting. Evaluation can suggest which of several alternative educational strategies is the most efficient and which steps have an effect on the behavior specified. Evaluation provides accountability for time spent. Results usually offer a sense of accomplishment to staff and consumers or sponsors of the program.

Formative and Process Evaluation

Formative evaluation is the earliest phase of **process evaluation.** Formative evaluation refers to preliminary assessments of the appropriateness of materials and procedures before beginning the program. Process evaluation refers to continuous observation and checking to see whether the program activities are taking place with the quality and at the time and rate necessary to achieve the stated objective. Sources of data for formative evaluation usually include pretesting of materials for their readability and acceptability to the target audience. Process evaluation requires ongoing sources of data that often include budget reports on monthly expenditures in specific categories where rate of expenditures would indicate amount of program activity relevant to achievement of objectives.

Professional consensus usually provides the source of the standards of acceptability in formative and process evaluation. The data for process evaluation often come from routine records kept on encounters with consumers, patients, or clients. These might include, for example, clinic attendance records tabulated weekly or monthly for total numbers of patients. Staff can tabulate systematic samples of the records in more detail to estimate progress on such variables as broken appointment rates, sources of referral, and trimester of first visit for pregnant women. Another type of data available for process evaluation is administrative records. Administrators can tabulate personnel records to assess the number of home visits attempted, the number completed, the number of group sessions conducted, and the time allotted for various educational functions.

Supervisors should conduct periodic reviews of personnel to review staff performance. Time should be set aside on the agenda of staff and community meetings for consideration of strengths, weaknesses, and adaptation of ongoing programs. There should be a plan for charting records over time or comparing progress statistics with other programs or standards.

Outcome Evaluation

Outcome evaluation, sometimes referred to as **summative evaluation,** assesses the achievement of objectives by measurement of expected outcomes. The more precisely the planners stated the objectives, the more meaningful the evaluation. Planners or evaluators should obtain baseline information on a period prior to the program's inception for comparison with similarly gathered data during the program or following the program.

Impact or outcome evaluation asks the following questions: What are the measurable results of program efforts in the promotion of health behavior? Has there been any change in the attitudes of the clients toward recommended actions or change in their ability to carry out the recommended action, or change in the resources and social support for such actions in the community?

The evaluation of a specific educational component (e.g., a pamphlet or a group discussion) should not depend on the comparison of people who receive only that method with people who receive nothing. The comparison should be between a group receiving a comprehensive health education program and another group receiving everything *except* the component to be evaluated. The outcome statistics (knowledge, attitude, and behavioral outcomes) should be better on subgroups exposed to the entire program than for those exposed to everything except for specific methods or materials of interest. If the evaluation finds no significant difference it would suggest ways to reduce costs and increase efficiency by eliminating those methods or procedures.

Evaluators should report on progress or outcomes to the affiliated organizations, agencies, and institutions participating in the program and to the clients and general public. Reports can encourage their continued participation by noting their contribution to, or influence on, the program. Finally, practitioners should seek to publish case histories and reports in professional journals and newsletters for use by other departments, programs, or projects and to contribute to the advancement of professional knowledge, practice, and policies.

U.S. Objectives for the Nation to Enhance Educational and Community-based Programs, by the Year 2000

Objectives target increasing years of healthy life, increasing the high school graduation rate, achieving access to developmentally appropriate preschool programs, increasing quality school health education, increasing health promotion programs at postsecondary institutions, increasing worksite health promotion activities, increasing worksite health promotion for hourly workers, increasing health promotion programs for older adults, increasing family discussion of health issues, establishing community health promotion programs, increasing health promotion programs for racial and ethnic minority groups, increasing patient education and community health promotion programs, increasing partnerships between television networks and community organizations, and increasing the proportion of people who are serviced by a local health department that is effectively carrying out the core functions of public health.

THE HEALTH EDUCATION SPECIALIST

The person assigned the responsibility for the community health education program ideally has training in public health or community health education and experience in a community health agency or institution. Competencies tested for the Certified Health Education Specialist (CHES) include the following:

1. Planning at the community level including epidemiological and sociological research methods, community organization, and health services administration
2. Assessment and adaptation of communications to attitudinal, cultural, economic, and ethnic determinants of health behaviors
3. Educational evaluation within the context of community health (as distinct from formal curriculum evaluation), including biostatistics, demography, and behavioral research methods

When these skills are not available within the staff of a community health agency, consultation for the planning and preparation stages of health education programs may be obtained from other organizations. Continuing education and in-service training are important to maintaining up-to-date knowledge and skills in all community health staff.

SUMMARY

Human behavior accounts for approximately half of the years of an average person's life lost prematurely in Western societies. Behavior develops through learning processes. Programs in health education seek to empower people to take control of their own health and adapt their behavior to protect their health. In addition, health promotion (see chapter 12) can build further supports for health behavior through organizational, economic, and environmental adaptations in the community. The planning and implementation steps outlined in this chapter apply to most of the following chapters.

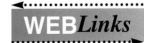

WEB*Links*

http://www.aahperd.org/aahe/aahe.html
Association for the Advancement of Health Education

http://www.emerson.edu/acadepts/cs/healthcom/Resources/HOME.HTM
Health Communication Links

http://www.ihpr.ubc.ca
Institute of Health Promotion Research (includes bibliography of over 600 publications applying the PRECEDE-PROCEED model)

QUESTIONS FOR REVIEW

1. Identify a trend you have noticed in your community or among your friends in health behavior and health concerns. Can you find objective data to support your observations? If not, how would you go about verifying your subjective view of the trend in health behavior?

2. Identify a national or community health campaign or program spanning a number of years. How do you account for the public concern with different health problems at different times? What were the major features of the health education component of the program? Why have different programs or problems at different times required different health education methods?

3. Among the demographic groups (geographic location, age, sex, etc.) of a population (students, patients, workers, residents), whose quality of life must a health agency try to improve? How would you involve the members of the population in identifying their quality-of-life concerns?

4. What health problems are related to the quality-of-life concerns identified in your population?

5. How would you rate (low, medium, high) each health problem according to (1) its relative importance in affecting the quality-of-life concerns and (2) its potential for change?

6. How would you justify your ratings of health problems as having high priority in terms of their prevalence, incidence, cost, virulence, intensity, or other relevant dimensions?

7. What evidence supports your priorities on health problems in question 5? Refer to the success of other programs or to the availability of medical or other technology to control or reduce the high-priority health problems you have selected.

8. How would you write a program objective for the highest priority health problem, indicating who will show how much of what improvement by when?

9. In relation to the highest priority health problem identified in your program objective in question 8, what specific behaviors in your population might be causally related to the achievement of that objective?

10. How would you rate (low, medium, high) each behavior in your inventory according to its (1) prevalence, (2) epidemiological or causal importance, and (3) changeability?

11. How would you write a behavioral objective for your population (who) showing what percentage (how much) will exhibit the behavior or change the behavior (what) by a given date or amount of time from the beginning of a program (by when)?

12. For one of the high-priority behaviors you selected, what are the predisposing, enabling, and reinforcing factors you can identify?

13. How would you rate each factor believed to cause the health behavior according to each of two criteria: importance and changeability?

14. How would you write educational objectives for the three highest priority determinants of the health behavior: one objective for a predisposing factor, one for an enabling factor, and one for a reinforcing factor?

15. For the population and health problem you have analyzed, what three educational methods would appear to be most appropriate?

16. How would your program affect and be affected by other programs and units within a health agency or educational institution?

17. What interorganizational coordination would be required to achieve the objectives of your program?

READINGS

Gilbert, G. G., and R. G. Sawyer. 1994. *Health education: creating strategies for school and community health.* Boston & London: Jones & Bartlett Publishers.
This textbook on selecting health education methods fills a gap between books on needs assessment and those on evaluation.

Glanz, K., and B. Rimer B. 1995. *Theory at a Glance: A Guide for Health Promotion Practice.* Bethesda: National Cancer Institute, NIH Pub. No. 95–3896, Public Health Service, U.S. Dept. of Health and Human Services.
This monograph summarizing major theories used in health education is free from NCI, Bethesda, MD; call Cancer Information Service at 1-800/4-CANCER.

Green, L. W., and C. J. Frankish. 1994. Theories and principles of health education applied to asthma. *Chest* 106(4, Suppl.): 219S.
Reviews the development of theories of behavior used in patient education and parent education for families with asthma. Also applies these theories to the behavior of physicians and other health care personnel.

Houle, C. O. 1992. *Literature of Adult Education: A Bibliographic Essay.* San Francisco: Jossey-Bass Publishers.
This review of the general literature of adult education includes commentaries on the utility of the Precede-Proceed model to general field of adult education, on pp. 233 and 274–275.

Timmreck, T. C. 1994. *An Introduction to Epidemiology.* Boston: Jones & Bartlett Publishers.
This textbook on epidemiology shows how the Precede-Proceed model applies in the use of epidemiology as a health education planning tool.

BIBLIOGRAPHY

Airhihenbuwa, C. O. 1995. *Healthy culture: decolonization of health and education.* Newbury Park, CA: Sage.

Breckon, D. J., J. R. Harvey, and R. B. Lancaster. 1994. *Community health education: settings, roles, and skills for the 21st century.* 3d ed. Gaithersburg, MD: Aspen Publishers, Inc.

Daniel, M., and L. W. Green. 1995. Application of the Precede-Proceed model in prevention and control of diabetes: a case illustration from an aboriginal community. *Diabetes Spectrum* 8:80.

Danigelis, N. L., N. L. Roberson, J. K. Worden, and B. S. Flynn. Breast screening by African-American women: insights from a household survey and focus groups. *Am J Prev Med* 11:311.

Davis, D. A., M. A. Thomson, A. D. Oxman, and R. B. Haynes. 1995. Changing physician performance: A systematic review of the effect of continuing medical education strategies. *Journal of the American Medical Association* 274:700.

Dignan, M. B, R. Michielutte, H. B. Wells, and J. Bahnson. 1995. The Forsyth County Cervical Cancer Prevention Project—I. Cervical cancer screening for black women. *Health Education Research* 9:411.

Earp, J. A., M. Alpeter, L. Mayne, C. Viadro, and M. L. Omalley. 1995 The North Carolina breast cancer screening program—Foundations and design of a model for reaching older, minority, rural women. *Breast Cancer Research & Treatment* 35(1):7–22.

Farley, C., S. Haddad, and B. Brown. 1996. The effects of a 4-year program promoting bicycle helmet use among children in Quebec. *American Journal of Public Health* 86(1):46–51.

Farthing, M. 1994. Health education needs of a Hutterite Colony. *The Canadian Nurse/L'Infirmiere Canadienne* 90(7):20–26.

Green, L. W., K. Glanz, G. M. Hochbaum, G. Kok, M. W. Kreuter, F. M. Lewis, K. Lorig, D. Morisky, B. Rimer, and I. M. Rosenstock. 1994. Can we build on, or must we replace, the theories and models in health education? *Health Education Research* 9(3):397.

Grueninger, U. J. 1995. Arterial hypertension: lessons from patient education. *Patient Education and Counseling* 26:37.

Grueninger, U. J., F. D. Duffy, and M. G. Goldstein. 1995. Patient education in the medical encounter: How to facilitate learning, behavior change, and coping. In *The Medical Interview: Clinical Care, Education, and Research,* edited by M. Lipkin, Jr., S. M. Putnam, and A. Lazare. Bern, 1995, Mack Lipkin, Jr., MD.

Hiddink, G. J., C. A. Maarssen, J. G. J. A. Hautvast, C. M. J. van Woerkum, C. J. Fieren, and M. A. van't Hof. 1995. Nutrition guidance by primary-care physicians: perceived barriers and low involvement. *European Journal of Clinical Nutrition* 49:842.

Johnson, C. C., C. R. Powers, W. Bao, D. W. Harsha, and G. S. Berenson. 1994. Cardiovascular risk factors of elementary school teachers in a low socio-economic area of a metropolitan city: the Heart Smart Program. *Health Education Research* 9:183–191.

Keintz, M. K., L. Fleisher, and B. K. Rimer. 1994. Reaching mothers of preschool-aged children with a targeted quit smoking intervention. *Journal of Community Health* 19:25–40.

Kloos, H. 1995. Human behavior, health education and schistosomiasis control—A review. *Social Science & Medicine* 40:1497.

Kristal A. R., R. E. Patterson, K. Glanz, J. Heimendinger, J. R. Hebert, Z. Feng, and C. Probart. 1995. Psychosocial correlates of healthful diets: baseline results from the Working Well study. *Preventive Medicine* 24:221–228.

Kroger, F. 1994. Toward a healthy public. *American Behavioral Scientist* 38:215–223.

Lefebvre, R. C., L. Doner, C. Johnston, K. Loughrey, G. I. Balch, and S. M. Sutton. 1995. Use of database marketing and consumer-based health communication in message design: An example from the Office of Cancer Communications' 5 a Day for Better Health program. Chap. 12 in *Designing Health Messages: Approaches from Communication Theory and Public Health Practice.* Thousand Oaks, London, New Delhi: Sage Publications Inc.

Lorig, K. 1996. *Patient Education: A Practical Approach.* 2d ed. Thousand Oaks, London, New Delhi: Sage Publications. See esp. pp. 216–223.

Mansour, A. A., and S. A. Hassan. 1994. Factors that influence women's nutrition knowledge in Saudi Arabia. *Health Care for Women International* 15(3): 213–223.

McGowan, P., and L. W. Green. 1995. Arthritis self-management in Native populations of British Columbia: An application of health promotion and participatory research principles in chronic disease control. *Canadian Journal on Aging* 14(Suppl.1):201–212.

Miilunpalo, S., J. Laitakari, and I. Vuori. 1995. Strengths and weaknesses in health counseling in Finnish primary health care. *Patient Education and Counseling* 25:317–328.

Morrison, C. 1996. Using PRECEDE to predict breast self-examination in older, lower-income women. *American Journal of Health Behavior* 20:3–14.

Morrison, S. D. 1994. PRECEDE model as a framework for using health education in the prevention of diarrhea infant mortality in rural Mexico. *The Eta Sigma Gamma Monograph Series* 12(1):41–49.

Nguyen, M. N., R. Grignon, M. Tremblay, and L. Delisle. 1995. Behavioral diagnosis of 30 to 60 year-old men in the Fabreville Heart Health Program. *Journal of Community Health* 20:257–269.

O'Loughlin, J., G. Paradis, N. Kishchuk, K. Gray-Donald, L. Renaud, P. Finés, and T. Barnett. 1995. Coeur en santé St-Henri—a heart health promotion programme in Montreal, Canada: design and methods for evaluation. *J Epidem Community Health* 49:495–502.

Oxman, A. D., M. A. Thomson, D. A. Davis, and R. B. Haynes. 1995. No magic bullets: A systematic review of 102 trials of interventions to improve professional practice. *Canadian Med Assoc J* 153: 1423–1431.

Paradis, G., J. O'Loughlin, M. Elliott, P. Masson, L. Renaud, G. Sacks-Silver, and G. Lampron. 1995. Coeur en santé St-Henri—a heart health promotion programme in a low income, low education neighbourhood in Montreal, Canada: theoretical model and early field experience. *J Epidem Community Health* 49:503–512.

Parcel, G. S., P. R. Swank, M. J. Mariotto, L. K. Bartholomew, D. I. Czyzewski, M. M. Sockride, and D. K. Seilheim. 1994. Self-management of cystic-fibrosis—A structural model for educational and behavioral variables. *Soc Sci Med* 38:1307–1315.

Reed, D. B. 1996. Focus groups identify desirable features of nutrition programs for low-income mothers of preschool children. *J Am Dietetic Assoc* 96:501–503.

Rimer, B. K. 1995. Audience and messages for breast and cervical cancer screenings. *Wellness Perspectives: Research, Theory and Practice* 11:13–39.

Selby-Harrington, M., J. R. Sorenson, D. Quade, S. C. Stearns, A. S. Tesh, and P. L. N. Donat. 1995. Increasing Medicaid child health screenings: The effectiveness of mailed pamphlets, phone calls, and home visits. *Am J Public Health* 85:1412–1417.

Simons Morton, B. G., W. H. Greene, and N. H. Gottlieb. 1995. *Introduction to Health Education and Health Promotion*. 2d ed. Prospect Heights, IL: Waveland Press, Inc.

Thompson, R. S., S. H. Taplin, T. A. McAfee, M. T. Mandelson, and A. E. Smith. 1995. Primary and secondary prevention services in clinical practice: twenty years' experience in development, implementation, and evaluation. *J Am Med Assoc* 273:1130–1135.

Turner, L. W., M. Sutherland, G. J. Harris, and M. Barber. 1995. Cardiovascular health promotion in North Florida African-American churches. *Health Values: J Health Behav, Educ & Promotion* 19:3–9.

U.S. Department of Health and Human Services. 1996. *Planned Approach to Community Health: guide for the local coordinator*. Atlanta, GA: U.S. Department of Health and Human Services, Centers for Disease Control and Prevention, National Center for Chronic Disease Prevention and Health Promotion.

Weiss, J. R., N. Wallerstein, and T. MacLean. 1995. Organizational development of a university-based interdisciplinary health promotion project. *Am J Health Promotion* 10(1):37–48.

Zuckerman, M. J., L. G. Guerra, D. A. Drossman, J. A. Foland, and G. G. Gregory. 1996. Health-care-seeking behaviors related to bowel complaints—Hispanics versus non-Hispanic whites. *Digestive Dis & Sciences* 41: 77–82.

Part Two

COMMUNITY AND POPULATION HEALTH THROUGH THE LIFE SPAN

Promoting the health of populations means developing and supporting the will and capabilities of people to address their own special health needs. Different health problems or needs will be of primary concern to the various segments within the population. Many health problems are common to expectant mothers, infants, children, adolescents, adults, and the elderly, but each category has special aspects of these common problems and its own unique problems. Whatever the objective epidemiological data may indicate about the health problems of any specific population, these data must be cast in social perspective by consulting with the population itself at the community level. Community measures to promote the health of the whole population often apply to the needs of all groups. Community attention to the specific needs of a particular segment of the population will serve to protect and promote the health and general well being of that group. This principle of specificity applies to age groups and to ethnic, occupational, residential, and socioeconomic groups, and other divisions of the population. Public health traditionally has given priority to the needs of the highest-risk populations and to the problems that affect the greatest number of people. Community health must address these problems and the less dramatic, everyday health concerns of people who are well and at average risk.

The following chapters in part 2 specify high-priority problems for disease prevention and health promotion, based on national and international assessments. From these assessments, objectives for entire nations, states or provinces, and communities can be proposed. This book adapts such objectives for the United States, which represents some twenty-five developed nations so far as its vital rates are near the average for other English-speaking and European countries. The objectives for the United States in disease prevention and health promotion are positive expressions of what the nation should be able to achieve by the year 2000 if it applies the knowledge and technology available. No assumptions are made about new breakthroughs in research, such as new cures for cancer or new immunizations. The objectives for 2000 are based in part on the highest levels of health or the lowest morbidity and mortality rates already achieved in certain other countries or in certain communities or populations.

These objectives are contrasted with the situation in developing countries and with the situation in North America through rates for different ethnic or socioeconomic groups. The intent in formulating the objectives for the nation was to challenge public- and private-sector organizations at national, state or provincial, and local levels to work toward the elimination of disparities between the haves and the have-nots, between regions or communities, and between races and cultural groups. It is hoped that you might feel challenged to adapt the objectives to populations within the communities in which you live or work.

Chapter *5*

Reproductive, Infant, and Child Health

W*ell begun is half done.*

—Horace

Objectives

When you finish this chapter, you should be able to:

- Identify the leading health issues, trends, and needs as they relate to reproduction and to infants and children as populations within a community

- Describe strategies to improve reproductive, infant, and child health
- Understand the role of family and social structures in reproductive, infant, and child health

From a community and population health perspective, reproductive health includes the social, personal, and biological preparation for the responsibilities of pregnancy and parenthood. While Western society has traditionally focused this preparation on married men and women, reproductive health is increasingly of concern with youth, some barely of reproducible age, and new social constructions of the family. Maternal, infant, and child health (MCH) encompasses community preventive care and education of infants, children, mothers, and families before and after delivery. It includes education of parents about immunization, dental care, nutrition, family planning, childcare and child abuse, substance misuse, physical fitness, and stress. Special attention is given in this chapter to preventive health services and health promotion approaches that should be incorporated into preparation for parenting, infant

and child health, and school health. International child survival figures are included to put North American issues in a global perspective.

REPRODUCTIVE HEALTH

Good reproductive health involves choice related to preparation for parenthood, maintenance of sexual health, family planning, pregnancy, and safe and healthful childbearing. Children that are planned and wanted start life with an advantage that include health benefits (see figure 5-1). How an individual functions from preschool through adolescence and into adulthood depends, in part, on his or her experiences before the age of three. The high number of unintended pregnancies in North America suggest that for many, particularly adolescents, reproduction does not involve conscious choice. For reproductive choice to occur, it

· · · · · · · · · · · · · · · · · ·

Figure 5-1

Planned children start life with a health advantage, although the traditional two-parent family is declining. (*Source:* PhotoDisc, Inc.)

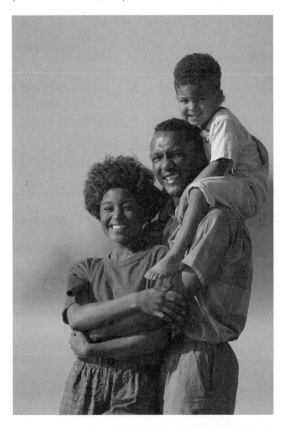

takes more than knowledge. It requires concern about the health and well-being of all involved and social support from the broader community.

Family Structure and Health

Family composition is changing. Formally, **family** is defined as a group of two or more people related by birth, marriage, or adoption residing together in a household. This definition does not include many extended families in Western societies or many of the new forms of cohabitation that have developed. The number of two-parent families has steadily declined in the West. By the mid-1990s, almost half of all children in the United States can expect their parents to divorce during their childhood. In Canada, 13 percent of all families are headed by a single parent. In the United States over a quarter of all births are to unmarried mothers. As laws change to allow single sex adoptions or as grandparents step back into parenting roles, the family next door may have a different structure than the traditional ideal. Changes in structure are important because families shape individual health. It is in families that an individual first learns to make choices that promote personal, community, and population health. Health conditions are likely to be affected by other social circumstances, notably gender, class, and race. Nearly one quarter of American children aged six years and younger live below the federal poverty level. The rates are higher still for African American and Hispanic families and single-parent families, many of which are headed by a single, female parent. Although these families may offer important nurturing, they are more likely to be economically and educationally disadvantaged. Across all ethnic groups and family structures, more children under three live in poverty than do older children, adults, or the elderly. Even families with two parents face pressures at work, which means they have less time with their young children. More than half of mothers with infants work outside the home, which means that more than 5 million children under age three are in the care of other adults. These social circumstances affect infant mortality rates, prenatal care, and the risk of developing other health problems for children.

Family Planning

Family planning provides individuals with information and services needed to make informed choices about whether and when to become parents. Achievement of family planning goals requires information, motivation, exercise of personal responsibility, access to a wide range of comprehensive services, community support, and effective means of family planning. Communities, through their multiple institutions, such as

Community Goals for Reproductive, Infant, and Child Health

- Pregnancy will occur by choice and under circumstances of lowest risk, and unwanted fertility will be eliminated.
- Every pregnant woman will receive appropriate reproductive health services, and every expectant mother will maintain good health, learn the art of child care, and bear a healthy infant.
- All couples anticipating parenthood . . . [and] all infants and children . . . will participate in a comprehensive health program that emphasizes preventive care.
- Child abuse and neglect will be eliminated.
- The incidence of preventable injuries and deaths occurring among children will be reduced.
- All children, including those with chronic handicaps, will function at their optimal level.
- Indicators for the health of any racial, ethnic, socioeconomic, or geographic subgroup will not be significantly more adverse than those for the entire community.

Healthy Communities 2000: Model Standards (1991)

U.S. Objectives for Family Planning

- By the year 2000 reduce to no more than 30 percent the proportion of all pregnancies that are unintended. Baseline: in 1988 56 percent of pregnancies in the previous 5 years were unintended.
- By 2000 increase to at least 60 percent the proportion of primary care providers who provide age-appropriate preconception care and counseling.
- By 2000 increase the effectiveness with which family planning methods are used, as measured by a decrease to no more than 5 percent in the proportion of couples experiencing pregnancy despite use of a contraceptive method. Baseline: approximately 10 percent of women using reversible contraceptive methods experienced an unintended pregnancy in 1982.

Healthy Communities 2000: Model Standards (1991)

government, schools, churches, and voluntary agencies, influence individual choice among acceptable family planning methods, such as adoption, abstinence from sexual activity outside of a monogamous relationship, use of contraceptive methods, natural family planning, and treatment of infertility. New and innovative forms of contraception can be researched, while providing a full range of family planning services when birth control efforts fail. Community influence can encourage males to participate in family planning decisions, not casting off these decisions as "her responsibility." The priority and program emphasis of these viable methods of family planning differ among communities and with changes in governmental leadership.

Intended and Unintended Pregnancies

Fifty-six percent of pregnancies in the United States and 80 percent of teenage pregnancies are unintended, either occurring too soon or when unwanted. The percentage of unintended pregnancies varies with age and socioeconomic status. Approximately every minute a teenage girl gives birth. Despite concerted attempts, only limited success has been realized in efforts to reduce pregnancy rates among adolescents, to convince teenagers to delay sexual activity, and to reduce repeat pregnancies. In addition to the social and psychological costs of unintended pregnancies for adolescents and their children, the economic costs to society are staggering. Over $25 billion is spent annually in the United States on social, health, and welfare services to families begun by adolescents. It is estimated that for every dollar invested in family planning, $4.40 in welfare and medical service expenditures is avoided. Health education plays a role in family planning by providing learning experiences that enable choice concerning reproduction. U.S. objectives for family planning are to reduce all unintended pregnancies to no more than 30 percent (see box titled "U.S. Objectives for Family Planning"); the mid-decade status of these objectives is found in figure 5-2.

·····················

Figure 5-2

Status of year 2000 national objectives for family planning (*Source:* Public Health Service, U.S. Department of Health and Human Services.)

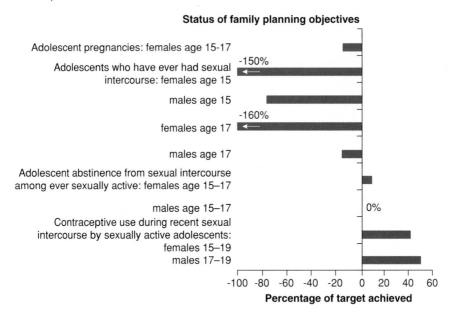

Status of family planning objectives

Birth Control Methods

Over 57 percent of unintended pregnancies were of women who were not using a contraceptive method. The most common contraceptive methods used to decrease the number of unintended pregnancies are shown in table 5-1 on pp. 122–123. These methods vary in their popularity and their estimated effectiveness, risks, benefits, convenience, availability, and cost. Health education and clinical service programs need to consider these facts, and the cultural, social, and political acceptability of these methods to selected subpopulations. Other methods, such as RU-486 ("morning after pill") are controversial in the United States, but are used in other countries as viable methods of birth control.

Infertility

Infertility affects an estimated 2.4 million married couples and an unknown number of potential parents among unmarried couples and singles. Common factors affecting infertility include problems in ovulation, blocked or scarred fallopian tubes, endometriosis, and low sperm count. The estimated 20 percent of infertility that arises from sexually transmitted diseases is the most preventable. The year 2000 objective for infertility is to reduce the prevalence of infertility from 7.9 percent to 6.5 percent of married couples with wives aged 15 to 44 years. Milestones in test-tube reproduction date back to the early research with animals (see box).

TRENDS IN MATERNAL MORTALITY AND MORBIDITY

Rates

A 1996 study released by the World Health Organization, reported that 585,000 maternal deaths occur in the world each year; 99 percent of these deaths occur in developing countries. Maternal deaths are those associated with deliveries and complications of pregnancy, childbirth, and **puerperium.** Rates are based on number of mothers

Milestones in Test-Tube Reproduction

1799	Pregnancy reported from artificial insemination
1944	First attempt at in-vitro fertilization
1949	Researchers discover that glycerol can be used to freeze sperm for later use
1950	First calf produced using frozen semen
1951	Frogs cloned from the cells of tadpoles
1952	Frozen sperm used for human artificial insemination

1959	Live rabbit offspring from in-vitro fertilization
1972	Live offspring from frozen mouse embryos
1973	First calf produced from a frozen embryo
1978	First test-tube baby, Louise Brown, born in Britain
1979	Cattle embryos cloned
1983	A baby is born to a mother from an embryo formed by her husband's sperm and a donor's egg

1984	Australian girl named Zoe born from a frozen embryo
1993	George Washington University researchers clone human embryos
1997	Scottish laboratory announces it has cloned a sheep named Dolly from the cell of an adult ewe

dying per 100,000 live births occurring in a given year. The lowest national figures are in Norway, Sweden, and Switzerland and the highest in Sierra Leone, where one of every seven women dies of pregnancy-related complications.

Causes

The causes of **maternal mortality** have altered, reflecting the relative decline in the instances of hemorrhage, infection, and toxemia. Anesthetic misadventures are relatively more common now, since other causes have decreased and since the number of patients receiving anesthesia for childbirth has increased. Paradoxically, advances in medicine have provided challenges in obstetrics: women with congenital heart disease and juvenile diabetes are able to become pregnant, but their safe delivery demands skill. **Abortion** as a cause of maternal mortality has declined with safe, legalized abortions replacing clandestine, septic abortions.

DES   Women were exposed to the drug diethylstilbestrol (DES) when their mothers took the drug during pregnancy from the 1940s into the 1970s for pregnancy complications. These DES daughters are at increased risk of cancer of the vagina and cervix. DES daughters are also more likely to have problems in their pregnancies. The rate of

Historical and Comparative Perspectives

Consider maternal health conditions at the turn of the century, when the population in the United States was about 76 million. More than 20,000 women died in childbirth each year. Some 90 years later, with a population of more than 230 million—three times the number of people at risk—the yearly number of deaths of women resulting from complications of childbirth has been reduced to fewer than 400. The chances of a woman's surviving childbirth in the United States and in most other developed countries are about 8,999 out of 9,000, and the survival rate continues to improve. How do you account for this dramatic reduction in the risks of childbearing in the more developed countries? Why do the maternal mortality rates for the least developed countries remain at levels as high as those in the United States at the turn of the century?

unfavorable birth outcomes for a group of women exposed to DES was nearly twice that of unexposed women, where *unfavorable birth outcome* was defined as a miscarriage, a stillbirth, or an ectopic pregnancy.

Table 5-1

Frequency of Use, and Pros and Cons of Selected Contraceptive Methods

	Condom	Diaphragm with spermicide	IUD	Birth control pills	Birth control implant	Vasectomy (male sterilization)	Tubal ligation (female sterilization)
Estimated Effectiveness	64–97%	80–98%	95–96%	97–99%	99%	99%+	99%+
% of users	6.7%	4.5%	4.0%	15.6%	<1%	25.7%	25.7%
Risks	Rarely, irritation and allergic reactions	Rarely, irritation and allergic reactions; bladder infection; constipation; very rarely, toxic shock syndrome	Cramps, bleeding, pelvic inflammatory disease, infertility; rare perforation of the uterus	Blood clots, heart attacks and strokes, gallbladder disease, liver tumor, water retention, hypertension, mood change, dizziness and nausea, not for smokers	Menstrual irregularity; headache, nervousness, depression, nausea, dizziness, appetite change, breast tenderness, weight gain, enlargement of ovaries and/or fallopian tubes, excess body and facial hair	Pain, infection; rare possibly psychological problems	Surgical problem; some pain or discomfort; possibly higher risk of hyersterectomy later in life

Non-contraceptive Benefits	Some protection against STDs, including herpes and HIV/AIDS	Spermicides may give some protection against some STDs	None	Less menstrual bleeding and cramping, lower risk of fibrocystic breast disease, ovarian cysts and pelvic inflammatory disease; protects against cancer of the ovaries and lining of the uterus	Less menstrual bleeding, contains no estrogen	None	None
Convenience	Applied immediately before intercourse	Inserted before intercourse; can be left in place 24 hours, but additional spermicide must be inserted if intercourse is repeated	After insertion, stays in place until physician removes	Pill must be taken on daily schedule, regardless of intercourse frequency	Effective 24 hours after implantation for approx. 5 years; can be removed by physician at any time	One-time procedure	One-time procedure
Availability	Non-prescription	Rx	Rx	Rx	Rx;minor outpatient surgical procedure	Minor surgery	Surgery

Source: Food and Drug Administration, U.S. Depart. of Health and Human Services, 1991.

Cesarean Deliveries   Cesarean delivery rates in the United States increased through the 1980s to a high of 24.4 per 100 deliveries in 1989. This contrasts with 1970 figures in which only 5.5% of deliveries were cesarean. In these deliveries the baby is removed surgically through the abdominal wall of the mother, rather than vaginally. 1990 was the first year in the two decades in which the rate *dropped* to 22.7 percent. The rate is still considered high, especially since there is no evidence to suggest that such deliveries have improved maternal or child health for their $1.3 billion price tag. Reasons for the high rate include misdiagnosis, widely varying physician practices, convenience to mothers and physicians, increased revenue from deliveries, and physician's concerns about malpractice suits. The slight decrease in 1990 is attributed to better patient education and organized programs to reduce the occurrence of such deliveries. The objective for the year 2000 is to reduce the cesarean delivery rate to no more than 15 per 100 deliveries.

Ectopic Pregnancies   An ectopic or tubal pregnancy occurs when the mass of cells that develops from the fertilized egg fails to move through the fallopian tube to attach to the wall of the uterus, where it is supposed to grow; instead, it attaches to the wall of the fallopian tube. Ectopic pregnancies are the leading cause of maternal mortality during the first trimester in the United States; the relative risk of death from an ectopic pregnancy is 10 times greater than from childbirth and 50 times greater than from a legal abortion. Dramatic increases in the number of women delaying pregnancy until after age 35 and in diseases and procedures affecting the fallopian tubes have increased the rate of ectopic pregnancy. In 1992, ectopic pregnancies accounted for approximately 2 percent of reported pregnancies, and ectopic pregnancy-related deaths accounted for 9 percent of all pregnancy related deaths.

Pelvic Inflammatory Disease (PID)   PID causes damage to the fallopian tubes. This can lead to infertility and can cause a pregnancy to be ectopic.

PID is an infection of the uterus and the fallopian tubes caused by sexually transmitted disease or sometimes by postsurgical infection. If the disease is treated quickly, damage to the reproductive structures can be prevented. Although progress has been made toward year 2000 goals for PID, the challenge is to narrow the gap in infection rates between the total population and among adolescents and certain racial and ethnic minority groups.

Abortions   Abortion may be spontaneous or artificial. A spontaneous abortion, also called a miscarriage, occurs when a pregnancy ends spontaneously before the beginning of the twentieth week of pregnancy. A miscarriage is due to the separation of the developing fetus and the placenta from the inner wall of the uterus. Usually the cause is unknown.

A pregnancy that ends artificially is also called an abortion, but the medical term is termination of pregnancy. In 1973 the United States Supreme Court ruled in *Roe v. Wade.* that women have a constitutional right to abortion for any reason during the first twenty-four weeks of pregnancy and, after that, if the pregnancy endangers the mother's life. In 1969 abortions were legalized in Canada if performed by a doctor in an approved hospital and medically certified that continuation of the pregnancy would likely endanger the life or health of the mother. In 1993, 1.3 million legal induced abortions were performed in the United States; in 1990 there were approximately 71,000 abortions in Canada. From 1972 through 1980, the national U.S. abortion rate increased each year, then stabilized during the next decade. Since 1990 the number of reported abortions has decreased each year. Factors possibly contributing to this decrease include changes in reduced access to abortion services, changes in contraceptive practices, attitudinal changes concerning the decision to have an abortion or to carry a pregnancy to term, aging of the baby boomers, and a possible decline in the number of unintended pregnancies. In the United States, states are free to restrict abortion, as long as they do not place an "undue burden" on a woman.

········

Figure 5-3

Antiabortionists and proabortionists have a standoff near the clinic at Vancouver General Hospital. (Photo courtesy *Vancouver Courier,* Eike Schroter.)

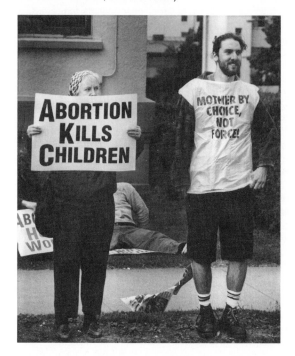

Despite its legal status, abortion remains controversial (figure 5-3) and is not equally available to all women. With increased restrictions and violence directed at clinics access to abortion services depends on judges, doctors who may or may not choose to perform them, lawmakers who decide on public funding for abortion services, and a woman's willingness to tolerate the threat of violence to receive services. Although the medical community overwhelmingly favors abortion rights, in practice few doctors perform abortions and the number of abortion providers is decreasing. A 1988 survey found 2,582 establishments offered abortion; in 1992, the number was 2,380. Disparity also exists between countries in Europe and in Latin America. For example, over 4,000 women from Ireland cross the Irish Sea each year to have legal abortions in England because they cannot obtain them in Ireland.

Strategies to provide abortion services could include counseling a woman facing an unintended pregnancy to apprise her of her options; starting freestanding clinics in more populous regions; encouraging physicians in hospitals to provide the services; and establishing clinics in county hospitals, with satellite clinics providing services to smaller communities at a distance from the main facility.

PROMOTING MATERNAL HEALTH

Successful birth outcomes and a healthy first year of life are strengthened by a planned and wanted child and by good maternal care during pregnancy. Couples have choices available in planning for children by means of contraception, termination of unintended pregnancies by abortion, prenatal care, continuation of schooling or work during and following maternity leave, and services for safe delivery. The community role lies in assuring access to these services, in making potential users aware of their options, in providing services and counseling in a culturally and linguistically sensitive manner, and in counseling as to appropriate choice.

Prenatal Care

Prenatal care (or **antenatal care**) should be sought early in pregnancy. Approximately one in four infants born in the United States, however, are born to mothers who receive late or no care (see box titled "Barriers for Prenatal Care"). Adequate care is defined as care in the first trimester and nine or more visits during a full-term pregnancy. Infants of women who received no prenatal care are more likely to have low birth weight and have about ten times the risk of dying in the first months of life. Prenatal care is also a bargain. Every dollar spent on prenatal care for low-income, poorly educated women saves about $3 in intensive care for infants born with birth defects.

The major purposes of prenatal care include health education, early detection of abnormalities, and identification of the high-risk mother and infant. At the first visit a complete medical, surgical,

ISSUES AND CONTROVERSIES
Prochoice and Prolife Controversy

Abortion is a highly controversial meeting ground for legal, political, economic, religious, social, and public health interests. Women who find themselves with unintended pregnancies meet health care workers whose decisions and actions are pulled by many interests. A woman exercising her legal right to choose an abortion may face a gauntlet of prolife supporters who believe that her choice constitutes murder. Health care workers who support a woman's right to choose found themselves "gagged" in 1988 by a federal rule that prohibited abortion counseling in federally funded family planning clinics. A physician in the south-

eastern United States who offered abortion services in several unserved counties was murdered in 1993 by a prolife supporter, a clinic worker in Boston was murdered in 1995, a clinic security officer died in a 1998 bombing in Birmingham and in Vancouver, BC a gynecologist was shot eating breakfast in his own home.

The abortion debate continues at national and local levels in North America. In 1988 the Supreme Court of Canada overturned the 1969 amendment legalizing abortions. The Court's decision left Canada without an abortion law. Shortly after his inauguration, President Clinton approved by execu-

tive order new policies that lifted federal abortion limitations imposed by the previous Republican administrations. These included lifting the "gag rule"; eliminating a ban on federal fetal tissue research; and forcing a decision on the ban to import RU-486, the "abortion pill."

How are political changes in North America likely to affect the prochoice and prolife controversy? Why is access to abortion services of concern to public health? What are the options for health care workers who find their personal beliefs at odds with professional requirements? How have abortions affected maternal mortality?

U.S. Objectives for Maternal and Prenatal Care

- By 2000 reduce the maternal mortality rate to no more than 3.3 per 100,000 live births. Baseline: in 1989 the overall rate in the United States was 7.9. Despite declines in maternal death rates for both whites and blacks, the rate for black women in 1989 was 18.4, more than three times the rate for white women, 5.6.
- By 2000 increase abstinence from tobacco use by pregnant women to at least 90 percent and increase abstinence from

alcohol, cocaine, and marijuana by pregnant women by at least 20 percent. Baseline: in 1985 75 percent of pregnant women abstained from tobacco use.
- Increase to at least 90 percent the proportion of all pregnant women who receive prenatal care in the first trimester of pregnancy. Baseline: in 1989 76 percent of all women who had live births met this objective. Baseline rates were lower for blacks—60.4 percent, American

Indian/Alaska Native women—60.5 percent, and Hispanic women—61.2 percent.
- By 2000 reduce iron deficiency to less than 3 percent among women of childbearing age. Baseline: 5 percent for women aged 20 to 44 years. For black, low-income women in the third trimester the baseline rate is 41 percent.

Healthy Communities 2000: Model Standards (1991).

Barriers for Prenatal Care

Important barriers to women seeking prenatal care include costs, available services, and public understanding of the importance of such care. The greatest barrier is financial. More than 14 million American women of reproductive age have no insurance to cover medical care. A growing shortage of obstetric providers, attributed to rising malpractice insurance rates, contributes to service delivery issues for all women. This is a particular problem for poor women who face inadequate facilities or clinical practices, such as long waits and poor interpersonal skills of staff, that make clinic visits difficult or unpleasant.

Although congressional mandates have expanded Medicaid, making more women eligible for prenatal and postpartum care, difficulties remain in getting eligible women into care. Lack of understanding about the benefits of prenatal care, along with transportation problems, personal or cultural beliefs, and lack of childcare, may deter these women from accessing services.

Figure 5-4

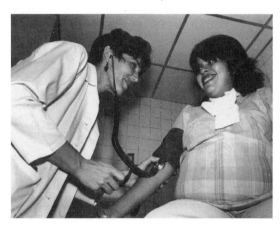

Prenatal care confers advantages to the fetus and the mother. (Photo by Marsha Burkes, courtesy University of Texas Health Center at Houston.)

obstetric, and genetic history is obtained, and a physical examination is performed (figure 5-4). Routine laboratory data are obtained, including blood type and Rhesus (Rh) factor determination; urinalysis; complete blood count; rubella titer; tests for syphilis, gonorrhea, and abnormalities of hemoglobin synthesis (sickle cell); and cervical smear. A social worker or genetic counselor may interview the woman or the couple and discuss available community resources or potential birth defects.

Health Education

Community information campaigns about the importance of prenatal care can be directed to the groups least likely to seek care. These include teenagers, especially those who already have children; low-income and uninsured women; women over age thirty-five; recent immigrants; and high-risk minorities. One-shot, short-lived campaigns seldom have much impact on public attitudes or personal health behavior.

The prenatal visits provide an opportunity for counseling and education about health-related behavior, including dental care, avoidance or reduction of alcohol and cigarette smoking, use of seat belts, balanced exercise, infection, exposure to irradiation, and rest. A supportive, nonjudgmental, warm, sympathetic climate is maintained so that communication and cooperation between patient and provider is enhanced and responsibility is shared. For high-risk groups (defined by medical history), exposures to physical abuse and harmful substances signal the need for more counseling (figure 5-5).

Education for childbirth should start at school in human biology studies. During pregnancy the most effective education is in peer group sessions, when experienced mothers can lead others. Removing fear is a great benefit, and the attendance of fathers is valuable. Visiting the hospital's delivery and newborn suites and meeting the staff can benefit the apprehensive woman. Various professional and lay groups endorse different plans of preparation for and practices during childbirth, but the common thread is open discussion, question

. . . .

Figure 5-5

Drug abuse invades the lives of users and often the lives of others, including the unborn. (*Source:* National Institute on Drug Abuse, U.S. Department of Health and Human Services.)

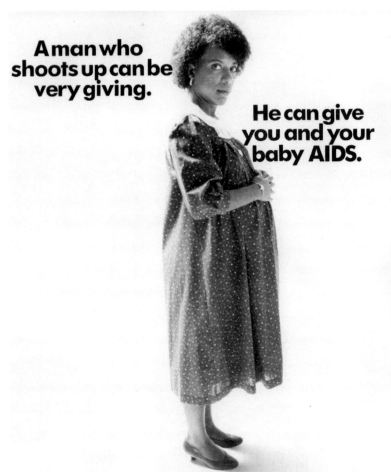

A man who shoots up can be very giving.

He can give you and your baby AIDS.

Most babies with AIDS are born to mothers who shot drugs or who sleep with men who have.

Babies with AIDS are born to die.

If you're thinking of having a baby you and your partner need to get tested for AIDS. Only get pregnant when you're sure both of you aren't infected. Until then help protect yourself and your partner by using condoms.

And if your man shoots drugs, help him get into treatment now. It could save three lives, his, yours and your baby's.

STOP SHOOTING UP AIDS.
GET INTO DRUG TREATMENT.
CALL 1-800 662 HELP.

A Public Service of the National Institute on Drug Abuse, Department of Health and Human Services.

and answer, and removal of fear. Partners in such programs enjoy the emotional experience of pregnancy and delivery. Studies have shown reductions in the amount of analgesia and anesthesia used by women who participated in childbirth classes and shortened labor.

Nutrition

A strong relationship exists between pregnancy weight gain of the mother and birth weight of an infant. The infant's birth weight is a determinant of potential for survival and future development, therefore recommended weight gain for the mother is important to achieve. In general, women who are normal weight or slightly overweight have better pregnancy outcomes than those who are underweight. Weight gain during pregnancy needs to consider not only caloric intake but also nutritional quality. Other factors influencing weight gain include smoking, strenuous physical work, and chronic illness. The social pressure on women to be thin may make it difficult for some to allow themselves adequate weight gain during pregnancy.

Pregnancy is an ideal time for nutritional counseling for women and their families. It provides an opportunity to educate women not only about their own nutritional needs during pregnancy but also about the future needs of their infants, themselves, and their families. Counseling can inform expectant mothers about the latest research, such as the studies showing that folic acid can protect against spina bifida or help prevent oral and facial birth defects, such as a cleft palate. Nutritional counseling needs to consider the recommended balance of food and should be sensitive to the cultural preferences and economic circumstances of the mother. If necessary, women may need referral to appropriate governmental or voluntary agency programs for assistance with their nutritional needs.

Detection of Abnormalities and Risk

High-risk pregnancies should be identified so that these cases can be given special care. Predictors are age, particularly under fifteen years or over thirty-five years; previous obstetric difficulty, such

as unexplained stillbirths, premature deliveries, and spontaneous abortions; women who attend clinics for sexually transmitted diseases, have multiple sex partners, a history of prostitution, or sexual partners who were IV drug users; and women who are under sixty inches tall or those who smoke cigarettes daily or use alcohol or drugs. Many procedures during pregnancy relate more to the health of the fetus and newborn than to the health or safety of the mother, but in the final analysis these considerations are inseparable.

Amniocentesis provides the means to assess many previously undetectable genetic abnormalities in the fetus. A sample of amniotic fluid, drawn from the expectant mother's uterus by means of a hypodermic needle, can be cultured in the laboratory and tested for biochemical and chromosomal defects. Genetic counseling and amniocentesis detect and provide the opportunity to prevent abnormal or defective births. Estimates of the incidence and prevalence of genetic diseases and congenital abnormalities vary. Some 36 percent of spontaneous abortions are caused by gross chromosomal defects (amounting to more than 100,000 per year in the United States). At least 40 percent of all infant mortality results from genetic factors, and genetic defects are present in 5 percent of all live births.

Many serious genetic disorders can be detected from the fourteenth to the twentieth week of pregnancy when therapeutic abortion is medically feasible and legally permissible in most states. If the fetus has abnormalities, the prospective parents can choose not to terminate the pregnancy but still gain from the time to prepare for the birth. Increasingly, medical science offers the potential to correct some problems in utero. Negative tests provide relief from fear and anxiety for prospective parents with any reason to suspect a genetic or congenital abnormality.

One type of screening that has become a standard of care for women is maternal serum alpha-fetoprotein (MSAFP) testing. This test can be used to detect neural tube defect in fetuses, twin pregnancy, central wall defects, Down syndrome, and fetal demise. Early prenatal care is essential because

· · · · · · · · · · · · · · · · · ·

Figure 5-6

Reproductive and perinatal mortalities are based on numbers of fetal and infant deaths in each of eight periods, some of which overlap.

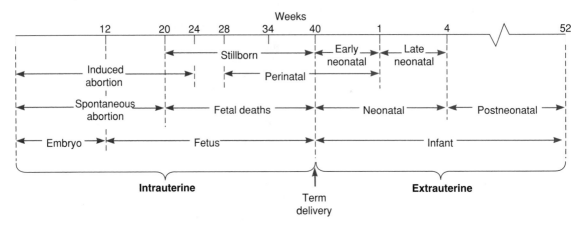

the test is not informative other than in the fifteenth to eighteenth week of pregnancy. In the long run, the total cost to the community of caring for the diseases and disabilities of children with genetic and congenital defects far outweighs the cost of prenatal counseling, screening, diagnosis, and abortion. The cost-benefit ratios run as high as $20 saved for every dollar spent on these procedures.

PROMOTING PERINATAL HEALTH

At the other end of the spectrum from **perinatal** health is perinatal mortality. Such mortality is the number of late fetal deaths (stillbirths) from the twenty-eighth week of pregnancy plus the number of deaths in the first week of life per 1,000 live births (figure 5-6). This reproductive index includes intrauterine and extrauterine deaths and is a measure of the quality and efficiency of obstetrical and neonatal services. Perinatal mortality is most heavily influenced by low birthweight, formerly called the **prematurity rate,** which is the percentage of babies born who weigh 2,500 grams (5 pounds, 8 ounces) or less. The rate of survival of such infants is naturally lower than that of term-sized infants, mainly because the respiratory system of premature infants

is not sufficiently mature to adapt to extrauterine life. Advances in neonatology, through the use of intensive care nurseries or prematurity centers, have been tremendous, so the survival rate is improving for all birthweight ranges.

Although national objectives are to reduce perinatal mortality (see box titled "U.S. Objectives for Perinatal and Neonatal Health"), mortality decline is limited by the low-birthweight rate, which has remained constant since 1950 in the United States. It was thought that the low-birthweight rate would fall in response to improved social conditions, but a complex interaction of factors has been operating. A high proportion of births now derive from adolescent mothers and those in lower socioeconomic strata. Mothers age fifteen years or less have a prematurity rate twice that of other mothers, and black babies are twice as likely as white babies to be born prematurely. Low-birthweight infants include newborns who are born too early and those whose intrauterine growth is retarded. Risk factors for low birthweight include (1) previous history of a low-birthweight infant, (2) younger and older maternal age, (3) low socioeconomic status, (4) low educational level, (5) late entry into prenatal care, (6) low pregnancy

U.S. Objectives for Perinatal and Neonatal Health

- By 2000 reduce the **fetal death rate** to no more than 5 per 1000 live births plus fetal deaths. Baseline: 5.5 per 1000 live births plus fetal deaths in 1989. For blacks and others, the baseline was 11.4 in 1989.
- By 2000 reduce the incidence of fetal alcohol syndrome to no more than 0.12 per 1000 live births. Baseline: 0.22 per 1000 live births in 1987. American Indians and Alaska Natives are a special population target. Their baseline rate of 4 in 1987 was 33 times higher than whites. The year 2000 target for this population is 2.
- By 2000 increase to at least 95 percent the proportion of newborns screened by state-sponsored programs for genetic disorders and other disabling conditions and to 90 percent the proportion of newborns testing positive for disease who receive appropriate treatment. Baseline: for sickle cell anemia, approximately 33 percent of live births were screened in 1989.

Healthy People 2000, 1991.

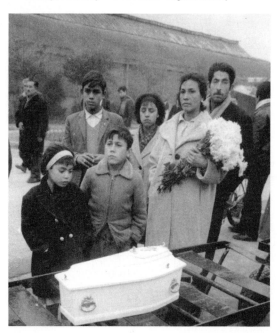

Figure 5-7

The baby's coffin and the faces of the mourning family tell the tragic story of infant mortality. (Photo by P. Almasy, courtesy World Health Organization.)

weight gain or low pregnancy weight, and (7) smoking and substance abuse. These factors are interrelated and are amenable to community influence through nutrition, family planning, health education, and more general socioeconomic support and improvement.

PROMOTING INFANT HEALTH

Infant Mortality

Infant mortality is the number of deaths of children under one year of age per 1,000 live births. It is an important measure of a nation's health and worldwide indicator of health status. Compared with other industrialized nations, the United States ranks twenty-fourth in infant mortality. Deaths in the first week of life contribute to rates for perinatal and infant mortality (figure 5-7).

At the beginning of this century about 100 of every 1,000 infants born in the United States died in the first year of life. This figure has progressively declined to 29.0 per 1,000 infants in 1950, 20.0 in 1970, and 8.5 in 1992. Continuing decline in infant mortality is a national objective (see box titled "U.S. Objectives for Infant Health"). Although infant mortality dropped to the lowest rate ever recorded in the United States in 1994, the gap between black and white newborns is increasing. Black infants have a mortality rate 2.4 times that of white infants (figure 5-8).

Infant mortality can be divided into neonatal and postneonatal mortality. **Neonatal mortality** occurs in the first twenty-eight days after birth, which largely reflects prenatal and perinatal circumstances and events. Neonatal mortality accounts for more than two-thirds of infant deaths, and it is in this category that the largest gains were being made until 1985. The best strategies to reduce neonatal deaths

· · · · · · · · · · · · · · · · · ·

Figure 5 - 8

Infant mortality rates by race, United States, 1980 to 1990 (*Source:* National Center for Health Statistics, National Vital Statistics System.)

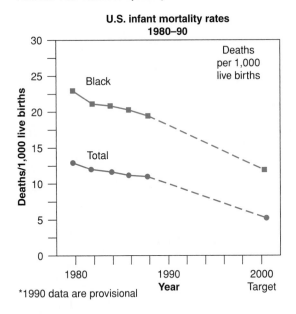

U.S. infant mortality rates 1980–90

Deaths per 1,000 live births

*1990 data are provisional

U.S. Objectives for Infant Health

By 2000 reduce the infant mortality rate to no more than 7 per 1000 live births. Baseline: 10.1 per 1000 live births in 1987. Blacks, American Indians, and Puerto Ricans have infant mortality rates substantially higher than the United States average.

Infant mortality per 1000 live births	1987 Baseline	2000 Target
Blacks	17.9	11.0
American Indians/Alaska Natives	12.5	8.5
Puerto Ricans	12.9	8.0

- By 2000 reduce low birthweight to an incidence of no more than 5 percent of live births and very low birthweight to no more than 1 percent of live births. Baseline: 6.9 percent and 1.2 percent, respectively, in 1987.
- By 2000 reduce the incidence of fetal alcohol syndrome to no more than 0.12 per 1000 live births. Baseline: 0.22 per 1000 live births in 1987. American Indians and Alaska Natives are a special population target. Their baseline rate of 4 in 1987 was 33 times higher than whites. The year 2000 target for this population is 2.

are family planning, prenatal care with risk assessment and management, obstetrical technology, breast-feeding, and newborn intensive care. **Post-neonatal mortality,** occurs between 28 days and 365 days of age (figure 5-6). It is more dependent on parenting and other aspects of the infant's environment; therefore other strategies are more appropriate such as educating parents on the care and feeding of infants, illness surveillance and care, and use of pediatric services.

International Rates Infant mortality in advanced countries is mostly influenced by deaths in the first month of life, which make up 70 percent of the deaths in the first year. This high proportion results from the reduction in deaths caused by infectious diseases, which earlier in the twentieth century contributed to the high infant mortality. Reduction of infant mortality depends on reducing

deaths immediately following birth, which in turn means reducing the low-birthweight rate. Countries that have low infant mortalities for example, Norway and Sweden, have low-birthweight rates of about 3.0 percent, which compares with an overall U.S. rate of 6.9 percent (5.6 percent for whites, 12.4 percent for blacks). Weight for weight, babies have a high survival rate in the United States relative to most countries because of advanced neonatology. However, the United States must contend with relatively more low-birthweight babies, which adversely affects reproductive indexes.

Improvements in the survival of infants will also stem from reduction in the needless waste of infant lives caused by injuries, infectious diseases, and other causes. One of the successful programs to reduce infant mortality has been directed at Sudden Infant Death Syndrome (SIDS). Community

Figure 5-9

Status of year 2000 national objectives for maternal and infant health (*Source:* Public Health Service, U.S. Department of Health and Human Services.)

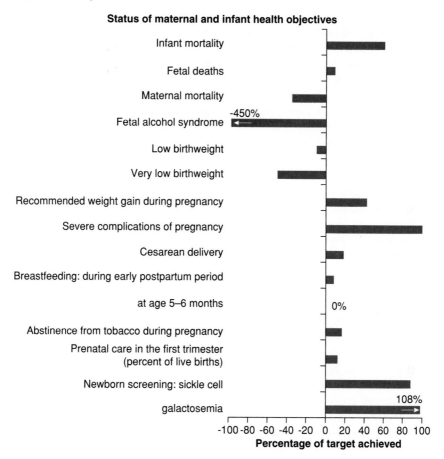

Status of maternal and infant health objectives

education programs promoting placement of infants on their backs when sleeping has contributed to a 25 percent reduction in the SIDS rate. Other types of community action are effective in providing a safe environment, for example requiring infant car seats by legislation; immunization programs; reduction of burns, alcoholism, and child abuse; and education of mothers to bring their children to a physician early in illness when infectious disease may be successfully treated. Adequate community resources to provide alternate childcare facilities for working mothers is imperative.

Breast-feeding

National objectives for breast-feeding are moving in the right direction, as 56 percent of mothers were breast-feeding in 1993, a 2 percent gain from the 1988 baseline data (figure 5-9). Breast milk alone, without supplements, is the optimal choice for feeding full-term infants for the first year. Mother's milk contains an ideal balance of nutrients, enzymes, immunoglobulin, anti-infective and anti-inflammatory substances, hormones, and growth factors that protect the infant and encourage growth. Breast milk changes over time to match the changing needs of the infant. For the mother, breast-feeding facilitates the physiological return to the prepregnant state and offers hygienic and economic benefits over bottle-feeding. For infant and mother, breast-feeding confers an intense opportunity for bonding and interaction. Breast-feeding is not recommended for women with the HIV/AIDS, those who abuse drugs or alcohol, and those receiving certain kinds of therapeutic agents, such as chemotherapy.

Breast-feeding rates are highest among women who are older, well-educated, relatively affluent, and who live in the western United States; they are lowest among low-income, black women under twenty years of age living in the southeastern United States. However, gains among racial and ethnic minorities are closing the gap. In early postpartum, breast-feeding was found among 31 percent of black mothers, 56 percent of Hispanic mothers, and 51 percent of American Indian/Alaska Native mothers.

Barriers to breast-feeding include the public portrayal of bottle-feeding as the norm, busy schedules of working mothers, and lack of information about the advantages and techniques of breast-feeding. As natural an act as breast-feeding is, sometimes mothers need help and support to initiate and sustain it. Voluntary groups such as the La Leche League can provide such assistance free of charge. Other barriers include work policies and facilities that discourage breast-feeding and societal attitudes about women's bodies that lead to the inappropriate perception that breast-feeding in public is an inappropriate act.

COMMUNITY HEALTH PROGRAMS FOR CHILDREN

Basic health services for the prevention of disease and the early identification of illness or disability should be available to all children. Well-child clinics providing assessment of growth and development, nutrition information, nurturing and anticipatory guidance, and immunization for children should be available. Well-child care should be at

regular intervals and may be performed by allied health personnel other than physicians. Competent pediatric nurse practitioners, experienced public health nurses, and physician's assistants working in tandem with psychologists and educators can assess the progress of a child, interpreting the steps already taken and the next steps to be expected for the person caring for the child.

Parent-infant bonding and anticipatory counseling to prevent problems will enable the child to grow up in a healthful and well-structured atmosphere. Early recognition of social and psychological problems will permit early and simple correction of adverse circumstances. School health is an essential component of community health.

Status of Child Health

Children are healthier than ever before, certainly as measured by the usual morbidity and mortality indicators. However, there are different threats to the health of children and youth, often characterized as the "new morbidity," for which environmental (social, physical, familial, and economic) and behavioral factors have been identified as causative or contributive. Some special childhood problems of concern to those who will work with these age groups are learning disorders, inadequate school functioning, behavioral problems, speech and vision difficulties, mental retardation, child abuse and neglect, and injuries. These new threats to morbidity, along with threats from falling immunization rates, are seen in the national objectives for childhood health (see box titled "U.S. Objectives for Childhood Health").

The family has profound effects on the health and educational status of its members. The national goals to improve the health of children and youth and to prevent consequences of the new morbidity are highly dependent on the family environment. However, the family is no longer seen as the sole agent of children's socialization; the emerging understanding is that the child and the family are affected by every institution of society. The focus is on children in the context of living in a complex world of family interactions, mass

U.S. Objectives for Childhood Health

- By 2000 90 percent of children under 2 years of age will have the basic immunization series. Baseline: 70 percent to 80 percent estimated in 1989.
- By 2000 increase to at least 90 percent the proportion of all children entering school programs for the first time who have received oral health screening, referral, and follow-up for necessary diagnostic, preventive, and treatment services.
- By 2000 reduce iron deficiency to less than 3 percent among children aged 1 through 4 years. Baseline: 9 percent for children aged 1 through 2 years. For low-income children aged 1 to 2 years the baseline is 21 percent.

media, and other societal forces. The attention to the impact of families and school on children's health will make children targets to an increasing degree for delivery of health, educational, and other community programs.

Child Abuse Prevention

The third National Incidence Study of Child Abuse and Neglect in 1996 estimated that the number of abused and neglected children in the United States grew from 1.4 million in 1986 to more than 2.8 million in 1993. The number of children seriously injured quadrupled in the same time period. The study found that children of single parents and those from families with annual incomes below $15,000 were more likely to experience abuse. Girls are sexually abused three times more often than boys, while boys are at greater risk of emotional neglect and serious injury than girls. No significant race/ethnicity differences in maltreatment incidence were found. To better protect children, community services need to focus on prevention and urge families to use such services early before a child ends up in the hospital, on the street, or dead. Policies toward children need to be proactive and not simply reactive to emergencies.

Education for parents needs to strengthen skills in coping with stress and risk factors. Violence prevention will be further discussed in chapter 9.

Immunization Programs and Procedures

There are eight diseases for which routine vaccination is widely recommended; seven (diphtheria, measles, mumps, pertussis, polio, rubella, and tetanus) through vaccination of all children in the first years of life and one (influenza) through routine annual vaccination of individuals at high risk of complications or death from influenza infection. Many infectious diseases stimulate the production of protective **antibodies** that usually confer long-lasting, even lifelong, protection against reinfection. Vaccines and toxoids stimulate production of these antibodies without causing disease. Decisions to recommend routine use of immunizing agents are typically based on the risk of acquiring the disease, the severity of the disease or its consequences, the efficacy of the vaccine, the safety of the vaccine, and the number of doses required for initial immunization or boosters.

Progress   From the 1950s through the mid-1970s remarkable progress was made in the reduction of vaccine-preventable diseases throughout the world. Historically, immunization programs have focused primarily on the protection of children against the childhood diseases, which only thirty years ago produced extensive mortality and residual disability in even the most advanced countries. In the United States the 1955 Poliomyelitis Vaccine Assistance Act, later expanded by the Vaccine Assistance Act of 1962, supported extensive growth in state-level programs to provide children with immunizations against the major childhood vaccine-preventable diseases. As more vaccines were developed, the list of diseases to be combated was expanded, and the number of reported cases fell as the vaccines came into wide use. As the incidence of disease fell, however, efforts to immunize all children did not receive priority, and levels of immunity to many of these diseases crested and, in some places, declined.

Strategy Nationwide immunization campaigns in the United States periodically must raise the percentage of children fully protected against these diseases back up to 90 percent. Although an effective national assessment of the preschool population has not been developed, the immunization level is believed to be approximately 70 percent to 80 percent with certain pockets of the population having levels lower than 50 percent. Special efforts need to be made to reach black and Hispanic populations who have substantially lower immunization levels than the general population. Particular attention must be paid to the gap between immunization levels in affluent communities and those in low-income areas and to the differences in levels between school-age and preschool children.

Canada has less of a problem in maintaining high immunization levels because its universal health care system provides access for all income groups to child-care services, including immunizations. Canada also has maintained controls on the pricing of drugs, including vaccines. President Bill Clinton tackled the U.S. drug industry's pricing of vaccines in his first week in office. The components of vaccines recommended for a two-year-old child increased dramatically in cost between 1982 and 1992.

The federal taxes were levied by Congress in 1986 to create the Vaccine Injury Compensation Fund, providing no-fault compensation to children suffering severe side effects from vaccines. The liability of drug companies to pay such compensation before 1986 had driven several drug companies out of the business of manufacturing vaccines. Liability suits have also had the effect of causing some parents to fear the vaccines, but the actual risks of side effects remain lower than the risks of disease complications. Another factor in the price increase has been research financed largely by the drug companies. Since 1982 this research has resulted in the two new vaccines for bacterial meningitis and hepatitis B.

The same set of vaccines costs the public sector less because the state and federal governments buy in bulk at a discount of over 50 percent. Government programs alone, however, have not been adequate to achieve the immunization targets. Many public health clinics require a physician's referral or a complete physical examination before they will administer a vaccination. In the eleven states that purchase all vaccines for free administration to all children, regardless of income, the increase in immunization rates over the national average of 58 percent is only to 61 percent. The problem then is not just price. Community coordination such as that achieved during the 1960s with the "Oral Polio Sundays" is needed with support from a variety of national and community organizations.

Coordination Many states have stepped up enforcement of school entry immunization laws and have expanded the requirements to include more diseases. All fifty states and ten Canadian provinces have school immunization statutes that will help ensure that North American children are protected against vaccine-preventable childhood diseases. One of the missing ingredients to coordinate national efforts is a childhood immunization registry. Central ideas that have emerged from several national efforts to create such a system are shown in figure 5-10. Such a system can help improve immunization rates by prompting parents when to take children for immunizations, by allowing health care providers to monitor immunization status of children, and by enabling health planners to identify populations at risk for delayed immunizations.

Schedule of Vaccines The generally recommended age to begin routine immunizations is two months. The first vaccines given are diphtheria and tetanus toxoids combined with pertussis vaccine, or **DPT,** and oral poliovirus vaccine, OPV. Measles vaccine for rubeola is most effective when given after one year of age. However, in some populations where natural measles occurs frequently in the first year of life, it is preferable to administer the rubeola vaccine as early as six

Figure 5-10

Recommended childhood immunization schedule, United States, January, 1995 (*Source:* Centers for Disease Control.)

A star ★ means your child is due for an immunization

Age ▶ Vaccine ▼	Birth	2 mos	4 mos	6 mos	12-15 mos	4-6 yrs	11-12 yrs
Hep B Hepatitis B	★	★		★			
DTP Diphtheria, tetanus, and pertussis		★	★	★	★	★	★*
Hib *H. influenzae* type b		★	★	★	★		
OPV Polio		★	★	★		★	
MMR Measles, mumps, and rubella					★	★ or ★**	

Note: Recommended ages are flexible, and some doctors may use slightly
   different schedules.
   Combined DTP and Hib vaccines are available.

*Td (tetanus and diphtheria toxoids for adult use) is given at this age.
**MMR may be given at 4-6 years of age or 11-12 years of age depending on
state school laws.

months of age. If this is necessary in a community, a repeat dose of measles vaccine needs to be given after the age of one year to immunize any infants whose earlier vaccine response had been blocked by passive immunity.

Selected Screening Programs

Among successful community screening programs for children are those directed at reducing lead poisoning in children. Approaches included door-to-door screening in high-risk areas and screening required as part of Medicaid and the Early and Periodic Screening, Diagnosis, and Treatment program. Screening was part of broader health promotion actions, which included legislation directed at sources of lead and continuing education for health professionals to detect and treat high lead levels in children. Despite the progress, the threat still exists for many families living in houses where chipping and dust-producing lead-

based paint makes serious health risks unavoidable, where the soil has been polluted by lead, and where drinking water may contain lead pollution from old plumbing.

Screening for tuberculosis should be performed routinely prior to rubeola vaccination. In addition, a hematocrit for anemia should be done on all children during the first six months of life. This is particularly important in the low-birthweight infant who has grown quickly. Other diseases screened will depend on the community and the population at risk. Thus, screening for sickle cell anemia, Tay-Sachs disease, thalassemia, and other genetic diseases should be done if the population is of the corresponding ethnic group at risk.

Screening for illness should be carefully performed prior to placement in daycare centers. It should be repeated for the preschool and school physical examination, and hearing, speech, and eye examinations should be performed. Trained paramedical personnel can perform these routine screening. Dental evaluation and fluoride therapy for the prevention of caries are also necessary.

Health Services for Chronic Diseases

Special health services for children with chronic diseases and disorders such as cerebral palsy, epilepsy, and congenital malformations require careful planning within the community. Various health professionals need to be involved. Continuity and comprehensiveness of care are essential to afford the child the best quality of life possible. Much of the care may be given by nonmedical providers, particularly in the school setting and in other areas in the community. Unfortunately, because of the large number of U.S. programs that provide services for problems, attempts to obtain care may reveal a fragmented and frustrating maze. Many programs provide only part of the full care needs for each child, and each program may have different eligibility rules and a separate point of entry that is often difficult to locate. The comprehensiveness of Canada's health care system overcomes many of these difficulties.

In the case of complicated congenital deformities, such as meningomyelocele, children frequently require the services of more than one program or need a service that is not provided within the community in which they live. There is no greater deterrent to the effective and efficient care of children with chronic diseases than the fragmentation of services as a result of the isolation of categorical programs. For example, rehabilitation programs for children with orthopedic deformities may not be available for children damaged by trauma. Confusing eligibility and elimination rules may result in children slipping through the cracks between programs that are narrowly defined and poorly coordinated. Health education can help families by providing information not only on community resources, options, and requirements but also on strategies for negotiating among them. Such strategies may include clarifying needs, identifying questions to be answered, training in childcare, and identifying key decision makers.

Organization of Health Services

Many programs have been developed by the federal governments and by the states and provinces of the United States and Canada to provide health services for children. These programs have had a major role in improving the health of the nations' children, but for a number of reasons some of them are less effective. The U.S. Federal Maternal and Child Health (MCH) and Crippled Children's Services (CCS) programs of Title V of the Social Security Act, for example, were created in 1935 to provide national leadership in the field of maternal and child health and to direct the state MCH and state CCS programs. Thus the state MCH programs remain the major providers of basic health services for mothers and children, and the state CCS programs remain the major public system for providing the special health services required for children with chronic diseases and disorders. The legislation that created these programs did not link them to community health programs and services.

Other categorical programs created by Congress have independent organizational structures at the federal, state, and community levels; these include Title I programs, the Developmental Disabilities program, the Early and Periodic Screening, Diagnosis and Treatment (EPSDT) program, and the Supplemental Food Program for Women, Infants, and Children (WIC). Some of these function at the national, state, and community levels parallel to, or even in open competition with, each other and with the MCH and CCS programs. The result is a duplication of services, inefficiencies in administration, and increased costs. More important, the fragmentation of service results in some children receiving suboptimum care or not receiving needed services. Table 5-2 suggests new models and ways that these programs could overcome their problems of coordination and fragmentation.

Some states and different communities have established special units in their mental retardation programs for the identification and care of such children. Mental health programs for children frequently dovetail with the adult services,

Table 5-2

Future Models at a Glance for Child Health

Future models will focus on	Rather than
a whole-life approach to health	specific symptoms
health investment strategies	band-aid solutions to problems
strengthening the capabilities of children and youth to increase their choices and their ability to continuously improve their lives	changing problem behaviors
constellations of success measures identified by the young people, the adults who are involved, and organizations	needs assessments
success measures that legitimize a young person's personal experience, intuitive deductions, and inner perceptions	statistics and indicators that measure external factors
organizations and ministries structured around human investment	structures that primarily serve institutions/systems/professionals
unusual partnerships to find innovative solutions	single discipline/sector approaches
resources to build young people's capacity to pursue their own lives	funding for institutions and high-tech procedures first
lessening the number of children living in poverty	spending millions to research one disease
the importance of family and friends	individual counseling
supporting informal play and group interaction	policies that prevent access to community facilities
involving children and youth in creating solutions and making decisions	doing what is best for them from an adult perspective

Source: British Columbia Ministry of Health.

and some function through the schools. Psychological services may be obtained through mental health programs or the school system. Each community must determine the organization of its own community child health services. The purposes of such services should be strongly influenced by national and state or provincial goals, and adapted by the community after careful study of that community's needs. The organization of local child health service should be the responsibility of the community. Thus the number and type of health services provided will vary a great deal. Certain services and programs, for example those concerned with teenage pregnancy and abortion counseling, sexually transmitted disease, and child abuse, should be available for all children who need them.

CHILD DAYCARE PROGRAMS

As more women enter the work force, the need for accessible, affordable, quality daycare for children has risen. Approximately 67 percent of married women who have children under 18 years of age work outside the home in the United States; nearly 70 percent of Canadian women with children under 16 years of age do the same. Many European countries have passed laws that guarantee

U.S. Objectives for Child Care Centers

- By 2000 95 percent of children in licensed child care facilities and kindergarten will have the basic immunization series. Baseline: 94 percent for children in licensed child care and 97 percent for children entering school.
- By 2000 reduce infectious diarrhea by at least 25 percent among children in licensed child care centers. Children in licensed child care centers have three to four times as much diarrheal disease as do those not in child care.
- By 2000 increase to at least 90 percent the proportion of child care food services with menus that are consistent with the nutrition principles in the *Dietary Guidelines for Americans* (or the *Canadian Food Guide*).

Source: Healthy People 2000; and Midcourse Review, 1996.

Figure 5-11

Child care provides for the development of social skills, but also brings the greater risks of communicable disease transfer. (*Source:* PhotoDisc, Inc.)

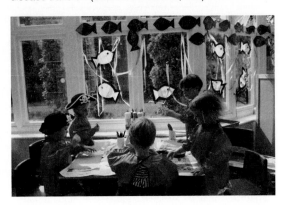

working mothers and sometimes fathers time off and wage replacement after delivery to care for their infants. In Canada women are guaranteed 15 weeks off work with 60 percent replacement of their salaries. The Family Leave Bill in the United States helps families care for seriously ill children.

Children of working families are cared for in a variety of ways (figure 5-11). Parents themselves provide care for 28 percent of working mothers, other relatives 19 percent, commercial daycare 28 percent, and neighborhood daycare 20 percent. Studies show that poor childcare practices, whether by parents or others, are linked to violence, crime, illness, depression, and immature moral development. Childcare centers are targeted with special objectives for the nation's health with regard to immunization levels, food service, and infectious diarrhea. Health education strategies directed at families can clarify childcare options and identify criteria for selecting among options. Health education strategies directed at childcare workers need to focus on year 2000 objectives.

Head Start programs in the United States have been found in long-term studies to have saved $4.75 in reduced costs of special education, public assistance, and crime for every dollar invested in quality preschool education. Fewer than half of the disadvantaged four-year-old children eligible for Head Start participated in the program in 1990. This was increased to 55 percent in 1991. The year 2000 target is 100 percent.

SCHOOL HEALTH PROGRAMS

Comprehensive school health programs that educate children about physical activity, sexuality, personal hygiene, substance abuse, physical abuse, nutrition, mental health, and the environment should be instituted on a communitywide basis. These programs should be supported by health services and environmental protection within the school setting and in the community. Although the U.S. national objectives is that 50 percent of schools provide comprehensive school health education at elementary and secondary levels by the year 2000, states vary in whether and what kind of school health education is provided (figure 5-12).

····················
Figure 5-12

States and territories requiring school health education as of 1990, with content varying by grade level (*Sources:* National Association of States Boards of Education, Council of Chief State School Officers, AIDS, HIV, and school health education; State policies and programs, 1990, Alexandria, VA 1991, National Association of State Boards of Education.)

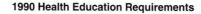

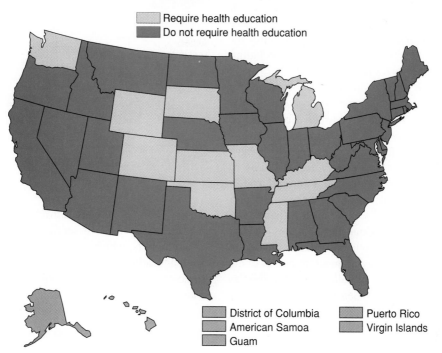

1990 Health Education Requirements

Require health education
Do not require health education

District of Columbia
American Samoa
Guam

Puerto Rico
Virgin Islands

Children and youth who spend most of the day in school are a captive audience during school hours. Teachers provide instruction and experiences that can help young people make decisions that promote health and prevent disease. School counseling personnel and administrators share responsibility for the early identification and treatment of physical and emotional health problems and in the building of a physical and social environment that is conducive to health growth and development. Parents enhance the opportunities for good health for their children by fostering healthful personal habits and by ensuring availability and use of appropriate childhood health services.

Comprehensive school health education requires intersectoral and multidisciplinary collaborations and must include coalitions and team building at the community level. Coalitions provide shared responsibility and resources and the development and strengthening of broader power bases. A broader community power base can provide political advocacy for the health of children and youth, who cannot vote for themselves. Without such collaboration schools are a convenient scapegoat for community problems such as drug abuse, teenage pregnancies, and highway injuries and deaths among youth. They have been criticized and blamed for many things pertaining to the generation gap, including the decline of reading and writing skills, couch-potato television viewing, and the decline of physical fitness in youth. Recognizing their accountability for the decline of reading and writing skills, schools are resistant to accepting any new responsibilities for the education of children and youth with respect to health and safety, sexuality, and substance abuse. Where they have accepted educational responsibility for these, they often have drawn the line excluding their accountability for behavior.

Part of the debate on schools between the health and educational sectors has centered on the question of responsibility. The health sector has had limited opportunity—given its current structure—to reach well children. Health professionals have assumed that it was the school's responsibility to provide most of the health and safety education and to provide many health services and health protection needs. The schools in turn have seen most of these needs as outside their purview and have repealed the responsibility to parents. Parents, then, can avoid paying much attention to the health and safety needs of their children as long as the children are well. When their children suffer illnesses, injury, or dysfunction, they look to the health sector for help or relief, thus completing the circle of transferred responsibility. The way out of this cycle is to share and coordinate the responsibility among schools, parents, and health agencies, while developing the knowledge and skills of children, so that they can assume a greater role in protecting themselves and promoting their own health.

The dramatic shift in child and youth health priorities suggests the need for the reassessment of health strategies, services, and policies organized for the enhancement of health and the prevention of disease. This includes a role for the community health sector in not only facilitating shared responsibility between schools and parents, but in empowering youth. What about the adequate labeling of foods so that even children could use the labels? What about advocating the availability of healthful food choices in restaurants frequented by

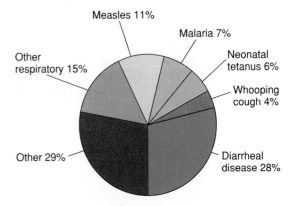

Causes of child deaths worldwide

Measles 11%
Malaria 7%
Neonatal tetanus 6%
Other respiratory 15%
Whooping cough 4%
Other 29%
Diarrheal disease 28%

children and possibly the restriction of permissible fat content in standard servings such as in triple cheeseburgers, which contain 15 teaspoons of fat? Such education and nutrition goals are reflected in some of the national health objectives directed toward school health.

INTERNATIONAL CHILD SURVIVAL

In the next hour, 1,700 children will die of illness and malnutrition. Television has brought many of these starving faces into our homes on the nightly news. Most of these children live in developing countries. The number of deaths amounts to 40,000 a day—15 million a year. Many millions more will live out their lives with mental and physical handicaps. The causes of many of these deaths are preventable (figure 5-13). Less than 100 years ago, when the United States was a developing country, children were ravaged by the same diseases that now prevail in the Third World, and its infant mortality rate was as high.

Education and socioeconomic development, improved sanitation and other public health measures in Europe, North America, and a growing number of countries in the Western Pacific, have

Ten Objectives for the World's Children

- Raise immunization coverage to at least 80 percent
- Eliminate neonatal tetanus
- Reduce measles deaths and cases
- Eradicate polio in key areas
- Increase the use of oral rehydration therapy to 80 percent to help control diarrhea
- Make maternity hospitals "baby friendly" by supporting breast-feeding, and end free and low-cost supply of breast-milk substitutes to health care systems as defined by the International Code.
- Achieve universal iodization of salt
- Virtually eradicate vitamin A deficiency
- Virtually eliminate guinea-worm disease
- Ratify the Convention on the Right of the Child in every country

Source: The World Health Organization and the United Nations Children's Fund, 1995

enabled over 95 percent of their children to survive through the preschool years. In developing countries as many as 25 percent of all children die before their fifth birthday. The techniques to save at least half of these children are available, even without immediate improvements in socioeconomic development (see box titled "Ten Objectives for the World's Children").

Growth Monitoring

Recording a child's weight gain once each month and using a chart that costs only 10 cents can indicate malnutrition before it causes serious damage to a child's health. At this early stage, a community health worker can educate a family on ways to improve a child's nutritional health, even when food and money are scarce.

Oral Rehydration Therapy (ORT)

Of the annual toll of 15 million, 5 million of these children die of dehydration from diarrhea. It is the single biggest killer of young children. Preparation of a simple mixture of sugar, salt, and water from a 10-cent packet can enable a child to absorb 25 times more fluid and salts than before. However, only 15 percent of families in the world know of this ORT method so far, although ORT is saving half a million children each year.

Breast-feeding

Infant formulas marketed in developing countries are often mixed with contaminated water. The baby has not yet developed immunities against the organisms found in the water. Therefore, infants receiving these formulas have as much as three times greater risk of dying in infancy than babies who are breast-fed. Breast milk provides the best possible nutrition. It also provides natural immunities against childhood diseases during the first six months of feeding.

Immunization

Six diseases—measles, whooping cough, tetanus, polio, tuberculosis, and diphtheria—account for over 3.5 million preventable childhood deaths yearly. Only 10 percent of children in the developing world receive immunizations against these diseases. The cost of the full set of immunizations is only $5.

Education, Food Supplements, and Family Planning

Health education can make these techniques readily available to families with little dependence on improved access to medical facilities or personnel. More general education for women can also make them more willing and able to take advantage of new innovations. The level of a mother's education is the single most influential factor in the health of her children.

Food supplements of only a few hundred calories a day for chronically malnourished women who are pregnant can reduce low-birthweight deaths by 50 percent. A 2-cent megadose of vitamin A every six months or a daily handful of leafy green vegetables can prevent the deficiency that causes vision impairment in 10 million young children and blindness in more than a quarter million children each year.

Spacing of births allows couples to provide more care and family resources to each infant, thereby assuring its survival with greater certainty. Spacing also gives the mother more time to regain her strength and to resume her education or career before the next pregnancy. Education for family planning remains a high priority for public health in the Third World.

SUMMARY

Mortality of mothers, infants, and children does not tell the entire story of reproductive, infant, and child health, but knowledge of what causes deaths at the various fetal, infancy, and childhood stages should be of benefit in any community health program. Specific death rates point out where specific emphasis must be placed if we are to save the lives of mothers, infants, and children.

To propose that all of these deaths could be prevented is unrealistic, but to say that at least half of them could be prevented with our present knowledge and means is a reasonable objective for the United States. Certainly injury deaths, which loom so prominently in the statistics of childhood, can be reduced. Deaths from infectious diseases can be controlled better than is indicated in the statistics. The health of mothers and children in all countries can be further improved.

Reproductive, infant, and child health care programs are the foundation of community and population health programs because they are the basis for health education, immunization, early diagnosis and treatment, and the development of health habits that sustain later health habits. In the spirit of disease prevention and health promotion, reproductive health is essential to successful infant health outcomes, which in turn provide the foundation for successful community health programs directed at children, youth, adults, and eventually the elderly.

WEB Links

http://www.familiesusa.org
Families USA Foundation

http://www.cfc-efc.ca/
Child and Family Canada

http://kidshealth.org/
Includes sections for kids, parents, and professionals

http://www.parentsoup.com/library/organizations/
bpdm018.html
Association of Maternal and Child Health Programs

QUESTIONS FOR REVIEW

1. If good reproductive health depends on choice, what factors affect such choice?
2. How does the changing structure of the family affect maternal and infant health?
3. What is the reciprocal obligation of expectant parents and society?
4. How can new models of child health programs contribute to the new morbidity issues for children?
5. What economic factors in your community are significant in maternal health?
6. What is one of the leading causes of infant deaths, and what are some measures for reducing the number of infant deaths from this cause?
7. Where are the best places in the field of infant health to invest time and funds for research?
8. What were the causes of infant deaths in your community during the past five years? How do these compare with worldwide causes of infant mortality?
9. What are the contributions of voluntary agencies to the infant health program in your community?
10. How would you educate parents about the advisability of taking apparently healthy children to their family physician, pediatrician, or child health clinic for a checkup at regular intervals?
11. What are some of the special social and mental health problems associated with disability in childhood, and what is a community's responsibility in dealing with these problems?

12. Does the school assume the role of the parent when it concerns itself with the pupil's health?

13. What official and voluntary agencies are available in your community for helping a family with a special needs child?

READINGS

Brown, S. S., and L. Eisenberg. 1995. *The best intentions: Unintended pregnancy and the well-being of children and families.* Washington, DC: National Academy Press.

This book provides specific recommendations to prevent unintended pregnancy, the clearest goal being that all pregnancies should be intended—clearly and consciously desired at the time of conception. It considers the effectiveness of pregnancy prevention programs, summarizes the health and social consequences of unintended pregnancy, and explores the complex web of influences on decisions about sex, contraception, and pregnancy.

Carnegie Corporation of New York. 1994. *Starting points: Meeting the needs of our youngest children.* New York: Author.

In no other period do such profound and rapid changes occur as during the first three years of life when the newborn grows from a completely dependent human to one who walks, talks, plays, and explores. This report provides a framework of scientific knowledge and offers an action agenda to ensure the healthy development of children from before birth to age three.

Committee on School Health, American Academy of Pediatrics, and P. R. Nader. 1993. *School health: Policy and practice.* 5th ed. Elk Grove Village, IL: American Academy of Pediatrics.

There is increasing recognition of the interdependence of health and educational services in attempting to optimize the potential and development of all children. This book provides health professionals and others with a framework and guidelines for developing comprehensive health-related programs for school-age children in a broad range of community settings.

Oberg, C. N., A. B. Nicholas, and M. L. Bach. 1994. *American's children: Triumph or tragedy.* Waldorf, MD: American Public Health Association.

America's children are increasingly represented in the poor and disadvantaged. The authors propose a solu-

tion to this plight in the form of an "Integrated Children's Network," which includes economic security, medical care, shelter, proper nutrition, childcare, and early education. Specific recommendations are provided on how current mechanisms can be improved.

BIBLIOGRAPHY

American Public Health Association and American Academy of Pediatrics. 1992. *Caring for our children: national health and safety performance standards for out-of-home child care programs.* Washington, DC: American Public Health Association.

B. C. Ministry of Health, Community Care Facilities Branch. 1992. *Preventing illness in childcare settings.* Victoria: Author.

Brett, K. M., K. C. Schoendorf, and J. L. Kiely. 1994. Differences between black and white women in the use of prenatal care technologies. *Am J Obstet Gynecol* 170(1 pt. 1):41–6.

Claire, M. 1995. *The abortion dilemma: Personal views on a public issue.* London: Plenum.

Field, P. A., and P. B. Marck. 1994. Uncertain motherhood. Thousand Oaks: Sage.

Fisher, E. B., R. B. Strunk, L. K. Sussman, C. Arfkin, R. K. Sykes, J. M. Munor, S. Haywood, D. Harrison, and S. Bascom. 1996. Acceptability and feasibility of a community approach to asthma management. *J. Asthma* 33:367.

Garbarino, J. 1995. *Raising children in a socially toxic environment.* San Francisco: Jossey-Bass.

Greenberg, L. W. 1991. Pediatric patient education: the unanswered challenge to medical education. *Patient Educ Couns.* 17:3.

Hawks, S. R. 1993. Fetal alcohol syndrome: implications for health education. *Health Educ* 24:22.

Heatherington, S. E. 1990. A controlled study of the effect of prepared childbirth classes on obstetric outcomes. *Birth* 17:86.

Hogue, C. J. R., and M. A. Hargraves. 1993. Class, race, and infant mortality in the United States, *Am J Public Health* 83:9.

Institute of Medicine Subcommittee for a Clinical Applications Guide. 1992. *Nutrition during pregnancy and lactation: an implementation guide.* Washington, DC: National Academy Press.

Kamerman, S. B., and A. J. Kahn. 1995. *Starting right: How America neglects its youngest children and what we can do about it.* Oxford: Oxford University Press.

Klerman, L. V. 1991. Alive and well? *A research and policy review of health programs for poor young children.* New York: National Center for Children in Poverty, Columbia University School of Public Health.

Keintz, M. K., L. Fleisher, and B. K. Rimer. 1994. Reaching mothers of preschool-aged children with a targeted quit smoking intervention. *J. Community Health* 19:25.

Malloy, M. H. H. J. Hoffman, and D. R. Peterson. 1992. Sudden infant death syndrome and maternal smoking. *Am J Public Health* 82:1380.

Mesters, L., R. Meertens, H. Crebolder, and G. Parcel. 1993. Development of a health education program for parents of preschool children with asthma. *Health Educ Res* 8:53.

Minkler, M. and K. M. Roe. 1993. Grandmothers as caregivers: raising children of the crack cocaine epidemic. Newbury Park, CA: Sage.

Parker, J. D., K. C. Schoendorf, and J. L. Kiely. 1994. Associations between measure of socioeconomic status and low birth weight, small for gestational age, and premature delivery in the United States. *Ann Epidemiol* 4(4): 271–8.

Read, J. 1995. *Counseling for fertility problems.* Thousand Oaks: Sage.

Reed, D. B. 1996. Focus groups identify desirable features of nutrition programs for mothers of preschool children. *J Am Dietetic Assoc* 96:501.

Rifkin, S. B. 1990. *Community participation in maternal and child health/family planning programmes: an analysis based on case study materials.* Geneva: World Health Organization.

Sciarillo, W. G., G. Alexander, and K. P. Farrell. 1992. Lead exposure and child behavior. *Am J Public Health* 82:1356.

Shane, P. G. 1996. *What about America's homeless children?* Thousand Oaks: Sage.

Siskind, V., C. Del Mar, and F. Schofield. 1993. Infant feeding in Queensland, Australia: long-term trends. *Am J Public Health* 83:103.

Stewart, D. D. 1993. Child passenger safety: current technical issues for advocates and professionals. *Fam Community Health* 15:12.

Sussman, S., C. W. Dent, D. Burton, A. W. Stacy, and B. R. Flay. 1995. *Developing school-based tobacco use prevention and cessation programs.* Thousand Oaks, Sage.

Weisz, V. G. 1994. *Children and adolescents in need: A legal primer for the helping professional.* Newberry Park: Sage.

Wortel, E., G. H. deGeus, G. Kok, and C. van. Woerkum. 1994. Injury control in pre-school children: a review of parental safety measures and the behavioural determinants. *Health Educ Res* 9:201.

Chapter 6

Adolescent Health

We abandon the young people at adolescence at the time when the negative peer group cultures are beginning to pull in ways that can be very troublesome. During that time, young people do tell us to go away, but they do not mean too far.

—James P. Comer

Most people who are going to smoke are hooked by the time they are 20 years old.

—M. Jocelyn Elder

If you think education is expensive, try ignorance.

—Derek Bok

Objectives

When you finish this chapter, you should be able to:

- Assess the special health problems and needs of the adolescent population of a community

- Identify programs appropriate to health promotion and disease prevention in these populations

---

Approximately 20 percent of American and Canadian adolescents suffer at least one serious health problem. In the United States, 25 percent of teens are at high risk for school failure, delinquency, early unprotected sexual intercourse, or substance abuse. In increasing numbers adolescents are poorly housed, poorly fed, and poorly educated. Such risks do not distribute evenly among the population. Roughly 51 percent of black teens, 45 percent of Hispanic teens, and 17 percent of white teens are "at risk." Teenagers in both countries are getting fatter and are less fit. Their 1995 to 1996 rates of tobacco, alcohol, and other drug use increased after more than a decade of declines. The rate of female sexual intercourse before grade ten has increased. With all these problems or risks, adolescents still seek health care less often than do other age groups. In the United States, they are more likely than any other age group to be underinsured or uninsured. The changing family structure has made parental guidance and nurturing less accessible to adolescents.

The community must fill these voids if it is to depend on this generation to become the adults

· · · · · · · · · · · · · · · · · ·

Figure 6-1

The potential of a child or adolescent to contribute to the community declines with the failure to intervene early, and the cost of treating or reversing problems increases with neglect. (*Source:* Oregon Legislative Committee on a Positive Future for Children and Families, 1993.)

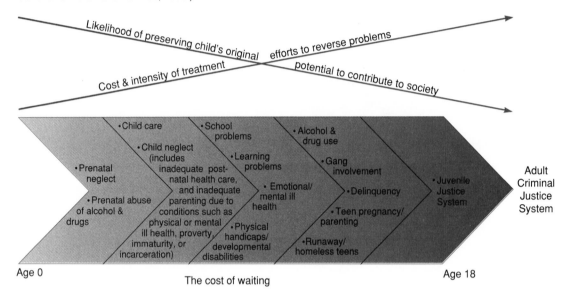

who must take responsibility for the community's health and well-being in the years ahead. The community must pick up the pieces of neglected needs and missed opportunity for community supports for adolescent development and a positive, preventative approach. Indeed the consequences of neglected needs in early prenatal care and early childhood development described in chapter 5 accumulate into adolescence. The cost to the community of waiting too long to intervene is that they get worse and increasingly hard to change. They sometimes lead, if uncorrected, to behavior and health problems that spill over into the community's well being in such forms as school disruption, delinquency, and crime, as illustrated in figure 6-1.

LIFE-SPAN TRANSITIONS

At the threshold between childhood and young adulthood, usually between ages ten and fourteen, teenagers become adolescents by virtue of **puberty.**

This is a time when new hormones are racing through the body, creating some emotional confusion, mood swings, and sexual awakening. Maturation to adult roles and characteristics brings with it a search for greater independence, new relationships, and new freedoms. This places the young adolescent at particular risk of making decisions and behavioral choices at times of vulnerability to unaccustomed feelings, often without the needed adult guidance and understanding. Some of the behavioral decisions, such as smoking or alcohol use, can lead to addictions; some can permanently injure the mind or body. Some place friends, family, or community at risk of injury or damage. These turbulent years set the stage for later adolescence, when still greater independence will take a greater toll if the earlier developmental process has led to self-destructive, self-indulgent, or self-demeaning behavior patterns.

Adolescents age twelve to fourteen are quite different from those ages fifteen to nineteen. The

Table 6-1

Examples of Issues for Health Promotion Related to Life-Span Transitions

Developmental transitions	Major tasks of coping and adaptation	Health consequences
Infant→child	Avoidance of hazards	Safety and injury control
Preschool→school	Selection of foods	Dental caries, obesity, nutritional deficiencies
Elem.→jr. high (early adolescence)	Resistance to peer pressure; changing bodily functions	Smoking, alcohol, drugs, pregnancy
Jr. High→high school (middle adolescence)	Development of autonomous identity and confidence	Substance abuse, pregnancy, auto accidents, sexually transmitted diseases
High school→work or higher education	Development of autonomous function and role; coping skills; uprooting	Suicide, homicide, alcoholism, addictions
Single→married and/or pregnancy and parenthood	Curtailed freedom and increased responsibility for life-style; uprooting	Congenital defects, infant mortality, low birth weight, obesity, stress
Young adult→middle age ("midlife" transition) Parent→"empty nest"	Reduced parenting roles, changing bodily function, reduced activity	Hypertension, digestive disease, atrophy, obesity, alcoholism
Working adult→retired adult or widowed	Reduced social roles; sedentary living; bereavement	Loneliness, reduced self-esteem, atrophy, loss of reasons for living and the will to live, or zest for living

Reproduced with permission from Green LW: Modifying and developing health behavior, *Annu Rev Public Health,* vol 5, © 1984 by Annual Reviews, Inc.

transitions from elementary to middle or junior high school and from there to high school are momentous changes in the lives of young people. The transition from high school to work or college is also stressful and sometimes fraught with new threats to health if not to life. The mortality risks for the broad age groups tell only part of the story of life-span variations in health. The problems of coping and adaptation to life span transitions have additional health consequences that are more pervasive than mortality risks at that age.

Transitions in the Life Span

Anticipating the potential health problems of populations so that they can be educationally prepared for them requires prediction. The best predictor of potential health problems in populations is age. Transitions from one age range to another could be the most propitious times to intervene for purposes

of primary prevention of problems anticipated in the next developmental stage in the life span.

As suggested in table 6-1, each transition in the life span has one or more major tasks of coping with challenging changes and adaptation associated with it. The life-span transitions mark important events affecting most people as they age. The tasks of coping and adaptation associated with those events or transitions lead to positive health consequences if they are carried out successfully. If the individual fails to cope or adapt effectively, they lead to negative consequences.

Other Transitions

The adolescent and adult years bring an increasing number of challenges to problem solving and adaptation in addition to life-span transitions. Transitions from one status, role, or circumstance to another also require adaptations of life-style. They present problems of stress and coping similar to those of the life span. For example, the high degree of mobility in North American life poses to communities the problems of uprooting, discontinuity of social support, isolation, confusion, stress, and economic insecurity. Unemployment clearly represents a challenge to coping and adaptation with known health consequences. These transitions, then, account for some of the typical or prevalent health problems and causes of death found in the adolescent and adult populations of most communities. Community and population health seek to design strategies to intervene effectively and preventively in relation to these transitions.

COMMUNITY INTERVENTION APPROACHES

The foregoing paragraphs suggest that communities should be able to organize a social history of intervention that anticipates critical transitions and prepares individuals for them.

Transition-Based Programs

The advantage of the life-span perspective is that it allows community health professionals to identify whole populations at risk using readily available demographic markers. Examples of such existing records related to age transitions in most communities are graduation, application for driver's license or marriage licenses, birth certificates, and applications for unemployment compensation. Other populations at risk of maladaptation to critical transitions can be identified from vital records. These may include divorce and death certificates and social agency records on newcomers to the community, disaster victims, school dropouts, and applicants for welfare or medical assistance. Clusters of transitions for an individual or for populations signal potential problems of coping with loss, bereavement, uprooting from social ties, and adaptation to new circumstances.

Being able to use such demographic markers to identify high-risk populations within the community means health agencies need not wait for the problems to surface as patients, clients, or victims before taking some action. This precept is fundamental to any preventative approach at the community level. In the prevention of childhood communicable diseases, it was possible to obtain nearly 100 percent coverage by requiring immunization of all children before they could enter school. Efforts toward the prevention of adolescent health problems resulting from life-style (see table 6-1) cannot be quite so regulatory or coercive.

Justification for Intervention

Communities could justify legal coercion in the prevention and control of communicable diseases on the grounds that they were protecting the population at large from the negligence or carelessness of individuals. With most life-style diseases and disabilities, the individual often is harming only his or her own health, so that coercive measures are difficult to justify in a democratic society. One can advance the argument that the harm people do to themselves usually spills over into the lives of others, especially family and friends.

That argument can be persuasive to the point of justifying coercive legislation prohibiting such individual behavior as drunk driving, child abuse, and other violent behavior. It can even carry over to more subtle infringements on the well-being of others, as addressed by the passage of "clean air" acts prohibiting smoking in crowded workplaces and restaurants. Legislative acts raising the age of driver's licensing and of alcohol purchasing also have successfully reduced overall automobile injury rates, especially alcohol-related injuries in the fifteen to nineteen age group.

For most of the individual life-styles influencing health, however, the justification for intervention must be based on a more generalized or collective notion of the well being of the community. These may include perceptions of social and economic health, quality of life, and responsibility. Such value-laden notions require that interventions remain largely noncoercive in their offering and voluntary in their selection. Restated from a different perspective, the individual retains the freedom to engage in the potentially harmful practice. The community then must find ways to minimize the damage done by practices that place a burden on the health and social resources of the community and ultimately on its quality of life and development.

The life-transitions approach to health promotion has the major advantage of not limiting itself to any particular disease. Each application anticipates a great number of potential problems known to compromise host resistance and resources and to produce risk factors for most of the leading causes of death and disability. It is a model, in short, that applies broadly to the range of behaviors and life circumstances posing threats to health. These may include smoking, alcohol and drug misuse, overeating, inactivity, reckless or violent behavior, and other dysfunctional ways of coping with stress or changing the conditions producing stress.

DEMOGRAPHY AND EPIDEMIOLOGY OF ADOLESCENT HEALTH

The subtle differences between psychosocial **maturation** and biological maturation blur the lines between childhood and adolescent status and between adolescence and young adult status. Psychosocial maturation concerns mental, emotional, moral, and social development. The ability of an adolescent to move through the life tasks associated with these ages signals psychosocial maturation (see table 6-1). Biological maturation for this age group centers on physical growth and development such as height and weight and on a set of sexual characteristics such as menstruation for females and voice change for males.

Psychosocial and biological maturation may occur at different rates, making it difficult to characterize the adolescent population by the usual developmental or chronological criteria. For example, biologically mature youth may lack the emotional maturity their physical size suggests; biologically immature youth may try to perform work or social roles their physical size does not

Figure 6-2

Adolescent modeling of behavior of adults and older teens creates challenges of coping with the consequences of the behavior beyond their psychosocial or physical maturity. (*Source:* Partnership for a Drug-Free America.)

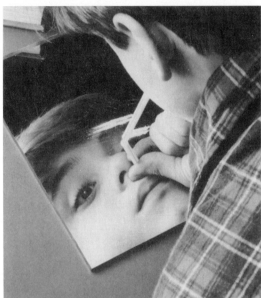

support. Biologically mature youth may experiment with behavior that seems to justify their physical size or maturity when their psychosocial maturity leaves them highly vulnerable to consequences of the behavior (figure 6-2).

Demographic Trends

The proportion of adolescents in most Western countries relative to the general population is on the decline, having reached a peak in the mid-1960s,

Objective for High School Graduation Rates

By 2000 increase the high school graduation rate to at least 90 percent. Baseline: 79 percent in 1988

when the post World War II babies, the "baby boomers," reached their teens. In 1980, 10- to 19-year-olds made up 17 percent of the U.S. population; by 1990, their percentage decreased to 14 percent. With an increase in the percentage of children under 5 years of age, resulting from the 1980s "baby boomlet," the percentage of younger adolescents is rising again in the 1990s.

The adolescent population of North America mirrors the increasing cultural diversity of Canada and the United States. Although whites comprise the largest proportion of adolescents, their overall percentage in the North American population fell relative to Hispanics, blacks, Native populations, Inuit or Alaskan natives, Asians, and other races during the 1980s. The number of Asian and Pacific Islander youth more than doubled between 1980 and 1990 in the United States and Canada. The percentage of adolescents living in poor or near-poor families also varies with race and ethnicity. The overall U.S. dropout rate for high school is 12.6 percent. This varies from 12.4 percent for whites, to 13.8 percent for blacks, and 33 percent for Hispanics. These demographic changes have implications for school health curriculum, community health activities, and community health services.

Epidemiological Trends

The overall U.S. death rates for those 15 to 24 years of age have decreased dramatically since the beginning of the century when there were nearly 600 deaths per 100,000 population. Communicable diseases were then among the leading causes of death. In 1983 the long-term decline in the

death rates for children 1 to 14 years of age continued, exceeding the 1990 objective for the nation by 1985 (figure 6-3A), but for 15- to 24-year-olds, the death rates reversed (figure 6-3B). This age group experienced increases for much of the remainder of the decade. Differences among races continued, and the leading causes of death changed. This is the only age group that has sustained a reversal in its death rates in recent decades.

In 1990 the United States saw another 4 percent increase in the death rate for the 15 to 24 age group. Declines in death rates for cancer and heart disease (6 percent and 1 percent, respectively) were offset by increases for injuries and homicides (up 4 percent and 25 percent, respectively). Motor vehicle crashes are the leading cause of death for youth in this age group, with rates twice as high in 1993 as those for the total population. They account for 78 percent of the injury deaths in 1990; over one-half are associated with alcohol. Homicide is the leading killer of black adolescents and young adults. The homicide rate increased from over 13 percent in 1980 to 20 percent in 1990. These deaths, too, are associated with alcohol and other drugs. Most suicides, the third leading cause of death, are among white males, although females attempt suicide approximately three times more often.

The corresponding comparisons for black and white U.S. adolescents ages 10 to 14 and 15 to 19 are shown in figure 6-4 for each of the leading causes of death. The three leading causes of death in these age groups—injuries, homicide, and suicide—are amenable to health-promotion strategies. In later sections we will show how the increases in these types of deaths are caused by another set of social, behavioral, and health problems, including alcohol and drug misuse, stress, and family disruption. For now, it will suffice to say that the inequities in life chances for survival and health take dramatic shape with the homicide experience of blacks compared to whites in the teenage years.

• • • • • • • • • • • • • • • • • •

Figure 6-3

A) Death rates for children 1 to 14 years of age, United States, 1977 to 1990, and 1990 goal. B) Death rates for adolescents and young adults 15 to 24 years of age, United States, 1977 to 1990, and 1990 goal. (*Source:* National Center for Health Statistics, National Vital Statistics System.)

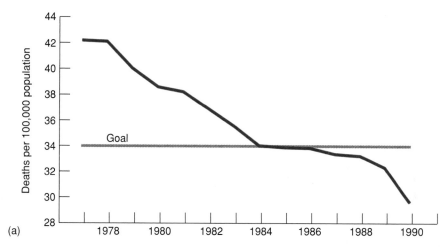

(a)

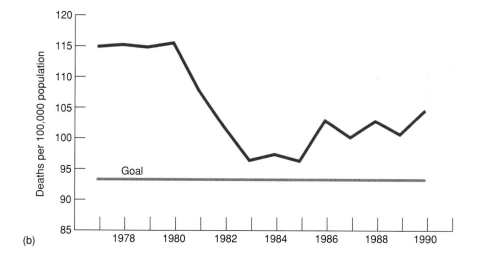

(b)

ADOLESCENT HEALTH CARE

A broad definition of adolescent health includes aspects of more traditional definitions, such as presence or absence of physical disease and disability. In addition, it includes consideration of developmental changes, social competence, health enhanc-ing or compromising behaviors, perceived quality of life, and social and physical environments. Most important, a definition of adolescent health needs to go beyond a view of adolescence *solely* as a transitional period between childhood and adulthood. Adolescence is to be lived, not lived through.

. . . .

Figure 6-4

Percent mortality attributable to seven leading causes of death for black and white U.S. adolescents ages 10 to 14 and 15 to 19. (*Source:* Office of Technology Assessment, 1991.)

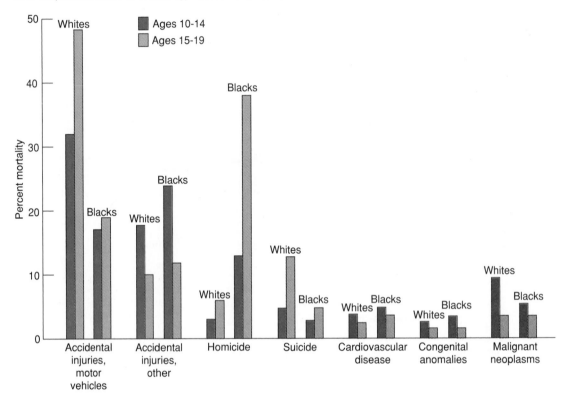

Recommendations for Preventive Services

The U.S. Preventive Services Task Force, building on the work of the Canadian Task Force on the Periodic Health Examination, recommends a specific set of screening, counseling, and selected other clinical procedures for adolescents. Table 6-2 shows the specific clinical services recommended for ages 13 to 18. Within the table are 15 high-risk ("HR") categories associated with some procedures. Table 6-2 identifies these as HR1 through HR15. Table 6-3 defines each of the high-risk groups. Screening and counseling for all adolescents should include history and current status of health behaviors and measures of physical growth

and blood pressure. Selected high-risk groups such as intravenous (IV) drug users and those with multiple sex partners should receive additional laboratory tests and counseling. Getting accurate information on such sensitive topics is important to planning health promotion strategies, but these groups may perceive the questions as intrusive and withhold the information.

Access to Health Care

Despite recommendations for preventive screening and counseling, 22 percent of American 16- to 24-year-olds had no private or government health insurance in 1990. These 7 million adolescents and young adults have limited or no access to health

Table 6-2

U.S. Preventive Services Task Force Recommendations for Clinical Prevention Procedures for Adolescents and Young Adults (Ages 11–24)

Screening

History	Physical exam/screening	Laboratory/diagnostic procedures

Dietary intake
Physical activity
Tobacco/alcohol/drug use
Sexual practices
	Height and weight
	Blood pressure
	Assess for problem drinking
	HIGH-RISK GROUPS (see table 6-3)
	    Complete skin exam (HR1)
	    Clinical testicular exam (HR2)
		HIGH-RISK GROUPS
		    Rubella antibodies (HR3)
		    VDRL/RPR (HR4)
		    Chlamydial testing (HR5)
		    Gonorrhea culture (HR6)
		    Counseling and testing for HIV (HR7)
		    Tuberculin skin test (PPD) (HR8)
		    Hearing (HR9)
		    Papanicolaou (Pap) smear (HR10)[4]

Counseling

Diet and exercise	Sexual practices	Dental health
Limit fat (especially saturated fat), cholesterol Adequate calcium intake[2] Caloric balance Selection of exercise program	Sexual development and behavior[3] Sexually transmitted diseases; partner selection, condoms/female barrier with spermicide Unintended pregnancy and contraceptive options	Daily tooth brushing with fluoride toothpaste, flossing Regular visits to dental care provider

Substance use	Injury prevention	Other primary preventive measures

Avoid tobacco use
Avoid alcohol and illicit drugs
Driving/other dangerous activities while under the influence
Treatment for abuse
HIGH-RISK GROUPS
    Sharing/using unsterilized needles and syringes (HR12)
	Lap/shoulder belts
	Safety helmets
	Violent behavior[5]
	Safe storage of firearms[5]
	Smoke detector
		HIGH-RISK GROUPS
		    Discussion of hemoglobin testing (HR13)
		    Skin protection from midday ultraviolet light (HR14)
		    Folic acid (HR16)
		    HIV screen (HR7)

Immunizations & chemoprophylaxis

Hepatitis B vaccine Tetanus-diphtheria (Td) booster [1] Folic acid for females planning/ capable of pregnancy, with multivitamins	Influenza vaccine HIGH-RISK GROUPS Daily fluoride supplements (HR15)	Hepatitis A vaccine (HR8)

Remain alert for:

Depressive symptoms Suicide risk factors (HR11)	Abnormal bereavement Tooth decay, malalignment, gingivitis	Signs of child abuse and neglect

This list of preventive services is not exhaustive. It reflects only those topics reviewed by the U.S. Preventive Services Task Force. Clinicians may wish to add other preventive services on a routine basis, and after considering the patient's medical history and other individual circumstances. Examples of target conditions not specifically examined by the Task Force include: Developmental disorders; Scoliosis; Behavioral and learning disorders; Parent/family dysfunction.

1. Once between ages 14 and 15. 2. For females. 3. Often best performed early in adolescence and with the involvement of parents. 4. Every 1-3 years. 5. Especially for males.

Source: This table is based on the original U.S. Preventive Services Task Force Report, with some modifications based on the second edition, 1996.

Table 6-3

Ages 13–18 High-Risk Categories for Clinical Prevention Services in Table 6-2

HR1 Persons with increased recreational or occupational exposure to sunlight, a family or personal history of skin cancer, or clinical evidence of precursor lesions

HR2 Males with a history of testicular atrophy

HR3 Females of childbearing age lacking evidence of immunity

HR4 Persons who engage in sex with multiple partners in areas in which syphilis is prevalent, prostitutes, or contacts of persons with active syphilis

HR5 Persons who attend clinics for sexually transmitted diseases; attend other high-risk health care facilities (e.g., adolescent and family planning clinic); or have other risk factors for chlamydial infection (e.g., multiple sexual partners or a sexual partner with multiple sexual contacts)

HR6 Persons with multiple sexual partners or a sexual partner with multiple contacts, sexual contacts of persons with culture-proven gonorrhea, or persons with a history of repeated episodes of gonorrhea

HR7 Persons seeking treatment for sexually transmitted diseases; homosexual and bisexual men; past or present intravenous (IV) drug users; persons with a history of exchanging sex for money or drugs, or multiple sexual partners; women whose past or present sexual partners were HIV-infected, bisexual, or IV drug

users; persons with long-term residence or birth in an area with high prevalence of HIV infection; or persons with a history of transfusion between 1978 and 1985

HR8 Household members of persons with tuberculosis or others at risk for close contact with the disease; recent immigrants or refugees from countries in which tuberculosis is common (e.g., Asia, Africa, Central and South America, Pacific Islands); migrant workers; residents of correctional institutions or homeless shelters; or persons with certain underlying medical disorders

HR9 Persons exposed regularly to excessive noise in recreational or other settings

HR10 Females who are sexually active or (if the sexual history is thought to be unreliable) aged 18 or older

HR11 Recent divorce, separation, unemployment, depression, alcohol or other drug abuse, serious medical illnesses, living alone, or recent bereavement

HR12 Intravenous drug users

HR13 Persons of Caribbean, Latin American, Asian, Mediterranean, or African descent

HR14 Persons with increased exposure to sunlight

HR15 Persons living in areas with inadequate water fluoridation (less than 0.7 parts per million)

HR16 Women with prior pregnancy affected by neural tube defect who are planning pregnancy

Source: U.S. Preventive Services Task Force, with modifications based on second edition, 1996.

services. Although this age group makes proportionally fewer visits to healthcare providers, health status indicators do not suggest that adolescents and young adults have the least need for health care.

ADOLESCENT HEALTH BEHAVIOR

Adolescent behavior is often of greater concern to the community than adolescent health. The health-related behavior of greatest emotional and political concern, although it does not show up directly in the mortality statistics, is the increase in sexual activity among teenagers. The associated consequences of adolescent pregnancy and sexually transmitted diseases, including HIV/AIDS, produce high emotional and social costs not accounted for in most vital statistics (figure 6-5).

Teenage Sex and Contraceptive Use

Since the 1970s sexually transmitted diseases, unintended pregnancies, and other problems that result from sexual activity have increased among adolescents in Canada and the United States. Among American students in grades 9 to 12 in 1995, 53 percent reported having had sexual intercourse. Male students were significantly more likely than female students to have had sexual intercourse, with 81 percent of black male students, 67 percent of black female students, 49 percent of male and female white students, and 58 percent of Hispanic students reported having had sexual intercourse. In Canada the rates are reported by age, with one-third of 15-year-old girls, more than one-half of the 17-year-olds, and nearly three-fourths of the Canadian 19-year-olds reporting they had engaged in sex.

Figure 6-5

This magazine ad for condom use was sponsored by the National AIDS Network, the American Foundation for AIDS Research, and the Advertising Council.

ANY WOMAN WHO WANTS TO HAVE A BABY SHOULD USE THEM.

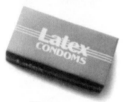

If you plan on having a child someday, you should be using latex condoms when you have sex now.

It's the best protection a sexually active woman has against the AIDS virus. A virus that has a 50-50 chance of passing from an infected mother to her child during pregnancy or birth.

And babies with AIDS rarely live to see their second birthday.

So take steps to make sure you don't get infected. Until you're ready to get pregnant, use a latex condom with spermicide. Use them every time, from start to finish, according to the manufacturers' directions.

Don't make exceptions. And don't start next week or next month.

Because no matter when you plan on having your baby, you have to start being a good mother right now.

HELP STOP AIDS. USE A CONDOM.

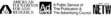

Photo: Jerry Friedman ⓒ1988, The Ad Council.

Among sexually active American students in 1995, approximately 54 percent used a condom. Seventeen percent had been using (or their partner had been using) birth control pills before their last sexual intercourse. The methods reportedly used by adolescents, such as birth control pills, condoms, and withdrawal, vary in effectiveness (see chapter 5, table 5-1). White female students were significantly more likely to use contraception than black or Hispanic female students. During sexual intercourse, alcohol or drug use by 25 percent of sexually active high school students can be expected to compromise the effective use of contraceptives or safe sex methods.

National objectives related to adolescent sexuality for the year 2000, developed during the late 1980s, include abstinence, combined method contraception (using more than one form of birth control during intercourse), and parent involvement. At the local level, nearly all school-based clinics provide counseling to students about choices related to sexual activity and birth control methods. Many of these clinics do not prescribe contraceptives, however, because of community resistance. Many school-based clinics operate in areas servicing low-income, minority adolescents who have limited access to other sources of health care. In addition to family planning, these clinics provide services such as physical examinations, immunizations, and nutrition counseling. Some colleges and universities have more boldly made condoms freely available to students and without requiring the perceived barrier of clinic visits in which students expect to have to register their names (figure 6-6).

Teenage Pregnancy and Childbirth

Teenage mothers face more complications in childbirth than women in their 20s, and their children are at greater risk for low birth weight, death in the first year of life, and developmental problems. Adolescent childbearing is a major concern for its social and economic consequences as much as for its health effects. From 1990 through 1995, the rates of births per 1,000 mothers age 15 to 19 were nearly 7 times higher in Canada than in Japan and 15 times higher in the United States (figure 6-7).

· · · · · · · · · · · · · · · · ·

Figure 6-6

Some more aggressive school-based clinics provide contraceptives for students in addition to family-planning services, examinations, and counseling. (*Source:* World Health Organization, Photo by Zafar.)

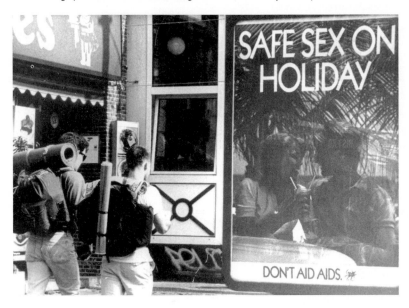

· · · · · · · · · · · · · · · · · ·

Figure 6-7

Adolescent birth rates for selected industrialized countries between 1990-1995. Births per 1,000 mothers age 15 to 19. (*Source:* United Nations Population Division, *World Population Prospects,* 1994.)

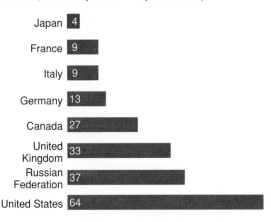

Japan	4
France	9
Italy	9
Germany	13
Canada	27
United Kingdom	33
Russian Federation	37
United States	64

The U.S. rate of 64 per 1,000 was the highest among industrialized countries, and four times higher than the average for the 15 countries in the European Union, which averaged 15 per 1,000.

The birth rates for U.S. females aged 15 to 17 years showed a steady decrease between 1970 and the mid-1980s. Between 1986 and 1989, however, the birth rate for black teenagers increased by 18 percent as did the birth rate for white teenagers. A second downturn then occurred between 1991 and 1996 with an overall decline each year from 1991 through 1995, from a high of 62.1 births per 1,000 females ages 15 to 19 to 56.9. Experts attribute these declines to better condom use; a plateau in previous increases in sexual activity rates; and the use of new, effective birth control methods. The birth rates are still higher than 20 years ago, and the rates of sexual activity are not declining.

Of the 1.1 million 15 to 19 year-olds in the United States who become pregnant each year, an estimated 84 percent do not intend to get pregnant.

· · · · · · · · · · · · · · · · · ·

Figure 6-8

What happens following sexual intercourse among U.S. adolescent males and females? (*Source:* Estimated from various sources by U.S. Congress, Office of Technology Assessment, 1991.)

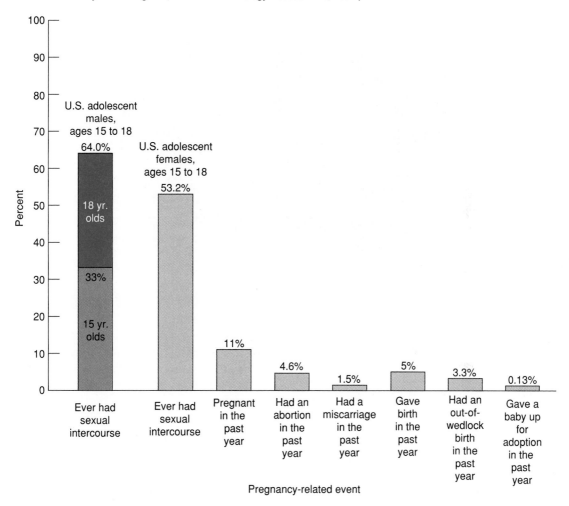

About one-half of these adolescents obtain abortions and about one-half of them give birth (figure 6-8). Black 15- to 17-year olds are almost five times more likely to have a second baby and seven times more likely to have a third baby than white females in the same age group.

The costs of adolescent pregnancy are high to young women and to the community. Besides the

Objective for Adolescent Pregnancy Rates

By 2000 reduce pregnancies among girls aged 17 and younger to no more than 50 per 1,000 adolescents. Baseline: 71.1 pregnancies per 1,000 girls aged 15 to 17 in 1985.

· · · · · · · · · · · · · · · · · · ·

Figure 6-9

Nurses provide much of the counseling to young mothers and teenagers of migrant families, requiring language skills and sensitivity to cultural perspectives. (Photo courtesy National Council for International Health.)

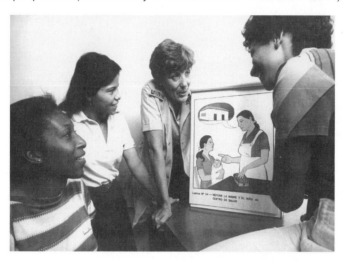

higher risks of low birthweight for infants born to very young mothers, teenage mothers face probable discontinuance of their education at an early age. This, in turn, diminishes employment prospects and increases the probability of welfare dependence. The Center for Population Options estimates that U.S. taxpayers spent $25 billion in federal dollars to assist families begun by a birth to a teenager. From 1989, through Aid to Families with Dependent Children (AFDC) and food stamps, support for these families increased by 16 percent to $3.5 billion in 1990. The additional risks of transmitting HIV infections from mothers to their babies will be discussed in the next section.

The causes of adolescent pregnancy are more complex than the simple stereotypes often used to characterize them. The debate too often begins and ends with the need for abstinence or to provide more accessible contraceptive services. Programs require greater understanding of adolescent attitudes, beliefs, values, and social influences in their choices about sexuality (figure 6-9). We will explore programs, services, and strategies more in the last section of this chapter.

Objectives for Adolescent Family Planning

- By 2000 reduce the proportion of adolescents who have engaged in sexual intercourse to no more than 15 percent by age 15 and 40 percent by age 17.
- By 2000 increase to at least 90 percent the proportion of sexually active, unmarried people aged 19 and younger who use contraception, especially combined-method contraception, that both effectively prevents pregnancy and provides barrier protection against disease.
- By 2000 increase to 85 percent the proportion of people aged 10 through 18 who have discussed human sexuality with their parents and/or have received instruction from them.

Sexually Transmitted Diseases and HIV/AIDS

Besides their risk for pregnancy, sexually active adolescents are also at risk for human immunodeficiency virus (HIV)/acquired immunodeficiency syndrome (AIDS) and sexually transmitted diseases

∙∙∙∙∙∙∙∙∙∙∙∙∙∙∙∙∙∙∙∙

Figure 6-10

Uptake of first use of selected drugs by age, United States, 1996. (*Source:* Centers for Disease Control and National Institute on Drug Abuse, U.S. Department of Health and Human Services.)

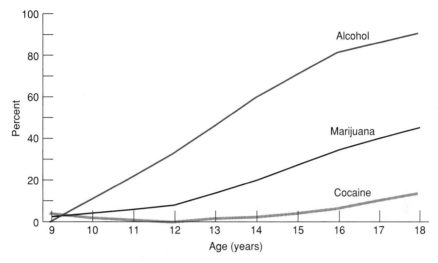

*Unweighted sample size = 11,631 students.

Objectives for Sexually Transmitted Diseases

- By 2000 increase to at least 60 percent the proportion of sexually active, unmarried 15- to 19-year-old women who used a condom at last sexual intercourse. Baseline: 25 percent used a condom at last sexual intercourse in 1988.
- By 2000 include instruction in sexually transmitted disease transmission prevention in the curricula of all middle and secondary schools. Baseline: 95 percent of schools in 1988.

(STDs). These infections spread by transfer of organisms from person to person during unprotected sexual contact. By age 21 approximately one out of every five young Americans has required treatment for an STD. Only some teenagers are sexually active, therefore this amounts to a rate of at least 25 percent among all adolescents who are sexually active and over 40 percent in the older teens. The number of AIDS cases nationally among American adolescents ages 13 to 19 doubled in the two years between 1993 and 1995 and has become the sixth leading cause of death for 15- to 24-year-olds.

About one out of three newly reported gonorrhea cases and 10 percent of newly reported syphilis cases in the United States occur among 10- to 19-year-olds. These and other STDs can cause serious complications, including pelvic inflammatory disease, sterility, ectopic pregnancy, and blindness.

Alcohol, Tobacco, and Illicit Drug Use

The use of alcohol, marijuana, and cocaine by high school seniors decreased throughout the 1980s. The use of tobacco, however, remained relatively constant. Beginning in the 1990s, teen use of these substances began to rise again. By age 18 over 90 percent of adolescents have tried alcohol, over 40 percent have tried marijuana, and over 10 percent have tried cocaine (figure 6-10). Use of these substances in adolescent years has the potential to set patterns for future behaviors that have an impact on health beyond the adolescent years.

Objectives for Adolescent Alcohol Use

- By 2000 reduce deaths among people aged 15 through 24 caused by alcohol-related motor vehicle crashes to no more than 18 per 100,000. Baseline: 21.5 per 100,000 in 1987.
- By 2000 reduce the percentage of 12- to 17-year-old youth who have used alcohol in the past month to 12.6 percent. Baseline: 25.2 percent in 1988.

Alcohol Use Alcohol use is lower in high school students than in the early 1980s, but alcohol remains the major drug of choice for adolescents. In 1996, over 80 percent of U.S. students in grades 9 through 12 have had at least one drink of alcohol. European countries have concentrated on preventing harm from drug and alcohol use rather than on preventing use. The American and Canadian programs have emphasized preventing initiation and decreasing overall use. This strategy has had little impact on alcohol use. Drinking in North America is more prevalent among those aged 18 to 24 than in any other age group. Alcohol use by adolescents that impairs judgment has serious consequences for injuries and homicides. One-half of motor vehicle accidents for 15- to 24-year-olds involve alcohol. Laws that make it illegal to sell alcohol to minors discourage but do not prevent adolescents from obtaining alcohol. Educational and other interventions intended to reduce alcohol use by adolescents need to address not only youth themselves, but also their families, friends and those who give or sell alcohol to them (figure 6-11).

Tobacco Use The Youth Risk Behavior Survey by the Centers for Disease Control in 1996 showed that 71 percent of all students in grades 9 through 12 had tried cigarette smoking. The percentage of students who tried cigarette smoking increases significantly between grades 9 and 12. The percentage of high school seniors currently smoking declined until 1992, but has increased

Figure 6-11

A partnership of a voluntary association and a federal agency, together with the Ad Council, sponsored this public service magazine spot as part of a national campaign on teenage alcoholism. (*Source:* Advertising Council, New York.)

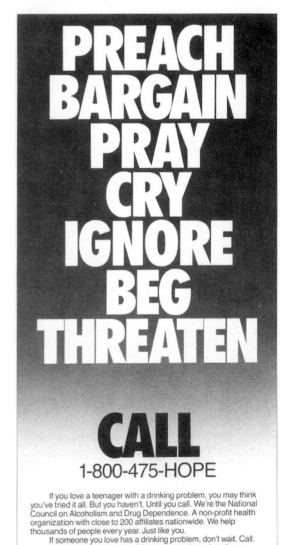

Figure 6-12

College student smoking has shown signs of inheriting the increases in teen smoking. (*Source:* Office on Smoking and Health, Centers for Disease Control and Prevention, U.S. Department of Health and Human Services.)

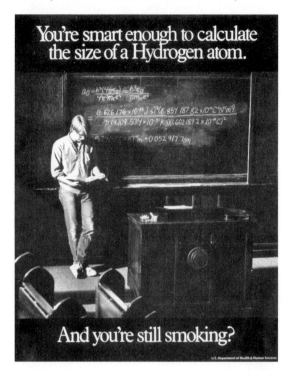

Figure 6-13

Smokeless tobacco, popular with teenage males, especially in rural areas, carries most of the risks of smoking plus added risks of cancer in the oral cavity. (*Source:* National Institute for Dental Research and National Cancer Institute, National Institutes of Health, U.S. Department of Health and Human Services.)

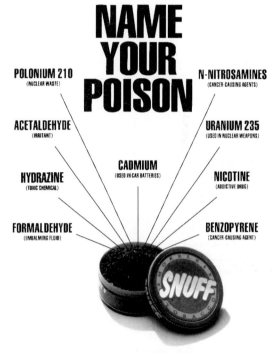

since then. Seniors who smoke show up in increased college smoking rates (figure 6-12). Smokeless tobacco use (chewing tobacco or snuff) was reported by over 11 percent of all students in the 1996 Youth Risk Behavior Survey. This rate is higher in rural areas. Significantly more males than females are likely to use this form of tobacco. Although cigarettes are associated with damage to the respiratory system and lungs, smokeless tobacco causes damage to the mouth, lips, and tongue. Both forms of tobacco are associated with increased cancer rates (figure 6-13).

Illicit Drug Use   The use of illicit drugs such as marijuana, cocaine, inhalants, hallucinogens, heroin, or nonprescription use of psychotherapeu-

tic drugs (sedatives or stimulants) appears to be far less common among adolescents living at home than the use of alcohol or tobacco. The percentages of high school seniors who had tried marijuana or cocaine in the previous month were more than halved during the 1980s to 14 percent and 2 percent, respectively, by 1990. Since 1990, however, rates have more than tripled for ever-use of marijuana and cocaine to 42 percent and 7 percent in 1996. White students are three times more

Objectives for Teenage Smoking Reduction (U.S. *Healthy People 2000*)

By 2000 reduce the initiation of smoking by youth to no more than 15 percent as measured by the prevalence of smoking among people ages 20 through 24. Baseline: 29.5 percent in 1987.
What needs to be done in communities to support the continuing reductions?

Objectives for Illicit Drug Use Reduction

By 2000 reduce the percentage of 12- to 17-year-olds who used marijuana in the last month to 3.2 percent. Baseline: 6.4 percent in 1988.
By 2000 reduce the percentage of 12- to 17-year-olds who used cocaine in the last month to 0.6 percent. Baseline: 1.1 percent in 1988.

Objectives for Tobacco Use Reduction by Adolescents (1996 Revision)

- By 2000 reduce the initiation of cigarette smoking by children and youths so that no more than 15 percent have become regular cigarette smokers by age 20. Baseline: 30 percent of youths had become regular cigarette smokers by ages 20 to 24 in 1987.
- By 2000 reduce smokeless tobacco use by males aged 12 to 24 to a prevalence of no more than 4 percent. Baseline: 6.6 percent among males aged 12 to 17 in 1988.

likely than black students to have used either drug in the previous month. Some black youth who may daily see the crime and horror of drug use in their communities have compelling reasons for turning away from illegal drug use, but their economic circumstances may make drug dealing seem the only viable alternative for financial success.

Diet and Physical Fitness for Adolescents

Dietary Patterns Dietary patterns established during youth may extend into adulthood and increase the risk for cancer and other chronic diseases. Diets that are high in fat and low in fruit, vegetables, and grain are of particular concern to future health. In 1996, only 28 percent of high school students were eating five or more servings of fruits and vegetables, the recommended daily intake. The 1996 national Youth Risk Behavior survey also showed that 40 percent of students were eating more than two servings daily of food high in fat content, such as hamburgers, hot dogs, sausage, french fries, potato chips, cookies, doughnuts, pie, or cake. Male students had better fruit and vegetable consumption rates, but worse fat consumption, than female students.

Weight and Physical Activity Physical activity and dietary patterns of adolescents contribute to problems of obesity. In 1996, more than one-fourth (28 percent) of high school students in the United States thought they were overweight. Females were more likely to identify themselves as overweight than males. Close to 55 percent of American youth between 5 and 17 years are actually of average weight in proportion to their height. Another 38 percent are overweight, and the remaining 8 percent are underweight. There is almost a linear relationship between family income and the probability of being overweight. Poor children are almost three times as likely as children in families with higher incomes to be overweight. Black children, regardless of sociodemographic characteristics, were the most likely to be overweight and the least likely to be underweight. More than twice the proportion of black children was reported as overweight compared with Hispanic children and white children.

Steroids Public health and school officials view with increasing alarm the use of steroids among

Objective for Physical Activity for Adolescents

By 2000 increase to at least 75 percent the proportion of children and adolescents aged 6 to 17 who engage in vigorous physical activity that promotes the development and maintenance of cardiorespiratory fitness 3 or more days per week for 20 minutes or more per occasion. Baseline: 6 percent for youth aged 10 to 17 in 1984.

Objective for Weight Control for Adolescents

By 2000 keep overweight to a prevalence of no more that 15 percent among adolescents aged 12 to 19. Baseline: 15 percent in 1976–80.

Objective for Steroid Use Reduction

By 2000 reduce to no more than 3 percent the proportion of male high school seniors who use anabolic steroids. Baseline: 4.7 percent in 1989.

Objective for Adolescent Abuse and Neglect Reduction

By 2000 reduce rape and attempted rape of women aged 12 to 34 to no more than 225 per 100,000. Baseline: 250 per 100,000 in 1986.

adolescent athletes and body builders. Approximately 1 million Americans, one-half of them adolescents, use black-market steroids. Countless others are choosing from among more than 100 other substances, legal and illegal, to enhance physical size and performance. The problem received worldwide attention during the 1988 Olympics when Canadian runner Ben Johnson had to forfeit his gold medal because of steroid use. The risks of steroid use are considerable, including damage to muscles, sex organs, and the nervous system. In addition to its physical dangers, steroid use can lead to aggression, violence, and a vicious cycle of dependency. The encouragement to use steroids comes from a personal competitive desire, peers, some coaches, and even parents. Over one-half of the teens who use steroids start before age sixteen, sometimes with the encouragement of their parents.

Mental Health of Adolescents

Abuse and Neglect   Child abuse and neglect includes physical or mental injury, sexual abuse or exploitation, negligent treatment, or maltreatment

of a person under the age of 18 by a person responsible for the child's welfare. Nearly 1 million American children nationwide experience demonstrable harm as a result of maltreatment, and 1.5 million experienced abuse or neglect. Abuse can be physical, emotional, or sexual, the latter remaining the least frequent type of abuse. Neglect includes physical, educational, and emotional failure to provide for a child or adolescent's basic needs. A 1992 study in Canada reported that teenagers and children comprised a larger proportion of victims of sexual assault than adults. Four out of every 10 sexual assault victims were under 12-years-old, 4 between 12- and 19-years old, and 2 over 19-years-old.

The reasons for abuse and neglect are multiple and include individual characteristics of parents or children, family interactions, and environmental conditions (see figure 6.14). An adolescent's race, ethnicity, and geographic location have no significant impact on the incidence of maltreatment, but small family size decreases and large family size increases the possibility. Females experience more abuse than males.

The maltreatment of children and adolescents is a community problem. No single agency, individual, or discipline has the necessary knowledge,

· · · · · · · · · · · · · · · · · · ·

Figure 6-14

Advice to parents and guardians on how to control their impulse to abuse their children was made specific in this national campaign on prevention of child abuse. (*Source:* Advertising Council, New York.)

12 alternatives
to lashing out at your kid.
The next time everyday pressures build up to the point where you feel like lashing out—STOP! And try any of these simple alternatives.

You'll feel better . . . and so will your child.

1. Take a deep breath. And another. Then remember <u>you</u> are the adult . . .
2. Close your eyes and imagine you're hearing what your child is about to hear.
3. Press your lips together and count to 10. Or better yet, to 20.
4. Put your child in a time-out chair. (Remember the rule: one time-out minute for each year of age.)
5. Put yourself in a time-out chair. Think about why you are angry: Is it your child, or is your child simply a convenient target for your anger?
6. Phone a friend.
7. If someone can watch the children, go outside and take a walk.
8. Take a hot bath or splash cold water on your face.
9. Hug a pillow.
10. Turn on some music. Maybe even sing along.
11. Pick up a pencil and write down as many helpful words as you can think of. Save the list.
12. Write for prevention information: National Committee for Prevention of Child Abuse, Box 2866L, Chicago, IL 60690.

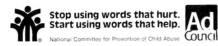

Stop using words that hurt. Start using words that help.
National Committee for Prevention of Child Abuse   **Ad Council**

Objective for Adolescent Suicide Rates

By 2000 reduce suicides among youths aged 15 to 19 to no more than 8.2 per 100,000. Baseline: 11.3 per 100,000 in 1988.

adjustment and stress reactions. The 1996 Youth Risk Behavior Survey by the Centers for Disease Control found that 24 percent of American students in grades 9 through 12 reported they had thought seriously in the past year about attempting suicide. Female students were significantly more likely than male students to report they had thought seriously about suicide and made an attempt that required medical attention. Black students reported lower levels of suicidal thought than white or Hispanic students.

Delinquency and Homelessness   The number of U.S. adolescents confined to public and private juvenile facilities for delinquent acts has been increasing. Most of the increase has apparently been due to an increase in the number of adolescents confined for minor offenses. Adolescents may be homeless, either on their own or with their families. Estimates for the United States range from 700,000 to as many as 1 million homeless and runaway adolescents each year (figure 6-15).

Anorexia Nervosa and Bulimia   Anorexia and bulimia are compulsive eating disorders with consequences similar to those of malnutrition. Both disorders involve the depletion of nutrients. Both have taken on epidemic numbers in adolescent and young women in North America. Societal pressures on women to be thin, especially media images, contribute to the problem for adolescents. The fixation on being thin causes the anorexic to starve herself and the bulimic to "binge and purge" (eating compulsively, then regurgitating). The bulimic person, male or female, also suffers from upper intestinal and oral tissue damage from the

skills, resources, or societal mandate to provide the assistance needed by those who are abused or neglected.

Suicide   Rates for suicide among adolescents 15- to 19-years of age more than tripled from 3 per 100,000 in 1950 to over 10 in 1988. They have continued to rise from 10.2 in 1989 to 10.9 in 1993. Suicide is the third leading cause of death among adolescents. Attempted suicide is a potentially lethal health event, a risk factor for future completed suicide, and an indicator of other health problems such as substance abuse, depression, or

Figure 6-15

Teenage homelessness affects all classes of runaway and shut-out adolescents, not just the poor. It relates to problems of crime, prostitution, and substance abuse. (*Source:* Advertising Council, New York.)

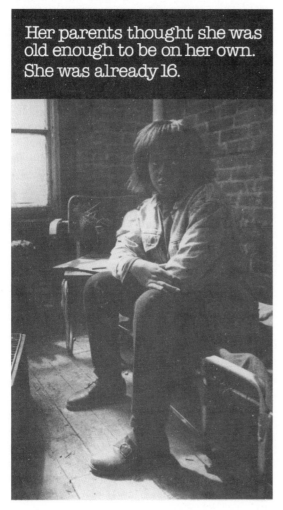

Her parents thought she was old enough to be on her own. She was already 16.

Every year hundreds of thousands of kids are thrown away. Put out onto the streets. With no job, no money and nowhere to go. But now there is a number for kids to call. The Covenant House Nineline helps kids with food, clothing, a place to sleep and, most of all, someone to talk to.

To get help in your hometown call our Nineline 1-800-999-9999. It's free.

Nineline
1-800-999-9999
Anytime.
Anywhere.

Objectives for Violence Among Adolescents

By 2000 reduce by 20 percent the incidence of physical fighting among adolescents aged 14 to 17. Baseline: not currently available.
By 2000 reduce by 20 percent the incidence of weapon carrying by adolescents aged 14 to 17. Baseline: not currently available.

frequent exposure of the throat and mouth to stomach acids. Dentists are often the first to detect the bulimic, recognizing their pattern of tooth erosion.

Adolescent Health Education and Services

School health education and school health services provide the best opportunities for the community to address the health needs of its teenage population. A major responsibility of community health education and ambulatory care services in the community is to recognize the special needs of adolescents beyond the classroom and the school. Peer pressure and parental disapproval present often conflicting and confusing expectations for adolescents in relation to their individual values and their decision-making ability. This confusion may preclude their seeking help before they begin using alcohol or become sexually active.

The personnel of ambulatory (walk-in) clinics and programs need to be aware that teens who are seeking services will have different levels of information, education, and experience. Adolescents vary in their knowledge levels, attitudes, cultural background, and behavior, therefore no single program activity can meet all of their needs. Teens may or may not be living with their parents or attending school, and regardless of the family's income they may be unable to pay for medical services. Health services staff members must deal with these variations in developmental levels, social situations, the teenagers' degree of communication with the parents, their ability to plan, and their willingness to recognize the risks of alcohol, drugs, or sexual activity. Ultimately, community health programs and services must find ways to help adolescents take preventive actions against unprotected sex, drunk driving, and other potential consequences of risky behavior. They must also walk a fine line between that obligation and the recognition that an important part of development at that stage of life is risk taking.

The guidelines that follow suggest specific considerations and strategies for adolescent health services and community projects.

- Adolescents often have vague and sometimes incorrect knowledge of drugs and sex. There is a need for open discussion of their ideas and beliefs about sex and reproduction; services should involve both members of a couple when possible. Teenagers need clear, unambiguous information about the possible results of alcohol or drug misuse and of sexual intercourse without moralizing. Group discussions sometimes help adolescents gain necessary information but should not replace individual counseling. Media and outreach programs should inform adolescents that the ambulatory care clinic or service will protect their privacy, maintain the confidentiality of their records, and provide free-of-charge education and counseling.

- Services and programs must give teenagers sufficient information at their level of understanding to make responsible decisions on key threats to health. Adolescents must know at least the basic ways to protect themselves against engaging in sexual activity that may lead to pregnancy or sexually transmitted diseases, and how to choose effective birth control methods. They must know the possible side effects and contraindications of use of the various contraceptive methods. They must become thoroughly aware of the physical, emotional, and social consequences of sexual activity for both participants, their families, and their communities.

- Risk taking with alcohol, drugs, or sex often results from, or leads to, other teenage problems. Health care providers can assist by referring teenagers to employment agencies, alternative school programs, and agencies dealing with drug or alcohol control. Counseling services must be available to a teenager in urgent need of discussing problems. Delay in getting to "talk to somebody" can cause the person to change his or her mind about asking for help.

- A project should identify the resources of the community and other resources available under state or province and federal programs that are potential sources of assistance and cooperation. Projects can also use the materials and experience of national groups (e.g., Red Cross, National Organization for Women, Salvation Army) that are also dealing with the problem of teenage pregnancy. Services and programs for adolescent populations should involve the local chapters of those organizations in the project's planning and execution.

- Community programs and services must find effective ways to reach the teenage population. They must select techniques and means of contact uniquely for the population; these might include teen-oriented radio stations, television, bulletin-board notices at teen hangouts, school group activities, and youth groups. Organizations such as the Parent-Teacher-Student Association, local school boards, churches, and Big Brother and Big Sister organizations have an interest in helping teenagers. Working with them can help to develop a broad base of support in the community. Working with the schools together with community groups can promote educational programs to alert teenagers and their parents about health issues related to smoking, drugs, drinking, and adolescent sexual activity (figure 6-16).

Develop Community Awareness   Projects should develop a plan for community education to increase awareness of adolescent pregnancy and health problems. Community programs and service agencies can do this by:

- Publicizing the scope and implications to the community of teenage sexual or substance

....

Figure 6-16

National campaigns on substance abuse or other teenage problems often provide a vehicle of mass media reminders to parents that can support the special efforts of schools in relation to these problems. (*Source:* Partnership for a Drug-Free America.)

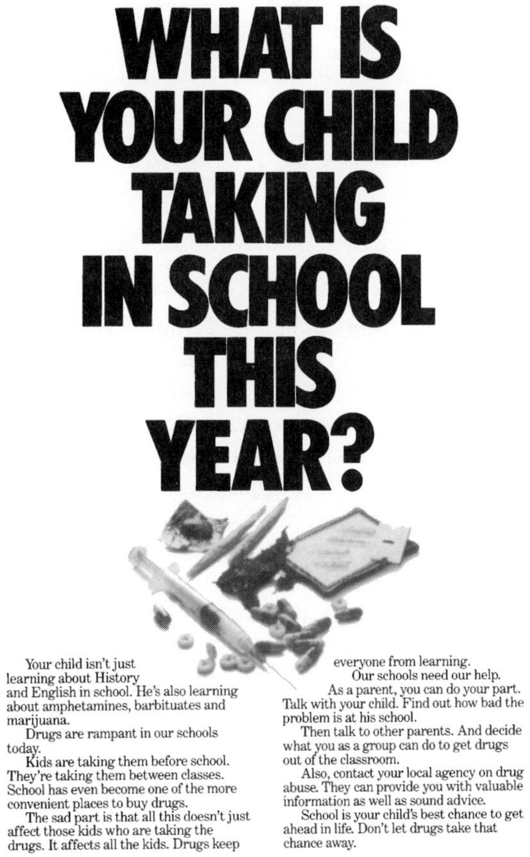

WHAT IS YOUR CHILD TAKING IN SCHOOL THIS YEAR?

Your child isn't just learning about History and English in school. He's also learning about amphetamines, barbituates and marijuana.

Drugs are rampant in our schools today.

Kids are taking them before school. They're taking them between classes. School has even become one of the more convenient places to buy drugs.

The sad part is that all this doesn't just affect those kids who are taking the drugs. It affects all the kids. Drugs keep everyone from learning.

Our schools need our help.

As a parent, you can do your part. Talk with your child. Find out how bad the problem is at his school.

Then talk to other parents. And decide what you as a group can do to get drugs out of the classroom.

Also, contact your local agency on drug abuse. They can provide you with valuable information as well as sound advice.

School is your child's best chance to get ahead in life. Don't let drugs take that chance away.

misuse activity (e.g., number of school dropouts due to pregnancy, number of teens with out-of-wedlock births, number of teen abortions, sexually-transmitted disease rates, the spread of HIV/AIDS, number of births to teenage women, number of automobile injuries and deaths involving alcohol). National media and data can serve to support or develop such information.

- Identifying community leaders and groups who can help to make contact with teens and remove barriers to their receiving services and continuing their education. These people could be school board members, social service workers, or youth workers. Parent groups can be highly effective in the review of materials and in initiating public action and may not have the same constraints as school administrators and teachers.

- Developing programs to educate parents about the extent of teenage sexual or drinking activity, the knowledge and guidance teens may need, and where they can get information and help (figure 6-16).

- Providing a central source of information, resource material, and personnel. This need not mean starting a new resource. Libraries and bookstores usually welcome help to acquire accurate and acceptable references. Community fairs and exhibitions welcome community agencies willing to set up a booth or to supply materials for community service booths or exhibits. Providing speakers for community groups takes advantage of the special relationship those groups have with specific teen constituencies. Notifying newspapers or radio and television stations of the availability of any of these resources can achieve more than starting new resources.

Develop Adolescent Awareness   Teenagers face adapting to the norms of a rapidly changing society. Although lacking sufficient life experience in their developmental years, they have to make decisions that can greatly affect their adult lives. Community health services and programs must adapt to the varying levels of knowledge and education of the adolescents who come to them for services. Individuals need appropriate information about human reproduction, contraception, alcohol, drugs, or other topics of concern. Sexually active teens need information about the specific services available to them. The following activities suggest effective ways to reach teenagers, whether in the

ISSUES AND CONTROVERSIES
Historical Perspective on Teenage Sex

At the turn of the century, girls had their first period at an average age of fifteen. Today, the average age at which menstruation begins is twelve. In 1900, menstruation began at the age when most girls were about to complete their education, marry, and begin their families. Society's norms were more closely coordinated with nature's biological clock.

Today, because of improved nutrition, the biological clock ticks faster, offering sexual and reproductive maturity at a younger age. However, social organization has delayed the other rights and responsibilities of maturity. With improved educational and employment opportunities, marriage and childbearing are delayed, leaving an ever-increasing gap between the age at which sexual maturity occurs and the age of first intended pregnancy.

How does this historical perspective bear on today's teenage pregnancy and abortion rates?

---

community or in family planning or adolescent health clinics, or in general ambulatory care services and teenage centers.

- Identify all access points of contact with adolescents (for example, schools, homes, recreation centers, shopping malls, employment agencies, local hangouts, teen-youth programs, and radio and television).
- Devise strategies to reach teenagers at their locations. The most effective way of reaching specific groups is to form discussion groups for church or other organizations and youth clubs. Another is to educate adults working with teens about availability of counseling and referral. Less influential methods but ones with greater reach because of their mass appeal include furnishing spot announcements regarding family planning clinics for use by radio and television stations. Another mass media method is sending flyers to other health and social service agencies. The most common mass media method is to put up posters at public places such as sports arenas.
- Use audiovisual materials suitable to adolescents of different ages and different environments. Project developers can use many materials available from national sources. These include the National Clearinghouse for Family

Planning Information, the National Health Information Clearinghouse, the National Clearinghouse for Smoking and Health (figure 6-17), Health Canada, and national clearinghouses for alcohol information. Materials developed locally should be age appropriate and easily understood. The information should strive to assist teenagers' decision making: whether to have sexual intercourse, how to choose a contraceptive, where and when to get tests for sexually-transmitted disease or pregnancy, and ways to resist peer pressure. Teenagers can help with the preparation of some materials and can act as valuable "reviewers."

- Make special efforts to reach teens who are not in school. One approach is to identify popular "hangouts" such as bowling alleys, video parlors, beaches, and swimming pools and then establish rapport with the informal leaders.
- Publicize the availability of services in terms that are meaningful to teenagers; teens may not know that family planning clinics, community health centers, or other ambulatory care projects are relevant to their needs. Teens need to know that family planning services are not only for adults or married couples. They need to know that some other services and programs are designed specifically for teens, or even better, *by* teens.

· · · · · · · · · · · · · · · · · · · ·

F i g u r e   6 - 1 7

Teenagers' responsiveness to peer pressure and their perception of the expectation or norms of attractive young adult role models make public service materials helpful in offsetting the use of the same strategy by tobacco industry advertising to young people. (*Source:* Office of Smoking and Health, National Clearinghouse for Smoking and Health, Centers for Disease Control and Prevention, U.S. Department of Health and Human Services.)

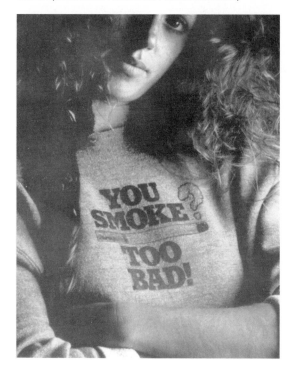

Counseling   Counselors and educators should have thorough training in adolescent growth, development, and behavior patterns. The hiring of paid staff and selection of volunteers should include screening for their ability to relate to teenagers. The first concern of the counseling process is to impart sufficient knowledge to help the individual make a responsible and intelligent choice about smoking, alcohol, drugs and sexual intercourse and, if indicated, about a birth control method. The second is to instill the necessary

motivation and skill to enable the individual to follow through with the decision to use birth control or not to smoke or use alcohol or other drugs.

Crisis counseling should be available to teenagers in urgent need of discussing their problems. Teens need more counseling than adults usually receive. Many teens who come to the clinics are uncertain or worried about the risks they are taking. Staff should encourage teens to include their sex partners or friends in the counseling sessions. If males, for example, refuse to participate in a counseling session, staff should send educational materials to them through the counseled partner.

Services   Any program or ambulatory care service should evaluate its usefulness and attractiveness to adolescents. Many teenagers coming to the facility lack knowledge about many things. They need reassurance and specific information on confidentiality of services, medical procedures, cost of services, and necessary follow-up of a positive pregnancy or test results for any disease or deficiency. To accept the project services, teenagers need special assurance that staff will honor the confidentiality of their record. To honor their concern with privacy, services should permit anonymity, either with clinics made available through multipurpose health centers or with separate entrances or hours established for teen use. Appointments should be available on short notice. Staff should see drop-ins if the project has sufficient personnel. Teens should receive pregnancy testing or treatment for sexually transmitted infections, as quickly as possible.

Teenagers need to know that project services are free or low-cost, and if there is a charge, they may make deferred payments. The inability to pay for services, regardless of family income, is a serious deterrent to their seeking help. Many will pay for services if they can do so in installments and without being billed at home.

Pregnancy testing services are highly attractive to teenagers. Studies have shown that a pregnancy scare is often a prime motivation for a teenager to attend a clinic. Providers wishing to attract

Table 6-4

The Youth Risk Behavior Surveillance System Collects Surveys from the States on High School Students in Grades 9–12. These Results are from the 1996 Reports.[1,2]

Unintentional and Intentional Injuries

22%	Rarely or never used safety belts
39%	Rode with a drinking driver during past month
20%	Carried a weapon during past month
39%	Were in a physical fight during past year
9%	Attempted suicide during past year

Alcohol and Other Drug Use

52%	Drank alcohol during past month
33%	Reported episodic heavy drinking during past month
25%	Used marijuana during past month
2%	Ever injected illegal drugs
20%	Ever sniffed or inhaled intoxicating substances

Sexual Behaviors

53%	Ever had sexual intercourse
18%	Ever had four or more sex partners
38%	Had sexual intercourse during past three months
46%	Did not use a condom during last sexual intercourse[3]
83%	Did not use birth control pills during last sexual intercourse[3]

Tobacco Use

71%	Ever smoked cigarettes
35%	Smoked cigarettes during past month
16%	Smoked cigarettes on 20 or more days during past month
11%	Used smokeless tobacco during past month
78%	Not asked proof of age for purchase of cigarettes[4]

Dietary Behaviors

72%	Ate <5 servings of fruits and vegetables yesterday
39%	Ate >2 servings of high-fat foods yesterday
28%	Thought they were overweight
41%	Were attempting weight loss
5%	Took laxatives or vomited to lose or maintain weight during past month

Physical Activity

64%	Participated in vigorous physical activity during past week[5]
21%	Participated in moderate physical activity during past week[6]
40%	Were not enrolled in physical education class
75%	Did not attend physical education class daily
30%	Exercised <20 minutes in an average physical education class[7]

1 1995 data
2 Among high school students only
3 Among students who had sexual intercourse during the past 3 months
4 Among students <18 years of age who currently smoked cigarettes and who purchased cigarettes in a store
5 On ≥3 of the 7 days
6 On ≥5 of the 7 days
7 Among students enrolled in PE class

Source: MMWR 45:(55–4), 1996; and Kann L, Warren CW, Harris WA, et al.: Youth risk behavior surveillance—United States, 1995. *J School Health* 66:365, 1996.

teenagers should provide easily accessible pregnancy testing services and should not turn away or refer a teenager who requests only a pregnancy test and declines birth control assistance.

Those working with teenagers should be sympathetic and sensitive to various teen-specific needs. They must avoid ambiguous language. For example, they should not assume that sexual activity is understood by a teen to mean sexual intercourse. Teenagers need to know what will happen at the clinic and should be told what to expect during the physical examination.

Training Drug and alcohol counselors, family planning workers, nutrition and health professionals who provide care or counseling to teenagers should have training that is specific to teenage needs and issues of growth and development. Besides content knowledge, staff members may need special training in health education and counseling or may need to supplement their skills by working with counselors who are alert and sensitive to the concerns of teenagers.

People outside the medical service disciplines who have contact and good rapport with adolescents can help disseminate information about adolescent health services and can counsel in areas beyond the mandate of health agencies. Some experienced providers suggest that the training of people who are not medical professionals and who can communicate well with young people is an excellent way of increasing teen use of available services. Training for counseling should be thorough in all phases, with emphasis on the ability to communicate at the teenager's level of comprehension. It may be advantageous to have counseling given by a young person or one who appears young. Many adolescents will not express themselves or listen to an individual whom they do not regard as a contemporary. The training of volunteer peer counselors (other teens) is a technique that recognizes adolescent communication patterns. Teen counselors can be an important resource in the community, but they cannot be a replacement for professionally trained staff who must supervise and monitor their work.

Parents also should receive education and discussion sessions on a community-wide basis so that they are better informed about reported teen behaviors, table 6-4. Although much teen learning comes from peers, parents are key to the development of their children's values, attitudes, and sense of responsibility. Professionals should see them as important members of the team. Teenagers can also play a role in supporting their parents in managing adult health problems; they will soon encounter such problems themselves. This brings us to adult health, the next chapter.

SUMMARY

Adolescents must cope with a most tumultuous period of life. Challenges to health from the adaptation to growing independence from adult authority are compounded by social trends making adult support and guidance more problematic than in

times past. Communities must help fill this gap through the organization of services, programs, and projects in schools, clubs, and recreational environments. The most important behavioral, social, and attitudinal issues for youth are reflected in table 6-4, summarizing the statistics reviewed in this chapter.

This chapter has concluded with specific guidelines and strategies for working with adolescent populations in the community and in program or clinical services to address these behavioral, social, and attitudinal issues with sensitivity to the special and varied circumstances of adolescence.

WEB*Links*

http://www.safersex.org
Information on safer sex for teens.

http://www.troom.com/index2.html
Information for young women on issues such as puberty and menstruation.

http://www.healthtouch/com/level1/leaflets/102504/1 02601.htm
Tips for teens about alcohol and drug abuse.

http://education.indiana.edu/cas/adol/mental.html
Mental health risk factors for adolescents.

http://www.cyberisle.org
Local Canadian site for teens with a strong research base and a variety of target audiences.

QUESTIONS FOR REVIEW

1. Why is it important to consider adolescent health to be on a life-long health continuum of growth and development rather than an isolated, discrete stage?
2. In what ways might prevention efforts for adolescents be the same as those for children and adults? In what ways might they be different?
3. How do biological and psychosocial maturation affect health differently? The same?
4. What factors account for adolescents as the only age group that has sustained a reversal in death rates in recent decades?

5. Review table 6-1. How can health education programs use the major tasks of coping and adaptation for adolescents to address health consequences faced by this age group?

6. What implications do demographic changes among adolescents have for school health curriculum, community health activities, and community health services?

7. In which leading causes of adolescent ill health is alcohol use involved? How would alcohol use by adolescents be addressed differently through health promotion, health protection, and health service efforts?

8. What are the costs of adolescent pregnancy to the infant, the teenage mother, significant others, and society at large?

9. What are the pros and cons of arguments about placing condoms in schools for easier access by adolescents?

10. How did health education contribute to the decline in adolescent female smoking in the 1980s? What forces might account for the increases in the 1990s?

11. What are the multiple factors that converge to make suicide the third leading cause of death for adolescents?

12. What existing services and facilities in your community meet the needs of adolescent health? What additional services are needed?

READINGS

Alexander, C. 1995. *The Health of Maryland's Adolescents.* Baltimore: Johns Hopkins Center for Adolescent Health Promotion and Disease Prevention.

This booklet provides a model of state-level analysis of the conditions and progress in addressing the problems of adolescents. It is available from the author at the Hopkins Center, phone (410) 614-3953 or fax (410) 614–3956.

Brown, S. S., and L. Eisenberg, eds. 1995. *The best intentions: unintended pregnancy and the well-being of children and families.* Washington, DC: National Academy Press.

This book reflects the findings and recommendations of a committee of national experts appointed by the Institute of Medicine to examine the issues of unintended pregnancies, many of which occur among adolescent mothers.

Kann, L., C. W. Warren, W. A. Harris, J. L. Collins, B. I. Williams, J. G. Ross, and L. J. Kolbe. 1996. Youth risk behavior surveillance—United States, 1995. *J School Health* 66:365.

The 1996 estimates of the prevalence of sexual intercourse, dietary practices, suicide attempts and thoughts, tobacco and alcohol consumption, and illegal drug use from a national sample of U.S. high school students reported in this chapter.

Lowry, R., L. Kann, J. L. Collins, and L. J. Kolbe. 1996. The effect of socioeconomic status on chronic disease risk behaviors among US adolescents. *J Am Med Assoc* 276:792.

Further analyses of the Youth Risk Behavior Survey examine the effect of educational level of the responsible adult and family income on five risk behaviors for chronic disease among adolescents: cigarette smoking, sedentary lifestyle, insufficient consumption of fruits and vegetables, excessive consumption of foods high in fat, and episodic heavy drinking of alcohol.

BIBLIOGRAPHY

Allensworth, D. D., and B. Bradley. 1996. Guidelines for adolescent preventive services: a role for the school nurse. *J Sch Health* 66:281.

Alteneder, R. R., J. H. Price, S. K. Telljohann, J. Didion, and A. Locher. 1992. Using the PRECEDE model to determine junior high school students' knowledge, attitudes, and beliefs about AIDS. *J Sch Health* 62:464.

American Medical Association. 1991. *Healthy youth 2000: national health promotion and disease prevention objectives for adolescents.* Chicago: Department of Adolescent Health, The Association.

Carnegie Council on Adolescent Development. 1989. *Turning points: preparing American youth for the 21st century.* New York: Carnegie Corporation of New York.

Colyer, E., T. Thompkins, and B. Barlow. 1996. Can conflict resolution training increase aggressive behavior in young adolescents. *Am J Public Health* 86:1028.

Contento, I. R., D. G. Kell, M. K. Keiley, and R. D. Corcoran. 1992. A formative evaluation of the American Cancer Society *Changing the Course* nutrition education curriculum. *J Sch Health* 62:411.

Copeland, L. A., J. T. Shope, and P. F. Waller. 1996. Factors in adolescent drinking/driving: binge drinking, cigarette smoking, and gender. *J Sch Health* 66:254.

Cornelius, L. J. 1991. Health habits of school-age children. *J Health Care Poor Underserved* 2:374.

Cottrell, R. R., E. Capwell, and J. Brannan. 1995. A follow-up evaluation of non-returning teams to the Ohio Comprehensive School Health Conference. *Journal of Wellness Perspectives* 12(1):1.

Dijkstra, M., H. deVries, and G. S. Parcel. 1993. The linkage approach applied to a school-based smoking prevention program in the Netherlands. *J Sch Health* 63:339.

Edet, E. E. 1991 The role of sex education in adolescent pregnancy. *J R Soc Health* 111:17.

Gerstein, D. R., and L. W. Green, ed. 1993. *Preventing drug abuse: what do we know?* Washington, DC: National Academy Press.

Gfellner, B. M., and J. D. Hundleby. 1995. Patterns of drug use among native and white adolescents: 1990–1993. *Can J Public Health* 86:95.

Gordon, T. E. 1996. The need for adolescent health education and training among health professionals. *Am J Public Health* 86:889.

Health and Welfare Canada. 1993. *The health of Canada's youth: views and behaviours of 11-, 13- and 15-year-olds from 11 countries,* Ottawa: Health and Welfare Canada.

Hechinger, F. M. 1992. *Fateful choices: healthy youth for the 21st century.* New York: Hill & Wang.

Hofford, C. W., and K. A. Spelman. 1996. The community action plan: incorporating health promotion and wellness into alcohol, tobacco and other drug abuse prevention efforts on the college campus. *Journal of Wellness Perspectives* 12(2): 70–79.

MacDonald, M., and L. W. Green. 1994. Health promotion and adolescent health. *Barlliere's Clinical Pediatrics* 2:227.

Mathews, C., K. Everett, J. Binedell, and M. Steinberg. 1995. Learning to listen: formative research in the development of AIDS education for secondary school students. *Soc Sci Med.* 41(12): 1715–1724.

Mosure, D. J., S. Berman, and E. Halloran. 1996. Predictors of chlamydia trachomatis infection among female adolescents: a longitudinal analysis. *Am J Epidem* 144:997.

Parks, C. P. 1995. Gang behavior in the schools: reality or myth? *Educational Psychol Rev* 7: 41–68.

Ploeg, J., D. Ciliska, and S. Hayward 1996. A systematic overview of adolescent suicide prevention programs. *Can J Public Health* 87:319.

Raphael, D., I. Brown, and P. Hill-Bailey. 1996. Adolescent health: moving from prevention to promotion through a quality of life approach. *Can J Public Health* 87:81.

Spruijt-Metz, D. 1995. Personal incentives as determinants of adolescent health behavior: the meaning of behavior. *Health Educ Res* 10:355.

Stivers, C. 1994. Drug prevention in Zuni, New Mexico: creation of a teen center as an alternative to alcohol and drug use. *J Community Health* 19: 343–359.

U.S. Preventive Services Task Force. 1996. *Guide to clinical preventive services.* 2d ed. Baltimore: Williams & Wilkins.

Villas, P., M. Cardenas, and C. Jameson. 1994. Instrument development using the PRECEDE Model to distinguish users/triers from non-users of alcoholic beverages. *Wellness Perspectives: Res, Theory & Prac* 10:46–53.

Wechsler, H., and E. R. Weitzman. 1996. Editorial: community solutions to community problems—preventing adolescent alcohol use. *Am J Public Health* 86:923.

Windom, C. S., and J. B. Kuhns. 1996. Childhood victimization and subsequent risk for promiscuity, prostitution, and teenage pregnancy: a prospective study. *Am J Public Health* 86:1607.

Worden, J. K., B. S. Flynn, L. J. Solomon, R. H. Secker-Walker, G. J. Badger, and J. H. Carpenter. 1996. Using mass media to prevent cigarette smoking among adolescent girls. *Health Educ Quar* 23:453.

Chapter *7*

Adult Health

*O*f all the anti-social vested interests the worst is the vested interest in ill health.

—George Bernard Shaw

Objectives

When you finish this chapter, you should be able to:

- Assess the multiple determinants of health
- Apply multiple perspectives of health to leading causes of adult morbidity and mortality
- Identify programs appropriate to health promotion and disease prevention for adults

More than once the preceding chapters have adjusted the lens through which you have been asked to view community health. The beginning of this chapter will review some of the dominant perspectives as an introduction to the subject of adult health (figure 7-1). Keep in mind that these perspectives apply to each of the age groups and to each of the health promotion, health protection, and health service chapters to follow. Following an overview of the perspectives, they will be applied to the two leading threats to adult health in North America—cardiovascular disease and cancer. The focus on these two threats to adult health enable an analysis of the multiple determinants of health, including lifestyle, genetics, race and ethnicity, gender, socioeconomic status, and the environment. This chapter closes with a review of diabetes and chronic disabling conditions, which are amenable to community health intervention. Other leading threats to adult health are discussed elsewhere in this book, including suicide in chapter 9, AIDS in chapter 11, and accidents and homicides in chapter 13.

SHIFTING PERSPECTIVES ON ADULT HEALTH

Developmental and Historical Perspectives

Developmental and historical perspectives look at trends in adult health across time, space, and context. Where as much attention has been paid to the stages of development in childhood and adolescents, those aged eighteen and older are lumped as adults. Research on development during the adult years has taken various forms including stages, transitions, or passages, such as childbirth, marriage, divorce, and death; or research on roles, such as parent, partner, or employee. Various chronological subpopulations are nested in the larger adult population, including those popularly labeled as Generation X (those born between 1973 and 1979) and the Baby Boomers (those born between 1946 and 1964), who represent nearly one-third of the U.S. population. These developmental and chronological differences are compounded by gender, cultural, geographical, and socioeconomic ones.

· · · · · · · · · · · · · · · · · · ·
Figure 7-1

The main features of the several perspectives from previous chapters are summarized.

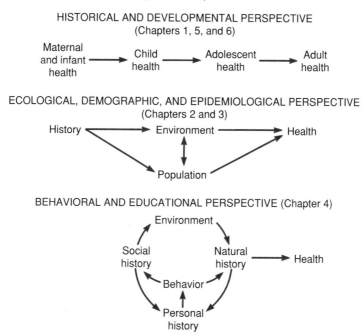

The health needs of this large and diverse population require tailored interventions that fit individual and community circumstances. Recommended preventive care for adults from eighteen to 75 and over includes a series of test, physical exams, immunizations, and health guidance at varied intervals (figure 7-2). A review of these recommendations portends the kinds of challenges to adult health, dominated by the chronic diseases.

At the beginning of this century, when community health professionals concentrated their efforts on the prevention and control of communicable diseases, their emphasis was on the school-age child. It soon became apparent, however, that effective health measures required earlier interventions with the preschool child. Eventually attention shifted to infant health. A truly preventive approach to infant health required increasing attention to prenatal factors, therefore intensified efforts in maternal health resulted. This legitimized

some shift in resources from infant and child health to adolescent and adult health, at least for females. Prevention efforts, which enter the life cycle at different points, affirm that health in all stages of life are linked.

With the advances in communicable disease control and the prevention of death in the early years of life, greater proportions of the population survived through **adolescence** to **adulthood** and into old age. The chronic and degenerative diseases, usually most prevalent in adulthood, became the leading causes of death and disability (figure 7-3). These changes led the health professions to expand their approach to the health of the adult population. These changes also signaled that further advances in health were not something that the health professions and medical care could do alone. Multisector—health, education, economics, political, social—approaches within and across communities and populations were needed.

· · · · · · · · · · · · · · · · · ·
Figure 7-2

Adult preventive care timeline: recommendations of major authorities. (*Source:* Put Prevention Into Practice, U.S. Public Health Service, 1994.)

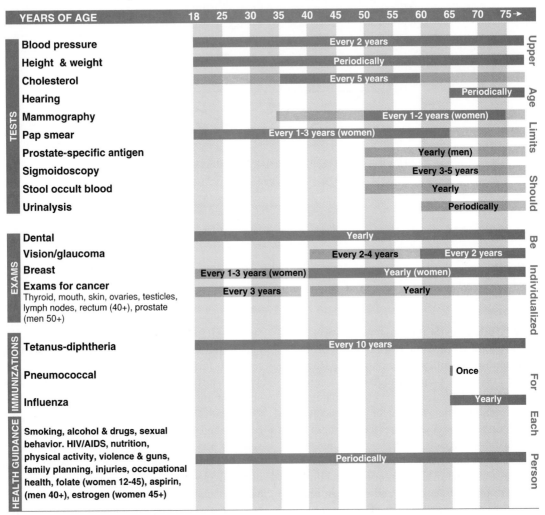

Adult preventive care timeline: recommendations of major authorities

YEARS OF AGE	18	25	30	35	40	45	50	55	60	65	70	75→	
TESTS Blood pressure							Every 2 years						Upper
Height & weight							Periodically						
Cholesterol							Every 5 years						Age
Hearing											Periodically		
Mammography							Every 1-2 years (women)						Limits
Pap smear					Every 1-3 years (women)								
Prostate-specific antigen								Yearly (men)					
Sigmoidoscopy								Every 3-5 years					Should
Stool occult blood								Yearly					
Urinalysis								Periodically					
EXAMS Dental							Yearly						Be
Vision/glaucoma						Every 2-4 years				Every 2 years			
Breast	Every 1-3 years (women)						Yearly (women)						Individualized
Exams for cancer Thyroid, mouth, skin, ovaries, testicles, lymph nodes, rectum (40+), prostate (men 50+)	Every 3 years						Yearly						
IMMUNIZATIONS Tetanus-diphtheria							Every 10 years						For
Pneumococcal										Once			
Influenza										Yearly			Each
HEALTH GUIDANCE Smoking, alcohol & drugs, sexual behavior. HIV/AIDS, nutrition, physical activity, violence & guns, family planning, injuries, occupational health, folate (women 12-45), aspirin, (men 40+), estrogen (women 45+)							Periodically						Person

Key ▬▬ Recommended by all major authorities.
▨▨ Recommended by some authorities.

Demographic, Epidemiological, and Ecological Perspectives

Demographic Perspective No variable relates more consistently to mortality and morbidity than age. Age is such a powerful correlate of mortality

and morbidity that crude death rates and cause-specific incidence and prevalence rates are difficult to use for comparative purposes without adjustment for age, as we have seen in chapter 3. Age serves as a convenient marker for program planning

· · · · · · · · · · · · · · · · · · ·
Figure 7-3

The "diseases of civilization" have almost reversed their position relative to the infectious diseases as causes of death since 1920 in the more industrialized countries. AIDS and HIV infections have brought a slight increase in the deaths due to communicable diseases relative to chronic diseases since 1981.

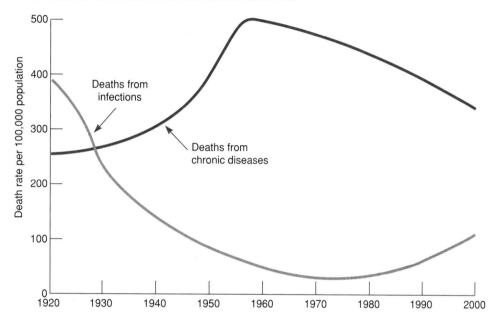

because it is so consistently associated with morbidity and mortality. A community can set its priorities for intervention on the problems of specific subpopulations defined by age. Differences in leading threats to the health of younger and older adults exemplify this point in figures 7-4 and 7-5.

Epidemiological Perspective The mortality of those in their later adult years are most threatened by cancer, heart disease, and stroke. These current leading causes of death contrast with those in 1900, tuberculosis, pneumonia, and gastroenteritis. Where as heart disease mortality has declined dramatically over the past 25 years, cancer mortality in the United States has been relatively stable. Worldwide deaths from noncommunicable diseases, such as cardiovascular disease and cancer, are expected to represent 73 percent of deaths by 2020, up from nearly 56 percent from 1990. This increase is primarily attributed to the aging of the

population and tobacco use. The current threats to adult health require comprehensive analysis.

Agents and Hosts Revisited One approach to the analysis of adult health, relative to that of other age groups, combines developmental, epidemiological, and behavioral perspectives to focus on transitions in the life span. Recall the epidemiological concepts of host, agent, and environment discussed in chapter 3. The ideal intervention in community and population health is one that anticipates potential problems or requirements for the health and prepares the "host" population—adults—to resist the problem or to provide for the need. Unfortunately, the "agents" of the new leading causes of morbidity and death are pervasive and are tightly woven into the fabric of modern living, such as rich foods, alcohol, drugs, sedentary work and leisure, stress, guns, and automobiles and other machinery. Few societies or communities have

....

Figure 7-4

Death rates for selected causes of death among persons 25 to 44 years of age by sex: United States, 1993. (*Source:* National Center for Health Statistics, Centers for Disease Control and Prevention, Public Health Service, U.S. Department of Health and Human Services.)

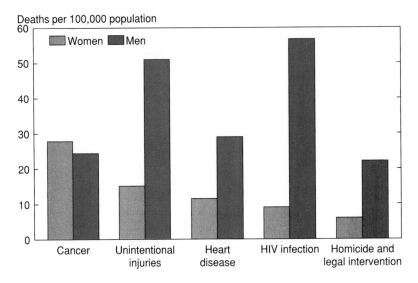

....

Figure 7-5

Death rates for selected causes of death among persons 45 to 64 years of age by sex: United States, 1993. (*Source:* National Center for Health Statistics, Centers for Disease Control and Prevention, Public Health Service, U.S. Department of Health and Human Services.)

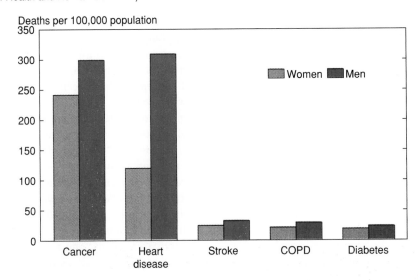

been willing to turn back the clock on such agents. Although some can be controlled through environmental regulation of their distribution, pricing, taxation, and public use, most of these agents are used privately. There is little choice, then, but to supplement organizational, economic, and environmental strategies with educational interventions that build host—in this case, human—resistance.

Risk Factors   Major epidemiological studies conducted in the 1950s and 1960s provided evidence for defining the risk factors associated with chronic illness and for developing intervention strategies to reduce morbidity. A **risk factor** is a habit, trait, or condition in a person that is associated with an increased chance (or risk) of developing a disease. Today many of the leading causes of adult death are associated with risk factors related to lifestyle. Risk can be divided into two types: nonmodifiable and modifiable. Nonmodifiable factors are those that cannot be changed through prevention measures, including age, sex, family history, and personality type. Modifiable factors are those that are amenable to prevention measures and include high blood pressure, overweight, cigarette smoking, and physical inactivity.

The government has addressed these risk factors with various programs. Smoking, diet, high blood pressure, and exercise are examples of risk factors. For example, it is estimated that 30 percent of all cancers are associated with smoking and that 35 percent may be linked to poor eating habits. In 1964 the U.S. Surgeon General's report on smoking and health was a bold step to address this major contributor to heart disease and cancer. Efforts by communities to reduce smoking and improve nutrition continue to expand and have produced positive results. Government sponsored research and education have supported these efforts. Risks due to high blood pressure have received considerable attention and are addressed later in this chapter. Through promoting the positive effects of physical fitness government programs have addressed the problems of inactivity. These efforts have had some impact. One third of

adult Americans exercise regularly, and the percentage of nonsmokers increased from 57 percent in 1974 to 74 percent in 1994.

Ecological Perspective   The risk factors for individuals needs to be considered in the broader social, economic, and political contexts that impact on individuals. Communities can encourage all public places to become smoke-free; thereby, reducing the risks of second-hand smoke and sending clear messages to youth about tobacco effects. They can also help make worksites healthier by discouraging tobacco use, while encouraging physical activity or stress reduction. Community partnerships and coalitions can be formed to support healthy lifestyles. Health care providers can integrate prevention messages into client contact, use screening effectively and efficiently, and advocate for prevention screening. Local and national governments can develop coordinated and consistent prevention policies and enable access to prevention services.

Behavioral and Educational Perspectives

From the behavioral and educational perspectives, adult health develops out of the cumulative historical, demographic, and epidemiological forces just described, combined with the attitudes, values, beliefs, and behavior of individuals, as described in chapter 4. These individual, cultural, and sociopsychological factors make up the personal history that each person brings to bear on the natural history of health, the social history of health, and the environment. The behavioral and educational perspectives are interwoven in this chapter and highlighted in chapter 12 on health promotion.

Educational programs for adults need not only to be well planned and targeted, they need to be part of broader community and population efforts to address the determinants of health. One-size-fits-all educational programs are inadequate to address the leading causes of adult morbidity and mortality. The twenty-something black woman who lacks access to mammography, the thirty-something immigrant who does not prefer and cannot afford low-fat chicken breasts to serve a large family, the forty-something white adult whose long-term obesity has demolished his or her confidence to change, the fifty-something Asian male who has repeatedly tried to stop smoking, and the sixty-something Hispanic male who is diagnosed with prostate cancer each need targeted health education and health promotion interventions. Such education needs to predispose these adults toward health while enabling and supporting individual actions and providing services and circumstances that contribute to health.

Adults often not only are responsible for their own health, but that of their children and aging parents. The middle years are sometimes referred to as the "sandwich" years because of these roles. In their domestic roles and the roles of worker and community participant, adults can be reached through educational interventions, such as those at the worksite, community organization, or adult education classes. Education aimed at one generation can often include another. For example, childhood immunizations provide an opportunity to discuss adult immunization needs with parents. Diabetic education for an aging parent can include risk factor information for the adult caregiver. Adults often serve as the gateway to the health of others, therefore they can be reached in ways to enable and support their own health.

PRINCIPAL THREATS TO ADULT HEALTH

Cardiovascular Health

Over the past twenty-five years, dramatic improvements have been made in reducing the death toll from heart disease and stroke. Over half of cardiovascular deaths are attributed to **coronary heart disease.** This disease causes reduced blood flow to the heart and results in damage to the heart muscle. A heart attack occurs when the damage to the heart muscle is permanent and may result in death. Nearly a quarter of heart attacks result in sudden death (within two hours). Two-thirds of heart attack victims survive their first attack, but

Objective for Adult Health

By the year 2000, reduce the death rate for adults by 20 percent to no more than 340 per 100,000 people aged 25 to 64. Baseline: 423 per 100,000 in 1987.

most of the fatalities occur before the patient can reach the hospital.

Strokes are a leading cause of death for adults and a leading cause of disability related to the nervous system. A stroke occurs when the blood supply to the brain is interrupted, either gradually or abruptly. This may happen when a blood clot forms in a cerebral artery, when a clot forms elsewhere in the body travels to the brain and the blood supply is cut off, or when a blood vessel or aneurysm ruptures. Statistics show that smoking can double or even triple the risk of a stroke and blacks are 60 percent more likely than whites to suffer a stroke.

Even this quick review of coronary heart disease and stroke should give you some clues about where community and population programs can intervene in cardiovascular health for adults, such as rapid response to a cardiovascular event, education programs aimed at risk factors, and targeted interventions for subpopulations. By the time you finish this section, other kinds of environmental and social interventions will have been noted.

Trends

Death rates from heart disease and stroke declined by 49 percent and 58 percent respectively in the 1980s and 1990s. Drops in high blood pressure and high blood cholesterol have contributed to these decreases through earlier and increased screening, detection and management, coupled with self- or provider-initiated changes in diet and other lifestyle improvements. Progress has been made on many of the heart disease and stroke objectives in the mid-decade review (figure 7-6).

· · · · · · · · · · · · · · · · · · · ·

Figure 7-6

Mid-decade status of Year 2000 Heart Disease and Stroke Objectives. (*Source:* National Institutes of Health, Public Health Service, U.S. Department of Health and Human Services.)

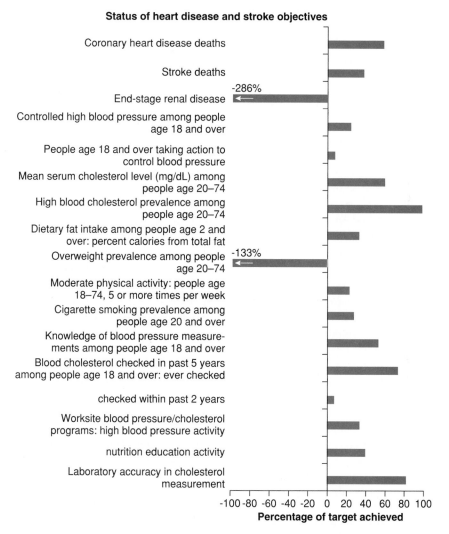

Despite these improvements, much remains to be done. For 25- to 64-year-olds, heart disease is the second leading cause of death. Approximately 7 million Americans are affected by coronary heart disease; 500,000 die each year; and annual costs to the nation are estimated at $190 billion as measured in health care expenditures, medication, and lost productivity due to disability and death. Between 400,000 and 500,000 Americans suffer nonfatal strokes each year. Heart and stroke disease remain the leading cause of death in Canada, claiming 75,000 lives each year. Downward trends in cardiovascular disease in the West are reversed in much of the less industrialized world. In some central and eastern European countries, for example, there have been sharp increases (30 percent to 80 percent) over the last 20 years. It is predicted that by the year 2005 cardiovascular death will have doubled to 20 million, with 13 million from developing countries and eastern Europe.

Demographic Factors

Major disparities in cardiovascular health exist among racial and ethnic groups, geographic regions, and gender with a disproportionate burden of morbidity and mortality in minority and low-income populations. For example, black Americans have nearly twice as many strokes, 10 to 18 times more kidney failure, and 3 to 5 times more heart failure related to high blood pressure. The "Stroke Belt" in the southeastern United Stated has an age-adjusted mortality from stroke more than 10 percent higher than the national average.

Gender differences have been found in cardiac care. Women less often undergo intensive or invasive evaluations and treatments for cardiac diseases than do men with symptoms of similar or lesser severity. Women are more likely than men to have chest pain misdiagnosed as a symptom of depression and anxiety. One study, which followed men and women after exercise stress tests and heart scans, found that within a year 14 percent of the women and 6 percent of the men had a heart attack or died from coronary heart disease. These kinds of racial, geographic, and gender differences point out the importance of studying not only broad populations, but subpopulations.

Social and Economic Factors

Changes in lifestyle and risk factor reduction were major contributors in the North American declines. Community action in reducing deaths from heart disease and stroke has a long history, during which the role of prevention has continually increased in emphasis compared with that of treatment. During the last decade, a global effort has been initiated to improve cardiovascular health.

The increase of cardiovascular disease in some countries can be attributed to different social and cultural norms, lack of access to primary care, and deterioration of living conditions that lead to psychosocial stress. The inequality of death due to tobacco use also can be attributed to tobacco companies aggressively targeting Third World markets as more developed countries succeed in limiting smoking. For example, it is estimated that sales of tobacco projects in the Asian-Pacific region will increase by 33 percent in the 1990s.

The transfer of the tobacco habit among countries necessitates an international, cooperative effort to decrease the inequalities that exist in the burden of heart disease and the resources to combat this modern epidemic. The Second International Heart Health Conference in 1995 identified prevention assets that can be used with existing resources to improve cardiovascular health: (1) the existing, extensive knowledge base on cardiovascular disease prevention; (2) the infrastructure through which this knowledge base may be applied; (3) the partnerships and coalitions that may already exist or that can be established; and (4) the applicable public policies. Barriers to implementing these assets include aversions or resistance to change, gaps between scientific knowledge and its applicability, conflicting commercial and marketing interests, and lack of collaboration. Successful policy to overcome these barriers requires linkages between policy and resources among governmental and nongovernmental organizations at three levels: international and regional, country, and local.

Nonmodifiable Risk Factors

Nonmodifiable risk factors for cardiovascular disease are those that cannot be changed through prevention measures, including age, sex, family history, and personality type.

Age The incidence rates for heart attacks rise steeply from age thirty-five to fifty-five years and then fall as those susceptible to the disease are lost.

Sex Males below fifty years of age are afflicted by coronary heart deaths in a ratio of 4:1 compared to females. After fifty years of age, the preponderance of male victims is markedly reduced but still persists. This suggests some hormonal factor. For women in menopause, some cardioprotective benefits have been shown from hormone replacement therapy (HRT).

Family History There is a strong familial tendency toward coronary heart disease, particularly on the male side. Families share many habits and customs of exercise, diet, and lifestyle; thus this familial predisposition reflects a combination of genetic and environmental causes.

Personality Type This is included as a nonmodifiable risk factor, for it has not been proved that it can be changed. People with a striving, time-conscious behavior pattern are identified as having a type A personality. They are involved in a chronic struggle against time or other people. There is no limit to the number of events these persons squeeze into a day. They have an intrinsic drive toward some goal, and the achievement of this goal is opposed by time, persons, and things. Consequently, persons with type A personality often suffer frustration, are constantly in a hurry, and have free-floating hostility. Type A personalities with hostility suffer higher rates of heart attack than those persons with the converse, type B, or type A without hostility.

Modifiable Risk Factors

Modifiable factors are those that are amenable to prevention measures. They include high blood pressure, high blood cholesterol, overweight, cigarette smoking, and physical inactivity. While progress has been made on smoking and high blood cholesterol, overweight has increased in prevalence (figure 7-7). Any one of these risk factors increases an individual's chance of developing heart disease; taken together, they may greatly increase heart disease risk by perhaps ten times or more.

High Blood Cholesterol About one in four adults has high blood cholesterol, a condition that puts a person at greater risk for angina, heart attack, and stroke. Cholesterol comes from two sources: what we eat and what the body itself produces. Pure cholesterol is an odorless, white, waxy, powdery substance. You cannot taste it or see it in the foods you eat. It is found in all foods of animal origin.

To carry cholesterol through the blood, the body wraps it in protein packages. This combination is called a "lipoprotein." Cholesterol is found in the major lipoproteins, including the low-density lipoproteins (LDLs)—the "bad" cholesterol—and the high-density lipoproteins (HDLs)—the "good" cholesterol. High LDL levels promote the deposit of cholesterol on artery walls; HDL is thought to carry cholesterol away from the arteries to the liver for excretion.

Over the past century cholesterol levels have gone up dramatically because of higher animal fat consumption. It has been estimated that a 1 percent drop in a population's cholesterol level will result in a 2 to 3 percent drop in heart disease. Average total cholesterol levels have shown a decline over the last thirty years (figure 7-8). There have also been declines in average levels of LDLs; in the percentage of individuals with high total cholesterol levels (240 mg/dl or greater); and in the percentage of adults requiring dietary therapy for high blood cholesterol. Community screening programs have contributed to an increased number of adults becoming aware of their cholesterol level (figure 7-9).

The declines in cholesterol levels are attributed in part to a two-pronged national strategy: (1) a high-risk or clinical approach that promotes detection and treatment of individuals whose elevated cholesterol places them at significantly increased risk for coronary heart disease; (2) a population approach that promotes reduced intake of saturated fat, total fat, and cholesterol, with increased physical activity and weight control. Guidelines for detection and treatment of high blood cholesterol urge adults age twenty and older to have their

. . . .

Figure 7-7

Prevalence of modifiable risk factors for heart disease and stroke: United States, selected years and year 2000 targets. (*Sources:* For cholesterol and overweight data, Centers for Disease Control and Prevention, National Center for Health Statistics, National Health and Nutrition Examination Survey: for smoking data, Centers for Disease Control and Prevention, National Center for Health Statistics, National Health Interview Survey.)

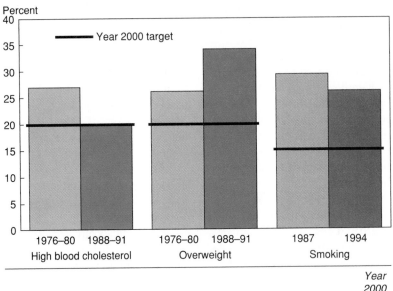

	1976–80	1988–91	1987	1994	Year 2000 targets
High blood cholestrol.........................	27	20	---	---	20
Overweight	26	34	---	---	20
Smoking	---	---	29	26	15

--- Data not available.

total and high-density lipoprotein cholesterol levels measure at least once every five years and to know their numbers. The cholesterol level is determined by a blood test. In adults a total blood cholesterol level of about 240 mg/dl warrants medical attention. Levels above 200 mg/dl also increase the risk of heart disease and may require further evaluation.

Hypertension Blood pressure is the force exerted by the blood against artery walls. The pressure the heart creates as it pumps blood is measured in two numbers: the top number (systolic pressure) measures the maximum pressure with

which blood pushes against the arteries during a heartbeat; the bottom number (diastolic pressure) gauges pressure against the arteries as the heart rests. Healthy blood pressure is in the 120/80 range; if the reading regularly hits 140/90, a person is said to have high blood pressure or **hypertension.** Elevated pressure means the heart is working harder than normal and the arteries are under greater strain. Hypertension is the single most important risk factor for strokes and heart disease.

Chronic hypertension is widely prevalent in the United States. It is often called the "silent killer" because 75 percent of those who have the condition

. . . .

Figure 7-8

Trends in age-adjusted mean serum total cholesterol. (*Source:* Centers for Disease Control and Prevention; NCHS; NHES I; NHANES I, NHANES II [Phase 1, 1988–91]

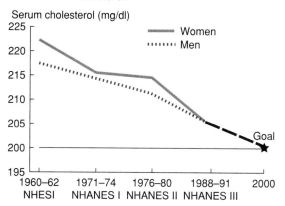

Trends in age-adjusted mean serum total cholesterol

. . . .

Figure 7-9

Community campaigns to control serum cholesterol levels have emphasized screening to make people aware of their readings. (*Source:* National Heart, Lung, and Blood Institute; National Institutes of Health; Public Health Service; U.S. Department of Health and Human Services.)

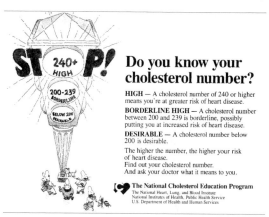

are without symptoms. Getting people without symptoms to have their blood pressure checked and to take action to control their blood pressure is an important objective of health education and health promotion interventions. When symptoms do occur, they are manifested by damage to the heart, brain, kidneys, and eyes. The cause of hypertension is unknown in 90 percent of cases. There is often a family history of hypertension, and relatives of hypertensive persons have been shown to be more likely to be hypertensive (especially children of two hypertensive parents). Black Americans have almost a 33 percent greater chance of having high blood pressure than whites (figure 7-10). It has been estimated that hypertension costs the nation more than $8 billion per year in medical care costs, lost productivity, and lost wages.

Lifestyle modifications have been found to lower blood pressure. Obesity and salt consumption are correlated with hypertension, and both of these factors are modifiable. Studies have found that people who fail to eat enough folic acid—commonly found in green vegetables such as

spinach and broccoli—face a great risk of clogged blood vessels and heart disease. The use of oral contraceptives may increase blood pressure also. Smoking and high blood cholesterol are not associated with development of hypertension, but contribute to a poor prognosis for those who have hypertension. A great advance has been made in the treatment of hypertension with the introduction of effective drug therapy and advances in diet, relaxation, and exercise therapy.

Interaction of Risk Factors   Risk factors for coronary heart disease, including high blood pressure and high blood cholesterol, interact with each other. Stress has been named as another possible risk factor. Stress is difficult to measure either as a source or as a result of emotional tension. Nevertheless, a period of severe stress or excessive fatigue is identified as having preceded a heart attack in many cases. In those who practice regular exercise the outcome of a heart attack is more favorable than in those who do not. The benefits of regular exercise are many and may include reductions in other risk factors such

. . . .

F i g u r e   7 - 1 0

Community high blood pressure control programs use public service materials from the National High Blood Pressure Education Program or similar national programs in other countries. Success of this program is credited with part of the remarkable reduction of strokes and other cardiovascular diseases in the United States. (*Source:* National Heart, Lung and Blood Institute; National Institutes of Health; Public Health Service; U.S. Department of Health and Human Services.)

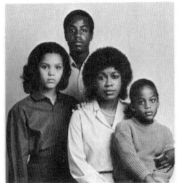

My husband took good care of us. If only he'd taken care of his high blood pressure.

Looking back at it all, it just doesn't make any sense. We have everything we need except a husband and a father.

If you have high blood pressure, take your pills, watch your weight and the salt. And if you think that is too much trouble... well...you just don't know about the trouble you could be leaving behind.

HIGH BLOOD PRESSURE
Treat it for life.

The National High Blood Pressure Education Program
The National Heart, Lung, and Blood Institute, National Institutes of Health
Public Health Service, U.S. Department of Health and Human Services

Cardiovascular Education Programs

A National Program Federally funded studies in the United States in the late 1960s and early 1970s clearly demonstrated that educational programs could impact the cardiovascular health of adults. One such program is the National High Blood Pressure Education Program. This national program demonstrated that cooperation among government agencies, private industry, voluntary health associations, and professional groups was effective in decreasing the proportion of undetected cases of high blood pressure. Further, the proportion of those under treatment whose blood pressure is controlled has also increased. The reductions in deaths from heart disease and stroke can at least partially be attributed to the success of the effort to control high blood pressure.

Hypertension lends itself well to community control, because community surveys can be performed to identify people who have high blood pressure and do not know it. People can visit centers in their community and have their blood pressure recorded, after which they can be referred for treatment if needed (figure 7-11). (There are some 2,000 locally organized hypertension programs in the United States.) Once the cases are identified, the problem then lies in patient education to effect compliance in taking the drugs to maintain normal levels of pressure. The increase in the number of hypertensive persons whose blood pressure has been brought under control because of efficient drug therapy has resulted in reduced mortality and morbidity. This reduction is reflected in a decrease in the number of heart attacks in which hypertension was a factor and also, more importantly, a decrease in the number of cerebrovascular accidents or strokes.

A Local Program An increased number of restaurants across North America focus on diet and nutrition, another cardiovascular risk factor. They aid diners in healthy food choices by marking menu items low in fat and sodium. One such effort is the Heart Smart Restaurant Program sponsored by the Heart and Stroke Foundation of British Columbia. Participating restaurants identify healthy

as high blood pressure, cholesterol, and stress, and more direct effects on reduced rate of heart attack. Obesity is associated with increased frequency of heart attacks, particularly in the markedly obese. The difficulty is that such patients are frequently hypertensive, of sedentary habit, or diabetic, and it is difficult to identify which risk factor is operative.

. . . .
Figure 7-11

Blood pressure measures are essential in part because the person cannot rely on any other symptom of high blood pressure, as the poster in the background of this clinical scene implies with the blank space following the colon. (*Source:* Photo by Marsha Burkes, courtesy University of Texas Health Science Center at Houston.)

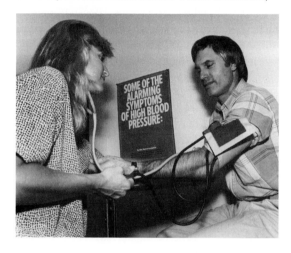

menu items by the use of a heart symbol to help aid in customer's food choices. Local and federal guidelines are aligned on which menu items are low in fat and sodium. Restaurants also offer information about other health choices and agree to make serving changes, such as offering salad dressings on the side or baked potatoes instead of French fries.

Community Mobilization Educational programs combined with medical and preventive interventions can help reduce mortality due to heart attacks. Millions of people in North America have been trained in cardiopulmonary resuscitation (CPR) procedures. If performed properly and early enough, CPR can keep 25 to 30 percent of the normal blood flow to the brain, enough to ensure that brain does not begin to suffer damage immediately. It is estimated that CPR can save as many as 120,000 lives each year. Other kinds of action that can reduce damage, especially to heart muscle, if

Heart Attack Warning Signs

1. Chest pain, usually in the center, perhaps with a squeezing sensation or a burning feeling that might be mistaken for heartburn. Heart attack pain usually doesn't stop on its own.
2. Radiation of pain to the lower jaw, neck, either shoulder or arm
3. Sweating, nausea, shortness of breath, weakness, or fatigue.

Some people having a heart attack do not have typical signs (especially women) or may deny they are uncomfortable. If you even suspect that you or someone else might be having a heart attack, do not delay: Call your local emergency number immediately.

administered quickly enough are the new "clot buster" drugs. To have these medical advances work, however, ordinary citizens need to be educated about heart attack symptoms and the urgency of the "golden hour" following symptom onset for themselves or others. They need to be supported by community services that enable speedy transportation to medical care.

CANCER

Cancer is found in all races and ages of human beings and in all other animal species. It is a leading cause of morbidity and mortality in North America. Cancer is a group of diseases characterized by uncontrolled and disordered growth of abnormal cells that displace or destroy normal cells. Usually the body's defenses target and destroy abnormal cells, but cancer occurs when abnormal cells manage to overcome these defenses. Cancer cells typically form a malignant tumor. Some of the cancer cells may spread to other parts of the body through the blood vessels and lymph channels. In some cancers the cells grow rapidly and spread early; in others they grow slowly and spread late or not at all. This means there is likely no single cure for cancer and prevention messages need to be targeted. The signs and symptoms of cancer are preceded by years of exposure that offer opportunities for prevention intervention, including communication strategies across communities, particularly in minority and underserved populations. When prevention fails, early diagnosis becomes the primary objective of community cancer control programs.

Trends

In contrast to cardiovascular disease, which has shown dramatic decreases in the last twenty-five years, the burden and consequences of cancer have increased. Cancer may surpass cardiovascular disease as the leading cause of death in the twenty-first century. In 1992, the overall rate of cancer mortality was 134 deaths per 100,000 population—a slight increase over the baseline. The mid-decade review of national objectives in cancer shows positive improvements, as illustrated in figure 7-12.

Different types of cancer have had different rates of success in terms of early detection, treatment, or prognosis. Five cancer sites account for about two-thirds of new cases of cancer. For males, these sites are prostate, lung, colorectal, bladder, and non-Hodgkin's lymphoma. For females, the leading five cancers are lung, breast, colorectal, ovarian, and uterine. Although mortality rates for lung and prostate cancer have increased, there have been decreases in colorectal, stomach, and breast cancer deaths. The cervical cancer rate has shown only slight improvement.

Demographic, Social, and Epidemiological Factors

Long-term trends in cancer progress vary according to many factors, including age, race and ethnicity, gender, and socioeconomic status. Cancer is predominantly a disease of middle and old age; it is not common in children and young adults. Persons age seventy and over account for a higher number of cases than any other age group. The risk of developing cancer increases with age. The chance of a person who is less than twenty-years-old developing cancer sometime during his or her lifetime is about one in four.

Racial and ethnic differences in cancer rates are evident, with the black population at relatively high cancer risk. For example, the five-year relative survival rate for those diagnosed with cancer for the total population is 53 percent; for blacks this rate is 39.4 percent. Other differences are found, for example, in breast cancer mortality rates. Black, white, and native Hawaiian women have breast cancer mortality rates about 25 per 100,000; Hispanic, Chinese, Filipino, and Japanese women have annual rates at or below 15 per 100,000. Among the reasons cited for these differences are higher incidence rates, access to screening and early detection, treatment and medical follow-up, and supportive care. National objectives, specific to problems of late detection, were set to increase the proportion of black women who have received a clinical breast exam and mammogram in the past one or two years.

Cancer death rates vary by gender. Overall, the death rate for males exceeds that for females. Clearly, some type of cancer can occur only in men, such as prostate cancer, but other cancers, including breast cancer can occur in men and women. Unfortunately, the leading cause of cancer deaths in both sexes is shared—lung cancer. In 1930 the lung cancer death rate for females was approximately 3 per 100,000; by the 1990s it rose to 31. For males in 1930, lung cancer deaths were approximately 5 per 100,000; by the 1990s the rate soared to 73! By the early 1990s the lung cancer death rate for men was beginning to decline, but the rate for females continued on an upward curve. Though smoking rates have dropped, lung cancer death rates reflect higher smoking rates in previous decades. Much of the debt for increased smoking among females since World War II is yet to be paid. Men who were smoking more than women earlier in the twentieth century have already paid the heavy price. With increased sale of tobacco to developing countries, lung cancer rates are expected to soar internationally.

The variations in cancer rates across society demonstrate that the population does not evenly share cancer-causing factors. Income level, education, and

....

Figure 7-12

Mid-decade status of Year 2000 Cancer Objectives. (*Source:* National Institutes of Health, Public Health Service, U.S. Department of Health and Human Services.)

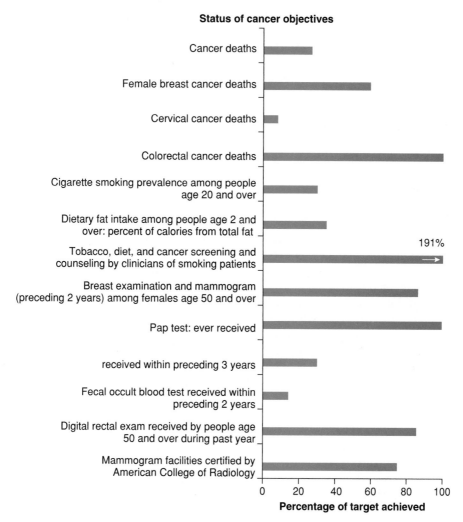

employment can influence cancer risk and outcomes. People with low incomes and little education tend to smoke more, drink more, and have a poorer diet than other groups. They also may work in jobs with more exposure to cancer-causing chemicals. The inequities within and across subpopulations must be considered in prevention efforts.

Risk Factors

Most cancers are associated with everyday things, including tobacco use, diet, occupation, and family history.

Tobacco   Tobacco is related to one-third of cancer deaths, therefore it is an important focus in prevention efforts. Smokers have higher rates of cancer for the tissues that are exposed to the **carcinogens** in tobacco smoke. These tissues include the larynx, oral cavity, esophagus, lung, and urinary bladder. Smoking accounts for 87 percent of lung cancer deaths. Overall, about 26 percent of Americans and 29 percent of Canadians smoke. There is a disproportionately high prevalence of smoking among blue-collar workers, military personnel, and American Indians and Alaska Natives.

Diet   It is estimated that about 20 percent of fatal cancers are related to diet. It seems to be an especially important factor in breast, bowel, and prostate cancers. Following dietary guidelines, and particularly reducing fat in the diet, can help reduce this risk.

Occupation   Risks for different types of cancer vary by occupation. For example, fire fighters have higher cancer risks because of their exposure to burning toxic substances; construction workers may be exposed to asbestos; outdoor work increases the risk of skin cancer; and industrial and medical workers exposed to old or faulty radio active devices may have increased risk for leukemia. Other factors may compound these risks, such as air pollution and smoking.

Family History   Risk factors for cancer include a familial tendency for the development of cancer, especially of breast, stomach, and large intestine. It is not known to what extent this is truly a genetic factor or to what extent it is caused by environmental factors such as diet, lifestyle, or occupation that may remain similar from one generation to the next. Research suggests that genetic make-up plays an indirect role, more likely influencing whether a person exposed to a cancer-causing substance goes on to develop the disease.

Early Detection of Cancer

The dominant factor in the prognosis for cancer patients is the stage at which treatment is first begun. The outlook is markedly improved if the cancer is treated when it is still localized, rather than spread to the neighboring lymph glands or to distant organs of the body. The most promising method of early detection is screening people who have no symptoms but who, by reason of their age, sex, occupation, ethnicity, or lifestyle, may be in a high-risk group. The validity of screening methods varies.

Cervical Cancer   The Papanicolaou (Pap) smear is an effective screening for cancer of the cervix, the entrance to the female uterus. This exam is sensitive and specific in detecting precancerous changes in the cervix. The test is reliable and painless and as a result has achieved wide use among health providers and patients. The five-year survival rate for the earliest, precancerous stage of cervical cancer is 100 percent. Nearly all women can be saved if the diagnosis is made at this early stage. The community problem is that certain groups of women, including the old, less educated, and low-income, do not seek out the screening test. Community efforts need to be directed toward identifying these women and encouraging them to avail themselves of this preventive procedure.

Breast Cancer   Breast cancer is the second leading cause of cancer deaths in women. The overall breast cancer rate for women has fallen about 5 percent. The age adjusted rates, however, show that the 6 percent drop in breast cancer rates for white women was offset by a 1 percent increase for black women. In 1997, 43,900 women in the United States died of breast cancer.

Methods of detecting breast cancer include breast self-examination, screening at physicals, and mammography. Monthly breast self-examination should be encouraged. The method is simple to learn and can be taught by demonstrations, films, television programs, and printed material. Fear of finding a "lump" and lack of experience with the technique are barriers to self-examination that health education can address. For some women, partner examinations may be preferable, if the partner is properly trained in the technique. Many physicians routinely do breast examinations during clinic visits for Pap smears.

Objectives for Pap Smear Screening

- By the year 2000 increase to at least 95 percent the proportion of women age 18 and older who have ever received a Pap test. Baseline: 88 percent had the test in 1987.
- By the year 2000 increase to at least 85 percent the proportion of women age 18 and older who received a Pap test within the preceding 1 to 3 years. Baseline: 75 percent within the preceding 3 years in 1987.

Mammography is an x-ray examination of the soft tissues of the breast to detect cancer in its early stages (figure 7-13). It can detect 85 to 90 percent of tumors in women over 50 and can discover a tumor up to two years before a lump can be felt. As of late 1994, U.S. mammography facilities are required by law to be certified by the Food and Drug Administration to ensure that the tests are safe and reliable. For women over 50 who have no symptoms of breast cancer and who are not at a higher risk for the disease, experts generally agree that screening should be done every one to two years. It is estimated such screening could reduce deaths from breast cancer by 30 percent. Experts do not agree on the usefulness of screening mammography for women in their 40s. For women at higher risk—which includes age, previous incidence of other cancers, close relative with breast cancer, first menstrual period at age 10 or earlier, no pregnancies, first live birth at age 30 or older, and previous benign breast disease—earlier or more frequent mammograms may be recommended. Any woman who has symptoms, such as a lump or change in the breast, should seek medical care immediately.

Prostate Cancer   Prostate cancer most often occurs in men in their 60s and 70s. In 1997 345,500 men in the U.S. were diagnosed with prostate cancer and 41,800 died from this type of cancer. For the United States the number of cases represents a

Figure 7-13

The mammogram compresses one breast at a time for better radiographic resolution of small lumps that would not be detected by physical breast examination (palpation). (Photo courtesy American Cancer Society.)

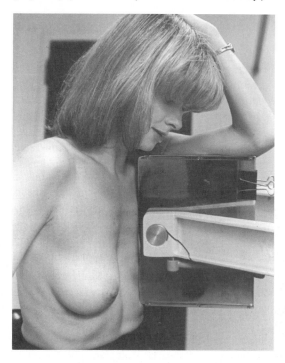

large increase from the 85,000 recorded cases in the 1980s. Research has narrowed the search for a prostate cancer gene, which holds promise for improved diagnosis and new treatments. With the incidence of prostate cancer exceeding lung cancer for men, recommendations have been made for screening. These include a blood test for prostate-specific antigen (PSA). The test is controversial, however, in that it does not appear to reliably distinguish between aggressive and slow growing forms of prostate cancer. While the PSA test has been helpful in identifying prostate cancer in some cases, in others it has resulted in anxiety, unnecessary treatment, and impaired quality of life following treatment complications. Health education messages about prostate cancer can enable men to

Objective for Lung Cancer

By 2000 slow the rise in lung cancer deaths to achieve a rate of no more than 42 per 100,000 people. Age-adjusted baseline: 37.9 per 100,000 in 1987.

make more informed choices about treatment and screening by providing them with current facts, identifying gaps in research and treatment knowledge, and providing updated information.

Lung Cancer   The gloomy outlook in lung cancer is slowly improving. Although we can identify persons of high-risk—namely, men and women over forty-five years of age who smoke more than one pack of cigarettes daily—it is still difficult to detect lung cancer early. This is because changes detectable by x-ray film occur late, and lung cancer cells are difficult to produce and interpret microscopically. Not all tumors exfoliate cells that may be coughed up and recognized as cancer cells under the microscope.

Colorectal Cancer   Colorectal cancer is highly curable, *if* detected early. Unfortunately, screening tests are unpleasant or embarrassing to many because they involve a direct examination of the bowels or stool (figure 7-14). Education programs need to address these issues. Colon and rectal cancers may be detected by the presence of blood in the stools. Sigmoidoscopy (an exam that allows direct vision of the lower bowel) and x-ray examination of the lower bowel are indicated if blood is present. The American Cancer Society recommends that sigmoidoscopy be done every three to five years in males or females over 50 on the advice of their physician. New, flexible scopes make this procedure more effective and comfortable. Stool sample tests are recommended annually for this group. Digital rectal examinations are recommended annually for males and females over 40 years of age.

Figure 7-14

Educational programs can help adults overcome the embarrassment of an exam for colon cancer, which if caught early is highly curable. (*Source:* American Cancer Society.)

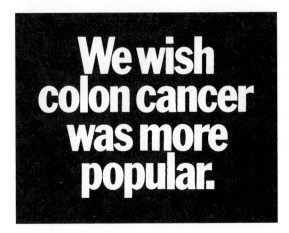

For good reason. Because of it was more top of mind, more people would know it's one of this country's top killers.

And more importantly, more people would know it's 90% curable if treated in its earliest stages.

If you're over 40, you're at risk. See your doctor and request a colorectal cancer checkup. Do it now.

We know its not the first thing on your mind. We just don't want it to be the last.

Learn more. Call the American Cancer Society at 1-800-ACS-2345.

Cancer Research

Cancer research has the following three thrusts: (1) to discover the causes of the cancer so that preventive measures may be taken; (2) to pioneer new screening and education programs for early detection and for reducing exposure to cigarettes and other risk factors; and (3) to improve results of treatment for persons with cancer. The public should not be persuaded to believe that if sufficient money is spent, the threat of cancer will be removed. Unfortunately, in cancers in which the cause has been discovered, the number of cases has actually increased. Lung cancer is the classic example. The cause is clearly identified as cigarette smoking, but prevention involves altering behavior, which is difficult to achieve. Many cancers may be prevented by the modification of lifestyle to avoid known hazardous customs and by the use of early detection methods already available. The community effort must be directed toward making people aware of this, rather than making them dependent on research results or cures at some future date.

DIABETES AND CHRONIC DISABLING CONDITIONS

Diabetes and other chronic disabling conditions lead to physical, emotional, social, and economic costs to individuals, families, and communities. While life expectancy at birth climbed steadily in the 1990s, years of healthy life have actually decreased. Diabetes is the seventh leading cause of death in the United States. Chronic disabling conditions cause major activity limitations for over 10 percent of the U.S. population. The percentage of minorities with chronic conditions is disproportionate and increasing.

Progress on the mid-decade national objectives for diabetes and chronic disabling conditions is mixed (figure 7-15). According to *Healthy People 2000 Midcourse Review,* this priority areas focuses on the need for prevention of disabilities; early diagnosis and treatment of chronic conditions; and provision of information, skills training, and support services to increase the ability of people to manage their conditions, to live independently, and to participate fully in their communities.

Diabetes

Diabetes is a vascular disease and a metabolic disorder. It is characterized by high blood glucose levels caused by a deficiency in insulin production, an impairment of insulin action, or both. Approximately 7 million people in the United States have been diagnosed with diabetes, and an additional 7 million may unknowingly have the disease. Diabetes is a risk factor for cardiovascular disease and the leading cause of lower extremity amputation, blindness, and end-stage renal disease.

High-risk populations for diabetes include blacks, Hispanics, Native Americans, obese people, people with a family history of diabetes, and women with previous gestational diabetes. The prevalence of diabetes in the U.S. black population is about 50 percent higher than in non-Hispanic whites, and the occurrence in Hispanics is about double that of non-Hispanic whites.

Lifestyle choices influence diabetic outcomes. For example, one study found that pack-a-day smokers are twice as likely as nonsmokers to get adult-onset diabetes, but moderate drinkers run a lower risk than teetotalers. The morbidity of diabetes is caused by its vascular complications. Coronary heart disease rates are increased by diabetes. Specific preventable complications of diabetes include renal disease; diabetic retinopathy and blindness if the retinal arteries are involved (figure 7-16); amputations necessitated when blood supply to the limbs is decreased, usually in the foot and calf, with resulting gangrene; and perinatal morbidity and mortality due to diabetes in birth mothers. Because of the role health education can play in these complications, one U.S. objective for the nation is to increase to 75 percent by the year 2000 the number and percentage of people with diabetes who have received formal patient education about their disease and resources to assist in the management of it.

One-half of diabetic persons may be treated by diet alone—one that is low in calories and fat. The remainder require insulin or oral hypoglycemic drugs. Community efforts are needed, for the prognosis in diabetes is related to the resources of the patients, their families, and the communities in which they live. Diabetics who are old, poor, or live alone tend to do poorly. The duties of the community toward persons with diabetes are similar to those toward persons with hypertension. Screening programs to uncover the disease early, before it is symptomatic, are of prime importance. After those with diabetes are identified, education is needed to ensure adherence to diet and drug regimens and other lifestyle modifications.

. . . .

Figure 7-15

Mid-decade status of Year 2000 Objectives for diabetes and chronic disabling conditions. (*Source:* National Institutes of Health, Public Health Service, U.S. Department of Health and Human Services.)

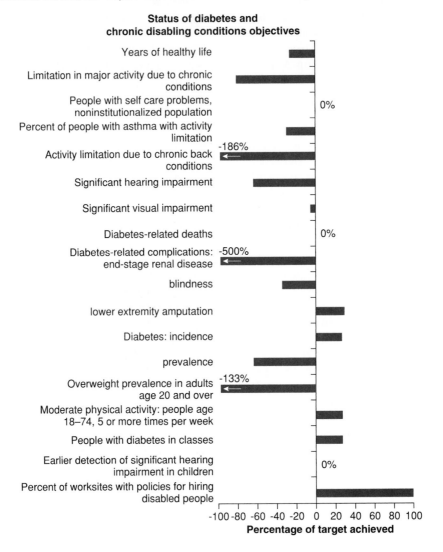

Status of diabetes and chronic disabling conditions objectives

Percentage of target achieved

Liver Disease

One of the ten leading causes of death for adults is liver disease, the most common of which is cirrhosis of the liver. Cirrhosis is a chronic disease that results in slow deterioration of the liver so that it is progressively less able to carry out its functions.

The most common cause of this disease in North America is alcohol abuse. Death from cirrhosis declined during the Prohibition Era when alcohol was illegal. Following Prohibition death rates from cirrhosis increased until 1973, when they again began to decline steadily with reductions in

. . . .
Figure 7-16

Among the complications of diabetes, retinopathy is the most common. Blindness can be prevented by adequate control of the blood-sugar level and self-management of the disease. (*Source:* National Eye Institute, National Institutes of Health, Public Health Service, U.S. Department of Health and Human Services.)

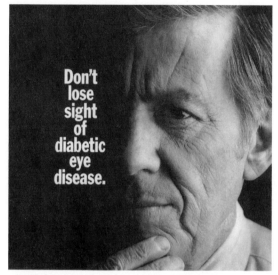

Don't lose sight of diabetic eye disease.

Almost *half* of all people with diabetes have diabetic eye disease—whether they know it or not. In fact, if you have diabetes, you're at increased risk for blindness. No matter how good you feel. No matter how well you're taking care of your diabetes.

With early detection and timely treatment, the risk of blindness can be greatly reduced. If you have diabetes, at least once a year, get a dilated eye examination in which drops are used to enlarge your pupils. This allows your eye care professional to see more of the inside of your

eye to check for diabetic eye disease. And, if you know anyone who has diabetes, ask him or her to get an eye examination, too.

For more information about diabetic eye disease, please write: National Eye Health Education Program, Box 20/20, Bethesda, MD 20892.

Get your eyes examined. NATIONAL EYE HEALTH EDUCATION PROGRAM

alcohol consumption. Community programs to reduce cirrhosis need to focus on efforts to reduce heavy drinking patterns, especially in high-risk subpopulations. Death rates for nonwhites remain almost 70 percent higher than rates for whites; the rates for Native American men are triple those of white men. These disparities may represent differential access to health care, differential drinking patterns, socioeconomic status or some combination of these and other factors.

Chronic Lung Disease

Chronic obstructive pulmonary disease (COPD) is characterized by permanent airflow obstruction to the lungs. Nearly 80,000 people die each year from this condition. Cigarette smoking accounts for 82 percent of those deaths. The death rate from this disease parallels that of lung cancer. Death from COPD often comes after an extended period of disability and many of those disabled by lung disease die from other causes. Community programs to reduce smoking rates will benefit reduction of this disease. With cessation of smoking, the rate of functional loss declines, but lost lung function cannot be regained. Timely smoking cessation can prevent the development of symptomatic disease.

Asthma

Asthma is one chronic lung disease that has increased in prevalence and in mortality rates, especially in the black population in the United States. Over 12 million Americans have asthma, a rise of 40 percent since 1982. It is estimated that ten Canadians die each week from asthma. Those most at risk include smokers and their children, those with a family history of the disease, and people with allergies. Experts are not sure why asthma is on the rise, but speculate that air pollution, airtight homes and sealed offices, secondhand smoke, viral infections, and poor living conditions have contributed to the increase. To help prevent or limit episodes the following can be useful: air filters and green plants to purify household air, humidifiers to lubricate air passages, and a vaporizer if an attack has begun.

Arthritis

Arthritis and rheumatic diseases are the most common cause of lost work days annually in most developed countries, although the respiratory diseases account for the greatest number of episodes of sickness. It is difficult to determine the prevalence of types of arthritis because of the range of symptoms and the variability of diagnostic standards. If major mobility limitations are used as the determining factor, the prevalence of some arthritic symptoms is 3 percent.

Rheumatoid arthritis is a systemic inflammatory disease with local joint manifestations, in which the small joints of the hands are often affected early. The disease pursues a chronic course marked by relapses and remissions. The sex ratio shows an excess of females, 2.5 to 1.0. Risk factors include lower socioeconomic status, infections, trauma, winter season, and social stress. The age of onset is young, between 20 and 45 years, commonly 30 to 40 years. In contrast, osteoarthritis affects older persons exclusively and occurs in larger, weight-bearing joints such as the hips and knees. Trauma and obesity are antecedent factors. The community role includes employers providing work for those arthritic persons who are able to work, which is a surprisingly high proportion. Transportation services from home to treatment facilities, home visits, and meals on wheels services are vital to these people.

As with each of the major chronic diseases (heart, cancer, diabetes, and lung diseases), the U.S. Congress has called for the establishment of regional comprehensive arthritis centers with two distinct purposes: (1) to develop and foster new methods for the prompt and effective application of available knowledge and (2) to develop new knowledge to combat arthritis. In response to this mandate the National Institute of Arthritis, Metabolism, and Digestive Diseases has developed a program of multipurpose arthritis centers, each of which engages in research, education, and community demonstration projects.

The Multipurpose Arthritis Centers have a national distribution ranging from Boston to Hawaii. Many of the projects underway in these centers could not have been started without the interaction of individuals brought together under their aegis. Examples of major efforts of the centers include research into the genetic basis of arthritis; new advances in health services research, such as cost effectiveness studies and analysis of disability; comprehensive education of allied health professionals; and research into the best methods of delivering arthritis health care and education to those least able to obtain it, such as the homebound individual and residents of the inner city.

IMMUNIZATIONS

While the preceding emphasis has been on chronic diseases as the leading causes of morbidity and mortality, adults also need protection against communicable diseases. Some immunizations are as important for adults as for children. There are eight diseases against which all or many adults need to receive immunizations (figure 7-17).

Influenza

The flu, or influenza, virus is a highly contagious disease with symptoms that include fever, chills, headache, sore throat, dry cough, runny nose, and body aches. Adults rarely have upset stomachs with influenza. This disease is spread by direct contact with an infected person or through contact with the airborne virus in crowded places such as theaters, store, and airplanes. A person becomes sick with flu soon after being exposed to it, usually within one to three days. Flu shots are especially important for people aged sixty-five or older and for people of any age with diabetes; chronic diseases of the heart, lungs, or kidneys; chronic anemia; or diseases that interfere with the body's immune system. Influenza viruses change often, therefore it is necessary for those at risk to get a flu shot every year. The best time of the year to get the shot is in November, ahead of the usual flu season.

Rubella

Although rubella, German measles, is often a mild disease it can cause serious birth defects in the unborn child if contracted by a mother during the first three months of pregnancy. It is estimated that as many as 12 million women of childbearing age are susceptible to rubella. Women of childbearing age can know they are protected against rubella either by receiving one immunization or by undergoing a simple blood test. Women should

Figure 7-17

Adults, responsible for the immunization of children, often forget their own needs for immunizations. (*Source:* National Immunization Program, Centers for Disease Control and Prevention, Public Health Service, U.S. Department of Health & Human Services.)

IMMUNIZATION
OF ADULTS

A Call to Action

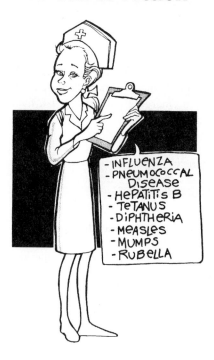

- INFLUENZA
- PNEUMOCOCCAL DISEASE
- HEPATITIS B
- TETANUS
- DIPHTHERIA
- MEASLES
- MUMPS
- RUBELLA

U.S. DEPARTMENT OF HEALTH & HUMAN SERVICES
Public Health Service
Centers for Disease Control and Prevention
National Immunization Program
Atlanta, Georgia 30333

September 1986
Revised September 1991
Revised May 1994

not receive the vaccine if they are pregnant or might become pregnant within three months.

Hepatitis B

Each year, up to half a million Americans are affected by one of the types of viral hepatitis that causes an inflammation of the liver. Hepatitis B virus is a serious form of this disease and accounts for half of all cases of hepatitis in the United States. The virus is transmitted by blood and sometimes other body fluids, such as saliva and semen. Approximately 10 percent of people infected become chronic carriers and about one-fourth of carriers develop chronic hepatitis that can result in severe liver damage. The vaccine to prevent hepatitis B is recommended primarily for those at highest risk including health care workers, people who have had sexually transmitted diseases, homosexually active men, and injecting drug users.

Tetanus

Tetanus occurs when soil contaminated with the tetanus bacteria gets into any break in the skin, such as a deep puncture wound or through small scratches, burns, and slivers. Once inside the wound, tetanus bacteria grow and produce toxin that attacks the body's nervous system. Unimmunized adults have only a 30 percent chance of surviving tetanus. Although many adults received tetanus immunization in childhood, a booster shot is required every 10 years for life. A simple way to remember the booster is to have the immunizations on the mid-decade birthday, ages 15, 25, 35, and so forth.

Other Vaccines

The four other diseases for which immunizations are recommended for adults include measles, mumps, diphtheria, and pneumococcus. In addition, it is best to contact a physician or public health department as early as possible when making plans for a trip abroad. Travel between the United States, Canada, Europe, Mexico, or the Caribbean requires no special immunizations.

ISSUES AND CONTROVERSIES
Is Culture Keeping Up with Changing Attitides toward Death?

Assisted suicide, euthanasia, people declining radiation or surgical therapies in their old age on the grounds that the cure is worse than the disease—these are signs of changing cultures of health, aging, and dying. As the baby-boom generation approaches retirement, the prospect of more old people with more chronic conditions because they have lived longer faces North American cultures with difficult questions. Organ transplant waiting lists grew nearly 300 percent from 1988, from just over 15,000 to nearly 45,000 in 1995. The number of donors has remained relatively constant, even declining. How can these issues of care and extended life for older people be faced by a society or community accustomed to applying whatever technology is available, at whatever cost? The majority of Americans disagree with a U.S. Supreme Court decision that there is no right to physician-assisted suicide, according to a 1997 poll. Oregon legalized it. Under what circumstances would you accept physician-assisted suicide in your family or community?

SUMMARY

Leading threats to adult health changed in the twentieth century from communicable to chronic diseases. Multiple factors contribute to the onset, morbidity, and mortality of the chronic diseases including lifestyle, socioeconomic status, heredity, race and ethnicity, and health services. Periodic health assessments and examinations contribute to adult health. Communities need to ensure access to such services for all citizens and provide education targeted to specific adult populations to enable informed use of services. Adults can contribute to their own health in many ways, including physical activity adapted to their capacity, stress management, rest, proper nutrition, tobacco avoidance, limited exposure to other harmful substances, prevention of disease, early treatment of disease and disability, promotion of life interests, and attainment of emotional stability. All are important in the promotion of a high level of health, the extension of the prime of life, and a greater life expectancy. Time, money, and effort must be devoted to health promotion and must be invested by communities and employers and by adults for themselves and their families.

The adult health program must concentrate on specific health problems and at the same time must promote general health education and coping skills. It must deal with the present, but also must project itself into programs anticipating future needs and emerging patterns of risk factors and risk conditions.

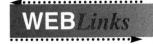

WEB *Links*

http://www.cdc.gov/diseases/diseases.html
Maintained by the CDC, this website contains diseases, health risks, prevention guidelines and strategies for specific diseases.

http://www.diabetes.com
Information on such things as diet, news, support groups, discussion groups, and complications of the disease.

http://www.amhrt.org
American Heart Association web site

http://www.cwhn.ca/
Canadian Women's Health Network

http://www.womens-health.com/main.html
Women's Health Interactive: An interactive learning environment that facilitates the exchange of information among participants; promotes learning; and motivates individual, proactive response.

http://www.cwhn.ca
The Canadian Women's Health Network: Product of
health care workers, educators, advocates, consumers
and others committed to sharing resources and strategies
to better women's health.

http://www.womenshealthalliance.com/
Women's Health Alliance: A membership organization
dedicated to giving all women reliable, up-to-date health
information.

QUESTIONS FOR REVIEW

1. How would the conquest of infection affect the incidence of the chronic diseases?
2. What is meant by a "disease of civilization"?
3. Why is it important that effort be extended toward
   research in the treatment and in the prevention of
   the chronic diseases?
4. In what ways are women likely to be treated differently than men in cardiovascular disease, and why?
5. In your experience, how have restaurants made
   healthy food choices easier or harder?
6. Why does the United States invest more money in
   cancer research than in cardiovascular research?
7. Provide examples of ways in which health education programs directed at children could also address the health of their parents.
8. How would you design a program for your community to decrease the incidence of cancer of the respiratory tract?
9. Why is it preferable to teach a respect for cancer
   rather than a fear of cancer?
10. Using only local funds and resources, how would
    you design a community program for early discov-
    ery of cancer through the regular medical examina-
    tion of nearly all adults?
11. If health is affected by so many different factors,
    how do we get a handle on what is "health" and
    what is not?
12. How would you design a program intended to
    discover all cases of diabetes mellitus in your
    community?
13. What are the services and facilities available in your
    community for the diagnosis and treatment of
    arthritis?
14. What additional services and facilities are needed
    by your community for an adequate adult health
    program?

READINGS

Devesa, S. S., W. J. Blot, B. J. Stone, B. A. Miller, R. E.
Tarone, and J. F. Fraumeni. 1995. Recent cancer
trends in the United States. *J Natl Cancer Inst*
87(3):175–82.
Cancer incidence rates have been reported to be increasing in the United States, although trends vary according to the form of cancer. This article identifies
cancers accounting for the rising incidence, quantifies
the changes that occurred from the mid-1970s to the
early 1990s, and contrasts incidence and mortality
trends to provide clues to the determinants of the tem-
poral patterns.

Green, L. W., and M. W. Kreuter. 1992. CDC's planned
approach to community health as an application of
PRECEDE and an inspiration for PROCEED *J
Health Educ* 23:140.
Describes how the PRECEDE model, introduced in
chapter 3 of this book, was used in the community
chronic disease prevention programs sponsored by
the U.S. Centers for Disease Control.

Lauzon, R. 1993. Heart disease prevention. In *Canada's
health promotion survey 1990: technical report,*
Health and Welfare Canada, edited by T. Stephens,
and G. D. Fowler. Ottawa: Minister of Supply and
Services Canada.
Reports on the 1990 national survey of Canadians
ages fifteen and over, their knowledge and perceptions of the causes of heart disease, and health behaviors people had taken to detect or control blood pressure or cholesterol, quit smoking, exercise, modify
diet, or maintain weight.

Manson, J. E., P. M. Ridker, J. M. Gaziano, and C. H.
Hennekens. 1996. *Prevention of mycardial infarction.*
New York: Oxford.
A state-of-the-art compendium of the scientific evidence on the efficacy of coronary disease prevention
that focuses on helping clinicians develop intervention skills to use available knowledge. Chapters by
leading authorities in cardiovascular epidemiology,
cardiology, cost-effectiveness analysis, and public
health translate the theory or preventive cardiology
into feasible implementation.

WHO Scientific Group. 1994. Cardiovascular disease
risk factors: New areas for research. Technical Report
Series, No. 841, ISBN 92-4-1208414. Geneva: World
Health Organization.

Specific research areas are reviewed that promise to yield better knowledge about risk factors for cardiovascular disease and the most effective strategies for prevention, including nutritional factors; the possible protective role of alcohol and physical activity; hormone replacement therapy; and the roles of genetic, social, cultural, and psychosocial factors.

BIBLIOGRAPHY

Allegrante, J. P., P. T. Kovar, C. R. MacKenzie, M. G. E. Petersen, and B. Gutin. 1993. A walking education program for patients with osteoarthritis of the knee: theory and intervention strategies. *Health Educ Q* 20:63.

American Heart Association. 1992. Statement on exercise—benefits and recommendations for physical activity programs for all Americans. *Circulation* 86:340.

Apter, T. 1995. *Women in the new midlife.* New York: W. W. Norton.

Battista, R. N., J. L. Williams, and L. A. MacFarlane. 1990. Determinants of preventive practices in fee-for-service primary care. *Am J Prev Med* 6:6.

Bertera, R. L. 1990. Planning and implementing health promotion in the workplace: a case study of the Du Pont Company experience. *Health Educ Q* 17:307.

Bertera, R. L., L. K. Oehl, and J. M. Telepchak. 1990. Self-help versus group approaches to smoking cessation in the workplace: eighteen-month follow-up and cost analysis. *Am J Health Prom* 4:187.

Biglan, A., and R. E. Glasgow. 1991. The social unit: an important facet in the design of cancer control research. *Prev Med* 20:292.

Braddy, B. A., D. Orenstein, J. N. Brownstein, and T. J. Cook. 1992. PATCH: an example of community empowerment for health. *J Health Educ* 23:179.

Brunk, S. E., and J. Goeppinger. 1990. Process evaluation: assessing reinvention of community-based interventions. *Eval Health Professions* 13:186.

Byrd, T. 1992. Project Verdad: a community development approach to health. *Hygie: Int J Health Educ* 11:15.

Canadian Heart Health Survey Research Group. 1992. Canadian heart health surveys: a profile of cardiovascular risk. *Can Med Assoc J Suppl.* June 1:1969.

Canadian Task Force on the Periodic Health Examination. 1991. Periodic health examination, 1997. *Can Med Assoc J* 145:15.

Cardiovascular disease mortality in the developing countries. 1993. *World Health Statistics quarterly* 46 (2).

Costanza, M. E. 1992. Physician compliance with mammography guidelines: barriers and enhancers. *J Am Board Fam Pract* 5:1.

Dignan, M. B., R. Michielutte, K. Blinson, H. B. Wells, L. D. Case, P. Sharp, S. Davis, J. Konen, and R. P. McQuellon. 1996. Effectiveness of health education to increase screening for cervical cancer among eastern-band Cherokee Indian women in North Carolina. *J National Cancer Inst* 88:1670.

Farquhar, J. 1992. Bridging the gap: science and policy in action. Declaration of the Advisory Board, Victoria: International Heart Health Conference.

Farquhar, J. W., S. P. Fortmann, and J. A. Flora. 1990. Effects of community-wide education on cardiovascular disease risk factors—the Stanford 5-city Project. *JAMA* 264:359.

Farr, L. J., and L. J. Fisher. 1991. "Bring your body back to life": the 1990 Western Australian quit campaign, *Health Prom J Austr* 1:6.

Gottlieb, N. H., C. Y. Lovato, R. Weinstein, L. W. Green, and M. P. Eriksen. 1992. Implementation of a restrictive work site smoking policy in a large decentralized organization. *Health Educ Quar* 19:77.

Klag, M. J., P. K. Whelton, and J. Coresh. 1991. The association of skin color with blood pressure in United States blacks with low socioeconomic status. *JAMA* 265:599.

Kumanyik, S. 1991. Behavioral aspects of intervention strategies to reduce dietary sodium. *Hypertension* 17:1190.

Lawrence, R. S. 1990. The role of physicians in promoting health. *Health Affairs* 9:122.

Leppik, I. E. 1990. How to get patients with epilepsy to take their medication: the problem of noncompliance. *Postgrad Med* 88:253.

Love, R. R., and J. E. Davis. 1991. Screening mammography in clinical practice: a complex activity. *Arch Intern Med* 151:19.

Mantel, J. E. A. T. DiVittis, and M. J. Averbach. 1997. *Evaluating HIV prevention interventions.* New York: Plenum Press.

McCoy, H. V., S. E. Dodds, and C. Nolan. 1990. AIDS intervention design for program evaluation: the Miami Community Outreach Project. *J Drug Issues* 20:223.

Nourjah, P., D. K. Wagener, M. Eberhardt, and A. M. Horowitz. 1994. Knowledge of risk factors and risk behaviors related to coronary heart disease among blue and white collar males. *Journal of Public Health Policy* 15:443–459.

Nutbeam, D., C. Smith, and J. Catford. 1990. Evaluation in health education: A review of progress, possibilities, and problems. *J Epidemiol Comm Health* 44:83.

O'Conner, A. 1993. Women's cancer prevention practices. In *Canada's health promotion survey 1990: technical report,* Health and Welfare Canada, edited by T. Stephens T, and Graham D. Fowler. Ottawa: Minister of Supply and Services Canada.

Reichelt, P. A. 1995. Musculoskeletal injury: ergonomics and physical fitness in firefighters. *Occup Med: State of the Art Reviews* 10:735.

Richard, L., L. Potvin, N. Kischuk, H. Prlic, and L. W. Green. 1996. Assessment of the integration of the ecological approach in health promotion programs. *Am J. Health Prom* 10:318.

Simons-Morton, B. G., W. H. Green, and N. H. Gottlieb. 1995. *Introduction to health education and health promotion.* 2nd ed. Prospect Heights, Ill.: Waveland Press, Inc.

Singer, J., E. A. Lindsey, and D. M. C. Wilson. 1991. Promoting physical activity in primary care: overcoming the barriers. *Can Fam Phys* 37:2167.

Walsh, J. M. E., and S. McPhee. 1992. A systems model of clinical preventive care: an analysis of factors influencing patient and physician. *Health Educ Q* 19:157.

Zapka, J. G., D. Hosmer, and M. E. Costanza. 1992. Changes in mammography use: economic, need, and service factors. *Am J Public Health* 82:1345.

Zuckerman, M. J., L. G. Guerra, D. A. Drossman, J. A. Foland, and G. G. Gregory. 1996. Health-care-seeking behaviors related to bowel complaints: Hispanic versus non-Hispanic whites. *Digestive Diseases & Sciences* 41:77.

Chapter *8*

Aging and Health of Older Populations

These are the soul's changes. I don't believe in aging. I believe in forever altering one's aspect to the sun. Hence my optimism.
—Virginia Woolf

Women over fifty already form one of the largest groups in the population structure of the western world. As long as they like themselves, they will not be an oppressed minority. In order to like themselves they must reject trivialization by others of who and what they are. A grown woman should not have to masquerade as a girl in order to remain in the land of the living.
—Germaine Greer

Objectives

When you finish this chapter, you should be able to:

- Assess the special health needs of a community's older population
- Identify community health programs and services appropriate to the needs of the elderly

- Anticipate future health needs of older populations

Gerontology and **geriatrics** study the aging process, including biological, psychological, and social change. Gerontology is concerned with the natural aging process and with pathological aging. Geriatrics deals with the care of the aged and is concerned primarily with enabling older people with illness or disability to live productively and enjoyably. The applied field of community health deals more with geriatrics than with gerontology; hence, this chapter will deal with health as an aspect of geriatrics. Health cannot be isolated from the total life of the community. Circumstances of

living indirectly related to health must also be considered, hence the use of *social* geriatrics in community health.

Healthy People 2000, the U.S. objectives for health promotion and disease prevention, suggests steps to maximize well-being at each stage of life. This chapter will review these from the perspective of older people. We must recognize, however, that many of the problems of old age—such as heart disease, stroke, and cancer—are rooted in circumstances and behavior found earlier in life. Health promotion and disease prevention are lifelong

Table 8-1
The Four Leading Causes of Death Are Notably Different for Each of Six Major Age Groups in the Life Span.

Rank	Infants	1-14	15-24	25-44	45-64	65+
1	Prematurity	Unintentional injuries	Unintentional injuries	Unintentional injuries	Cancer	Heart disease
2	Birth-related	Cancer	Homicide	Cancer	Heart disease	Cancer
3	Congenital defects	Congenital anomalies	Suicide	HIV infection	Stroke	Stroke
4	Sudden infant death	Homicide	Cancer	Heart disease	Injuries	Chronic obstructive pulmonary disease

concerns that can produce benefits at any stage of the life cycle, but their benefits for the elderly are cumulative.

This chapter concentrates on the three points of intervention represented by the models of the health field and community health promotion developed in previous chapters. First, we examine the natural history of health behavior among the aging population. We will then examine the social history of changes in the lives of aging persons that may support the processes of adaptation represented in figures 2-3 and 2-4 and in tables 6-1 and 8-1. You should review these figures and tables now. Discussion will concentrate specifically on three circumstances or transitions of the type implied by table 6-1: relocation, retirement, and **bereavement.** Finally, this chapter will suggest a number of health-promoting programs focused on these and other transitions and targeted to those elderly people most at risk in a community. It will suggest how you might be able to help mobilize community resources and the elderly themselves in support of such programs.

The Natural History and Demography of Aging

Aging begins with conception, but for practical purposes aging refers to that phase in life when body functioning begins to decline. Technically, then, one could describe everyone over the age of 30 as aging. The problem is with the particular health factors that are of special importance to a given age (table 8-1). Sixty-five is the most widely accepted age of eligibility for retirement benefits, therefore it is customary to think of anyone beyond this age as being in the classification of "aged." Yet a person of chronological age 55 could be older socially or physiologically than another individual of age 75. The arbitrary age of 65 epidemiologically marks off a segment of the population that has health needs different from those of other segments. Many of the health problems of the retired population could have been prevented at earlier ages or at least anticipated constructively with **preretirement counseling.**

The Life Span Perspective

One approach to the analysis of the health of older adults relative to that of other age groups, combining the developmental, epidemiological, and behavioral perspectives, is to use transitions in the life span. Recall the epidemiological concepts of host, agent, and environment discussed in chapter 3.

Host Resistance The ideal intervention in community health is one that anticipates potential problems or requirements for the health of populations and prepares the "host" population to resist the problem or to provide for the need. If we can structure the environment in such a way as to preclude the need for any action on the part of the host, so much the better. If we can isolate the agent and neutralize it, better yet. The pervasive agents of the new leading causes of morbidity and death, however, are parts of the fabric of modern living, not so easily isolated and neutralized. They include high fat foods, alcohol, tobacco and other drugs, sedentary work and leisure, stress, and automobiles. Communities are unwilling to give up the convenience and pleasures of such agents. We can control some or limit their negative impact on health by regulating their distribution, pricing, taxation, and public use. People use most of these agents privately. however, so we cannot control them entirely by restraints on public behavior. Educational strategies must therefore supplement environmental strategies to build host resistance or behavioral capacity to adapt to these conditions of living.

Life Span Risks No variable relates more consistently to mortality and morbidity than age. Age is such a powerful correlate of mortality, morbidity, and activity limitation that crude death rates and cause-specific incidence and prevalence rates must be adjusted for age, as seen in chapter 3. Age correlates so consistently with morbidity and mortality, therefore it serves as a convenient marker for program planning. A community can set its priorities for intervention on the problems of specific subpopulations defined by age. The four leading causes of death for each of six major age groups, for example, are different in each age group.

The Relativity of Health

Although health is a primary concern of the oldest adults, illness and age are not synonymous. Data from national surveys indicate that the majority of the elderly in Canada and the United States see themselves as well, not sick. **Functional health** refers to a state of general health emphasizing ability to perform activities of daily living. On a scale of one to five, over 88 percent of men and 83 percent of women have a high level of health (scoring four out of five, or 0.80 where 1.0 would be "per-

fect health"). This percentage declines with age, as shown in figure 8-1, but even among those over seventy-five years of age, more than half report good health by this measure. In assessing their health status, the elderly tend to compare themselves not with all people, but with their age cohorts, including those who live in institutions and those who have died. A high correlation exists between the negative evaluation of health status and the degree to which an elderly person feels economically stressed, lonely, alienated, or useless.

Older people who report that they have good to excellent health also more often report having a positive psychological attitude, feeling financially secure, having a high sense of the worth of things, feeling useful, and feeling personally secure. They also report fewer feelings of anger, tension, restlessness, and confusion.

Natural History

Aging is a natural process involving a number of physiological changes, many of them merely a decline in the rate of functioning. A reduction in the metabolic rate of about 7 percent occurs every ten years after the age of thirty. There is a retardation of the rate of cell division, cell growth, and cell repair. Tissues, including their cells, tend to dry out. A fatty infiltration usually occurs with cellular atrophy, and a decrease in the speed of muscular response and a decline in muscular strength result. With a reduction in the efficiency of circulation, endurance declines. Connective tissues suffer a decrease in elasticity, bones become more brittle as the amount of organic material becomes reduced, teeth lose their structural integrity, and functioning of the digestive system slows. Many people over age sixty produce no hydrochloric acid in their stomach. Some of the nutritional deficiencies of older people result from poor digestion and inadequate absorption rather as much as from poor diet. There is also a general decline in the functioning of the nervous system and special sense organs. Older people may experience longer periods of illness because of the body's delayed response to infection or any other disorder.

····················

Figure 8-1

Percentage of Canadians age 12 and over who rate their health at least 4 on a 5-point scale, by age and gender, 1994 to 1995. Besides age and gender, income and educational levels also contribute to the decline in functioning with age. Activity limitations are four times as common among people with eight years of education than among those with sixteen years or more. (*Source:* Statistics Canada: National Population Health Survey, analysis by Federal, Provincial and Territorial Advisory Committee on Population Health: *Report on the Health of Canadians: Technical Appendix,* Toronto, 1996, Ministers of Health.)

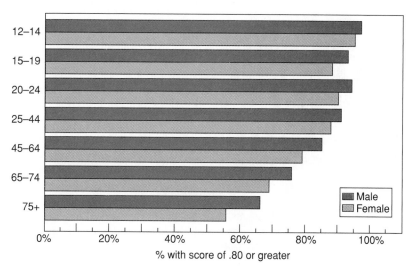

% with score of .80 or greater

Prevention of Faster Aging

Health science seeks to prevent premature death and to promote optimum health with the life span. Pathological aging refers to a hastening of the aging process by adverse factors affecting body functioning. Repeated insults to the body leave their mark. We could extend the prime of life as we know it and delay the disabling effect of aging if we could control the factors that produce pathological aging.

Chronic low-grade infection takes its toll on the body. Toxins from the environment also hasten the aging process. Extended critical illness from which an individual recovers may nevertheless hasten aging. Degenerative diseases such as hypertension, arthritis, and rheumatism tend to produce premature aging. Chronic tension, worry, and fatigue, associated with an inability to relax, can hasten the aging process. The stress syndrome masks a disturbance of biochemical functioning that can con-

tribute to premature aging. In addition, the use of multiple drugs commonly results in overdosages and toxicities that complicate the other factors.

Inactivity can be a factor in producing **atrophy** and pathological aging. The level of effectiveness that the circulatory system attains and the strength of the muscular and skeletal systems depend on regular activity. Marked nutritional deficiency that results in emaciation over an extended time has a recognized adverse effect on the retention of the prime of life. Inadequacy of vitamins, proteins, and minerals in the diet can also hasten premature aging. Cigarettes, excessive alcohol, and cholesterol are the most clearly isolated agents that contribute to early degeneration. If nutritional deficiencies account for premature aging in some poor communities and populations, food excesses such as dietary fat may account for as much in affluent communities and populations (figure 8-2).

• • • • • • • • • • • • • • • • •
Figure 8-2

The factors that accelerate aging do so in part through producing chronic diseases that shorten the life span. Dietary fat consumption has been implicated in at least these three diseases, plus diabetes and other conditions associated with obesity. (*Source:* The Henry J. Kaiser Family Foundation and the Advertising Council.)

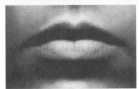

COLON CANCER, BREAST CANCER AND HEART DISEASE CAN ALL START IN THE SAME PLACE.

Too many people get into trouble because they open their mouths without thinking.
Unfortunately, the diet that most Americans eat may contain enough fat to increase the risk of certain cancers as well as heart disease.

But you can help reduce your risk by eating a low-fat diet containing lots of fruits, vegetables, whole grain foods, lean meats, fish, poultry and low-fat dairy products.
For a free booklet on low-fat eating, call 1-800-EAT-LEAN.

Remember, your brain is only a few inches from your mouth.
When you eat, we suggest you use it.

1-800-EAT-LEAN

A public service message from The Henry J. Kaiser Family Foundation.

Knowledge of these factors in hastening the aging process can guide the planning of programs to promote health in ways that will extend the years of quality life. Quality years mean added years with optimum functioning and vitality, not merely adding years to lives in which people will be disabled and too sick to enjoy them.

Demographic Trends

Age distributions of populations (see figures 3-11 and 8-3) are shifting toward the older groups. The number of people 65 years and older in the United States increased from 3 million in 1900 to ten times this number in 1990 (31.7 million). The number of people under 60 years old increased at only one-fourth this rate. The growth rate for the elderly population was somewhat slower in the 1990s when people born during the depression of the 1930s, constituting a relatively small cohort, reach the age of 60. As persons born during the "baby boom" years are reaching the age of 60 early in the twenty-first century, most of the growth in the Western populations will again occur in the older age brackets. Between 2000 and 2040, the oldest age group (85 years and over) in the United States is projected to triple (figure 8-3).

The elderly merit an organized community program for the promotion of their health. Concern for the health of the older age segment of the population has intensified with the rapid increase in the number of older people. Concern has been fueled by the costs associated with their increased burden of medical care. The growth of this segment of the population also produces a political force that has forced policy attention to the concerns of this age group. Health and the costs of health care have been their greatest concerns.

A 65-year-old man can expect, on the average, to live to 80; a woman of 65, to 85. By the year 2000, life expectancies for 65-year-olds may increase by another one or two years. The gain in life expectancy during the twentieth century represents an outstanding achievement, but it brings with it substantial changes in society as a whole and enormous challenges for communities. The "young-old" in their late 50s, 60s, and early 70s are retired, are relatively healthy and vigorous, and seek meaningful ways to use their time, either in self-fulfillment or in community participation. They challenge the community to use their talents to enrich their own lives and to improve society at large.

· · · · · · · · · · · · · · · · · ·
Figure 8-3

The rates of growth in the over sixty-five population in the United States and Canada have outpaced the nonelderly rates since 1900. This relative growth of older ages will continue through the middle of the twenty-first century. Most notable is the growth of the oldest-old, those eighty-five years and over. (*Sources:* Day, J. C.: *Current Population Reports,* P25-1104, Washington, DC, 1993, U.S. Bureau of the Census; Institute for Health and Aging: *Chronic Care in America: A 21st Century Challenge,* Princeton, NJ, 1996, The Robert Wood Johnson Foundation.)

Distribution of elderly population, by age groups, 1900–2040

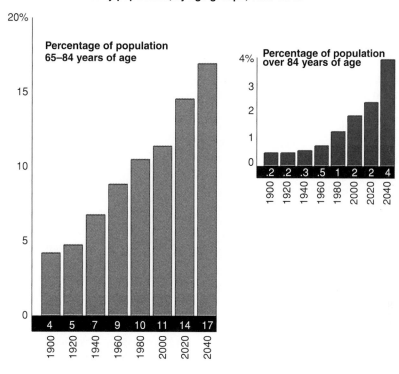

By the year 2000, 13 percent of our population will be over 65.
By 2040, the percentage over 65 will have grown to 21 percent.

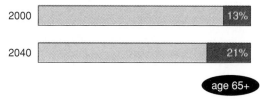

A second set of community issues stems from the even more striking increases in the numbers of the "old-old" persons in their mid-70s, 80s, and 90s. An increasing minority of the old-old remain vigorous and active, but the majority need a range of supportive and restorative health and social services. The old-old of the 1990s represent a disproportionately disadvantaged group. The reasons are several, for example, this group includes many immigrants who were poorly educated and who have spent their working years at low-paying jobs. Many have been unable to accumulate savings or to build sufficient equity in the Social Security system to sustain them adequately through their years of retirement.

Future populations of young-old and old-old persons will have different characteristics. They will have been better educated and will have received better medical care and nutrition throughout their lives. Their life experiences as a cohort will have been markedly different from those of the present population of older people, therefore their expectations of life, including their expectations of old age, will be different. As a result, programs suited to the young-old and old-old persons need continuous revisions if they are to serve the needs of future populations.

THE SOCIAL HISTORY AND EPIDEMIOLOGY OF AGING

Social norms and conditions produce for many older people the following sequence of related circumstances:

1. Biological changes, accompanied by loss of income and status, result in changes in social roles and an increased uncertainty about personal worth.
2. Insecurity associated with a feeling of inability to meet the demands of life, apprehension about health, difficulty in adjusting from a work routine to one of retirement, inability to find avenues of service that will provide personal gratification, difficulty in handling stresses created by social change, and limited incentive for social participation.
3. The changes in psychological security and functioning, combined with actual symptoms of health problems, lead to changes in health behavior.
4. The changes in health behavior may protect and promote health, but some may compromise health.
5. Changes in health result in further declines in biological functioning associated with aging.

These changes are summarized in figure 8-4.

Just as many of the health problems of minorities stem from racism, and some problems of women arise from sexism, so too are major problems of the aged related to **ageism.** A community approach to the health of the elderly therefore must concern itself with public and professional attitudes toward aging and stereotypes about the aged. Institutional prejudice also exists to the extent that our community services and institutions discriminate against the aged in ways that threaten their access to health care and other resources. Community health programs should attempt to adjust resources, communications, and organizational arrangements to meet the special needs of older people.

The community sees its older people irregularly and may assume that they are living more enjoyably and effectively or more unhappily than they really are. Rather than relying on assumptions, the community needs to make a critical appraisal of the status of its older members.

Compression of Morbidity and Active Life Expectancy

Longevity, or mean life expectancy at birth, has increased not because we have lengthened the life span, but because we delayed the premature deaths that were occurring within that biologically set life span. We have, in a word, compressed the *mortality* experience of the population into later and later stages of the life span, as shown in Scenario 1 of figure 8-5.

. . . .

Figure 8-4

The cycle of lifestyle transitions and aging. The cycle shows the natural history of change and points of intervention to modify: (1) the impact of biological aging on social roles and status; (2) the impact of changing social roles and status on psychological security or functioning; (3) the impact of psychological changes on human behavior; (4) the impact of behavior changes on health; and (5) the effects of changing health status on declining biological functioning. (*Source:* Adapted from Green, L. W. 1984. Some challenges to health services research on children and the elderly. *Health Serv Res* 19:793.)

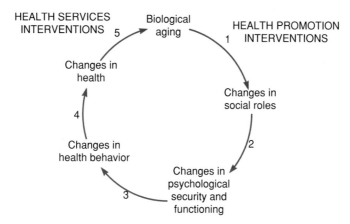

. . . .

Figure 8-5

Rather than merely extending the period of illness and disability by prolonging life, as in Scenario 1, health promotion for older adults seeks to compress the onset of illness and disability into the latest possible years, as in Scenario 2. (*Source:* Fries, J. F., L. W. Green, and S. Levine. 1989. Health promotion and the compression of morbidity. *Lancet* 1:105.)

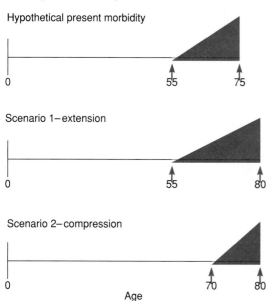

As we compress mortality tighter and tighter against the wall of the biological limit, there is less remaining gain to be sought in prolonging life or reducing mortality. Much remains to be gained, however, in delaying the onset of *morbidity,* as shown in Scenario 2 of figure 8-5. This is the task of health promotion.

The morbidity in question at these older ages is the manifestation of chronic and degenerative conditions that afflict us all. Most adults have some degree of atherosclerosis; hypertension or hypotension; osteoporosis; decreased lung function; and some loss of agility, sensory acuity, memory, suppleness, muscle endurance, and circulatory and metabolic efficiency. They are not diseases to be prevented. They are conditions to be slowed in their progression, limited in their impact, and adapted to as they relate to lifestyle, functioning, and the quality of life. This brings us to the second concept.

As we seek to compress morbidity against the far wall of our biologically determined maximum life span, we also seek to maintain active functioning in the years of waning biological functions. We might have to slow down in old age, but we

· · · · · · · · · · · · · · · · · ·

Figure 8-6

The three ways age operates to influence health status outcomes include the era in which people were born and experienced their developmental years, the biological aging process, and age combined with social determinants to affect health directly through life events and social or economic support and indirectly through behavior or lifestyle influenced by social norms for the age group. (*Source:* Green, L. W. and N. H. Gottleib. 1989. Health promotion for the aging population: approaches to extending active life expectancy. In *Health care for an aging society,* edited by S. Andreopoulos and J. R. Hogness. New York: Churchill Livingstone.)

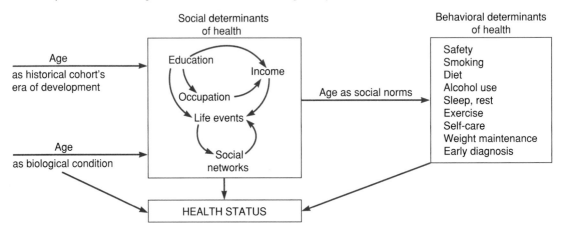

should not have to live too many years in pain, social embarrassment, inability to function independently, or incapacity to enjoy life. The concept of **active life expectancy** refers to the quality of the remaining years of *functional* well-being.

Historically, we have compressed mortality mainly by controlling infections and communicable diseases and more recently by reducing the death rate from cardiovascular diseases in middle-aged adults. The former we accomplished largely through environmental interventions, the latter largely through lifestyle changes. In the earlier case, the real gains in longevity came with the suppression of death rates at younger ages, not in the over sixty-five age groups. That was because the population was concentrated in those ages and more of the deferrable mortality occurred at those ages. The historical and demographic circumstances have changed.

In the decades ahead, the opportunities to compress morbidity and to increase active life expectancy appear likely to increase during the older

ages. The opportunity can be deceptive, however, for we have evidence that intervening late in the degenerative processes can make a significant difference in health for some conditions compromising active life expectancy, but not for others.

Health and the Three Functions of Age

Figure 8-6 illustrates the biological, social, and behavioral paths through which age influences health status. It indicates the variety of social and behavioral determinants of health status that require consideration in health promotion for the elderly population.

When considering the influence of age on health status, it is important to consider three meanings of age: (1) age as maturation or biological condition, (2) age as cohort or historical location, and (3) age as life course or a set of age-related social roles. These three functions of age are not independent of each other. One's cohort location (for example, those born and raised in the 1920s compared with those born and raised in the 1940s) influences the social norms or expectations held by society for behavior at different ages. The era in which the population cohort was born and spent their developmental years may also influence biological development. Improved nutrition and living conditions in succeeding generations have influenced biological aspects of aging. The Great Depression of the 1930s and the World Wars of other decades makes those people born or raised during those eras susceptible to some of the social and health consequences of economic upheaval and war.

Besides the compression of morbidity and active life expectancy, behavioral patterns and social transitions also produce key elements in improving the quality of life and self-reported health status of older adults. For each of these entities we can suggest intervention strategies for health promotion programs directed to the older population.

Behavior and Lifestyle as Points of Intervention

Lifestyle and behavior form a cornerstone of disease prevention and health promotion. As a function of age, the health status of elderly persons derives from their earlier personal health practices. Never smoking, moderate alcohol consumption or abstinence, regular physical activity, and weight maintenance have been associated with lower mortality rates overall. These also account for lower rates for specific diseases. These specific practices carry a high relative risk for death from several specific diseases. It is not clear (except for smoking among women) that current lifestyle practices among the elderly are associated (independent of age, health status, and income) with mortality. The evidence is clear, however, that these behaviors accumulate over a lifetime to influence overall quality of life and alter the course of various diseases and conditions among older adults. For example, stopping smoking after a myocardial infarction has been shown to reduce the mortality rate, and exercise among elderly persons increases the physical capacity to withstand illness and injury, increases flexibility, and improves cardiovascular functioning.

However, earlier cessation of smoking might have prevented the heart attack in the first place, and earlier exercise could have made a bigger difference in cardiovascular functioning.

National health interview surveys compare the prevalence of selected lifestyle health practices among the elderly and the total population (table 8-2). Such data based on self-report cannot separate the three functions of age as they influence health-related practices. For example, older persons may be less likely to engage in aerobic exercise because they are physically unable to do so. Or, they do not exercise because the primary socialization of their cohort was in an era when exercise was not popular. Or, they do not exercise because age-graded norms for exercise stereotype them as fragile, slow, and clumsy, and they are expected not to engage in "child's play."

ACTIVE LIFE EXPECTANCY APPROACH TO HEALTH PROMOTION FOR THE ELDERLY

Taking the task for health promotion to be the compression of morbidity would lead a community to intervene primarily in smoking, alcohol and drug misuse, exercise, and nutrition in the young and middle-aged populations. These precursors to morbidity have their genesis in early ages, and they are cumulative in their impact on morbidity. Taking the task also to be the extension of active life expectancy would lead the community to emphasize these same interventions plus some others, but more with the older age groups. We need to step back from the problems of a particular age group and ask what preceded that age that might have precipitated the problem. It is perhaps inherent in the concept of health promotion that intervention must precede the problem. To intervene before a problem manifests itself in symptoms or illness, we must anticipate the problem. We can only anticipate population health problems with probability estimates.

The probabilities used for most health planning are vital statistics and incidence rates. Prevalence

Table 8-2

Comparisons of Older (Age 65+) Populations of North America with All Adults (Age 18+ in the United States, 15+ in Canada) on Selected Health Promoting Behavior and Conditions, 1990 in Canada, 1995 in United States.

Parameter	Percentages 65+ years	All ages
Physical activity		
U.S.: Exercise strenuously 3 or more times per week	26	37
Canada: Vigorous physical activity	48	48
Usually 30 minutes or more		
Men	43	55
Women	29	42
Three or more times/week		
Men	61	52
Women	49	49
Stress		
U.S.: Experience high levels of stress at least several days a week	21	37
Canada: Perceive their lives as somewhat or very stressful		
Men	31	61
Women	33	60
Smoking		
U.S.: Do not smoke	88	74
Canada: Do not smoke	84	37
Men	82	69
Women	86	72
Alcohol		
U.S.: Do not drink alcohol	59	40
Canada: Lifetime abstainers and former drinkers	38	19
Men	34	15
Women	42	23
Seat belt use		
U.S.: Wear seat belt all the time in front seat of car	71	73
Canada: Always wear seat belt in car	86	79
Men	81	72
Women	90	86

Sources: The Prevention Index: a report card on the nation's health, Emmaus, PA, 1995; *Canada's health promotion survey 1990: technical report.* Ottawa, 1993, Health and Welfare Canada.

rates serve to inform health planning for purposes of allocating facilities and resources for the care of existing problems. To anticipate and plan for prevention, however, we need age-specific incidence rates. Unfortunately, incidence rates for the morbidities of old age are the least developed of all health statistics. They simply do not exist for most of the chronic and degenerative diseases because the onset of such conditions is undefined and, as noted earlier, most adults have some of these conditions to some extent.

Communitywide Approach

How then can we recognize and target health promotion interventions strategically and efficiently? One answer to this question is the communitywide approach to lifestyle modification. This approach rests on two theories, one epidemiological and the other sociological. The epidemiological theory is that by moving the average of population risk factor levels a small amount in an entire community, we achieve a statistically greater impact on mortality than if we reduced the average risk factor levels of high-risk groups a large amount. The sociological theory is that intervening on the community at large, behavioral and environmental changes happen on a more pervasive scale. This would produce a social influence or normative effect and set into motion a more permanent diffusion process. Both theories and the argument they support for communitywide interventions have merit, but with some limitations for the elderly.

Communitywide approaches are appropriate for reducing the risk of later morbidity and mortality in young and middle-aged populations. For programs directed at older age groups, however, these approaches are less applicable. The elderly represent a distinct community in only a few places, such as retirement villages, mobile home parks, and arguably nursing homes. Community organization and communitywide health education or screening methods are ideally suited to these situations, but they miss most elderly people. Communitywide programs intended for the elderly but applied to the community at large are costly and inefficient in reaching the elderly.

This situation, then, is the dilemma of health promotion for the elderly. Traditional medical approaches are often too late for purposes of prevention and active life expectancy. The traditional public health method of identifying high-risk groups on the basis of incidence rates fails to apply because the new morbidities have undefined onsets and therefore few meaningful incidence rates available. The promising new communitywide strategies for chronic disease prevention do not fit for this demographic group because the elderly seldom make up a geographic community of their own.

Research has demonstrated that it is possible to build a sense of community and self-reliance among even the low-income elderly residing in single-room occupancy hotels in an inner city area. It requires, however, a highly targeted, labor-intensive outreach strategy that engages and organizes unaffiliated elderly people in identifying and solving their own mutual problems. It is not the same as the media-oriented, communitywide interventions used in the general population. The solutions for health promotion for the elderly seem to lie with an open-ended strategy of involving the elderly in identifying their own needs.

Transitions in Aging

Most older individuals do encounter situational changes associated with aging. The most pervasive of these in their effects on lifestyle and health are relocation, retirement, and widowhood. These changes produce stress or bereavement. These in turn can make the individual susceptible to physical and psychological illness and even chronic disability.

Many older adults experience transitions without developing any subsequent pathological conditions. Others experience adverse outcomes as measured by health status indicators (nursing home admissions, hospitalizations, operations, acute illness) and psychosocial indicators (depression, psychosomatic illness, low morale, lowered life satisfaction). Factors that appear to influence adaptation or resistance include experiential, environmental, and social aspects of the individual and of the change. Stressors and protective factors that influence the adaptation process can be identified in the community for each of the three transitions: relocation, retirement and widowhood.

Relocation Relocation takes the form of various types of moves. These include moves from one home to another within the community, from one community to another, from home to institution, from one institution to another, or even within an institution. Studies of the effects of relocation on the elderly have detected changes in mortality rates; physical health status indicators; and social, economic, and psychological outcomes. The effects of relocation depend on the degree of support provided, the degree of preparation for the move, and the degree of environmental change involved. The effects also depend on the relocation's duration, its predictability, whether the move was voluntary or involuntary, and the degree of control felt by the elderly person.

Two factors seem most consistently to act as buffers for an individual's response to relocation stress: the degree of control over the event and the degree of predictability of the new environment. When the elderly perceive a move as voluntary and feel a sense of control or choice about the relocation process, they feel less stress and fewer negative physical or psychosocial consequences result. Similarly, the more radical the environmental change and the less predictable the new environment, the more negative the reaction in older populations.

Individuals respond to relocation stress depending on their characteristics prior to the move. These include their attitudes about the move, their degree of preparation for the move, and their degree of physical disability at the time of the move. Individual characteristics consistently associated with the adverse consequences of relocation include advanced age, poor physical health, psychiatric disturbances, and cognitive malfunctioning. Adverse consequences of relocation are also greater in males, those living alone, those having few social contacts with friends and kin, those in poor financial circumstances, those lacking access to various

social services, and those who lived in the same place a long time.

Finally, the degree and type of preparation for the move influence relocation outcomes. Uncertainties, and thus stress, diminish as predictability of the new environment increases through anticipatory counseling or preparatory education programs. The increased attention the residents receive as a result of participation in preparatory programs might cause a decline in negative outcomes immediately following the relocation. A protective effect associated with increased social support and attention prior to and immediately following relocation probably results in a delayed and possibly reduced peak in mortality rates among those relocated.

Retirement In the future a greater percentage of citizens over age sixty-five will receive Social Security and survivors' insurance benefits. Socioeconomic factors may even produce a retirement age of sixty for the general population. The earlier retirement age and the shrinking resources available from Social Security funds will pose additional problems unless better programs are promoted to prepare people for retirement. At least half the people over age sixty-five are potential members of the labor force, and many of them prefer to work. Frequently it is necessary for them to learn a new type of work. Some find that their skills and trades have become obsolete and for this reason have to find new types of employment. Many of these individuals have an adequate physical capacity and an adequate learning capacity to take up new jobs. Industries are reluctant to employ elderly workers because they believe them to be slower and to have higher rates of injury and absenteeism. The older worker, however, is generally meticulous, produces work of a high quality, and is extremely reliable. There is a need to lower work barriers for the elderly who are physically and mentally capable. Employment opportunities for elderly citizens capable of contributing to the community's economy can be created (figures 8-7 and 8-8). Part-time jobs have their merit, particularly

Figure 8-7

Volunteer work puts lifetime skills to useful applications and helps the retired person maintain a sense of self-worth and social value. (*Source:* Advertising Council, New York.)

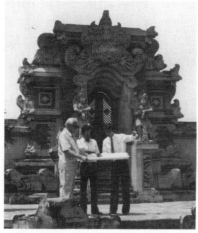

Turn your lifetime of experience into the experience of a lifetime.

IESC Volunteer Gordon Swaney, a retired U.S. manager, on project site in Indonesia.

We're looking for executives who know their way around the trenches as well as the front offices. Because if you're recently retired, there's a whole world out there desperately waiting to be taught what you spent a lifetime learning.

Through the International Executive Service Corps—the not-for-profit organization that sends U.S. managers to help businesses in developing nations—you can volunteer for short-term assignments in foreign countries where you're truly needed. Although you will not be paid, you and your spouse will receive all expenses, plus the personal satisfaction of teaching others while you discover more about yourself.

Think of it. Your experience can make a difference in a land much different from your own. Instead of ending your career, you could be starting the experience of a lifetime.

Send for more information today.

International Executive Service Corps

Ad Council
A Public Service of This Publication

YES, I'd like to share my lifetime of experience with others. I recently retired from my position as a hands-on manager with a U.S. company. I also understand that volunteers and their spouses receive expenses, but no salary. Please send me more information now.

Name_____

Address_____

City_____State_____Zip_____

Write to: IESC, 8 Stamford Forum, P.O. Box 10005, Stamford, CT 06904-2005. Or, for faster response, call this number: (203) 967-6000.

E2

Figure 8-8

In the first year of the Peace Corps only 83 of the 10,078 volunteers, less than 1 percent, were people 50 or over. In 1992, out of a total of 5,300 Peace Corps volunteers, 556 were 50 or older. The biggest increases were between 1988 and 1991, with more than a doubling of the proportion who were older volunteers. (*Source:* U.S. Peace Corps.)

Percent of peace corps volunteers over 50

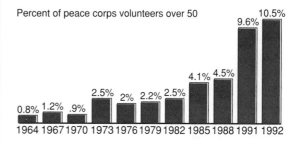

1964	1967	1970	1973	1976	1979	1982	1985	1988	1991	1992
0.8%	1.2%	.9%	2.5%	2%	2.2%	2.5%	4.1%	4.5%	9.6%	10.5%

when the elderly person supplements work with other community services and activities. Childcare roles for the elderly seem especially suited to the needs of some and to communities because of growing numbers of working women.

Preparation for successful old age ideally begins at about age forty, with the development of a wide range of interests and channels of community service. Elderly persons can accept change, cultivate a range of interests, maintain a willingness to learn, and participate actively in community affairs.

Some retire freely. Others experience compulsory retirement; but even among those who face compulsory retirement, some willingly retire, while others reluctantly give up the work role. Still others retire for health reasons, while some persons may face retirement after job loss. Given these varied conditions, retired people experience different physical and mental health outcomes as they pass from working to nonworking lifestyles.

Some possible phases in the natural history of the adaptation process might be the honeymoon phase, the disenchantment phase, the reorientation phase, and the stability phase. Such phases remain understandably undocumented, given the difficult task of measuring and verifying their manifestation, duration, and sequence. The notion of retirement adaptation as a transition process is important to health promotion so far as interventions could be targeted to phases. Different retirement outcomes might be predicted at specific time intervals for different groups of retirees (see table 6-1).

Widowhood and Bereavement A third common life transition of old age is widowhood. Like retirement, widowhood is a complex phenomenon that produces losses and changes beyond the loss of a spouse. For some it may mean the loss of dependable financial resources and a concomitant decline in economic status. For others it may mean a decline in social interaction and a concomitant decline in social status. Many widowed people suffer from stigma and deprivation, the stigma leading to altered self-concept and isolation and the deprivation to loneliness and depression.

Poor adaptation to the stresses produced by widowhood has been found to be associated with inadequate income, poor physical health, lack of a supportive reference group, and lack of alternative roles to substitute for the lost role of spouse. Such lost roles include employment or extended family involvement. These studies suggest that the association between widowhood and lower morale or depression may be attributed to factors other than the loss of a spouse. These other factors are the concomitant life changes that widowhood may bring. As with relocation and retirement, situational factors that occur along with widowhood rather than widowhood itself may be the causal agents of stress, adaptation, and lower morale among the widowed (figure 8-9).

Community Interventions in the Transitions

Considering each major transition separately and applying the model in table 6-1, what might be appropriate health-promoting interventions?

Relocation Less negative consequences of relocation result from a predictable postrelocation en-

....
F i g u r e 8 - 9

Widowhood comes more often to women than to men because men have higher mortality rates and because women are less likely to remarry. This leaves more women without partners in old age. (*Source:* Photo courtesy Kitsilano Community Centre, Vancouver, BC.)

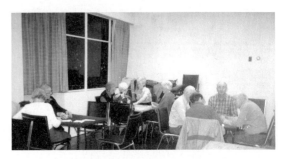

vironment and change perceived as voluntary and in one's control. While one may not be able to change the nature of a move, prerelocation preparation might help the relocated person better manage the new environment. In the case of an institutional setting, providing information as to what to expect in terms of new routines, new staff, and new time schedules might make the new environment more predictable and thus more manageable, even with a radical move.

Reality limits the control a resident has over an administrative move within an institution or even a move from the home setting into the institutional one. Education can at least provide understanding and can actively engage the resident in the relocation process. In this way, the resident perceives that he or she has some control over the relocation process. People of any age who believe that they have control over outcomes can better manage change and are more likely to adopt positive adaptive behavior, leading to a sense of competence and control that may motivate further adaptive behavior (figure 8-10).

Providing preparation for the move therefore appears to be an important factor in mediating the stress experienced by relocated persons. Group programs can provide the helpful social support

Figure 8-10

People who have control over their own selection of housing and social relationships enjoy greater emotional and physical health. (*Source:* Photo by Judy McLarty, courtesy University of British Columbia.)

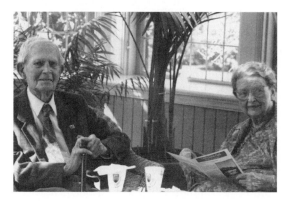

Figure 8-11

A retired engineer maintains interests in technical matters and turns increasingly to the use of his computer for writing and family matters. (*Source:* Photo courtesy of Raymond and Petey Ottoson.)

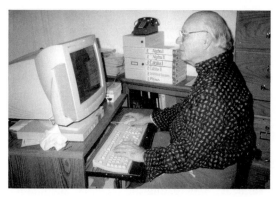

needed in times of uncertainty and change. Such support can serve as a protective mechanism against any stresses caused by the change. The group can offer support by mobilizing psychological resources to master emotional burdens, by sharing tasks, and by providing the skills and guidance to improve handling of the situation.

Retirement For many, the process of retirement is a normal, expected life event that in itself does not constitute a stressful transition, but rather calls forth changes in self-concept, self-identity, and social roles. While these changes do call for new adaptations, they are not necessarily traumatic. Successful adaptation to nonworking status seems to depend on a retiree's health and on the psychological, social, and financial resources he or she brings to retirement (figure 8-11).While many resources are fixed, such as finances, others are more amenable to change. Retirees' adjustment to their new roles depends in part on their ability to support consistent, coherent self-images despite major changes in their social system and on the degree of support provided in their social environment. Interventions aimed at helping the individ-

ual retiree find meaningful ways of maintaining a positive self-image may be oriented toward anticipatory socialization. This might involve identifying a variety of role options open to the retiree and preparing the retiree for the role chosen.

Bereavement The treatment of widowhood as a unitary phenomenon with similar outcomes for all is equally unsuitable. Communities can support interventions targeted toward building the knowledge and skills needed to cope with whatever unique sources of difficulty the widow or widower will experience. While some sources of stress may not be amenable to change, interventions might at least enable the bereaved to cope better with certain problems—for example, financial worries. Other situational factors of widowhood are more amenable to direct manipulation and change. If a widowed person lacks sufficient family interactions, programs can increase activity with peers. If difficulties result from lack of work involvement, efforts can be directed at securing employment. In other words, interventions should be tailored to meet individual needs. A number of programs have been established to ameliorate the loneliness and isolation experienced by the recently widowed. These "widow-to-widow" programs train widowed persons to serve as outreach workers for those more recently bereaved.

Major life events do not necessarily precipitate crisis reactions in the majority of the aged, but many elderly people experiencing these events are at high risk of mental and physical illness. Even for those who are adversely affected, it seems that the set of mostly controllable circumstances surrounding the event, not the event itself, constitutes the source of difficulty. Community programs can be directed at these situational factors. Such interventions can be regarded as health promotion insofar as they represent a primary prevention approach to the cycle of deteriorating lifestyle and health. By anticipating the potential adaptations required in transitions to come, health education can be combined with organizational, economic, and environmental supports for coping strategies and behavior conducive to health in the oldest members of communities.

HEALTH PRIORITIES OF OLDER ADULTS

Physical Health

Arthritis, rheumatism, hearing disorders, diseases of the heart, arteriosclerosis, and other degenerative diseases require far more medical care than the disorders of earlier years. Government must bear a larger proportion of the bill for the aged. Primary prevention is still in order for certain infectious diseases, such as influenza and pneumonia, and for injury control. Early detection and treatment (secondary prevention) of malignant neoplasms (cancer) and hypertension could give these older citizens several additional years of active life. Even individuals over age sixty-five who appear to be in excellent health should have a medical examination every year (table 8-3). Those who are at high risk should have checkups more frequently (table 8-4).

Two of the principal causes of disability in the aged, though not commonly a cause of death, are arthritis and rheumatism. They can usually be treated to relieve patients of much of their pain and enable them to extend their activities. Self-care education has been shown to improve many of the problems of arthritis.

Disorders of vision are common among the elderly (figure 8-12). Some degree of correction is usually possible even though the individual's vision with glasses may still not be normal. When the loss of vision has progressed to a state where the individual can no longer read, recordings are available that enable the blind or near-blind to enjoy hearing the literature or feature articles of the day that they would normally read.

Loss of hearing in the later years of life is also common. Hearing aids have been developed to the point where a much higher percentage of the hard-of-hearing are aided to hear adequately for customary needs. Deafness produces a feeling of loneliness. It can lead to social isolation and a consequent decline in social functioning. This emphasizes the need to develop programs to enable whatever level of hearing can be attained. Indeed, when asked to rank the importance of priorities for disease prevention and health promotion, the elderly gave highest priority to sensory deprivation control.

Mental Health and Mental Disorders

Definitions of health and disease change not only with biomedical advances, but also with social and historical factors—for instance, with changes in social attitudes toward deviant behavior. These changes apply especially to attempts to distinguish mental health and mental disorder, as the next chapter will show. For older people they pose growing social problems. It is estimated that 15 percent of persons over sixty-five suffer from mental disorders, 5 percent from severe disorders. Alcoholism and drug misuse appear to be increasing among older persons. One striking fact is that, while this age group constitutes only 10 percent of the total population, it accounts for over 30 percent of suicides. Criminal behavior, on the other hand, drops dramatically with age.

Table 8-3

Periodic Screening and Health Services Recommendations of the U.S. Preventive Services Task Force for People Sixty-Five and Over. (Leading Causes of Death: Heart Disease; Cerebrovascular Disease; Obstructive Lung Disease; Pneumonia/Influenza; Lung Cancer; and Colorectal Cancer)

Screening

History	Physical exam	Laboratory/diagnostic procedures
Prior symptoms of transient ischemic attack	Height and weight	Nonfasting total blood cholesterol
Dietary intake	Blood pressure	Dipstick urinalysis
Physical activity	Visual acuity	Mammogram[2]
Tobacco/alcohol/drug use	Hearing and hearing aids	Thyroid function tests[3]
Functional status at home	Clinical breast exam[1]	*HIGH-RISK GROUPS*
	HIGH-RISK GROUPS	Fasting plasma glucose (HR5)
	Auscultation for carotid bruits (HR1)	Tuberculin skin test (PPD) (HR6)
	Complete skin exam (HR2)	Electrocardiogram (HR7)
	Complete oral cavity exam (HR3)	Papanicolaou smear[4] (HR8)
	Palpation of thyroid nodules (HR4)	Fecal occult blood/Sigmoidoscopy (HR9)
		Fecal occult blood/Colonoscopy (HR10)

Counseling

Diet and exercise	Injury prevention	Dental health
Fat (especially saturated fat), cholesterol, complex carbohydrates, fiber, sodium calcium[3]	Prevention of falls	Regular dental visits, tooth brushing, flossing
Caloric balance	Safety belts	*Other primary preventive measures*
Selection of exercise program	Smoke detector	Glaucoma testing by eye specialist
	Smoking near bedding or upholstery	
Substance use	Hot water heater temperature	*HIGH-RISK GROUPS*
Tobacco cessation	Safety helmets	Discussion of estrogen replacement therapy (HR13)
Alcohol and other drugs:		Discussion of aspirin therapy (HR14)
Limiting alcohol consumption	*HIGH-RISK GROUPS*	Skin protection from ultraviolet light (HR15)
Driving/other dangerous activities while under the influence	Prevention of childhood injuries (HR12)	
Treatment for abuse		

Immunizations

Tetanus-diptheria (Td) booster[5]	Pneumococcal vaccine	*HIGH-RISK GROUPS*
Influenza vaccine[1]		Hepatitis B vaccine (HR16)

Remain alert for:

Depression symptoms	Changes in cognitive function	Malignant skin lesions
Suicide risk factors (HR11)	Medications that increase risk of falls	Peripheral arterial disease
Abnormal bereavement	Signs of physical abuse or neglect	Tooth decay, gingivitis, loose teeth

This list of preventive services is not exhaustive. It reflects only those topics reviewed by the U.S. Preventive Services Task Force. Clinicians may wish to add other preventive services on a routine basis, and after considering the patient's medical history and other individual circumstances. Examples of target conditions not specifically examined by the Task Force include: chronic obstructive pulmonary disease; hepatobiliary disease; bladder cancer; endometrial disease; travel-related illness; prescription drug abuse; and occupational illness and injuries.

*The recommended schedule applies only to the periodic visit itself. The frequency of the individual preventive services listed in this table is left to clinical discretion, except as indicated in other footnotes. See definitions of high-risk (HR) groups in table 8-4.

1. Annually. 2. Every 1-2 years for women until age 75, unless pathology detected. 3. For women. 4. Every 1-3 years. 5. Every 10 years.

Table 8-4

Ages Sixty-Five and Over High-Risk Categories for Preventive Services or Counseling (See Table 8-3).

HR1 Persons with risk factors for cerebrovascular or cardiovascular disease (e.g., hypertension, smoking, CAD,* atrial fibrillation, diabetes) or those with neurologic symptoms (e.g., transient ischemic attacks) or a history of cerebrovascular disease.

HR2 Persons with a family or personal history of skin cancer, or clinical evidence of precursor lesions (e.g., dysplastic nevi, certain congenital nevi), or those with increased occupational or recreational exposure to sunlight.

HR3 Persons with exposure to tobacco or excessive amounts of alcohol, or those with suspicious symptoms or lesions detected through self-examination.

HR4 Persons with a history of upper-body irradiation.

HR5 The markedly obese, persons with a family history of diabetes, or women with a history of gestational diabetes.

HR6 Household members of persons with tuberculosis or others at risk for close contact with the disease (e.g., staff of tuberculosis clinics, shelters for the homeless, nursing homes, substance abuse treatment facilities, dialysis units, correctional institutions); recent immigrants or refugees from countries in which tuberculosis is common (e.g., Asia, Africa, Central and South America, Pacific Islands); migrant workers; residents of nursing homes, correctional institutions, or homeless shelters; or persons with certain underlying medical disorders (e.g., HIV infection).

HR7 Men with two or more cardiac risk factors (high blood cholesterol, hypertension, cigarette smoking, diabetes mellitus, family history of CAD); men who would endanger public safety were they to experience sudden cardiac events (e.g., commercial airline pilots); or sedentary or high-risk males planning to begin a vigorous exercise program.

HR8 Women who have not had previous documented screening in which smears have been consistently negative.

HR9 Persons who have first-degree relatives with colorectal cancer; a personal history of endometrial, ovarian, or breast cancer; or a previous diagnosis of inflammatory bowel disease, adenomatous polyps, or colorectal cancer.

HR10 Persons with a family history of familial polyposis coli or cancer family syndrome.

HR11 Recent divorce, separation, unemployment, depression, alcohol or other drug abuse, serious medical illnesses, living alone, or recent bereavement.

HR12 Persons with children in the home or automobile.

HR13 Women at increased risk for osteoporosis (e.g., Caucasian, low bone mineral content, bilateral oopherectomy before menopause or early menopause, slender build) and who are without known contraindications (e.g., history of undiagnosed vaginal bleeding, active liver disease, thromboembolic disorders, hormone-dependent cancer).

HR14 Men who have risk factors for myocardial infarction (e.g., high blood cholesterol, smoking, diabetes mellitus, family history of early-onset CAD) and who lack a history of gastrointestinal or other bleeding problems, or other risk factors for bleeding or cerebral hemorrhage.

HR15 Persons with increased exposure to sunlight.

HR16 Homosexually active men, intravenous drug users, recipients of some blood products, or persons in health-related jobs with frequent exposure to blood or blood products.

*Coronary artery disease.
Source: U.S. Preventive Services Task Force.

· ·

Figure 8-12

Public service advertisements encourage black men over forty and older adults to seek screening examinations for glaucoma, the leading cause of blindness in adults over sixty. (*Source:* National Eye Institute, National Institutes of Health, Public Health Service, U.S. Department of Health and Human Services.)

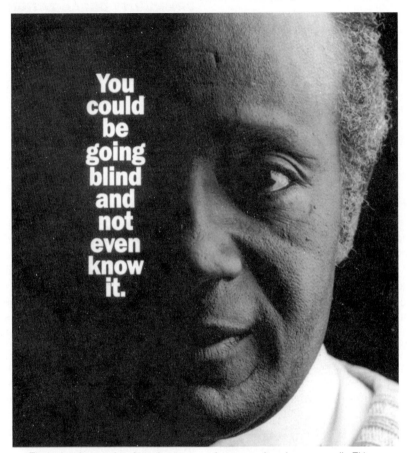

That's what glaucoma does. It sneaks up on you — gradually. Glaucoma is a leading cause of blindness among *all* adults over 60.

But it's especially common among African Americans. If you're Black and over 40, you're up to five times more likely to develop it.

Vision loss from glaucoma is permanent. But glaucoma can usually be controlled and the risk of blindness reduced if it's detected and treated early.

So, get a dilated eye examination in which drops are used to enlarge your pupils. This allows your eye care professional to see more of the inside of your eye to check for signs of glaucoma. It doesn't hurt, it's easy, and it could save your eyesight.

For more information, write: National Eye Health Education Program, Box 20/20, Bethesda, MD 20892.

Don't lose sight of glaucoma. NATIONAL EYE HEALTH EDUCATION PROGRAM

National Eye Institute, National Institutes of Health, Public Health Service, U.S. Department of Health and Human Services

Mental health depends on physical health, but even more on social factors. Such social issues as ethnicity, socioeconomic status, marital status, and rural or urban residence may contribute to the incidence, prevalence, cause, diagnosis, and treatment of mental disorders. For instance, industrialization and urbanization are often said to be producing greater social stresses and greater social isolation for older persons, and therefore more mental disorders. The nature of social stress is not well understood, and studies indicate that social isolation is as often an outcome as a cause of mental illness in older people.

Education and income are highly related to the type of mental illness suffered and also to the type of treatment offered by mental health professionals. There is a relationship also between education and the extent to which people seek help, either professional or nonprofessional. Western society has experienced a broadening range of problems for which people seek assistance and a rising level of expectation with regard to outcomes. As new cohorts of the old are increasingly well educated, their needs and expectations of the mental health system are likely to change.

The majority of functional psychiatric disturbances in old age (hypochondriacal states, paranoid reactions, and particularly depression) are responsive to appropriate treatment. Estimates of the prevalence of **Alzheimer's disease** in the over sixty-five population range from under 5 percent to over 11 percent. For the over eighty-five population, estimates average between 15 percent and 20 percent but range as high as 47 percent. Ten percent to 15 percent of organic brain syndromes are reversible (those due to coexisting physical illness or to drug intoxication, for instance). No cure has yet been found for Alzheimer's disease.

From the perspective of the mental health system as a whole, there have been striking changes in patterns of use of psychiatric facilities for different age groups. As mental health ideologies have changed, the mental health system has served a smaller proportion of older persons, with a great shift occurring after World War II from the use of mental hospitals to the use of nursing homes. These issues will be discussed further in the chapter to follow on community mental health.

COMMUNITY ORGANIZATION AND THE ELDERLY

Community provisions for the allocation of resources and social roles to the aged make a large difference in the quality of life and consequently in the health of the elderly.

Social Networks

To prevent feelings of isolation, older persons need continued involvement in various social networks (such as family, friendship, work, leisure, church, and organizational contexts). Dyadic or paired relationships (for example, a confidant) maintained over time seem to be of particular importance, but dyadic bonds have seldom been organized, except for the husband-wife relationship.

Older age brings a decline in number of social roles, amount of interaction, and variety of social contacts. Less active persons, however, are likely to be older, in poorer health, and in more deprived circumstances, so it is not clear to what extent the decline is a cause or a consequence of the aging process. It is probably both, creating an isolation-aging cycle. There is evidence that older people living alone more often become institutionalized, and that people with strong social networks survive and remain healthy more than those without frequent social contact.

Communities cannot ignore the impact on older adults of declining involvement in various social networks. Activity and morale are influenced by the extent to which social networks encourage or discourage continued participation. Therefore a distinction must be made between voluntary and involuntary withdrawal. Furthermore, quality of interaction is probably more important than the frequency.

Family Networks

Among social networks, the family remains paramount. Although social norms may stress nuclear family independence, older people remain linked to kinship networks. Most older people have close relatives within easy visiting distance; contacts are frequent; and it is children, particularly daughters, to whom older people turn for help.

The family has remained a strong and supportive institution for older people. Most older persons want to be as independent of their families as possible, but when they can no longer manage for themselves, they reasonably expect their children to come to their aid. Not only do such expectations exist, they are usually met. Patterns vary among social classes and ethnic groups, but most older persons see their children regularly, and a complex pattern of exchange of goods and services exists across generations, with ties of affection and obligation remaining strong. Furthermore, elderly parents appear to have attitudes and values remarkably similar to those of their children and grandchildren.

Trends toward separate households for older persons have developed (*family* is not synonymous with *household*). However the latest national data show that the older and sicker the individual, the more likely the person is to be found living with a child (the "sandwich generation")—more than twice as likely as to be living in an institution. The trend toward separate households will be affected by economic factors, housing policies, and the increasing number of families in which old-old persons have children who are old themselves. If more effective networks of supportive social and home health are built, more intergenerational households in which both generations are old may emerge.

Family structures have changed in other ways in the past few decades. A larger proportion of older men and women are married and living with their spouses. These couples mean decreases in the proportions of people widowed, divorced, or never married. At the same time, the absolute number of widows is increasing as the difference in longevity between the sexes grows greater. Whether these trends will continue will depend on a host of social and economic factors. Changing attitudes toward divorce and remarriage and toward nontraditional forms of family life, such as communal living for people in their later years, will influence these trends.

Friendship and Membership Ties

Friendship and membership ties complement kinship ties by relieving some of the burden of care from the family. The more characteristics neighbors have in common (such as socioeconomic status, marital status, and value orientations), the more integrated the friendship network. Voluntary membership in associations and participation in various organizations, including old-age clubs and senior citizen centers, depend to a considerable extent on styles established earlier in life.

More women have been assuming dual roles in the home and workplace. Women have increased the time spent in paid work and have somewhat decreased the time spent in family roles, although not enough to compensate for the increase in paid work time. The allocation of men's time to work and family roles, on the other hand, has remained relatively constant. It appears that as women's participation in the labor force increases, there is a net transfer of labor away from men and toward women. Many women are under considerable stress resulting from these dual roles, but their opportunities for social ties that will carry over into retirement have been multiplied.

Religion and Aging

Church attendance drops off among the very old, but it is not clear how much this relates to such factors as health, residential location, or socioeconomic status. Nor is it clear how age-related factors relate to historical factors in affecting patterns of church attendance or private devotions. In what ways does church attendance among older people reflect broader social trends? To what extent do private devotions replace church attendance? Related questions concern the church as a social institution in the lives of older persons. To what extent and for what subgroup does the church perform a supportive social and psychological function?

Civic Participation

Older people disengage from the fabric of society because of their displacement from their earlier roles, especially work and family. They are correspondingly more alienated from their community. Civic participation is a means of reestablishing this connection.

Within populations with a similar level of education, social class, and ethnic background, the political behavior, community organizational involvement, and volunteer activities of older people are not noticeably different from those of younger people. Voting behavior remains remarkably consistent far into old age; older people do vote, and they tend to vote for the party for which they have always voted. Participation in political activity other than voting is infrequent among older people, but lobby groups among older adults have increased in number, size, and effectiveness.

Retired people are overrepresented on community citizen boards and voluntary organization committees. Those who participate in community organizations appear to be a very select sample (who may represent their individual needs more than any constituency). Community organizations often select as representatives of the older population those who can be expected to go along with the organization's practices rather than those who might be critical or seek reform.

Age-Based Organizations

An age-based organization is one that depends on the existence of older persons for its activities. The elderly are its members, its direct or indirect consumers, or its subjects of special concern. Such organizations exist in industrialized nations throughout the world. A few are active in U.S. politics, such as the National Council of Senior Citizens, the Gray Panthers, and the American Association of Retired Persons. Such organizations can play a role in shaping the issues of public policy debate: they gain access to legislators, administrative officials, and political party organiza-

tions. They often seek to organize elderly voters as a block at the local or national level.

Aging as a Concern of Political Systems

The older aged population first became a major concern of governments in the late nineteenth century. The birth of the modern welfare state, with economic relief for older persons as a major feature, began with Bismarck, Germany in the 1880s, then spread to other industrialized countries. Relatively late, the United States enacted the Social Security program in 1935.

Income-maintenance policies have undergone innumerable expansions in the intervening decades. The range of efforts for helping older persons has broadened. It includes attempts to meet personal needs, such as shelter, medical care, and employment training, and group needs, such as better transportation and other community improvements. The evolution of governmental policies toward older people can be traced to factors ranging from the efforts of individual reformers to various societal changes brought about by long-term economic, demographic, and ideological trends. Organizations such as political parties, labor unions, and professional and commercial organizations have found reason either to advocate or oppose governmental action toward the aging. As they grow in number and in proportion to the total voting-age population, the political power of the aging grows. The costs of health and pension support for the elderly will grow concomitantly.

Canadian Pension Plan and U.S. Social Security System

Though not a community organization issue, the provisions for income security in old age has become a political issue with community implications. In Canada and the United States, social security funds are under siege with the growing numbers of older people to be covered by the Canada Pension Plan and the U.S. Social Security benefits. Canada was forced to dip into its Pension Plan surplus for the first time in 1994 and has raised pension contribution requirements of employers and employees every year since 1986. U.S. projections are for the Hospital Insurance Fund to be depleted in 2001 unless something is done to make the fund fiscally sound. By 2012, social security outlays will exceed income with increasing deficits each year until the system is bankrupt around 2030 if remedial action is not taken. These effects are partly the aging of the population, but also partly the trend toward earlier retirement. In 1956, for example, only 2 percent of Americans receiving Social Security took their benefits before age sixty-five. By 1993 that figure had climbed to 68 percent. The rate of applications for early retirement to the Canada Pension Plan increased by 8 percent in 1993.

The obvious remedial actions of raising Pension Plan contributions or Social Security taxes and decreasing the range or amounts of benefits have their obvious political liabilities. In a time of fiscal restraint by federal governments, raising any taxes has proved increasingly odious to the voting publics of the United States, Canada, Australia, and most European countries. On the other side of the ledger, the growing political influence of the lobby for retired citizens prevents most politicians from taking a strong stance on reducing benefits to the retired. Most retirees are receiving more from Social Security than what they paid into it as taxes when they were working. This is because the program began in 1935 after most of today's retirees were well into their working years and their contributions for many years were limited to 3 percent of their pay (plus another 3 percent from their employer). The current rate is a combined payroll tax of 15.4 percent. To repair the system, this rate would need to rise to at least 20 percent by the year 2020, and to as much as 40 percent by 2040.

The prospect of such high Social Security taxes or Pension Plan contributions frightens and angers younger workers who see their future being mortgaged. America's younger workers also face the prospect of higher income taxes to enable the federal government to pay back the $4 trillion it owes

Figure 8-13

Social Security, enacted in the United States in 1935 as a major source of income security for elderly people, also provides survivors' benefits for dependents and disability payments for injured workers. (*Source:* Social Security Administration.)

Just who is eligible for Social Security?

More people than you think. Because Social Security isn't just for retirement.

If a serious illness or injury prevents you from working, it can provide disability payments. If your life is cut short, it will pay survivors benefits.

Now you can find out what your benefits might be. Write to Dept. 74, Pueblo, Colorado 81009, to apply for your own Personal Earnings and Benefit Estimate Statement.

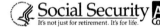 **Social Security** It's not just for retirement. It's for life. Ad Council

to Social Security. Social Security is their future security too, and it provides a form of life insurance ("survivor's benefits") and disability payments for injured workers (figure 8-13). The same applies to the Canada Pension Plan, as shown by the distribution of payouts from the CPP in figure 8-14. These facts make the political rescue of Social Security and Pension Plan funds virtually certain, but they also make the next generation of retirees, the baby boomers, less able to count on increased benefits or on help from their adult children as they grow more dependent. The only winners in these scenarios are the savers who have—or are—investing in private plans, RRSPs in Canada, IRAs and SEPs in the United States. These supplements to Pension Plans and Social Security offer financial and emotional tranquillity for those facing retirement.

······················

Figure 8-14

Like the U.S. Social Security funds, the Canada Pension Plan distributes its funds largely to retirement benefits, but also to worker disability and survivor benefits. (*Source:* Supply and Services, Canada.)

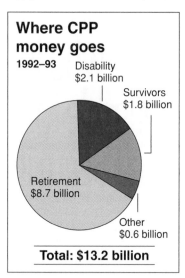

Where CPP money goes

1992–93   Disability $2.1 billion

Survivors $1.8 billion

Retirement $8.7 billion

Other $0.6 billion

Total: $13.2 billion

COMMUNITY HEALTH PROMOTION PROGRAMS

Programs that serve people with sensitivity to local cultures and circumstances can best be formulated on the community level. At more distant bureaucratic levels, planned programs often fail to touch individual older persons and their families. Of necessity, the national, state, or provincial program will be more removed from the individual and will be less sensitive to local variations in needs and perceptions.

Features of Community Programs for Older Populations

Community programs for older persons usually have three goals: (1) public education in the field of adult health, (2) integration of resources and forces in the community that have a service to offer

elderly persons, and (3) the acquisition and provision of necessary services that the community does not have available. A community health agency designated to determine health promotion needs and the approaches that should be used ideally serves as the coordinating focus. If the official community health center does not provide medical service, it may serve as a center for information, coordination, and health education.

Community programs must include public health education. The public needs to understand the nature of aging and the personal and social phenomena associated with it. The public should understand what can be done to prevent some of the premature deterioration of aging and should have an understanding of measures for the prevention of diseases and disabilities of the advancing years. The public needs to be informed of the importance of self-care and medical supervision and of the contribution that various individuals, agencies, and self-help groups have to make to the elderly citizens of the community. Perhaps most important, the public needs to adjust its perceptions of aging and of the elderly.

Community programs must also provide for the diagnosis, treatment, hospitalization, and rehabilitation of those older people who have some disability. It must provide for activities that elderly people can enjoy through participation. The program should also provide some means through which elderly people who are unable to pay for professional services may receive the services required.

Most older people in a community are self-sufficient or have members of their immediate family who can provide advice or assistance, but some have no such source of aid. These individuals would greatly benefit from an effective community health program for the older population.

Nutrition Programs for Older Populations

Community nutrition policies and programs promote better health among older people through health education, counseling, and the limited delivery of food services. Nutrition programs help reduce the isolation of older persons by offering them an opportunity to participate in community activities and to combine food and friendship.

Some elderly people do not eat adequately for reasons that may include: (1) insufficient income; (2) insufficient skills to select and prepare nourishing and well-balanced meals; (3) dental problems; (4) limited mobility; and (5) feelings of rejection and isolation that obliterate the incentive necessary to prepare and eat a meal alone. Such physiological, psychological, and social and economic changes can cause malnutrition and further physical, mental, and sensory deterioration.

Provision of meals in group settings by communities include schools, churches, community centers, senior centers, public housing, and other public and nonprofit facilities where additional supportive services may be available. Outreach programs identify those older persons most in need. Escort and transportation services bring participants to nutrition program sites.

Nutrition programs may provide home-delivered meals to participants who from time to time are unable to attend the meal service site. The program recognizes the need for a network of supportive services, including health services, information and referral, escort services, health and welfare counseling, and consumer education. Nutrition projects act as centers of activity, attracting older persons to a place where, in addition to getting a nourishing meal, they have the opportunity to receive these other services and advice on such important matters as legal rights, housing, shopping assistance, income maintenance, and crime prevention. Older persons also have the opportunity for socialization and recreation and for volunteer service to others. Under the terms of the Older Americans Act, states are encouraged to make nutrition program projects part of the system of services for the elderly.

Nutrition education can make older persons, project staff members, and volunteers aware of the relative values of food and its contribution to health and well-being. They can thereby influence selection, purchase, and preparation of food. Increased public and professional awareness can also lead to advocacy for policy changes at the local level and organization for advocacy at the state or provincial and national levels.

The government-sponsored community programs must give highest priority to low-income persons sixty years of age and over and their spouses and others who are determined to be in great need. These may include minorities, native populations, and persons who speak little English. Meal sites need to be located in urban and rural areas that have high proportions of older persons in these categories.

Community programs should give participants an opportunity to contribute to all or part of the cost of the meal. The nutrition program advisory council, which should contain a participant majority, establishes either a contribution schedule based on resources or a single flat sum as a guide to the size of contribution. Each participant determines what he or she is able to contribute. Contributions are received in such a manner that the amount given is known only to the contributor.

The quantity of food required by the person in the later years of life is not as great as in the earlier years, but the qualitative needs are just as important. Diversity of proteins and adequate vitamins and minerals should be included in each day's diet. Food should be attractive because the sense of taste becomes dulled with age. In the later years of life the output of digestive enzymes is reduced and the rate of digestion is much slower. For this reason, many elderly people prefer eating smaller but more frequent meals.

Other Health Promotion Programs

The benefits of smoking cessation and of increasing physical activity are more immediate and dramatic for the elderly than for other age groups (figure 8-15). A U.S. national objective for the year 2000 states that the proportion of adults sixty-five years and older who regularly participate in vigorous activities that promote the development and maintenance of cardiorespiratory fitness, for 3 or more times per week, 20 or more minutes per occasion should increase from 7.5 percent to 20 percent. Vigorous is defined as 60 percent or

• • • • • • • • • • • • • • • • • • • •

Figure 8-15

The benefits of increasing physical activity from a minimal (sedentary) level to a moderate level are notable even in old age. (*Source:* Photo courtesy M. Jane Ford, Health Director, Lincoln-Lancaster County Health Department, Lincoln, NE.)

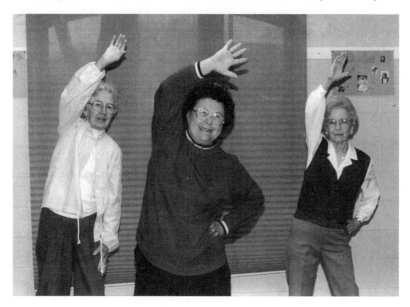

greater of maximal cardiorespiratory capacity. Inactivity increases with age. By age 75, about one in three men and one in two women engage in no extra physical activity.

The 1996 U.S. Surgeon General's Report on Physical Activity suggested various ways communities can support programs that will promote physical activity for older people (see box titled "What Communities Can Do to Support Physical Activity in Older Populations"). Efforts might include developing focal points, such as senior centers, to coordinate physical activity services to older citizens. Health care institutions such as hospitals and nursing homes should provide encouragement, equipment, and facilities to enhance the physical activity of their staff and clients. Designs for all multifamily housing should incorporate facilities such as exercise rooms or open spaces and gardens to provide physical activity options. More examples will be found in chapter 10.

Injury Prevention Programs

Injury and traumatic death rates increase in the old-age groups. Slowed reaction time, poor vision, and the inability to adjust readily to changing situations make the old person more injury-prone than younger individuals. Conditions in the home should be made as safe as possible. Living on one floor is an effective safety measure, because falls on stairs constitute a frequent cause of death for old people. Well-lighted rooms and hallways, and even the use of continuous dim light through the night, can be effective safety measures. Old people also have a high fatality rate in motor vehicle-pedestrian collisions. Loss of sensitivity in the skin can result in scalds and **hypothermia.**

Examples of injury prevention programs for the elderly and other high-risk groups will be presented in chapter 13.

What Communities Can Do to Support Physical Activity in Older Populations

The annual report of the Surgeon General of the United States was devoted in 1996 to physical aerobic activity and health. The report noted that older adults can benefit from moderate activity to increase cardiorespiratory endurance, and from muscle-strengthening activities. Stronger muscles help reduce the risk of falling and improve the ability to perform the routine tasks of daily life. Communities can:

- Provide community-based physical activity programs that offer aerobic, strengthening, and flexibility components specifically designed for older adults.
- Encourage malls and other indoor or protected locations to provide safe places for walking in any weather.
- Ensure that facilities for physical activity accommodate and encourage participation by older adults.
- Provide transportation for older adults to parks or facilities that provide physical activity programs.
- Encourage health care providers to talk routinely to their older adult patients about incorporating physical activity into their lives.

Plan community activities that include opportunities for older adults to be physically active.

MEDICAL AND LONG-TERM CARE SERVICES

Older people require proportionately more medical services than the general population. Most communities can provide the variety of medical skills necessary for the more complex problems of the aged by calling on the services of the various specialists available in the area. Interest in the health aspects of geriatrics has been rising, as evidenced by increasing numbers of physicians and other professionals who are members of geriatric or gerontological specialty societies. Unfortunately, medical and nursing students have shown resistance to working with geriatric patients.

Special geriatrics clinics have been established. Their goal has been to offer coordinated medical and social services to the population of independent, working elderly to aid them in retaining their independence. In addition to providing important diagnostic services to the elderly, the geriatrics clinic is able to formulate a continuing program of health supervision for its clients. These efforts and special projects are most laudable, but as yet most communities rely on the general hospital and medical services that are already available.

Nursing Homes

More than 1 million elderly people in the United States are in nursing homes, but it is encouraging that over 19 million are not. Most of the geriatric concern has been with the 5 percent who are institutionalized. This has tended to bias popular and professional perceptions of what old age is like.

Public health departments have been slow in licensing nursing homes in the United States. All fifty states have licensing laws, but their requirements are below the minimum standards recommended by national organizations (see table 8-5). The present situation still calls for legal action for providing desirable conditions through licensing of nursing homes.

Nursing homes should be affiliated with and should cooperate with general hospitals. In such an arrangement, physicians will have elderly patients moved from the general hospital to the less expensive nursing home, where they know the chronically ill can receive the necessary nursing care. Such an arrangement also means a greater likelihood that the majority of the patients in the nursing home will be under medical supervision.

Home Care

Physicians, nurses, occupational therapists, and social workers agree that the aging who are ill should be cared for in their own homes as long as possible. Obviously, certain situations make this impossible or undesirable. However when home conditions are acceptable, some chronically ill patients

Table 8-5

Community Surveillance of the Quality of Nursing Homes Will Be Tested by the Careful Examination Given to Them by Consumers Searching for a Place for Their Parents or Grandparents

When you visit a nursing home, you should carry this checklist with you. It will help you to compare one facility with another, but remember to compare facilities certified in the same category; for example, a skilled nursing facility with another skilled nursing home. Because nursing homes may be licensed in more than one category, always compare similar types of service among facilities.

Home A   **Home B**

	Home A YES	Home A NO	Home B YES	Home B NO
Look at Daily Live				
1. Do residents seem to enjoy being with staff?	☐	☐	☐	☐
2. Are most residents dressed for the season and time of day?	☐	☐	☐	☐
3. Do staff members know the residents by name?	☐	☐	☐	☐
4. Do staff respond quickly to resident calls for assistance?	☐	☐	☐	☐
5. Are activities tailored to residents' individual needs and interests?	☐	☐	☐	☐
6. Are residents involved in a variety of activities?	☐	☐	☐	☐
7. Does the home serve food attractively?	☐	☐	☐	☐
8. Does the home consider personal food likes and dislikes in planning meals?	☐	☐	☐	☐
9. Does the home use care in selecting roommates?	☐	☐	☐	☐
10. Does the nursing home have a resident's council? If it does, does the council influence decisions about resident life?	☐	☐	☐	☐
11. Does the nursing home have a family council? If it does, does the council influence decisions about resident life?	☐	☐	☐	☐
12. Does the facility have contact with community groups, such as pet therapy programs and Scouts?	☐	☐	☐	☐
Look at Care Residents Receive				
1. Do various staff and professional experts participate in evaluating each resident's needs and interests?	☐	☐	☐	☐
2. Does the resident or his or her family participate in developing the resident's care plan?	☐	☐	☐	☐
3. Does the home offer programs to restore lost physical functioning (for example, physical therapy, occupational therapy, speech and language therapy)?	☐	☐	☐	☐
4. Does the home have any special services that meet your needs? For example, special care units for residents with dementia or with respiratory problems?	☐	☐	☐	☐
5. Does the nursing home have a program to restrict the use of physical restraints?	☐	☐	☐	☐
6. Is a registered nurse available for nursing staff?	☐	☐	☐	☐
7. Does the nursing home have an arrangement with a nearby hospital?	☐	☐	☐	☐

continued

Table 8-5—*Continued.*

Look at How the Nursing Home Handles Payment

1. Is the facility certified for Medicare? ☐ ☐ ☐ ☐
2. Is the facility certified for Medicaid? ☐ ☐ ☐ ☐
3. Is the resident or the resident's family informed when charges are increased? ☐ ☐ ☐ ☐

Look at the Environment

1. Is the outside of the nursing home clean and in good repair? ☐ ☐ ☐ ☐
2. Are there outdoor areas accessible for residents to use? ☐ ☐ ☐ ☐
3. Is the inside of the nursing home clean and in good repair? ☐ ☐ ☐ ☐
4. Does the nursing home have handrails in hallways and grab bars in bathrooms? ☐ ☐ ☐ ☐
5. When floors are being cleaned, are warning signs displayed, or are areas blocked off to prevent accidents? ☐ ☐ ☐ ☐
6. Is the nursing home free from unpleasant odors? ☐ ☐ ☐ ☐
7. Are toilets convenient to bedrooms? ☐ ☐ ☐ ☐
8. Do noise levels fit the activities that are going on? ☐ ☐ ☐ ☐
9. Is it easy for residents in wheelchairs to move around the home? ☐ ☐ ☐ ☐
10. Is the lighting appropriate for what residents are doing? ☐ ☐ ☐ ☐
11. Are there private areas for residents to visit with family, visitors, or physicians? ☐ ☐ ☐ ☐
12. Are residents' bedrooms furnished in a pleasant manner? ☐ ☐ ☐ ☐
13. Do the residents have some personal items in their bedrooms (for example, family pictures, souvenirs, a chair)? ☐ ☐ ☐ ☐
14. Do the residents' rooms have accessible storage areas for residents' personal items? ☐ ☐ ☐ ☐

Other Things to Look For

1. Does the nursing home have a good reputation in the community? ☐ ☐ ☐ ☐
2. Does the nursing home have a list of references? ☐ ☐ ☐ ☐
3. Is the nursing home convenient for family or friends to visit? ☐ ☐ ☐ ☐
4. Does the local ombudsman visit the facility regularly? ☐ ☐ ☐ ☐

can be as well taken care of in the home as in the nursing home or the hospital. Visiting nursing services can be used to good advantage, especially when only part-time nursing service is necessary.

Home health care services can include part-time nursing care, physical therapy, home-delivered meals, transportation and escort services, and other programs of assistance and care. Families and professionals are well advised to explore home health care services available in the community before contracting with a nursing or custodial home (figure 8-16).

Day care programs for older people have become more common. Many of them include health services such as medication administration, podiatric services, rehabilitation therapies, dietary counseling, and mental and recreational services and programs.

Consumer Issues in Health Care for the Elderly

Nursing Homes   The Health Care Financing Administration, which is the U.S. agency with responsibility for Medicare and Medicaid, issued a 75-volume report in December 1988 evaluating the 15,000 American nursing homes then caring for the more than 1.5 million Medicare and Medicaid patients. For each home the report bluntly stated "not met" for criteria similar to those in table 8-5 if the nursing home was deficient on that standard. More than 40 percent mishandled food; 29 percent of them improperly dispensed medicines; and 25 percent fell short on isolation techniques to prevent the spread of infection. About 2,400 of the 15,000 met all of the 32 health, safety, and care standards. This "consumer guide" to nursing homes was helpful to communities seeking to improve their services and to people looking for a nursing home.

Health Insurance   The elderly as health care consumers also face an array of confusing and difficult choices with health insurance. A federal health insurance program was added to Medicare in 1989 to cover "catastrophic" illnesses, costing

Figure 8-16

The United Way in most communities seeks to support independent living for elders. Home health care expenditures have risen by more than twice the rate of increase in overall health care expenditures. (*Source:* United Way and Advertising Council, New York.)

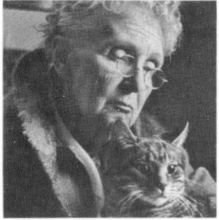

LIKE MOST PEOPLE HER AGE, SHE BELONGS IN A HOME. HER OWN.

For 30 years, it's been her home. But now, she could end up in a nursing home. Simply because she could use a hand shopping for groceries.

Who do you turn to when you're all alone?

She got help through a volunteer shopping program for the elderly. They got help from the United Way. All because the United Way got help from you.

You helped support a program that provides a volunteer to do the shopping for a 79-year-old woman. A woman who wants nothing more than to live out her life in the home she loves.

United Way

It brings out the best in all of us.

some elderly people an additional $800 per year as a federal income-tax surcharge. Many viewed this as a discriminatory tax on the elderly. Organizations in the following year succeeded in repealing the law.

Out-of-Pocket Health Costs The elderly spend approximately 18 percent of their income—an average of $2,566 in 1990—on health costs. The costs not covered by Medicare, Medicaid, private health insurance, or government amounts to 13 percent of the total. Elderly health care payments went up 12 percent per year between 1980 and 1990, while their income went up 7.1 percent per year.

Rehabilitation

Older people who are ill or disabled need more than custodial care. Chronic disease hospitals are not the answer, because they tend to create the conception of lifelong disability. The general hospital can usually provide the services necessary for the care and treatment of the elderly patient, without creating the impression of cold-storage institutionalization. Hospital patients should have a combination of medical care and rehabilitation to prepare them for their mode of living after they are discharged from the hospital. Nursing and social services are necessary before patients are transferred home. The elderly person may need some supervision to make a reasonable adjustment to a normal living routine. Even when the elderly person lives with other members of the family, social work services can be of value in aiding all concerned to understand how to meet the elderly person's needs.

COMMUNICATING WITH THE ELDERLY

Like all members of society, old people must be able to read and grasp the meaning of a great deal of printed and optically projected material if they are to maintain a self-sufficient lifestyle. However it is not recognized that older persons' lack of comprehension, when it occurs, may result from a sensory rather than intellectual failure.

Print Media

One aspect of this sensory failure is that type style, type size, and layout of printed materials affect an older person's reading speed, ease of reading, and interest in written materials. Older persons prefer and can read faster when shown roman rather than other styles of type. Roman type may be found in newspapers and many textbooks. Increasing the type size beyond a certain point does not facilitate reading for older people.

We know little about specific benefits or costs of the communications media used to provide information about social services. Isolation from communication flows sometimes accompanies physical isolation. Communication by print—flyers, pamphlets, notices, newspapers, and the like—is the least effective substitute for face-to-face contact between older people and those responsible for interpreting laws, regulations, eligibility, and entitlements.

Electronic Media

Communications other than face-to-face communication are not necessarily inferior. Modern communications media, including the telephone, allow telecommunications in place of transportation, sharing of valuable human resources among underserved populations, and other benefits. These media provide solutions ready and waiting to alleviate problems.

More than half the services provided to clients by public social service agencies are information exchanges of one sort or another and are directly amenable to enhancement by telecommunications. Older adults watch television, on the average, three hours per day—slightly less than the average for the total population. On the other hand, adult television viewing increases with age. A majority of old people consider television viewing as an important recreational activity; in fact, television viewing ranks first among all activities of the elderly, according to some surveys. It has been reported that old people prefer personal, nonfiction programs in which people like themselves play important roles, either as members of the studio audience or as contestants.

Radio and television have brought religious services into the home for elderly shut-ins, and the churches have supplemented this by providing

ISSUES AND CONTROVERSIES
Out of Sight, Out of Mind?

The older woman is far more likely than the older man to live alone. This isolation impairs communication, making both the diagnosis and the treatment of physical and mental illness more difficult in older women. Many women may be diagnosed as suffering from senile dementia or Alzheimer's disease when in fact they are lonely, isolated, and depressed. How do loss of vision or hearing, common health problems of the aged, lead to misunderstandings and misdiagnoses?

---

additional, more personal, services to the shut-ins. These personalized services need not be of a strictly religious nature. Church people are in a strategic position to give the type of personal service that will help the older shut-in to attain and maintain the frame of mind and general well-being so essential to physical and mental health.

Telephone Contact

Telephone reassurance provided by daily telephone contact with an older person who might otherwise have no outside contact for long periods of time can be an important service. Persons receiving telephone reassurance may be called at a predetermined time each day. If the person does not answer, help is immediately sent to his or her home; usually a neighbor, relative, or nearby police or fire station is asked to make a personal check. Such details are worked out when a person begins receiving this service. Telephone reassurance has been credited with saving many lives by the quick dispatching of medical help.

In one case, an alert caller noticed a slight slurring of speech in a client she talked with regularly. Although the client reported no difficulties, the caller reported the slurred speech to her supervisor, who sent someone to check the situation. The client had suffered a heart spasm and was rushed to the hospital in time. Telephone reassurance generally costs little and can be provided by callers of any age, from teenagers to older people themselves. It is sponsored by a variety of organizations and agencies in the United States ranging

from women's clubs to police departments. For example, in one community, residents of a home for the aged make calls to the elderly living alone. In another, older persons who cannot leave their homes are called daily by senior center members. In a third, a hospital auxiliary and the Business and Professional Women's Club make daily calls.

TRANSPORTATION

Older people require access to the services, facilities, resources, and opportunities necessary for existence. Transportation, whether for visiting and traveling, taking the individual to a health service or facility, or bringing a service provider to the individual, influences the effectiveness of other services for the elderly. Basic priorities and accompanying funding for transportation will remain inadequate, forcing communities to choose between improvements for the elderly or improvements for all travelers.

Mass Transit

Mass transportation systems have become increasingly important with the growing problems of the automobile as the primary mode of transportation. Automobile ownership declines with age. This decline is mostly a result of the lower incomes of the elderly, but it is also influenced by their decreasing physical or psychological ability to drive. Studies indicate a greater dependence on walking among the aged, but walking is limited by the inadequacy of pedestrian accommodations and security. Studies also indicate that public transportation is least adequate for those most in need of it: the physically frail, individuals with no friends or relatives to drive them, minority group members, and the poor.

Some communities and civic organizations offer various forms of assistance to help meet the transportation needs of the older population. In European countries, public transportation systems are far better suited to the needs of the elderly than those of North America.

Federal and State or Provincial Support

Canadian transportation policy resides with the provinces, and mass transit is more fully developed in most large cities in Canada than in the U.S. The U.S. National Mass Transportation Act of 1974 included a number of provisions that aided older riders. The act required that any public transit system receiving capital assistance funds from the Urban Mass Transportation Administration of the U.S. Department of Transportation charge half fare or less for the elderly. Other programs administered by the Urban Mass Transportation Administration include research and development grants to test innovative approaches to transportation problems and funding for capital assistance and the acquisition of vehicles and other needed equipment.

Several other avenues of assistance can be used to provide transportation services for the elderly. Under Title III of the Older Americans Comprehensive Services Amendments, which authorizes support for state and community programs, the U.S. Administration on Aging awards grants to the designated state agencies on aging to assist state and local agencies in the development of comprehensive and coordinated services to the elderly. The designated state or provincial agency can identify potential sources of funding for transportation, provide advice on how best to plan for and implement a project, and coordinate efforts with other agencies and organizations that might be involved in planning and supporting transportation projects.

Community Programs

Many communities operate transportation projects. Some are relatively inexpensive, using volunteer drivers in small towns and rural areas. Others use sophisticated demand-responsive or regularly scheduled transit vehicles, often designed to meet the special needs of the elderly.

Free or reduced fares on public transportation vehicles are enabling the elderly in many parts of North America and Europe to travel during midday, night, and weekend hours. Many areas that permit older people to ride free during off-peak transit hours also offer reduced fares during rush hours. One community mobilized service to the elderly and handicapped where little or none existed before. Eligible riders have access to specially equipped minibuses that offer door-to-door service; nominal fares; and transportation by advance reservation, weekly subscription, telephone request, and charter service.

LEISURE-TIME ACTIVITIES

Communities acknowledge the value of recreational and social participation, but for no group are these of greater health value than for older people (see chapter 10). With a great deal of newly found time on their hands, the elderly need activities that will occupy them profitably and enjoyably. Some have business interests, trade skills, voluntary association memberships, or a garden to occupy their attention and time, but many are in need of help in developing satisfying leisure-time activities. Most of the elderly seek and enjoy the companionship of others. A community can provide for individual instruction for recreation purposes, but provision for instruction and supervision on a group basis is usually more practical.

Small groups of elderly people can take up arts and crafts, music, dramatics, poetry, and creative writing. The mutual encouragement, the sociability, and the general elation that come from such participation can do more for many of these people than can the physician or the hospital. On the other hand, participation in social activities and associations cannot be offered as a substitute for health care.

Zest for living is extremely important in the health of the elderly. On a large-group basis, concerts, lectures, dancing, parties, excursions, and outings can be highly important in the lives of the elderly and can contribute measurably to their outlook. Checkers, chess, cards, and shuffleboard are popular games that can be organized and promoted among the elderly. Social action groups such as the Gray Panthers provide a vehicle for productive civic participation. Communities without such organizations should provide avenues for the development and promotion of a zest for living. This aids older people in their feeling of security, a primary need of every person, but it also brings returns to the community in the continuing participation of the aging in community life.

SUMMARY

Community responsibility for the health of the aging population encompasses concern for the citizen's total living. A community health program for the elderly should include or take into account medical services, hospital facilities, nursing home services, housing conditions, health education, health counseling, recreation programs, and individual and group participation in productive and enjoyable activities. The community health department alone cannot carry the whole program, but it can be the agency that integrates all community resources having a contribution for the elderly. Social service, education, communication, and transportation agencies can complement the health department and initiate action necessary for the promotion of the well-being of the elderly.

The compression of morbidity thesis and the goal of extending active life expectancy lead us to seek points of intervention for health promotion that will head off the downward, cumulative spiral characterizing the degenerative process. The most effective prevention, as usual, would be early prevention, but it is difficult to mount programs, capture resources, and sustain the attention and motivation of people who have yet no symptoms and for whom the benefits of the recommended actions are years away. Conventional public health strategies do not fit the needs of the elderly because the early onset of most conditions cannot be identified, incidence data are largely unavailable, and communitywide interventions are too costly and inefficient in reaching the dispersed elderly population.

Health promotion programs designed and evaluated to date have been directed primarily at more affluent people, leaving the search alive for approaches that use the development of community ties, and those that use early warning signs or life events as points of intervention. Clearly identified transition points such as retirement, relocation, and widowhood enable professionals to intervene in anticipation of the adaptations people and communities need to make in their lifestyles to adjust. Successful adjustment reduces the development of dysfunctional coping and the harm to health that usually follows. This anticipatory approach to transitions serves the primary prevention purposes of health promotion and the health enhancement purposes, strengthening the coping abilities of older people.

WEB*Links*

http://www.healthguide.com/livingoptions/
Education about living options for seniors.

http://www.ssa.gov
Social Security Administration—updates, information, services, research, questions, and current issues.

http://www.benefitscanada.com
Information on building retirement income, managed health care, and trends in Canada.

QUESTIONS FOR REVIEW

1. What are some signs of "ageism" in your community?
2. Why must gerontology concern itself with social, psychological, and physiological aging?
3. List ten persons of your acquaintance who are over sixty-five years of age. What percentage have good health, what percentage have fair health, what percentage are ill but up and around, and what percentage are disabled? What percentage have health impairments that could be corrected or at least reduced?
4. To what extent do changes in the economy affect the population age distribution of a state or province?
5. What factors are essential if an individual is to be relatively "young" at age 75?
6. What is the general social status of the elderly people of your community and what is the significance of their social status in terms of their health?
7. To what extent is the community health program for aging people primarily a program of curing illness rather than of promoting health?
8. What does your state or provincial health department have in the way of an agency and a program for the promotion of the health of the elderly?
9. What special activities in the interest of better health for the older population are carried on by your official community health department?
10. What are the voluntary health agencies of your community doing on behalf of the health of the older population?
11. What are the contributions of other institutions in your community, such as churches, to the health and well-being of older people?
12. How interested in and how well informed about matters relating to the health of older people is the general public in your community?
13. What would be a good routine of daily living for a man or woman of age 70 without impairments?
14. Why are sensory losses so important to older people?

READINGS

Institute for Health and Aging, University of California, San Francisco. 1996. *Chronic care in America: a 21st century challenge.* Princeton, NJ: The Robert Wood Johnson Foundation.

This book of charts and commentary on the growing burden of chronic conditions and societal responses to the needs for chronic care is available online through the Foundation's home page on the World Wide Web at http://www.rwjf.org.

Keith, J. 1994. *Age and culture: diversity and commonality in experiences of aging.* Newbury Park, CA: Sage.

Using anthropological methods in four countries, the author provides cross-cultural insights on the varying perspectives different communities and populations have on health and well-being, age and the lifecourse, and political economy and age, based on ten years of field observations.

McGowan, P., and L. W. Green. 1995. Arthritis self-management in native populations of British Columbia: an application of health promotion and participatory research principles in chronic disease control. *Can J Aging* 14(suppl. 1): 201.

This adaptation of the Arthritis Self-Management Program was developed in collaboration with native people in their own communities, applying the Precede-Proceed model introduced in chapter 4.

Stern, L. 1997. Can we save Social Security? *Modern Maturity* 40(1):28.

Social Security's threatened fund in the face of the soon retiring Baby Boomers forces some choices to avoid putting the entire tax burden on young workers.

BIBLIOGRAPHY

Advisory Committee on Immunization Practices, National Immunization Program, CDC. 1995. Assessing adult vaccination status at age 50 years. *Morb & Mort Weekly Rep* 44:561.

Baltes, M. M., and L. L. Carstensen. 1996. The process of successful ageing. *Ageing and society* 16:4.

Beresford, T., and E. Gomberg. eds. 1995. *Alcohol and aging.* New York: Oxford University Press.

Bureau of the Census. 1991. *Global aging: comparative indicators and future trends.* Washington, DC: Economics and Statistics Administration, U.S. Department of Commerce.

Canada pension plan, old age security act, and pension benefits standards act, with regulations. 1992. 9th ed. Don Mills, Ontario: CCH Canadian Limited.

Chatman, E. A. 1992. *The information world of retired women.* Westport, CT: Greenwood.

Erben, R., P. Franzkowiak, and E. Wenzel. 1992. Assessment of the outcomes of health intervention. *Soc Sci Med* 35:359.

Fries, J. F., L. W. Green, and S. Levine. 1989. Health promotion and the compression of morbidity. *Lancet* 1:105.

Gilleard, J. T. 1996. Consumption and identity in later life: toward a cultural gerontology. *Ageing & society* 16:489.

Glickstein, J. K., and G. K. Neustadt. 1992. *Reimbursable geriatric service delivery: a functional maintenance therapy system.* Frederick, MD: Aspen.

Golander, H., and A. E. Raz. 1996. The mask of dementia: images of 'demented residents' in a nursing ward. *Ageing and society* 16: 269.

Health Canada. 1996. *Seniors guide to federal programs and services.* Ottawa: Minister of Supply and Services Canada.

Institute of Medicine. 1990. *The second 50 years: promoting health and preventing disability.* Washington, DC: National Academy Press.

Kane, R. S. 1996. The defeat of aging versus the importance of death. *J Am Geriatrics Soc* 44:321.

Kannisto, V., J. Lauritsen, A. R. Thatcher, and J. W. Vaupel. Reductions in mortality at advanced ages: several decades of evidence from 27 countries. *Popul & Devel Rev* 20:793.

Leigh, J. P., and J. F. Fries. 1994. Education, gender, and the compression of morbidity. *Intl J Aging & Hum Devel* 39:233.

McDonald, P. L. 1991. *Elder abuse and neglect in Canada.* Toronto: Butterworths.

Minkler, M., and C. L. Estes, eds. 1990. *Critical perspectives on aging: the political and moral economy of growing old.* New York: Baywood.

Moschis, G. P. 1992. *Marketing to older consumers.* Westport, CT: Quorum.

Newcomer, R., C. Harrington, and R. Kane. 1996. Managed care in acute and Primary care settings. *Ann Rev Gerontol & Geriatrics* 16:1.

Nordin, R., A. M. Hamid, and W. A. W. Adnan. 1992. Preparing the young to look after the old. *World Health Forum* 13: 300.

Perks, T. T. 1995. The oldest old. *Scientific Amer* 272(1): 70.

Phillipson, C. 1996. Interpretations of ageing: perspectives from humanistic gerontology. *Ageing and society* 16:3.

Schaie, K. W., D. Blazer, and J. S. House, eds. 1992. *Aging, health behaviors, and health outcomes.* Hillsdale, NJ: Erlbaum.

Stone, R. I., and R. E. Katz. 1996. Thoughts on the future of integrating acute and long-term care. *Ann Rev Gerontol & Geriatrics* 16: 217.

Topp, R., and J. S. Stevenso. 1994. The effects of attendance and effort on outcomes among older adults in a long-term exercise program. *Res Nurs H* 17:15.

Troyansky, D. 1996. The history of old age in the western world. *Ageing and society* 16:233.

Wagner, E. H., A. Z. LaCroix, L. Grothaus, S. G. Leveille, J. A. Hecht, K. Artz, K. Odle, and D. M. Buchner. 1994. Preventing disability and falls in older adults: a population-based randomized trial. *Am J Public Health* 84:1800.

Walker, A., and C. Walker. 1996. Older people with learning difficulties leaving institutional care: a case of double jeopardy. *Ageing and society* 16:125.

World Health Organization. 1995. *Quality health care for the elderly: a manual for instructors of nurses and other health workers.* Ottawa, ON: Canadian Public Health Association for WHO Western Pacific Education in Action Series, No. 6.

Part Three

COMMUNITY AND POPULATION HEALTH PROMOTION

Part 3 outlines the strategies for health promotion in the community or in populations, beginning with community or population mental and social health, stress, and suicide prevention. Community recreation and fitness and the development and support of healthful lifestyles and policies round out this presentation of health promotion.

Health promotion goes beyond health education in its emphasis on social and evnironmental supports for invididual, organizational, and community action. It seeks to make the community conducive to health by altering the forces making it difficult for individuals to gain control over or to maintain their own health.

Chapter 9

Community Mental and Social Health

The only normal people are the ones you don't know very well.

—Joe Ancis

The only feelings that do not heal are the ones you hide.

—Henri Nouwen

Objectives

When you finish this chapter, you should be able to:

- Analyze and assess the mental health concerns and needs of a community

- Identify strategies appropriate to address those needs

- Identify resources in the community to support a comprehensive mental and social health program

As discussed in previous chapters, health is more than the absence of disease or limited to a concern about physical well-being. Community health is concerned also about the mental well-being of populations. Physical and mental health are linked. Like physical health, mental health is affected by characteristics of individuals and the broader socioeconomic environment in which they live. Some populations are disproportionately affected. Past efforts to deal with mental illness have swung from warehousing people in isolated mental hospitals to deinstitutionalizing them with little care or support.

Communities have learned to deal with less fear and superstition with mental health and mental disorders (figure 9-1). The prejudices once associated with "madness" have given way to more enlightened and tolerant perspectives on the full range of stresses in daily living, problems of coping, emotional setbacks during times of critical transitions and events, and minor neuroses and compulsions that afflict everyone at some time. The gradient from these common states of mind to peak performance and well-being at one extreme and the depths of psychotic disorientation and antisocial violence at the other reflects the distribution of mental health and mental illness in a community.

Research on the brain, the nervous system, and emotions can be applied to organize a highly effective community mental health program. Such a program first assesses the social problems or

. . . .

Figure 9-1

Reducing the stigma and fear associated with mental illness has been one of the success stories of mental health education over several decades, beginning largely in the 1950s. (*Source:* American Mental Health Fund.)

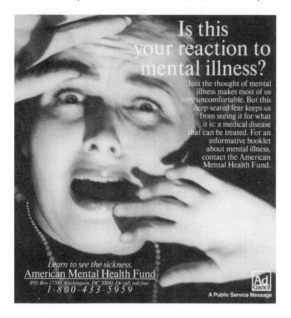

quality-of-life concerns of a community, considering what the people perceive to be their own priorities for improving the quality of their lives. Applying knowledge from the sciences of mental health and public health to the subjective concerns of a community is the essence of community mental and social health. Prevention within the mental health field means "intervening in a deliberate and positive way to counteract harmful circumstances before they cause disorder or disability," according to the landmark report, *The Prevention of Mental-Emotional Disabilities,* in 1986. This definition is controversial, however, in that it suggests that if treatment is given, prevention has failed. The concept of secondary and tertiary prevention noted in earlier chapters, seems to be precluded from this understanding of prevention in mental health.

In this chapter we will discuss the concept of mental health; the epidemiology of mental distress, illness, and disorder; issues in promoting mental health; the social pathology of divorce, suicide, and violence; resources for community action in mental health; and provisions for the rehabilitation of those who have been mentally ill. The control of stress and violence in the community, considered a priority objective of many health agencies, will be included. Community actions to control violence and the abuse of alcohol and drugs will be considered in chapters 12 and 13.

CONCEPTS OF MENTAL AND SOCIAL HEALTH

The term **mental health** refers to the emotional and social well-being and the psychological resources of the individual. This includes an individual's ability to negotiate the daily challenges and social interactions of life. Emotions are feelings with physiological and psychological components. Anger, for example, is more than a mental state; it evokes physiological responses, some of which are beneficial in preparing the individual to cope with circumstances. Over time, however, any chronic emotional state or stress becomes a strain on the body's organs and physiological systems. Thus, physiology contributes to mental health and is affected by it. Stress also underlies many of the other behavioral and immunological problems that account for much of the chronic disease and infectious disease in the community.

Stress and **coping** (the ability to adjust to stress) influence smoking, drinking, compulsive eating, resistance to infections, reckless driving, and various forms of violence. Interventions to reduce stress and to help people manage stress might represent a powerful program of primary prevention in relation to most of the leading causes of death and disability in modern society. There appears to be a strong, positive correlation between a person's perception of coping successfully and his or her health status.

Modern Definition of Community Mental Health

A community mental health perspective looks beyond the individual to social, economic, and political sources of well-being. The Canadian Ministry of Health and Welfare defines mental health as "the capacity of the individual, the group and the environment to interact with one another in ways that promote subjective well-being, the optimal development and use of mental abilities (cognitive, affective and relational), the achievement of individual and collective goals consistent with justice and the attainment and preservation of conditions of fundamental equality." This interactive definition moves mental health from an individual psychological perspective to a community social-psychological perspective.

This definition also minimizes the view of mental health as a static trait of the individual but, rather, recognizes it as a dynamic combination of energy, strengths, and abilities of the individual interacting effectively with those of the group, the family, and the community. It places mental health on a continuum from optimal to minimal, with the two ends of the continuum defined by the harmony and integration of individual, group, and environmental factors.

Social Health

Social health must be assessed by community criteria of productivity and quality of life. The goal of "Health for All by the Year 2000" has been declared by the World Health Organization (WHO) and the United Nations Children's Fund (UNICEF) to be a level of health such that all people are capable of working productively and participating actively in the social life of their community.

The breakdown of social health is signaled by problems of family breakdown through divorce or separation, the alienation of young people from community norms, racial and ethnic conflict, crime, high unemployment, homelessness, and growing or persistent poverty accompanied by conspicuous consumption and opulence in the same community. These reflect social pathologies

Spiritual Dimensions of Health

Spirituality may enhance health by providing:

- A personal system of belief or faith that includes and extends beyond the physical self, giving one a sense of belonging
- A locus of power and empowerment that provides opportunities for self-realization and community
- A system of unconditional meaningfulness and purpose that provides the self with a sense of positive direction and the possibility of fulfillment
- Peace and calm in the face of stressful life circumstances

that undermine the foundations for physical and mental health.

No person lives with perfect efficiency, nor does any person experience continuous happiness. The best that most people can do is attain happiness occasionally, and then only for short periods. It would not be fair to label an occasional lapse of "socially considerate behavior" a mental disorder. Imperfect people in an imperfect world means that even the highest level of mental health is not perfect health. Varying degrees of mental health are distributed broadly in the community in accordance with the normal curve characterizing the distribution of most natural phenomena. The goal of community mental health is to shift the average for the population toward more positive levels and to prevent, control, and alleviate suffering at the negative end of the curve.

EPIDEMIOLOGY OF MENTAL HEALTH AND ILLNESS

Mental illness is the most prevalent disease in America, more prevalent than cancer, heart disease, and lung disease combined. It is also indiscriminate, striking people from all walks of life. One in three adults in North America will suffer a diagnosable mental disorder in their lifetime. This

· · · · · · · · · · · · · · · · · ·
Figure 9-2

Mid-decade status of selected U.S. mental health and mental disorders objectives for the year 2000 (*Source:* Substance Abuse and Mental Health Administration, National Institutes of Health.)

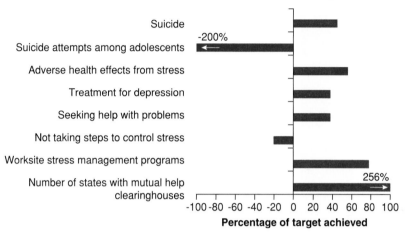

Status of mental health and mental disorders objectives

translates into 100 million adults who will have had a mental disorder at some time in their lives and several million children who suffer from mental and emotional disturbances. U.S. national mental health targets have had mixed success, as evidenced by the mid-decade review (figure 9-2). While the overall suicide rate has decreased since 1987, suicide attempts by adolescents have increased. The social and economic costs of serious mental illness are extensive as the limitations of such illness affects many aspects of a person's functioning.

A Mental Health Continuum

No two individuals are alike. Nevertheless, most of us, in terms of mental health, fit within the overall pattern or range accepted as **normal.** This allows for the wide span of individual differences to be found among persons whose conduct is regarded as quaint, faddish, eccentric, or avant-garde, but within accepted patterns. Within this range of mental health we find various points on a continuum.

At the extreme positive end, some individuals function efficiently on a high level and derive unusual enjoyment in their living. They encounter frustration, disappointment, and failure, but with a minimum of friction. They freely and effectively use their abilities in harmony with life's demands and gain a maximum of personal satisfaction in their accomplishments.

Another group of individuals, still a standard deviation or more from the population average, adjusts to frustration, disappointment, and failure and experiences only a moderate amount of disturbance from the friction they encounter in life. This is a desirable quality of mental health and perhaps should be rated as good mental health. Doubtless, many of the individuals in this group could attain an even higher level of mental health with better understanding and organized community efforts.

A third group constitutes a majority of people in some populations. These individuals do not have mental disorders, although they do experience occasional or even more frequent emotional upsets. Their distinguishing characteristic is that

· · · · · · · · · · · · · · · · · ·

Figure 9-3

Lifetime prevalence of psychiatric disorders among persons 15–54 years of age by sex: United States, 1990–92.
(*Source:* University of Michigan, Institute for Social Research, Survey Research Center, National Comorbidity Survey.)

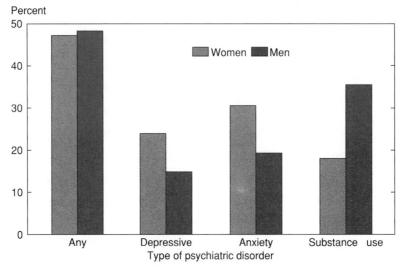

NOTES: The presence of a psychiatric disorder did not have to be formally
diagnosed for persons to be included as having had a disorder. The category
"Any Disorder" includes disorders not included in the specific types shown.

they seldom seem to reach a dynamic level of adjustment in which they attain considerable accomplishment with an accompanying great amount of enjoyment. They tend to operate in second gear and live rather uninteresting, uninspired, and passive lives. They drag through life, getting a half-measure of what life really has to offer. These individuals possess a fair level of mental health. Many of them, through understanding and community support, could enjoy life more.

At the negative end of the continuum, one or more functional disorders dominate the lives of some people. The prevalence of some psychiatric disorders varies among men and women, as noted in figure 9-3. Some of these disorders, such as depression, strike most people at some times, but for the chronically mentally distressed they persist and make it difficult if not impossible for the individual to carry out the functions of daily living. Functional incapacity strikes most notably in relation to those functions involving interaction with other people.

Changing Perspectives on Treatment

Long-term community care for the mentally ill has grown to a point where state hospitals play a minor role. Most states have proprietary hospitals that specialize in the care of the mentally ill, but these facilities are used by a small and declining percentage of mentally ill patients. The severely mentally ill need special medical and hospital services, and this is the province of the psychiatrist or the medical practitioner. **Psychiatry** concerns itself with the diagnosis, treatment, and cure of mental disorder.

The present psychosomatic approach to mental illness indicates that the physical and the psychological are interrelated and that mental disorders can have their genesis in a physiological disturbance. Mental illness, once regarded as primarily a problem of custodial care, is regarded as a problem of medical care. This change has come about because of the development of specific medication in the treatment of mental disorder and the concept that a mental hospital is a place where one can go for a short time for treatment. Cold-storage institutionalization has become obsolete, and mental illness is regarded as truly remediable. Advances in the 1980s indicated that a major breakthrough in the treatment and care of mental disorder occurred and that the problem was yielding to the united efforts of the many disciplines attacking it. The general public is not yet aware that the success of **chemotherapy** in dealing with the symptoms of mental illness represents a landmark in the progress of the public's health.

Epidemiology of Mental Illness

Epidemiology uses population-based rates to identify the incidence and prevalence of a specific condition, its distribution, and changes in the occurrence of phenomena; from these factors it infers the likely causes of the condition and suggests points of intervention in the natural history of its spread in the population. Such analysis helps identify that major mental illness affects more than 35 million Americans and costs more than $40 billion in direct care. Another $50 billion will accrue in the indirect costs of their mental illness, such as lost work time and wages (figure 9-4).

Whether mental disorder is on the increase in North America is difficult to assess. People are more inclined to use professional services and facilities. Medication has not reduced hospital admissions significantly but has shortened the length of stay and increased the use of outpatient services.

The Range and Symptoms of Mental Illness

Mental illness is not one disease but a broad classification of many. More than 13 million Americans suffer from anxiety disorders, over 9 million from depression, and over 2 1/2 million from schizophrenic disorder. Twelve million children suffer from autism, depression, hyperkinetic disorders, and other diseases. Drug and alcohol abuse, suicidal tendencies, obsessive-compulsive disorder, Alzheimer's disease, anorexia nervosa, and bulimia can all be classified as mental illness.

Many mental disorders have a biological origin. Schizophrenia and depression, for example, may result from chemical imbalances, chemical deficiencies, or structural abnormalities that can create a malfunction in the brain's signaling system. This awareness has led to new research and progress in the treatment of mental illness. Using advanced technologies, many chemical imbalances can be corrected, controlling the manifestations of many forms of mental illness. These advances have set the stage for new techniques in psychotherapy. With proper treatment, two out of three victims of mental illness can expect to get better and lead productive lives.

Despite these statistics, only one in five people with mental illness seeks professional help, because they do not understand the symptoms and the wide variety of treatments available to them. Sometimes inappropriate or extreme behavior can be a warning sign of mental illness (figure 9-5). Some of the common warning signs people can learn to recognize are:

- Marked personality change over time
- Confused thinking; strange or grandiose ideas
- Excessive anxieties, fears, or suspiciousness; blaming others
- Withdrawal from society, lack of friendliness; abnormal self-centeredness

··················

Figure 9-4

Prevalence of limitations due to serious mental illness among persons 25–64 years of age with these disorders, by sex: United States, 1989 (*Source:* Centers for Disease Control and Prevention, National Center for Health Statistics, National health interview survey.)

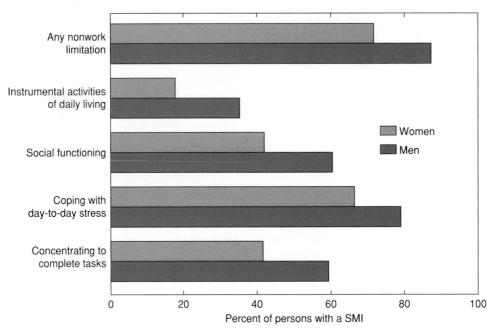

- Denial of obvious problems; strong resistance to help
- Thinking or talking about suicide
- Numerous, unexplained physical ailments; marked changes in eating and sleeping patterns
- Anger or hostility out of proportion to the situation
- Abuse of alcohol or drugs
- Growing inability to cope with problems and daily activities such as school, job, or personal needs

Types of Mental Illness

The four most common mental disorders in lifetime incidence and prevalence rates are substance abuse, anxiety disorders, severe cognitive disorders, and affective disorders. These categories were revised in the 1992 *International Classification of Mental and Behavioral Disorders,* as shown in table 9-1. Future statistical tabulations will increasingly classify mental and behavioral disorders as they appear in this table. Within each broader category is contained at least one subcategory associated with biological etiology and one subcategory associated more with environmental or developmental conditions.

Substance Abuse Substance abuse disorders are diagnosed in 16 percent of adults over 18 at some time during their lives. Alcohol abuse accounts by far for the majority of these disorders, with 13 percent of Americans likely to have an alcohol

. . . .

Figure 9-5

Recognizing the symptoms or warning signs of mental illness could help people get the help they need earlier and prevent some of the problems that arise from untreated mental illness. (*Source:* Courtesy American Mental Health Fund.)

Mental illness has warning signs, too.

Excessive anger. Withdrawal from social activities. Persistent sleeplessness. These could be the first warning signs of a mental illness. Unfortunately, most of us don't see the signs. Which is tragic. Because mental illness can be treated. In fact, 2 out of 3 people who get help, get better. For a free booklet about mental illness, write to or call:

American Mental Health Fund
P.O. Box 17700, Washington, DC 20041
1-800-433-5959

Learn to see the sickness.

Table 9-1

Structure of ICD-10 classification of mental and behavioral disorders

Organic mental disorders	
1. Organic and symptomatic disorders 2. Alcohol and drug disorders	**F0** Organic, including symptomatic mental disorders **F1** Mental and behavioral disorders due to psychoactive and other substance use
Psychotic mental disorders	
1. Schizophrenia and related disorders 2. Affective disorders	**F2** Schizophrenia, schizotypal, and delusional disorders **F3** Mood (affective) disorders
Neurotic, stress and personality disorders	
1. Neurotic and stress disorders 2. Adult personality and behavior disorders	**F4** Neurotic, stress-related and somatoform disorders **F5** Behavioral syndromes and mental disorders associated with physiological dysfunction **F6** Disorders of adult personality and behavior
Disorders of childhood, adolescence, and development	
1. Mental retardation 2. Disorders of childhood, adolescence, and development	**F7** Mental retardation **F8** Disorders of psychological development **F9** Behavioral and emotional disorders with onset usually occurring in childhood or adolescence

Source: World Health Organization: *The ICD-10 classification of mental and behavioral disorders,* Geneva, 1992, World Health Organization.

ISSUES AND CONTROVERSIES
Is Health Promotion Contributing to Anxiety Disorders?

The mass media have played on a commonly felt symptom. It is the symptom of the increased pace of living and increased levels of expectation for performance and appearance. The mass media share in the blame for setting these expectations for faster, more competent, and more glamorous living. Advertisers promote body images for women that adolescents strive obsessively to achieve until they find themselves in a cycle of self-starvation (anorexia nervosa) or bingeing and purging (anorexia bulimia). Has health promotion with its emphasis on low-fat eating, weight control, and fitness contributed to the distorted self-images of young women and their eating disorders? Consider the trade-offs between health promotion remaining silent in the face of the epidemic of obesity in children in North America and the anxiety disorders possibly produced in those who overcompensate in their effort to control calories, fat, and weight.

problem during their lives. This is more common than abuse of all other drugs combined. Chapter 12 will address the substance abuse disorders and community strategies to prevent them.

Anxiety Disorders   After substance abuse, anxiety disorders are the second most common lifetime mental illness, but they are the most common at any given time. These include phobias, panic disorders, and obsessive-compulsive disorders such as anorexia nervosa. These affect 15 percent of Americans during the course of their lives and 7 percent in any given month.

Severe Cognitive Disorders   Severe impairment of intellect is quite uncommon below the age of sixty-five, except in those with injuries to the head or congenital anomalies. It increases in incidence rapidly after age sixty-five as a result of strokes and dementia. For example, Alzheimer's disease results in loss of mental functioning and previous relationships.

Affective Disorders   Depression is the most common affective disorder. As one of the strongest risk factors for attempted and completed suicides, depression is a significant public health problem with potentially fatal consequences. Depression has also been found to coexist with smoking, alcohol abuse, and drug abuse. Chronic depression can be expected to affect 8 percent of Americans during their lives and 5 percent at any given time. Many people do not recognize that they have a treatable illness and do not seek treatment that can help the majority of people with depression to recover. New U.S. national objectives for depression were established in 1995 because of its importance. These included a new baseline and target for expanded diagnostic criteria for children and adolescents.

Etiology of Mental Illness

To be viable, prevention of mental-emotional disabilities requires the identification of risk factors amendable to intervention. Potential risk factors and situations contributing to mental illness include genetic heritage; family history; poverty; chronic illness; disruption of family stability; abuse and neglect; social isolation; substance abuse; or sudden stressful events such as divorce, bereavement, or unemployment. Continuing epidemiological research will help link these risk factors and situations more specifically to the symptoms and diagnoses of mental illness. George Albee, an early leader in prevention for mental health, proposed the following formula for the ratio of difficult life circumstances to available strengths and resources accounting for the incidence of psychopathology:

Incidence of psychopathology =

$$\frac{\text{Organic factors} + \text{Stress} + \text{Exploitation}}{\text{Coping skills} + \text{Self-esteem} + \text{Social support}}$$

A broad range of studies on psychopathology during the 1990s promoted the theory that most of the major psychoses stem from a combination of biogenetic and environmental factors. In other words, a genetic susceptibility to schizophrenia and manic-depressive psychosis induces vulnerability within the nervous system. This, together with multiple environmental factors (physical and social), triggers one of these two disorders, each of which affects 1 percent of the population.

Organic Factors Biological integrity can be compromised by genetic or congenital conditions before birth and by illness, trauma, malnutrition, lead poisoning, and abuse or neglect in childhood. Injury to the head and substance abuse at any point in life can cause permanent damage to mental capacities or neurological functioning. Strokes, sensory decline, and dementia later in life account for most of the adult deterioration in mental capabilities. Studies of adopted offspring and identical twins have strongly suggested genetic factors influencing schizophrenia and depressive disorders.

Stress Much of the research in reducing the incidence of preventable mental-emotional problems has focused on moderating the consequences of stressful life events. As noted previously in figure 9-2, stress is integrated into various national mental health and mental disorder objectives. Probably the most pervasive determinant of stress is the confrontation of situations over which the person has, or perceives to have, no control. The same situation will produce more or less stress for different people depending on how much control they have or feel they have over it. Thus a poor person or a person with a disability will encounter more

Objectives for the Nation for Mental Disorder Reduction

- By the year 2000, reduce to less than 10 percent the prevalence of mental disorders among children and adolescents. Baseline: 12 percent among youths <18 years in 1989.
- By the year 2000, reduce the prevalence of mental disorders (exclusive of substance abuse) among adults to less than 10.7 percent. Baseline: one-month point prevalence of 12.6 percent in 1984.

circumstances over which they have little control than will a person with more resources at his or her disposal. When the sources of such stress persist on a daily basis, the individual employs conscious and unconscious defense mechanisms. Chronic and habitual use of some defense mechanisms such as denial, repression, anger, or substance abuse, can lead to dysfunctional coping styles that spill into all areas of living and interacting with other people.

Social Conditions Stress derives from a combination of stressors and the absence of controls or buffers. Two people confronting the same source of stress can have quite different reactions, because one feels alone in dealing with the stress whereas the other feels the support of others. Social support can come immediately from coworkers or classmates in a supportive work or classroom situation or secondarily from a solid family and friendship network to fall back on. Self-help groups have been organized in many communities to provide social support for those who have common problems or needs. These have been especially beneficial for single people living long distances from family and long-standing friends. The average American moves twelve times in a lifetime, according to the Census Bureau. This makes for a nation of uprooted strangers, having few of the natural social supports traditionally provided by extended family and friendship networks. This, in turn, has made the work setting an increasingly important source of social support.

EPIDEMIOLOGY OF SOCIAL PATHOLOGY

Mental Disorder and Social Pathology

Many factors contribute to the **social pathology** of a community, but most seem to relate to a failure in human adjustment. In some instances psychosis, in some cases neurosis, and in other cases inadequate adjustment of an otherwise normal individual is fundamental to a particular social pathology. Mental disorder does not account for all crime, delinquency, alcoholism, drug misuse, narcotic addiction, divorce, child abuse, and suicide. Indeed, of these problems the greatest portion is caused by people who are regarded as normal. However, these individuals regarded as normal are people with explosive tempers, exaggerated feelings of inadequacy, and marked feelings of persecution, or people who are asocial or antisocial, highly suspicious, overly sensitive, impulsive, overly emotional, unstable, or unable to obtain self-gratification through the usual avenues of life.

Epidemiology of Social Disorder

A review of the extent of social pathology gives some indication of the magnitude of the problem in the United States.

- Approximately one out of every two marriages results in divorce.
- The United States has more than 2 million serious crimes each year.
- About 300,000 children between the ages of 11 and 17 appear in court each year.
- Over 30,000 suicides are recorded each year.
- In a national U.S. survey, 82 percent of those polled indicated that they "need less stress in their lives." Nearly one in five (18 percent) said they experience great stress almost every day.
- In recent years suicide has ranked as the eighth leading cause of death for all age groups. It ranks as the third leading cause of death among youths ages 15 to 24. Increasingly, it is also an important cause of death among the aged.
- It is estimated that 200,000 to 4 million cases of child abuse occur each year and that 2,000 children die each year in circumstances suggesting abuse or neglect.
- Hundreds of thousands of cases of violent, but nonfatal, assault occur each year. These include instances of spouse and child sexual abuse and rape.
- The death rate from homicide among black males ages 15 to 24 more than doubled in two decades. For black males 25 to 44 years the rate is 12 times the rate for the general population.

Whether these social pathologies are the consequence of many individuals suffering mental disorders, or whether they are causing the mental disorders of individuals can only be conjectured. Causation probably works in both directions, creating a vicious cycle of deteriorating mental and social health in a community.

Control of Stress

Stress is considered an inevitable condition of life. Stress is not necessarily an unhealthy phenomenon; for some people, it may lead to benefits and increased productivity. For others, however, it can have negative consequences by increasing the demands on their emotional resources. Stress is measured in different ways, one of which is the number and kinds of major life events experienced by individuals. In a survey of Canadians age forty-five and older a substantial proportion had experienced a significant life event in the previous year (figure 9-6).

Efforts to help individuals confront stress have been proactive and reactive. Proactive programs can help reduce the likelihood of stressful life events; reactive programs help people cope with stressful life events that have occurred.

Stress as a Risk Factor   Stress should be viewed as a risk factor for many health problems—

· · · · · · · · · · · · · · · · · ·
Figure 9-6

Major life events in previous twelve months, Canada, age forty-five and over, 1991 (*Source:* Health and Welfare Canada. Aging and Independence Survey, 1991.)

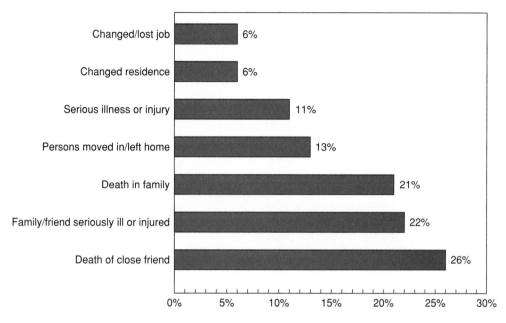

including hypertension, obesity, smoking, and alcohol and drug abuse—and as a direct contributing factor in violent behavior. Excessive and continuous stress can have serious physical and emotional consequences. It contributes to a variety of diseases and conditions, including depression, fatigue, gastrointestinal disorders, coronary heart disease, suicide, homicide, and other violent acts. The many causes of stress and its multitude of health-related outcomes complicate the task of identifying risk factors and reducing the consequences of excessive stress.

Stress and Violence Control   Stress should be recognized as leading to constructive, self-destructive, and violent behavior. Individual response to excessive stress is a complex and interactive process.

Objectives for Stress Reduction

- By the year 2000, reduce to less than 35 percent the proportion of people aged 18 and older who experienced adverse health effects from stress within the past year. Baseline: 42.6 percent in 1985.

Special target population	1985	2000
People with disabilities	53.5%	40%

- Decrease to no more than 5 percent the proportion of people aged 18 and older who report experiencing significant levels of stress who do not take steps to reduce or control their stress. Baseline: 21 percent in 1985.

Whereas some people react to stress by overeating or drinking too much, others react by abusing members of their family. Unfortunately, many of these coping activities in response to stress do greater damage to health than stress itself.

The degree to which stress contributes to most physiological and psychological dysfunction is largely unknown. There is general agreement, however, that homicide and suicide result from increased levels of stress. In the United States, suicide and homicide account for more than 50,000 deaths annually. Thousands of additional injuries and deaths of children are inflicted by parents, usually in response to stress. Mortality statistics, however, reflect only a small proportion of the actual incidence or severity of violent acts in society. For example, the ratio of murders to aggravated assaults is approximately 1 to 17, and estimates of the ratio of suicides to attempted suicides range from 1 to 10 to 1 to 100.

Stress reaches all segments of society (figure 9-7), as does violence. In general, however, the economically disadvantaged and certain age groups, such as children, adolescents, young adults, and the elderly, appear to be more vulnerable to violent outcomes of stress. Many of the U.S. national objectives for the year 2000 for control of stress and violent behavior are directed toward these high-risk groups. Other objectives are directed toward a better understanding of the behavioral objectives of stress and increased identification of factors linking stress to health disorders. The boxes in this chapter and in chapter 13 show high-priority objectives for the control of stress and violent behavior in the United States. Some progress toward objectives aimed at reducing the adverse health effects of stress has been achieved, but little change has occurred in adults who take action to reduce or control significant stress levels.

Stress in the Workplace   Much of the growing perception of a stressful life in Western countries has been attributed to economic conditions and the pressures these have placed on employers to

· · · · · · · · · · · · · · · · · ·
Figure 9-7

Stress affects all age groups. Exercise, relationships with others, and relaxation can help reduce stress. (*Source:* The President's Council on Physical Fitness and Sports.)

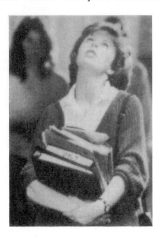

A TIP FOR TEEN

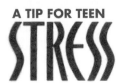

It's not easy being a teenager . . . Exercise can relieve some of the tension and improve your fitness. Exercise with a friend. You can talk about what's bugging you while you help each other get through your workout.

For more information, write to: Fitness, Dept. 84, Washington, DC 20001.

The President's Council on Physical Fitness and Sports

reduce the work force and demand more productivity and quality control from their smaller work force. A survey by Statistics Canada found that work stress is highest among employed teens and declines with age to reach its lowest value among employed seniors. There appeared to be an inverse relationship between work stress and satisfaction, with nearly no difference reported in work stress between employed men and women. Working conditions produce the greatest stress and physical manifestations such as back pain when the worker lacks autonomy or control over the pace of work. Those whose pace of work is driven by automatic electronic systems or by assembly line machines suffer the most.

Changes in work methods or routines, even when these are intended to increase worker efficiency, can create stress, especially if the workers have not participated in the introduction of the new methods. Computers and new software, for example, create demands for more rapid turnaround of information and expectations of higher productivity. The pressure to produce more work faster becomes a stressful condition. When combined with job uncertainty, poor supervision, or relationships with other workers; other automation and robotics controlling the pace of work; or physical aspects of the work area such as poor lighting, temperature, ventilation, furniture, high noise levels, or interruptions, these conditions add up to a stressed worker who likely comes home to a working partner who has suffered similar strains. Parenting responsibilities may then prevent them from taking the time they need to support each other or to look after their own needs.

Divorce and Reconstructed Families

Families set the stage for health and well-being of its members. The relationship between primary partners sets the stage for the mental well-being of the family. A successful marriage and partnership is partly a matter of personality adjustment. The individual who has difficulty adjusting to single life is ill-prepared to adjust to the complexities of married life. One needs only to go over the complaints of wives and husbands in divorce actions to recognize the extent to which inadequate personal adjustment is the basic factor. Husbands' complaints in divorce actions are revealing: wife's feelings are too easily hurt, wife criticizes me, wife is too nervous and emotional, there is a lack of freedom in the home, wife is quick-tempered, wife nags, wife tries to improve me, wife complains too much, wife is not affectionate, wife is too argumentative, we cannot agree on choice of friends. Wives, on the other hand, offer these complaints: husband is nervous and impatient, husband criticizes me, husband is argumentative, husband is quick-tempered, husband doesn't talk things over, husband is selfish and inconsiderate, husband is touchy, husband doesn't show affection, husband is too demanding, our marriage is too confining, husband criticizes my choice of friends. These comments, which were obtained from complaints filed in divorce proceedings, are an indication that personality, maturity, and adjustment are factors in marital stability.

Marriage counselors can provide a valuable service to a community for those individuals who are having difficulty in making an adequate marriage adjustment. More important is a community health service that assists people in problems of mental health before they are married. Of course, not all people in a community need mental health counseling, and not all married couples need the services of a marriage counselor. However, a community health department that provides mental health counseling for those who need such services will contribute, not only to the level of mental health, but also to the prevention of social pathology within the family.

The divorce rate increased steadily from 1958, when it was 2.1 divorces per 1000 population, to 1984 when it was 10.5 per 1000. It has since declined gradually, although half of marriages end in divorce (figure 9-8). The number of children involved in divorces also increased from 1953 until recently, when the delays in marriage and in childbirth after marriage, slight reductions in divorce rates, and the reduction in family size reduced the number of children affected by divorce.

• • • • • • • • • • • • • • • • • •

Figure 9-8

Divorce and family dissolution are related to multiple sources of stresses, including alcohol abuse. (*Source:* Alcohol and Drug Programs, Ministry of Labour and Consumer Services, British Columbia.)

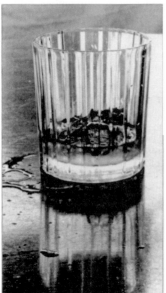

Last year, 1 in 4 marriages ended up on the rocks.

It's a sad fact that almost half of today's marriages end in divorce. But what's even sadder is that in over half of all divorce cases, alcohol is a major cause.

When an alcoholic drinks, the problem affects everyone. Spouses. Children. Friends.

Isn't it time we did something about it?

The Responsibility is Yours.

1-800-663-1441

Alcohol and Drug Programs
Ministry of Labour and Consumer Services
The Honourable Lyall Hanson, Minister

Criminal and Antisocial Behavior

Mental Illness Among Prisoners It is estimated that at least 10 percent of the 1 million people in jail in the United States suffer from serious mental disorders, mostly schizophrenia and manic depression. A study by the National Association for Mental Health in 11 state penitentiaries of 8,581 consecutive admissions revealed that 25 percent of the prisoners were psychotic and that 14 percent were borderline cases. As of 1995, only two states had established official protocols to prevent suicide by male inmates. An early recognition of

mental illness might have prevented some of the crimes in which these individuals were involved. In this respect, informed citizens of a community could be of service in recognizing abnormal behavior that could be associated with violence.

Violent and Reckless Behavior Individuals who have a tendency toward violent outbursts of temper, who are overly suspicious, who have delusions of persecution, who are antisocial, or who are quarrelsome are more likely to be involved in violent and destructive acts. Behind the wheels of automobiles a community will find people who are frankly psychotic and borderline cases. Antisocial drivers have little respect for the rights or welfare of others. Not only will they inconvenience others, but also their recklessness, impatience, carelessness, excitability, and lack of responsibility can be important factors in causing motor vehicle injuries. In terms of injury prevention, the driver's personality is more important than a mechanical ability to handle the car. This situation eventually may force communities to deny motor vehicle operator's licenses because of personality deficiencies and deficiencies in driving skills.

After a crime has been committed, courts properly refer the prisoner to a psychiatrist for determination of the prisoner's level of mental responsibility. A corollary of this program is the effort to determine irresponsibility in individuals before they become involved in serious crimes. It is not possible to predict all people who may engage in crime, but repeat offenders have identified themselves as possible chronic criminals and have indicated the need to determine whether they are mentally ill. Others who show marked deviation in their behavior should also be examined to determine the degree of mental and emotional competence they possess. Unfortunately, the legal machinery is frequently cumbersome and threats to civil rights so great that social workers and law enforcement officers are hesitant to initiate any action to provide for the psychiatric examination and counseling of citizens who could be possible

· · · · · · · · · · · · · · · · · · ·

Figure 9-9

Age adjusted rates for suicide: United States, 1987 to 1993, and year 2000 targets for selected objectives. (*Source:* National Center for Health Statistics, Centers for Disease Control and Prevention, Public Health Service, DHHS.)

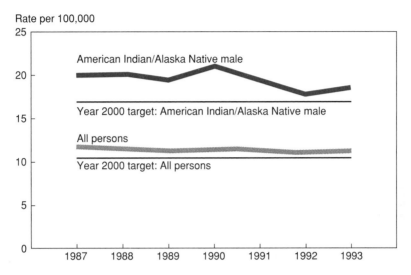

threats. A true program of prevention would protect the rights of the individual whose conduct appears deviant and the welfare of the children and adults in the community.

Suicide

Suicide is the eighth leading cause of death in the United States. For those who die by their own hand, suicide represents a permanent solution to what, in retrospective, may have been a less than permanent state of hopelessness or despair. For the families and friends left behind, the loss of a loved one from suicide leaves a painful mix of sorrow, anger, and guilt. The overall suicide statistics vary with population groups (figure 9-9). The rate among men is more than three times that among women. For adolescents and young adults, ages 15–24, suicide is the third leading cause of death. It is unclear if the increases in suicide attempts by adolescents is increasing because of improved reporting mechanisms, increased drug use, or other reasons. Suicide rates among the elderly are also high. For some groups, the suicide rate is low, in-

cluding Mormons, Roman Catholics, and blacks. These population differences suggest a range of social and developmental factors that affect suicide rates.

Factors   Most information on the mental state of people who attempt to take their own lives is obtained from those people who failed in a suicide

Objective for Sucide Reduction

- By the year 2000, reduce suicide to no more than 10.5 per 100,000 people. Age-adjusted baseline: 11.7 per 100,000 in 1987.

Special Population Targets	1987	2000
Youths aged 15–19	10.3	8.2
Men aged 20–34	25.2	21.4
White men 65+	46.1	39.2
American Indian/Alaska Native Men Reservation State	15	12.8

attempt. There is one successful suicide for every ten attempts, and about 5 percent of those who fail are repeaters. The conditions of an individual's life influence the suicide rate. Studies indicate that perhaps 30 percent of those who take their own lives are actually mentally disordered. The remaining suicides largely result from a decision that death is the best solution to a situation. For many of these situations there were coping possibilities that were not adequately realized or explored. When life has lost its purpose or has resulted in great frustration, loss of self-esteem, or depression, an individual who lacks good personality integration may attempt to escape from reality by self-destruction.

A substantial number of suicides could be prevented by increased recognition and treatment of persons with clinical depression and other treatable mental disorders. Helping individuals over the immediate crisis, together with counseling to help them see the problem and its solution, will at least prevent a present attempt, and also might prevent further attempts at self-destruction. People who threaten suicide often carry out their threats. Such threats indicate disturbance and the need for assistance. Most suicides can be prevented if people recognize individuals who are disturbed, take action to protect the individuals against themselves, and assist them in understanding and solving the situation. Those who suffer marked depression are particularly in need of guidance during the period of depression. Highly sensitive persons may take their own life to hurt others; these individuals are too sensitive for the rugged world in which they live. For these people, mental health counseling is long past due. It can be predicted conservatively that if a community has adequate mental health counseling and a considerable number of citizens who recognize the various factors indicating that a person is likely to attempt to take his or her own life, suicide can be cut to one-third of its present rate.

Adolescent Suicide   Suicide rates for adolescents 15 to 19 years of age quadrupled from 2.7 per 100,000 in 1950 to 11.3 in 1991. Data from earlier decades are not available to assess similar trends in rates of attempted suicide in this population. Attempted suicide is a potentially lethal health event, a risk factor for future completed suicide, and a potential indicator of other health problems such as substance abuse, depression, or adjustment and stress reactions.

The national school-based Youth Risk Behavior Survey (YRBS) periodically measures the prevalence of priority health-risk behaviors among American youth through comparable national, state, and local surveys. The school-based American YRBS obtains a representative sample of students in grades 9 to 12 in the 50 states, the District of Columbia, Puerto Rico, and the Virgin Islands. Students are asked whether they seriously thought about attempting suicide during the 12 months preceding the survey, whether they made a specific plan about how they would attempt suicide, how many times they had actually made a suicide attempt, and whether their suicide attempt(s) resulted in an injury or poisoning that had to be treated by a doctor or nurse.

For the 12 months preceding the 1990 survey, 27.3 percent of students in grades 9 to 12 reported that they had thought seriously about attempting suicide. Fewer students (16.3 percent) reported that they had made a specific plan to attempt suicide. About half the students who made a specific plan (8.3 percent of respondents) reported that they actually attempted suicide. Two percent of the students reported that they made a suicide attempt that resulted in an injury or poisoning requiring medical attention.

Gender, race and ethnic differences were found among adolescents. Female students were significantly more likely than male students to report that they had thought seriously about attempting suicide, had made a suicide plan, or had attempted suicide one or more times during the twelve months preceding the survey. Hispanic and white students reported higher levels of suicidal thoughts and behaviors than black students, although these differences were not always statistically significant.

A great number of suicides could be prevented by increased recognition and appropriate treatment of persons with clinical depression and other treatable mental disorders clearly associated with an increased risk of suicide.

FEDERAL AND STATE SPONSORED MENTAL HEALTH PROGRAMS

An agenda for mental health programs can be structured around three types of preventive interventions—universal, selective, and indicated. Universal interventions are designed for the general public or a population group. Selective preventive interventions focus on high-risk individuals or groups based on biological, psychological or social risk factors. Indicated interventions focus on high-risk individuals with detectable symptoms of behaviors that foreshadow a mental disorder or who have a biological predisposition to mental health problems.

Successful mental health programs are founded on a good understanding of the risks and problems encountered by the target group. One-size-fits-all programs do not work any better for mental health problems than they do for physical health problems. Successful programs also acknowledge the interaction among biological and psychosocial factors. For example, an inherited vulnerability to alcoholism may be influenced by poverty, the home environment, and learning experiences. Successful programs also emphasize protective factors, such as psychosocial competence and social support. The former includes skills in relating to others and capabilities to handle crises; the latter includes strengthening the natural support from family, community, or school settings.

Federal Agencies and Programs

At the federal level a new prevention branch in the Center for Mental Health Services is charged with coordinating prevention and developing prevention initiatives within the Alcohol, Drug Abuse and Mental Health Administration. Mental health programs at the federal level involve funding of

> ## Selected *Healthy People 2000* Mental Health Objectives
>
> * Reduce number of suicides
> * Reduce prevalence of mental disorders among children, adolescents, and adults living in the community
> * Reduce adverse health effects from stress
> * Increase number of people who seek help in coping with personal and emotional problems
> * Reduce uncontrolled stress
> * Increase worksite stress prevention programs
> * Establish mutual help clearinghouses
> * Increase routine reviews of cognitive, emotional, and behavioral functioning in adults and children by primary care providers

prevention research, sponsorship of national conferences and coalitions on mental health, and other efforts to help achieve national mental health objectives. A selected sample of these objectives are found in the box above.

State Agencies and Programs

Responsibility for the treatment and promotion of mental health occurs at various levels. In the United States, state governments direct and finance most mental health programs. Mental health promotion is a function of state and local health departments; treatment of severe mental disorders and care of the institutionalized mentally ill are functions of mental health professionals and hospitals for the mentally ill. Although 63 percent of people with health insurance coverage in the United States are enrolled in managed health care plans for mental health care services, cost-shifting from private to public mental health services occurs when individuals reach service limits within their insurance plans.

Functions of State Agencies   The division of mental health, or some similarly designated agency, has the primary responsibility for mental health promotion in many states and provinces. This division serves as the coordinating agency for statewide forces concerned with the promotion of the mental health of the general population. It co-operates with the various voluntary and official agencies in the state or province that are engaged in some phase of mental health. It also cooperates with the state department of education, prisons, law enforcement and social service agencies, hospital commissions, and hospitals. Its major concern is with the mental health of the general population, but it does provide assistance for the maladjusted—the alcoholic, the drug addict, the juvenile delinquent, the criminal—and for the physically handicapped, the aged, and other segments in the population having special mental health risks.

The official division of mental hygiene at the state or provincial level carries out legislation concerning mental health, makes statistical studies, provides library facilities, makes mental health education materials available, provides consulting service to agencies or communities, conducts workshops and seminars for professional personnel, sponsors special programs of mental health promotion, establishes and promotes mental health facilities, and otherwise serves as a mental health resource for other agencies and for communities.

States that have not enacted a specific mental health services act nevertheless have provided for the establishment of a statewide mental health program. A few states promote mental health as a component of existing programs, such as in the maternal and child health division of the state health department. An identifiable state mental hygiene agency within the state department of public health provides recognition of the importance of mental hygiene as a phase of public health service. For example, Maryland gave prominence to its mental health program by naming the state public health agency the Department of Health and Mental Hygiene.

Shifting State Responsibilities   One example of the changing approaches in mental health services

is the state's role in treatment of the mentally ill. In the twentieth century state responsibility for mental health shifted from the warehousing of the mentally ill in isolated institutions to mental health promotion. As states moved away from running large mental health institutions, the resulting deinstitutionalization brought problems of homelessness and lack of care for some. It also brought the need for greater cooperation between states and communities in dealing with the problems and care of the mentally ill.

Mental Hospitals   The treatment of the mentally ill was centered around the mental hospital from the mid-1800s to the mid-1900s, most often in state-run institutions. From 1880 to 1955 there was a steady increase in the average number of patients in state and county mental hospitals per 100,000 people in the United States. In 1955 the average daily census of the state and county mental hospitals in the United States was 559,000—54 percent of patients in *all* hospitals. In 1956 for the first time in the history of the United States, there was a reduction in the number of resident patients in the state and county mental hospitals: on December 31, 1956, there were about 7,000 fewer patients in these hospitals than on December 31, 1955. The decline was particularly significant when one considers that between the years 1945 and 1955 there was an average increase of 10,000 patients per year in these mental hospitals. In the years since 1956 there has been a further decrease in the year-end census of patients in mental hospitals in the United States.

Deinstitutionalization   Tales of abuse in large state mental hospitals in the 1950s and concern for the civil rights of the mentally ill in the 1960s led to increasing legislative restrictions making it difficult to commit people to hospitals against their will. At the same time the introduction of new drugs made it possible for more people to be discharged from state hospitals. State cost-cutting measures in the 1970s accelerated the **deinstitutionalization** trend, which brought the patient count in state institutions from 552,000 in 1955 down to 119,000 in 1990.

Many of the deinstitutionalized have not been able to cope with employment or other conditions, leading to financial instability and, for many, homelessness. Up to 30 percent of the estimated 500,000 homeless suffer from serious mental disorders, mostly schizophrenia and manic depression. Some of these may become special wards of integrated community mental health and social service agencies; others are without care on the streets. The dramatic decline of the hospitalized mentally ill has placed a greater burden on communities to provide halfway houses and other facilities to compensate for the deinstitutionalization of mental illness.

Further budget cuts in the 1980s and 1990s resulted in the failure to open halfway houses and other community facilities to help absorb and support the flood of liberated former mental patients. The system of most communities is left capable of responding only to episodic acute care, not chronic care. Some 70 percent of mental health dollars are spent for hospital rather than clinical or outreach services. Demonstration programs have shown that mentally disturbed people can lead safe, happy, and productive lives outside institutions given community support for monitored medications, specialized training, and stable housing.

COMMUNITY DIAGNOSIS AND RESPONSE TO MENTAL AND SOCIAL DISORDERS

A health matter becomes a community health problem when it is amenable to amelioration through collective action. Many aspects of the mental health problem can be dealt with most effectively through public action. The community needs mental health services just as it needs services that promote physical health. As with physical health, early intervention helps prevent more serious problems. Some people need the benefit of mental health counseling; some need guidance in special social and economic problems they may encounter; some need social support and a safe

place of shelter (figure 9-10). Every community needs to provide the means by which people showing indications of mental disorder will be directed to professional resources for diagnosis, treatment, and care. A community diagnosis of specific mental and social health needs determines what the mental health program should be in a particular community or for a population group.

Community Diagnosis

Some mental health needs are common to most communities, but specific factors that influence the mental health of subpopulations must be recognized and evaluated for each community. Socioeconomic neighborhood, and ethnic backgrounds; family relationships; child-rearing practices; community norms; and cultural values are such factors affecting the mental health program.

Mental and social health needs include problems for which people have a need for special assistance in the province of normal, everyday adjustment. Individual and family counseling services, marriage counseling, sessions for expectant parents, child study groups, parent discussions, employment services, guidance services for elderly citizens, promotion of cultural interests, recreation programs, and general health information services all address social needs in a community. No one agency will necessarily provide all of the services to satisfy these needs, but by means of an integrated community health and social service program, some agency or individual will provide for each of the various needs. The program will also be concerned with mentally disturbed people in hospitals, patients under physicians' care, patients who have been released from psychiatric hospitals and are in the process of rehabilitation, and individuals who have come to the attention of legal authorities and community agencies and are under the direction of these agencies.

Organization and Administration of Services

Effective community mental health programs require planning, organization, and direction. A

· ·

Figure 9-10

Communities can provide a variety of mental health supports, including shelter, for displaced adolescents. (*Source: Advertising Council, New York.*)

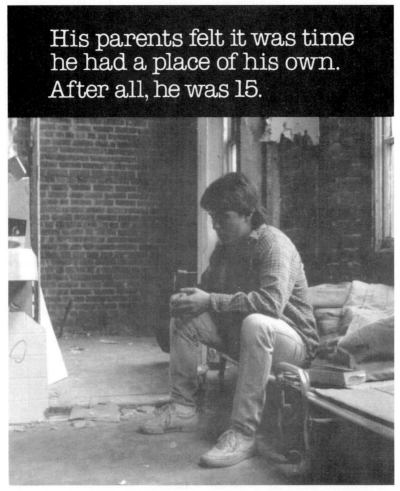

Every year hundreds of thousands of kids are thrown away. Put out onto the streets. With no job, no money and nowhere to go, these kids turn up in abandoned buildings, alleys and in morgues.

But now there is a number for kids to call. The Covenant House Nineline helps kids with food, clothing, a place to sleep and, most of all, someone to talk to.

To get help in your hometown call our Nineline 1-800-999-9999. It's free, and you can call from anywhere.
**Nineline 1-800-999-9999
Anytime. Anywhere.**

community may possess many resources for dealing with its manifold mental health needs. Unless some central agency exists that will assess and coordinate the various services available, however, many needs that could be fulfilled will be neglected, many services will be inadequately provided, and there will be unnecessary duplication of effort and even conflict in function. Setting up a central administrative agency does not mean that the various individuals, agencies, and services in the community will be hampered or otherwise obstructed in their functioning. Rather, it means a coordination of services available from the various agencies and individuals in the total program that will help reduce duplication and fragmentation of services.

Community Mental Health Centers

The U.S. Community Mental Health Centers Act of 1963 authorized the construction of community mental health centers, which formed the core of the U.S. national mental health program. Allotments to states continued to rise up to 1980, based on population, financial need, and the need for community mental health centers. Funds were provided on a matching basis. The centers were expected to include the following:

- Inpatient services
- Outpatient services
- Partial hospitalization, including day, night, and weekend care
- Emergency services
- Community services, including consultation with community agencies and professional personnel
- Diagnostic, screening, and follow-up services
- Precare and postcare community services, including foster home placement, home visiting, and halfway houses
- Alcohol and drug problem services
- Training
- Research and evaluation

The Mental Health Systems Act gave states greater authority over mental health grants, allowing funding of innovative programs, targeting of certain priority populations, and putting greater emphasis on prevention.

Mental Health Programs in Community Health Departments

Many county, district, and city health departments have had a mental health division or section. Indeed, this was once a standard unit in the local health department. More recently, separate departments of mental health provide this service. Frequently, the mental health program is organized as a clinic with a staff consisting of one or more psychiatrists, clinical psychologists, psychiatric social workers, health educators, and mental health nurse consultants. The staff provides consulting services for children and adults. Marriage counseling and family counseling are frequently included in the services.

The community mental health clinic provides diagnosis and recommends treatment. Although a limited amount of treatment may be provided, the program is not designed for complete care. In some instances, the mental health staff advises courts on matters relating to the mental competence of people before the court. The staff may recommend rehospitalization or may assist in rehabilitation of a patient who has been released from a mental hospital.

The importance of a mental health unit in the community health department lies in its value as a coordinating agency. The community public health department can point out mental health needs in the community that are not being met. It can assume the role of leader in obtaining necessary services to fulfill recognized needs, and it can provide for the fullest use of voluntary services that are available in the community. It can serve as the liaison between segments of the public and the special mental health services they need. Last, it can keep the community informed about matters of mental health, particularly in terms of services available and how these services may be used.

Outpatient Clinics

With the development of effective medications, about one-third of the patients treated in clinics would have been hospital patients but are able to remain at home. In addition, many patients hospitalized for chronic disorders can be released to return to their communities under the supervision of a clinic or a physician. Qualified authorities maintain that there should be one psychiatric clinic for every 50,000 people, a standard that would require nearly doubling the full-time clinics in the United States. With more successful treatment of the mentally ill and a declining population in psychiatric hospitals, the need for hospital staff becomes less, but the need for community workers becomes greater.

Voluntary and Community Agencies

Voluntary agencies, such as mental health associations, play an important role in providing leadership and understanding of mental health and a sincere interest in mental health promotion. Various professional organizations whose members deal with services and problems related to mental health have been of particular value in pointing out the need for more services in the mental health field and have provided leadership and support necessary for its attainment on a population scale. Frequently, it is a movement initiated by groups such as these that gives rise to the establishment of an official mental health agency in the state or province devoted to the promotion of the mental health of the general public. The value of the service provided by each agency in the community depends on the freedom each agency has to do its best work within the general community mental health program or organized mental health plan.

Self-Help Groups

More than 15 million Americans seek aid from a half million support groups that meet across the country. Traditionally, family and friends offered emotional support that could help a person cope with stressful situations, but changes in family and community have meant that these emotional support systems are less likely to be available.

A wide range of self-help groups exist in four broad categories: coping with a mental or physical problem (breast cancer, child abuse); recovering from addiction (alcohol or food abuse); surviving a crisis (death, divorce, rape); and coping with another person's behavior or illness (family of a batterer or Alzheimer patient). These groups offer low or no cost aid to individuals, not based on professional expertise, but the shared experience of group participants. The success of these groups can be attributed to helping members understand what they are going through and learning to identify causes of behavior and gaining ability to change undesirable patterns. Self-help groups vary in size, composition, activity, and sponsorship. Some groups are supported by national organizations, such as Alcoholics Anonymous or the Cancer Society; others are supported by local communities. Whatever the differences, the groups share a similar focus; offering mutual emotional or functional support to persons sharing common concerns. There are also two federal and eight state clearinghouses to facilitate mutual self-help activities and information for people and their family members experiencing emotional distress.

Health Professionals

Health professionals and those in related fields can play an important role in prevention by identifying patients at risk for mental-emotional disorder and referring them to appropriate agencies or community resources.

Objectives for Mental Health Services

- By the year 2000, establish mutual-help clearinghouses in at least 25 states. Baseline: 9 states in 1989. Only Ontario in Canada.
- By the year 2000, increase to at least 40 percent the proportion of work sites employing 50 or more people that provide programs to reduce employee stress. Baseline: 26.6 percent in 1985.

Medical Practitioners   Practicing physicians play an important role in the mental health of the community. About 50 percent of general medical and surgical patients in the United States are estimated to have some kind of emotional disorder. Serious mental and emotional illnesses are partly responsible for many physical complaints. Individuals who would be classified as having normal mental health often have minor or moderate mental health problems and look to a physician as their consultant in dealing with these mental and emotional disturbances. A citizen with a neurosis—under the supervision of a family physician who understands the patient's total background—can usually adjust reasonably well to his or her situation and live a nearly normal life.

The physician is frequently the first person consulted when a family suspects that one of its members is suffering from mental disturbance. Unfortunately, too few primary care providers are trained to recognize depression and the variety of disabilities associated with it. A 1992 survey of primary care providers on the extent to which providers routinely review a patient's mental functioning shows that counseling is not widespread. The results were most optimistic for pediatricians who inquire about cognitive development in children and least optimistic for obstetricians/gynecologists and family physicians working with adults. National objectives were set to increase physician involvement in mental health screening.

Other Professionals   Nurses, psychologists, health educators, and social workers usually have a background that gives them an understanding of the field of mental health, and their place in and contribution to the field. Nurse practitioners, for example, are more likely than family physicians or obstetricians/gynecologists to review their patients' cognitive functioning. Working in cooperation with psychiatrists, family physicians, and other medical personnel, nurses, psychologists, health educators, and social workers can make constructive contributions to community mental health through their understanding of various factors operating in the community and of the resources that can be drawn on to help the individual, the family, or the neighborhood.

Regional Resources

Many small communities with limited professional mental health resources can draw on the facilities available in a large neighboring community. A reasonably well-organized mental health program, even in a small community, will have complete information on facilities available in nearby communities, so that citizens in the smaller community can benefit from the services of the highly trained psychiatrists and other specialists who are most likely to be practicing in metropolitan areas.

An appraisal of available professional resources in mental health must include clinics and professional personnel available to the general public, and psychiatrists, nurses, and other personnel working in psychiatric hospitals. An accurate accounting of mental health services available to the general public is extremely difficult to make because of the number of human service workers who devote only a limited portion of their practice to the mentally disordered but who nevertheless contribute a very important service. Most studies are limited to those clinics and practitioners concerned primarily with the mentally ill.

Citizen Participation in Community Mental Health Programs

Community action groups can work to promote innovative services or programs, to change the goals and priorities of organizations as needed, and to expand the rate and effectiveness of participation by citizens. They can pressure for action through governments or for old and new organizations by lobbying and advocacy. Steps in an idealized model of community action might follow those introduced in chapter 3. Face-to-face visits among various community partnerships, such as health professionals, school teachers, the clergy, and businesspeople have been shown to be an effective activity. Community resources and needs must be understood before community development by mental health groups can be successful.

Typical community awareness surveys address mental health needs and problems in the community, knowledge about community resources, and attitudes toward mental health issues. Data concerning the physical and environmental status of minority groups are important for citizen boards to consider, for these often correlate with mental illness and should influence the selection of priority target areas. The use of, and resistance and accommodation to, mental health services by minority groups in the community are important considerations in programming and delivering services. Alienation from mental health agencies and services must be recognized among minority groups, if it exists; services should be designed to be attractive, responsive, and viable for all groups.

COMMUNITY MENTAL HEALTH PROMOTION

Mental health promotion provides people with the skills, energy, and courage to face life's problems and difficulties. People need to understand why they do certain things, what gives rise to certain emotions, what they must do to adjust to their emotional responses, and what personality qualities they need to fortify or develop. This is the area in which a community mental health program can provide its greatest service to the average citizen. People of the community need a better understanding of mental health, and this education can be provided through the various methods and devices available to community health personnel. Despite this need, few communities have well-organized, well-functioning programs for promoting the mental health of citizens. Large segments of the community's population have a vital interest in mental health promotion as it relates to their community, their neighborhood, their family, and themselves. However, few want to see a mental health facility located in their neighborhood.

Whose Responsibility?

Establishing a community mental health program means developing community support. Leadership can come from the local mental health association, the community health council, United Way, and other sources. Productive action usually requires long-range planning rather than a high-pressure "crash" program. Lay leadership is important, even though primary responsibility must rest with the official community public health agency. Interagency cooperation is necessary for the success of a mental health program and full cooperation can be obtained only with public understanding, interest, and support. These require continuing public education.

Not in My Backyard

Communities recognize the need for treatment facilities and halfway houses for the rehabilitation and reentry of those who have been institutionalized in state mental hospitals. The public understands that a large number of the homeless on the streets of their communities are people with mental illnesses who should be under care in decent facilities. However, the fear of mental illness leads most people to say they want the community mental health facilities located anywhere but in their own neighborhood. "Not in my backyard" has become the rallying cry for neighborhood resistance movements that have blocked, not only mental health clinics, but also youth centers; drug treatment facilities; halfway houses; and family planning clinics; and industrial, transportation, and waste management facilities. The wealthier neighborhoods have the greater power of resistance, so that such facilities too often end up in the poorest neighborhoods. These are sometimes the most dangerous areas of large cities and the areas least conducive to mental health.

The drive to overcome such public resistance requires public education to demystify mental illness. Some of the earliest mental health education campaigns successfully changed the public's perception of the mentally ill as shameful. This resulted in many people who would not have sought help being more willing to admit they had an emotional problem and going for counseling or psychotherapy. Fear and misunderstanding, however, continue to stigmatize the mentally ill. The American Mental Health Fund has undertaken a national "Anti-Stigma Campaign" to help the public "learn to see the sickness." Part of the campaign seeks to redirect the shame at those who make crude jokes about mental disorders that perpetuate stereotypes rather than seeing them as illnesses (figure 9-11).

Education for Mental Health

At the base of the pyramid of community mental health promotion is community education in mental health. Such a program is directed primarily to the mental health needs of the general population and high-risk groups. Its objectives are to promote constructive attitudes toward mental health (see figure 9-11). This is particularly important because continuing public stigmatization of mental disorders creates one of the greatest barriers to obtaining mental health care. Such programs can also help people understand themselves, to show people how to manage and control stress, to keep the community informed of the various mental health services and facilities available and how they are best used, to engage community leaders in support of mental health, and to reduce public prejudice against people who experience mental illness.

Administration   A community mental health education program will function effectively under the direction of an individual professionally prepared in community health education. An important function of the program director is to enlist and use the services of qualified people or organizations in the community who can contribute to mental health education. This means organizing and administering a continuous program that provides for the mental health education needs of the various segments of the population. Resourcefulness and ingenuity are demanded, particularly when necessary resource people or organizations are not available.

As in other categorical programs, the function of health education in community mental health is to identify behaviors requiring development or change, to analyze the factors influencing these behaviors, and then to select or develop communications, community organizations, and training methods to influence these factors. Examples of specific behaviors to which mental health education can be addressed are coping and clinic dropouts. It is estimated that approximately one-third of the patients of community mental health centers drop out of treatment without staff approval or recommendation.

Educational Strategies   To disseminate information, community mental health education programs use discussion groups, pamphlets, radio, television, films, posters, newspapers, journals, and other materials and aids. Personal contacts between the health department and individual residents in their homes are usually confined to visits by public health nurses for the purpose of conveying information or advising the individual where certain services may be obtained. The development and use of clinical facilities in most U.S. communities for temporary hospitalization and care of mentally ill patients require public education. Acquiring the necessary funds for the construction and maintenance of adequate community facilities depends on the understanding and the interest of the public. The proper use of such facilities similarly requires public education.

Multidisciplinary Approach   Responsible people in the community can be informed about the early indications of mental disturbance or possible mental illness. The popular misconception that a mentally disordered person dresses oddly, has weird mannerisms, is likely to be maniacal, or talks foolishly must be displaced by a more realistic view. People in the parahealth fields, such as teachers and social workers, could be better trained to recognize the early signs of mental disorder. When this nucleus of professional workers coming in daily contact with the public is aided by

Figure 9-11

Changing public perceptions of mental illness is one of the intents of mental health promotion interventions. (*Source:* Advertising Council, New York.)

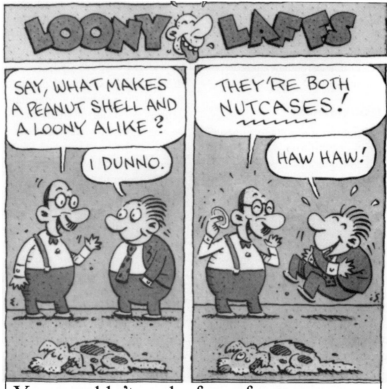

reliable citizens who understand the early indications of mental disturbance, then a community possesses a valuable means by which individuals likely to need diagnostic services and counsel are directed to services at an early stage when constructive and even preventive measures can be taken. In addition, such a group of informed citizens in a community can be the means by which tragedies such as child abuse and other forms of violence can be prevented.

Citizen Action and Support   Informed citizens can give responsible support to programs for providing hospital clinics and other services necessary for the proper care and treatment of the mentally disordered. They can advocate desirable legislation to promote an effective mental health program. They can support the necessary official agencies, including courts, in their programs to deal with the mentally disturbed. Most immediately in their family, work, and friendship circles they can offer understanding and support to those experiencing severe distress; bereavement; depression; anxiety; disorientation; extreme anger; fear; or difficulty with alcohol, drugs, or relationships.

The most immediate help people can offer a sick relative or friend is compassion, understanding, and support. Pretending that nothing is wrong or blaming the sick person for causing worry, embarrassment, or family problems only makes the problem potentially worse.

Mental illness is a medical condition that requires medical treatment. Willpower is not enough. Here are some other steps people can take on behalf of others.

- Seek help from trained professionals and accredited treatment centers.
- Be patient and persistent. After failing to make contact with the right agency or person after one call, try others. Every source offers different services.
- Describe the problem clearly and completely. All information is confidential and privileged.
- Change doctors if not satisfied. A good relationship between doctor and patient is critical.

- Support one another. Do not allow other family relationships to deteriorate. Seek help or counseling if needed for other family members. People who succeeded in making changes to improve their health, such as weight loss or reducing stress, report that the support of a family member or friend was important to realization of the intended change.
- Provide a secure, well-patterned environment for a mentally ill relative or friend. They need love, not stress. ("Tough love" is wrong in this case because it causes stress.)
- Learn as much as possible about mental illness and its treatments. There is no substitute for becoming well informed.

A word of caution: Everyone has a potential contribution to make to the community's mental health program. Unfortunately, individuals with a smattering of knowledge or with a morbid curiosity about mental health may be willing volunteers or even persistent participants, but the public is entitled to protection from the charlatans and the incompetent in mental health as in other areas of health.

Workplace Mental Health Promotion

The workplace has become an increasingly important site to address mental health issues because of the many ways it influences physical and mental health. It is estimated that job-related stress, anxiety, and depression lead to an average loss of 16 work days annually. Employers have supported such programs because they recognize that healthy workers are more productive workers. Approximately 37 percent of employers with 50 or more employees offer information, resource materials, group classes, or lectures to reduce employees' stress. Individual counseling is offered by 27 percent of employers.

Workplace mental health activities include the reduction of stress in the work setting through work design (how the work itself is structured), workplace design (ergonomics), health promotion programs such as stress management and employee assistance (figure 9-12), and surveillance of work-linked risk

· · · · · · · · · · · · · · · · · · · ·

Figure 9-12

Types of stress management activities offered by worksites reporting these activities (percent of worksites offering any of these activities), United States, 1990. (*Source:* U.S. Public Health Service: *Prevention Report,* March 1991.)

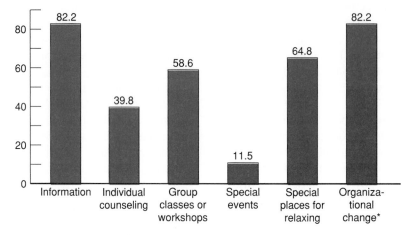

*Respondents were asked: "Does your worksite attempt to change the organization so that the empoloyees will experience less stress, such as training supervisors to handle problems more effectively?"

factors and psychological disorders in the workplace. Employee assistance programs were for many years concerned mainly with identifying alcohol abuse in employees and referring them for professional treatment outside the workplace. If they failed to heed the referral or to improve, they could then be disciplined or fired. Increasingly, these programs have looked to more progressive interventions to counsel or support workers in managing some of the work, family, or economic problems that underlie their alcohol or drug abuse.

Comprehensive School Health Education

Child and adolescent mental health services will be provided largely through the schools. In addition, most communities have other agencies that will provide for some of the mental health needs of children and adolescents. These needs include psychological testing and diagnostic services, counseling services for children, consulting services for parents of the youngsters, mental health guidance services for adolescents, remedial programs in the

school, an in-service mental health training program for teachers, mental health instruction as a phase of the basic health curriculum, and family life education. An effective, coordinated community-school mental health program should devote its major attention to the mental health of all youngsters but must also provide for the special mental health needs of the delinquent, the emotionally disturbed, the mentally retarded, the academically handicapped, the homeless, and children and adolescents who are having adjustment problems.

REHABILITATION

Rehabilitation is the restoration to the fullest degree of physical, mental, social, vocational, and economic usefulness of which an individual is capable. Total rehabilitation of persons who have recovered from mental illness may require only the services of their family physician or may require the well-integrated program of a rehabilitation team consisting of psychiatrist, psychologist, psychiatric social worker, nurse, occupational therapist, rehabilitation therapist, and family counselor.

The success of chemotherapy in the treatment of mental disorders has relieved the overcrowding in mental hospitals in North America but is increasing the need for rehabilitation services. With specific measures for the treatment of mental disorders, a mental hospital has become a place where one can go for a short time for treatment. This revolution in the treatment of mental disease means that custodial care is being replaced by medical treatment and deinstitutionalization. A patient who has been hospitalized for several years has a social adjustment to make besides a medical recovery. When the medication is effective in improving the patient's mental illness, the patient is permitted to visit a neighboring community under the guidance of a hospital attendant. After several escorted visits and observable improvement in adjustment to society, the patient is permitted to visit the community unescorted. When the patient's social adjustment and mental adjustment appear to be sufficiently advanced, the patient is permitted to return to his or her home, but only when adequate supervision is available. This means that medical and social supervision must be provided.

A family physician may accept responsibility for continuing the treatment the patient has been receiving, or medical supervision may be arranged through a psychiatric clinic in the patient's community. Rehabilitation services also are needed to assist the recovered or recuperating individual in making the necessary social, economic, and other adjustments that normal living requires. Getting a job, finding social groups and interests, adjusting to the tempo of community living, and finding leisure activities may require the services of specially prepared people. Statewide clinic systems are emerging in the United States from the community mental health centers. State hospitals that presently have a rehabilitation service are establishing links with centers throughout the state where former patients in need of assistance may obtain rehabilitation services conveniently and promptly.

RESEARCH

Research has not received the attention in mental health that it has in most other areas of health. The fifty states in the United States, which properly provide millions of dollars for hospitals for the care of the mentally ill, appropriate for research only 1.5 percent of their total mental hospital budgets.

Social and preventive psychiatry is concerned with the mental health of individuals and communities. Researchers in this discipline are investigating the social factors associated with the etiology, prevention, and consequences of mental disorders. Whereas neuropharmacology and psychology are concerned, respectively, with finding a specific drug or psychotherapeutic approach for treatment of a psychiatric disorder, research in social and preventive psychiatry explores the application of these approaches in prevention. These lay the groundwork for the development and assessment of specific psychosocial therapies and types of services apt to improve the mental state and quality of life of individuals with severe psychiatric disorders.

Social psychiatry relies chiefly on the methodologies of evaluative and epidemiological research. The emphasis of evaluative research is on developing tools with which to assess patient care needs. Those tools are subsequently used in epidemiological research to determine whether the assessed needs are being met and to establish policy for the planning of appropriate services.

Despite its enormous impact and cost to society, mental illness has been disgracefully neglected. The United States spent only $9 per patient on mental illness research in 1992. The same amount was spent to study tooth decay. Over one-half the money spent on cancer research comes from the private sector, but only 10 percent of the money used for research into mental illness comes from this source.

The most fruitful area of research would be in the prevention of mental illness. One benefit of such research has been the use of alkaloids, enabling many individuals to remain at home who otherwise would be kept in a psychiatric hospital for treatment. As important as preventive medication procedures are in dealing with mental illness, functional or psychological measures for the prevention of mental illness may be an equally productive field of research.

Research is also needed in the mental health of the normal individual. Advances in the health and medical fields in the United States in the past quarter century have included only modest progress in the understanding of the mental health of the normal individual. The motivation of human conduct, the genesis of emotional disturbance, the nature of mild deviations, procedures for improving and fortifying personality attributes, and measures by which a normal individual may cope with stress all warrant intensive study. New methods of research need to be developed, and more behavioral scientists should be prepared to do research in the mental health of the normal individual.

Research on methods of mental health education will become more urgent as other research findings accumulate. Community leaders, particularly those in the health professions, must take the lead in emphasizing the need for research in the field of mental health.

SUMMARY

The essence of community mental health, we have argued in this chapter, is to involve people in collective and mutually supportive efforts to address their quality-of-life concerns. Such concerns will relate to a wider range of issues than health alone. Some will relate to phobias and compulsive behaviors, such as fears of nuclear warfare and drug abuse. Some will relate to sources of stress, such as computers, loneliness, bereavement, divorce, and financial difficulties. Mutual self-help groups and institutional arrangements to support people in coping with these fears, compulsions, and stresses represent the best points for intervention for community mental health and the best primary prevention strategies in relation to other health problems, such as alcohol and drug misuse, smoking, obesity, and violence.

Social health is mental health in relation to community criteria of productivity and quality of life. The World Health Organization seeks, as a goal for the year 2000, levels of health so that all people are capable of working productively and participating actively in the social life of their communities.

Such goals are ideals, however; most communities find their mental health programs tied up in medical treatment programs for the psychotic and severely disturbed. Such medical treatment, thanks to modern drugs in particular, has succeeded in returning these mental patients from institutions to their homes and communities. Some of these are homeless or unemployed, or both. These persons become the special wards of integrated community mental health and social service agencies.

The future of community mental health will depend on the success of nations, states, and communities in accomplishing prevention and mental health promotion objectives, such as those for stress and violence control. It will depend on their investment in such programs as employee assistance and student counseling; these programs will permit early intervention in the problems of troubled employees and students that might lead to alcoholism, drug misuse, suicide, or prolonged depression and isolation. The future of community mental health will also depend on investments in research and evaluation to improve the effectiveness of interventions and support services in the community.

WEBLinks

http://nmha.org/
National Mental Health Association

http://www3.synpatico.ca/cmha.toronto
Canadian Mental Health Assocation

http://www.stressfree.com
Information to help manage and provide solutions to stress.

QUESTIONS FOR REVIEW

1. How have communities' attitudes about mental health changed over time?
2. Why is social health properly regarded as a dimension of mental health?
3. Why is public health education fundamental to a community mental health program?
4. What can a community mental health program do to assist people in improving their social personalities?
5. Why do citizens with marked aggression represent a special community mental health problem?
6. What are the drawbacks of having the staffs of the states' mental hospitals in charge of the total state mental health program in the United States?
7. What kind of mental health programs exist in your community?
8. In what ways does the environment effect mental health?
9. How would you describe the mental health needs of your community?
10. How can personality maladjustment be the true cause of a divorce?
11. If you had good reason to believe that one member of a family of your close acquaintance was in need of psychiatric service, what measures would you take to bring this about?
12. If you had good reason to believe that one member of a family you did not know was in need of psychiatric service, what measures would you take to bring this about?
13. To what extent is it correct to say that every person has his or her mental measles and emotional chicken pox?
14. How will research in the field of mental disorders create the problem of preparing professional specialists in the field of rehabilitation?
15. What research is needed in mental health?

READINGS

Cohen, P. and C. S. Hesselbart. 1993. Demographic factors in the use of children's mental health services. *Am J Public Health* 83:49.

Significant lags in mental health service use were found for youths 18 to 21 years of age, for rural and semirural residents, and for those in middle-income families.

De Girolamo, G., and J. H. Reich. 1993. *Epidemiology of mental disorders and psychosocial problems.* Geneva: WHO.

A state-of-the-art review of knowledge on the epidemiology of personality disorders. The book contributes to an understanding of the epidemiology of mental disorders and therefore facilitates the identification of risk factors, including social and cultural determinants.

Ghadirian, A. M., and H. E. Lehmann, eds. 1993. *Environmental and psychopathology.* New York: Springer.

Focuses on the effects of less studied environmental variables, such as nutrition and illumination—and natural and human-made catastrophes—on psychopathological manifestations.

Kinnier, R. T., A. T. Metha, J. S. Keim, J. L. Okey, R. L. Adler-Tabia, M. A. Berry, and S. W. Mulvenson. 1994. Depression, meaninglessness, and substance abuse in "normal" and hospitalized adolescents. *Journal of Alcohol and Drug Education* 39(2): 101–111.

High school students who viewed themselves negatively, were depressed, or had found little meaning in their lives were more likely to consider suicide and to abuse drugs. A strong mediating relationship was found between purpose in life with the precursor of depression and the consequent of substance abuse.

McColl, M. A., H. Lei, and H. Skinner. 1995. Structural relationships between social support and coping. *Soc. Sci. Med.* 41:3, 395–407.

Relationships between social support and coping were examined over a one-year period in a sample of (n=120) exposed to a specific stressor (i.e., spinal cord injury). The study provides evidence for the dynamic effects of social support on coping, depending on one's stage in the process of long-term adjustment.

Sheahan, S. L., and M. C. Latimer. 1995. Correlates of smoking, stress, and depression among women. *Health Values* 19:(January/February), 29–36.

Smoking among women is linked with stress and coping. Health care providers need to consider a woman's stress levels and socioeconomic status prior to initiating a smoking cessation program.

Warner, R. and G. de Girolamo. 1995. *Epidemiology of mental disorders and psychosocial problems.* Geneva: WHO.

A state-of-the-art review of knowledge about the epidemiology of schizophrenia. Emphasis is placed on studies that shed light on the etiology of this disorder and the social and biological factors that influence its onset.

BIBLIOGRAPHY

Avison, W. R., and I. H. Gotlib, eds. 1994. *Stress and mental health.* New York: Plenum.

Bagley, C. 1992. Changing profiles of a typology of youth suicide in Canada. *Can J Public Health* 83:169.

Bickman, L. and D. J. Rog, eds. 1995. *Children's mental health services: research, policy and evaluation.* Newbury Park: Sage.

Cole, R. F., and S. L. Poe. 1993. *Partnerships for care. Systems of care for children with serious emotional disturbances and their families.* Washington DC: Washington Business Group on Health, Mental Health Services Program for Youth.

Hirsch, B. G., and D. L. DuBois. 1992. The relation of peer social support and psychological symptomatology during the transition to junior high school: a two-year longitudinal analysis. *Am J Community Psychol* 20:333.

Institute of Medicine, National Academy of Sciences. 1993. *Reducing risks for mental disorders.* Washington, DC: National Academy Press.

Kelly, G. R. 1990. Medication compliance and health education among outpatients with chronic mental disorders. *Med Care* 28:1181.

Knight, S. M., K. Vail-Smith, and A. M. Barnes. 1992. Children of alcoholics in the classroom: a survey of teacher perceptions and training needs. *J Sch Health* 62:367.

Leslie, M., and C. K. Mikanowicz. 1992. The significance of cultural differences and characteristics in program development. *Wellness Perspec* 9:24.

Levy, L. H., and J. F. Derby. 1992. Bereavement support groups: who joins; who does not; and why? *Am J Community Psychol* 20:649.

Lustig, J. L., S. A. Wolchik, and S. L. Braver. 1992. Social support in chumships and adjustment in children of divorce. *Am J Community Psychol* 20:393.

MacFarquhar, K. W., P. W. Dowrick, and T. R. Risley. 1993. Individualizing services for seriously emotionally disturbed youth: a nationwide survey. *Administration and Policy in Mental Health,* 20:165–174.

Martin, S. L. and M. R. Burchinal. 1992. Young women's antisocial behavior and the later emotional and behavioral health of their children. *Am J Public Health* 82:1007.

National Advisory Mental Health Council. 1996. *Health care reform for Americans with severe mental illness: Report of the national advisory mental health council.* Rockville, MD: U.S. Public Health Service.

Neighbors, H. W., and J. S. Jackson, eds. 1996. *Mental health in black America.* Newbury Park: Sage.

Newton, J. 1992. *Preventing mental illness in practice.* London: Routledge.

Newton, T., with J. Handy, and S. Fineman. 1995. Managing stress: Subjectivity and power in the workplace. Newbury Park: Sage.

Norris, F. H., and K. Kaniasty. 1992. A longitudinal study of the effects of various crime prevention strategies on criminal victimization, fear of crime, and psychological distress. *Am J Community Psychol* 20:625.

Redman, S. 1991. Women and body image. In *Women and health,* edited by D. Saltmar. Sydney: Harcourt Brace Jovanovich.

Roberge, R., J. M. Berthelot, and M. C. Wolfson. 1995. Observed health differences by socioeconomic status in Ontario. *Health Reports* 7(October)2.

St-Amand, N., and H. Clavette. 1992. *Self-help and mental health: beyond psychiatry.* Ottawa: Canadian Council on Social Development.

Stein, C. H., M. Ward, and D. A. Cislo. 1992. The power of a place: opening the college classroom to people with serious mental illness. *Am J Community Psychol* 20:523.

Taggart, V. S., A. E. Zuckerman, R. M. Sly, C. Steinmueller, G. Newman, R. W. O'Brien, S. Schneider, and J. A. Bellanti. 1991. You can control asthma: evaluation of an asthma education program for hospitalized inner-city children. *Patient Educ Counsel* 17:35.

Vega, W. A. 1992. Theoretical and pragmatic implications of cultural diversity for community research. *Am J Community Psychol* 20:375.

Walker, B. R., and S. M. Wright. 1992. Whole people: putting personal and social issues into school health curricula—a case study from Australia. *Health Prom Int* 7:99.

Wilson, R. W. 1986. The PRECEDE model for mental health education. *J Human Behav & Learning* 3(2):34.

Ying, Y. W., and L. S. Miller. 1992. Help-seeking behavior and attitude of Chinese Americans regarding psychological problems. *Am J Community Psychol* 20:549.

Chapter 10

Community Recreation and Fitness

*W*e do not want in the United States a nation of spectators. We want a nation of participants in the vigorous life.
—John Fitzgerald Kennedy, President

*T*he exercise boom is not just a fad; it is a return to 'natural' activity—the kind for which our bodies are engineered and which facilitates the proper function of our biochemistry and physiology.
—Eaton, Shostak, Konner, 1988, p. 169

Objectives

When you finish this chapter, you should be able to:

- Identify the recreational and fitness needs of a community and its populations

- Describe how recreation and fitness contribute to physical, mental, and social health in a community or population

- Identify resources in a community to support the development of recreational and fitness opportunities

- Participate in planning and evaluating recreational and fitness programs

The term **recreation** implies a health benefit. To "recreate" means to revive or refresh after toil or exertion, to renew the mind, the spirit, and the body. Amusement serves these purposes, as does exercise. Together, they contribute to the promotion of health, the prevention of certain disorders, and the treatment of certain disabilities. Humor and mirth have healing powers. Most experts believe that the physical and mental benefits of **fitness** combine with the social and emotional benefits of recreation to give individuals, families, and communities a quality of life that produces greater resistance to infection and greater ability to cope with stress.

As an activity pursued during **leisure** time and one that is optional and pleasurable, recreation has its own immediate appeal. It is a behavior available in some degree to everyone. Recreation has come to be viewed also as an emotional state or condition that flows from feelings of mastery, achievement, exhilaration, acceptance, success, personal worth, and pleasure. As such it is not necessarily dependent on any physical or social activity.

Community health is supported by recreational and fitness programs that provide for a wide diversity of participation. With the trend toward participation in physical activities, the community finds it necessary to serve citizens who desire to occupy their leisure hours in more stimulating, and outdoor, pursuits. Recreation includes creative and aesthetic interests and those of a predominantly physical nature. The community enhances the quality of life and provides alternatives to drugs and alcohol as leisure pursuits by having an organized recreational program that meets many of the social, creative, aesthetic, communicative, learning, and physical needs of its varied population groups.

TRENDS IN RECREATION AND FITNESS IN NORTH AMERICA

Modern western attitudes toward fitness and recreation are influenced by the ancient Greeks who viewed athletic achievement as embodying physical and spiritual strength.

The history of recreation and fitness in the United States and Canada provides insight into these roots. Recreation, as it is recognized, is largely a reflection of four historical movements: the conservation movement, the urban parks movement, the recreation movement, and the fitness movement. Each has its own history. The first Surgeon General's report on *Physical Activity and Health* released in 1996 summarizes existing knowledge on the benefits of physical activity. Whether it ushers in a new "movement" remains to be seen through historical analysis.

The Conservation Movement

The conservation movement was based on a belief in the wise and balanced use of natural resources. The U.S. and Canadian governments played a leading role by helping to conserve large areas of open spaces and unique landscapes, beginning with the designation in 1864 of Yosemite Valley as the first national park. The establishment of a national park and national forest system was perhaps the most notable accomplishment of the movement.

The Urban Parks Movement

The urban parks movement was nineteenth century North American leaders' response to the effects of industrialization and immigration on the rapidly growing urban population. Landscape ar-

- By 2000 increase to at least 30% the proportion of people aged 6 years and older who engage regularly in light to moderate physical activity for at least 30 minutes per day. Baseline: 22% of people aged 19 years and older were active for at least 30 minutes five or more times per week in 1985.
- By 2000 increase to at least 20% the proportion of people aged 18 years and older and to at least 75% the proportion of children and adolescents aged 6 to 16 years who engage in vigorous physical activity that promotes the development and maintenance of cardiorespiratory fitness 3 or more days per week for 20 or more minutes per occasion. Baseline: 12% for people aged 18 years and older in 1985; 66% for youth aged 10 to 17 years in 1984.
- By 2000 reduce to no more than 15% the proportion of people aged 6 years and older who engage in no leisure-time physical activity. Baseline: 25% for people aged 18 years and older in 1985.

chitects, typified by Frederick Law Olmsted, created a new legacy of public green spaces among the bricks and grime of North America's maturing cities. Beginning with Olmsted's Central Park in New York City, the urban parks movement spread rapidly across the continent. By the early 1900s most big cities had large urban parks, and municipal governments had become well-established parkland providers.

The Recreation Movement

Unlike the conservation and urban parks movements, initial support for the recreation movement came largely from private and philanthropic sources rather than from the government and was specifically aimed at producing social reforms. The movement originated in private settlement houses of major cities where play programs, notably the "sandgardens" of Boston in 1885 and Jane Addams' model playground at Hull House in 1892, successfully provided organized recreational opportunities for children of immigrant tenement dwellers.

The recreation movement was also characterized in the 1920s and 1930s by the development of spectator sports and box office attractions. These were decades that created glamorous films and professional athletics. Leisure time was more plentiful with the eight-hour work day becoming a standard.

The park and recreation efforts expanded rapidly after World War II in response to population growth, large incomes, and new housing developments. By the late 1950s, however, the existing parks and programs could not satisfy the increased demand. In response, the U.S. Congress created the Outdoor Recreation Resources Review Commission in 1958, which stimulated a resurgence of federal interest in parks and recreation.

The 1960s brought expanded protection and development of natural resources and recreational services, as reflected in the creation of the Land and Water Conservation Fund and the National Wilderness, Wild and Scenic Rivers, and Trails Systems.

During the 1970s, recreation expenditures increased at all levels of government. In some cases, however, these funds were unable to keep pace with price escalations affecting recreational land acquisition, capital development, energy supplies, and staffing or programming. The 1980s and 1990s saw budgetary cutbacks and increased dependence on user fees to finance park and recreation facilities.

The Fitness Movement

The President's Council on Physical Fitness and Sports was established in 1956 by President Dwight D. Eisenhower. The council was an outgrowth of the President's Council on Youth Fitness, established out of concern about the poor performance of American boys and girls on standardized physical fitness tests. Subsequently, it was recognized that the fitness problem permeates all age groups. In 1963 the council was directed to begin promoting adult fitness. Today the Council addresses its efforts to all ages, including the elderly, and its activities are part of national preventive health efforts

under the direction of the U.S. Office of Disease Prevention and Health Promotion.

The United States, Canada, Australia, New Zealand, Japan, China, and some European countries engaged in a genuine exercise boom: more bicycles than automobiles were being bought; sports fashion and athletic footwear became major industries; and the number of runners, in-line skaters, skiers, and tennis players tripled in the United States. Joggers, backpackers, and bicycling commuters are commonplace in most communities in several Western countries. Commercial fitness centers and worksite fitness facilities have developed rapidly in Canada and the United States. Physicians increasingly prescribe recreation and fitness as ways to maintain and to enhance health and as accepted therapy for many heart patients and other patients.

Following the 1974 Lalonde Report on the Health of Canadians, a new agency was created to oversee the development of physical fitness programs in Canada in cooperation with provincial and municipal governments and with private industry. Fitness Canada makes use of extensive mass media campaigns, materials, and grants in support of local programs and federal support for national organizations developing specialized programs in physical fitness.

Participation rates in regular leisure-time physical activity gradually increased during the 1960s, 1970s, and early 1980s, but have remained approximately the same in recent years in the United States. The trend in physical activity during leisure time shows a steady decline since the late 1980s in Canada (figure 10-1). One concern is that the mass media presented messages about physical fitness through images such as Jane Fonda and Arnold Schwarzenegger. These images were impossible to either attain or maintain, not only for the average citizen, but the stars themselves, who age over time. Such images may have left some with the impression (or excuse) that if they could not achieve the media image of physical fitness, they would do nothing. Further, many did not know how to begin or sustain exercise programs. Just

· · · · · · · · · · · · · · · · · · · ·

Figure 10-1

Active leisure time physical activity, Canada, age fifteen and over, 1981 to 1995. (*Sources:* Fitness and Lifestyle in Canada, 1981; Well-being in Canada, 1988; National Population Health Survey, 1994-95; original analysis.)

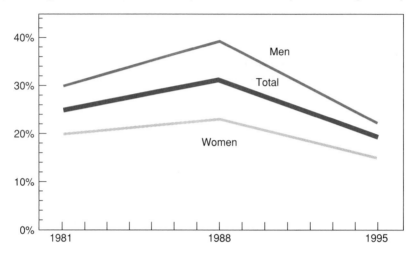

buying videos or signing up for health clubs was not enough. The physical fitness movement was one of many social trends.

Trends that Counter Physical Activity

Despite these advances, public apathy, urban growth, and the modern lifestyle continually threaten to neutralize physical fitness advances. Daily living no longer provides enough vigorous exercise to develop and maintain good muscle tone or cardiovascular and respiratory fitness. In homes and factories, and even on farms, machines have nearly eliminated the necessity for walking long distances, climbing stairs, or even bending and stretching. In 1850 human muscles supplied nearly one-third of the energy used by workshops, factories, and farms. Today the comparable estimate is less than 1 percent. Millions of North Americans and Europeans are willing victims of schemes that promise fitness in a few minutes a day, without sweat or strain. One-third of American children and about 26 percent of American adults are overweight.

As we move increasingly toward an "information age," more and more adults and youth sit in front of computer screens for endless hours on work and recreational pursuits. The most pervasive influence on fitness and recreational patterns has been television, which has substituted passive entertainment for creative recreation and sedentary recreation for physical activity. A study by the American Academy of Pediatrics found that from age 2 years on American children watch more than 22 hours of television a week. By the time a child is 70 years old, he or she will have watched 7 years of television.

Longer hours at work mean less of the leisure time once seen as the promise of a technologically advanced society. For example, in the 1850s Americans cut the average work week from 70 hours to fewer than 40. Today, American manufacturing workers are punching the clock an average of 42 hours a week, two hours more than they did in the 1970s. Further Americans increasingly give leisure time less priority. While 74 percent of Germans rate free time as important, only 40 percent of Americans do the same. This lower priority may result from economic insecurity, a return to work ethics, or other influences.

The continuing financial crisis of schools and the trend away from required subjects have caused the loss of many physical education programs. A simultaneous trend toward "elective" physical education often results in students taking courses that contribute little to fitness or development of progressive skills. Communities shy away from sport and leisure facilities for fear of long-term staff commitments, crime on community property, and potential lawsuits from accidents or injuries. The more society cocoons, the less pressure there is for publicly supported leisure and community sport facilities.

Economic disparity means that while the rich can afford to purchase such services privately, the poor increasingly do without. Public support for "midnight basketball" was highly criticized by some as a waste of public funds, while supported by others for its social and physical fitness goals.

Surgeon General's Report

In the midst of these trends and countertrends, the first Surgeon General's report to address physical activity and health was released by the U.S. Department of Health and Human Services in 1996. The report encourages moderate amounts of regular physical activity as a way to improve health and quality of life. The health benefits of physical activity generally correspond to the amount of activity performed. The vast majority of people who are mostly sedentary stand to gain the most by doing some activity rather than remaining sedentary. The recommendations for moderate intensity physical activity are intended to complement, not replace, previous advice urging at least twenty to thirty minutes of continuous aerobic exercise three times per week. While more vigorous exercise strengthens the heart, regular moderate activity can cut substantially the risk for disease.

Although exercise has long been encouraged, it was not until the later half of the twentieth century that a substantial amount of research accumulated to support this advice. The Surgeon General's report summarizes diverse research findings from a number of fields to emphasize the role of physical activity in disease prevention and debunks the notion that only vigorous physical activity has health benefits. One does not need to train like an Olympic athlete to experience the benefits of physical activity. Physical activity has been known most often for its cardiovascular and musculoskeletal effects. Research also supports the other benefits of regular exercise including functioning of the metabolic, endocrine, and immune systems.

EPIDEMIOLOGY OF PHYSICAL ACTIVITY

Epidemiological studies provide data on levels of physical activity undertaken by selected population groups in various geographical locations. To make sense of these studies, however, it is first necessary to have an understanding of the terminology used. **Physical activity** can be categorized in various ways, including type, intensity, and purpose. **Exercise** is a type of physical activity that is structured, repetitive, and intended to improve **physical fitness.**

Three levels of physical activity were studied in the Surgeon General's report on *Physical Activity and Health:* (1) physical inactivity during leisure time, in other words, no activity during leisure time during previous 2 to 4 weeks; (2) regular, sustained physical activity during leisure time, in other words, moderate activity with sustained, rhythmic muscular movements for at least 30 minutes at least 5 times per week or preferably daily; and (3) regular, vigorous physical activity during leisure time, in other words, rhythmic contraction of large muscle groups, performed at 50 percent or more of estimated age- and sex-specific maximum cardiorespiratory capacity, 3 times per week or more for at least 20 minutes per occasion. Populations vary in regard to physical activity at these levels.

Studies find that about one-quarter of adults in the United States and 13.7 percent of adolescents and young adults are physically inactive; about

Major Conclusions of the Surgeon General's 1996 Report on Physical Activity and Health

- People of all ages, male and female, benefit from regular physical activity.
- Significant health benefits can be obtained by including a moderate amount of physical activity, (e.g., 30 minutes of brisk walking or raking leaves, 15 minutes of running, or 45 minutes of playing volleyball) on most, if not all, days of the week. Through a modest increase in daily activity, most Americans can improve their health and quality of life.
- Additional health benefits can be gained through greater amounts of physical activity. People who can maintain a reg-

ular regimen of activity that is of longer duration or of more vigorous intensity are likely to derive greater benefit.
- Physical activity reduces the risk of premature mortality in general, and of coronary heart disease, hypertension, colon cancer, and diabetes mellitus in particular. Physical activity also improves mental health and is important for the health of muscles, bones, and joints.
- More than 60 percent of American adults are not regularly physically active. In fact, 25 percent of adults are not active at all.
- Nearly half of American youth 12 to 21 years of age are not

vigorously active on a regular basis. Moreover, physical activity declines dramatically during adolescence.
- Daily enrollment in physical education classes has declined among high school students from 42 percent in 1991 to 25 percent in 1995.
- Research on understanding and promoting physical activity is at an early stage, but some interventions to promote physical activity through schools, worksites, and health care settings have been evaluated and found to be successful.

22 percent of adults engage in regular, sustained physical activity; and 15 percent of adults engage in regular, vigorous physical activity (figure 10-2). More females than males were found to be inactive among adult and adolescent and young adult age groups (figure 10-3). Whites have a lower prevalence of leisure-time activity than other racial and ethnic groups. Physical activity is positively associated with higher levels of education and income, living in the western part of the country, and warmer months. The prevalence of physical activity was not consistently related to employment or marital status. In the 1990 Health Promotion Survey in Canada, just under half of Canadian adults were classified as high on the index of leisure-time physical activity.

Efficacy of Risk Reduction

Persons with moderate to high levels of physical activity or **cardiorespiratory fitness** have a lower mortality rate than those with sedentary habits.

Sedentary lifestyle has been linked to 28 percent of deaths from leading chronic diseases. Physical inactivity contributes to several debilitating medical conditions, including **coronary artery** disease, **stroke,** hypertension, cancer, noninsulin-dependent **diabetes** mellitus, osteoarthritis, osteoporosis, falling, obesity, and mental health. An increased understanding of the relationship between physical activity and health has lead to changes in health-related recommendations. For example, the 1990 Dietary Guidelines for Americans recommended that people "maintain health weight"; the 1995 summary guidelines recommend that people "balance the food you eat with physical activity; maintain or improve your weight."

In addition to the benefits of physical activity, research identifies its adverse effects including musculoskeletal injuries. Most injuries can be prevented by gradually working up to a desired level of activity or by avoiding excessive amounts of activity. Although serious cardiovascular events

....
Figure 10-2

The percentage of adults engaging in various levels of physical activity. Note the large percentage of adult who are either not regularly active or are inactive. (*Source:* CDC 1992 Behavioral Risk Factor Survey, Center for Disease Control and the President's Council on Physical Fitness and Sports.)

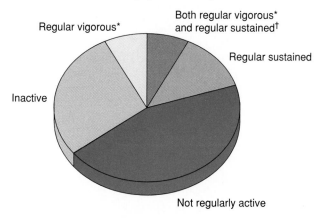

Adults and physical activity

*Regular vigorous—20 minutes 3 times per week of vigorous intensity
†Regular sustained—30 minutes 5 times per week of any intensity

....
Figure 10-3

Moderate and vigorous physical activity levels of adolescents and young adults vary by sex and decrease with increases in age. (*Source:* CDC 1992 National Health Interview Survey/Youth Risk Behavior Survey, Centers for Disease Control and the President's Council on Physical Fitness and Sports.)

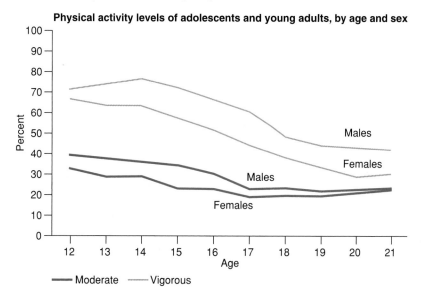

Physical activity levels of adolescents and young adults, by age and sex

Recommendations for Physical Activity and Health

The 1996 Surgeon General's report on *Physical Activity and Health* summarizes the relationship between physical activity on health and disease as follows:

CARDIOVASCULAR DISEASES

- Regular physical activity decreases the risk of **cardiovascular disease** mortality in general and of coronary heart disease (CHD) mortality in particular. Existing data are not conclusive regarding a relationship between physical activity and stroke.
- The level of decreased risk of CHD attributable to regular physical activity is similar to that of other lifestyle factors, such as not smoking.
- Regular physical activity prevents or delays the development of high blood pressure, and exercise reduces blood pressure in people with hypertension.

CANCER

- Regular physical activity is associated with a decreased risk of colon cancer.
- There is no association between physical activity and rectal cancer.
- Data is sparse or inconsistent on the relationship between physical activity and other kinds of cancers, such as breast, prostate, or ovarian.

NONINSULIN-DEPENDENT DIABETES MELLITUS

- Regular physical activity lowers the risk of developing noninsulin-dependent diabetes mellitus.

OSTEOARTHRITIS

- Regular physical activity is necessary for maintaining normal muscle strength, joint structure, and joint function. In the range recommended for health, physical activity is not associated with joint damage or development of osteoarthritis and may be beneficial for many people with arthritis.

FALLING

- There is promising evidence that strength training and other forms of exercise in older adults preserve the ability to maintain independent living status and reduce the risk of falling.

OBESITY

- Low levels of activity, resulting in fewer kilocalories used than consumed, contribute to the high prevalence of obesity in the United States.
- Physical activity may favorably affect body fat distribution.

MENTAL HEALTH

- Physical activity appears to relieve symptoms of depression and anxiety and improve mood.
- Regular physical activity may reduce the risk of developing depression.

can occur with physical exertion, the net effect of regular physical activity is a lower risk of mortality from cardiovascular disease.

Specific Forms and Levels of Activity

Physical activity cannot lower cardiovascular risk or provide other health benefits when performed only occasionally or seasonally. Moderate or vigorous activity performed regularly, long enough, and with sufficient intensity can produce health benefits. The intensity of exercise—how hard you exercise—can be determined by your pulse rate as shown in figure 10-4. Lighter activities can be beneficial as well if done more often and/or for longer periods of time. Rather than emphasizing a particular level of intensity or frequency of activity, the key to benefits from lighter activity is to be moving around, using muscles, and keeping the heart active.

The emphasis on regular, moderate exercise is welcome by many. Vigorous exercise may not be advisable for some individuals susceptible to injury or cardiovascular complications. Brisk walking, climbing stairs, gardening, and recreational activities with a modicum of movement appear to confer more benefits than previously thought, especially in the elderly, the sedentary, those who are hypertensive or obese, and others with low baseline fitness levels. Exercise classes for senior's have been shown to produce physical and mental health benefits. The most popular leisure-time physical activities among adults are walking

●●●●●●●●●●●●●●●●●●●●

Figure 10-4

Pulse rates during exercise in beats per ten seconds recommended for different ages and levels of training. These levels are shown as percentages of maximum heart rate in the legend. (*Source:* Fitness Section, Manitoba Health, Winnipeg, Manitoba.)

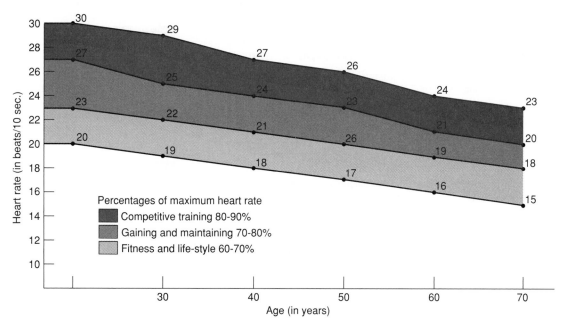

and gardening or yard work that can be enjoyed by all ages (figure 10-5).

The greatest health benefits appear to occur in the most inactive persons who make small increases in their activity levels. For example, increasing fitness through moderate exercise, such as a brisk 30- to 60-minute walk daily may reduce an unfit man's risk of early death by approximately 37 percent and an unfit woman's risk by nearly 50 percent.

NATIONAL GOALS
FOR PHYSICAL ACTIVITY

Progress toward the national goals for physical activity were reviewed mid-decade (figure 10-6). Progress was seen on the number of adults who engage in moderate and vigorous physical activity and on the number of employers offering worksite

●●●●●●●●●●●●●●●●●●●●

Figure 10-5

Walking is an exercise that can be engaged at moderate or vigorous levels by persons of all ages. It can fulfill different kinds of activity goals including physical exercise, social interaction when engaged in with others, and functional purposes such as walking to work or school. (*Source:* World Health Organization, Geneva, Switzerland.)

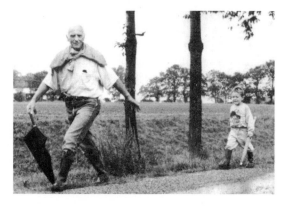

• • • • • • • • • • • • • • • • • • • •

Figure 10-6

Status of selected year 2000 U.S. national objectives for physical activity and fitness in 1995 (*Source:* Lead agency, President's Council on Physical Fitness and Sports.)

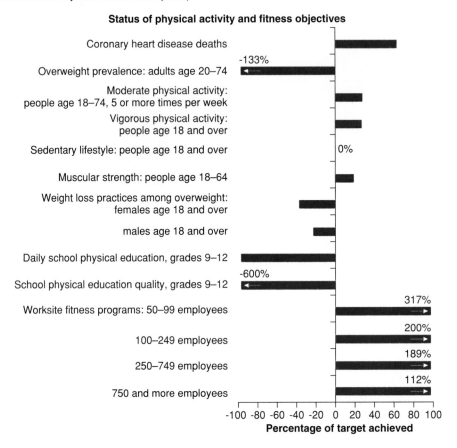

fitness programs. Lack of progress was seen on the number of overweight individuals, where nutrition and physical fitness goals are intertwined. Decreases were also found in the number of students engaging in daily school physical education.

Physical Inactivity Among Adults

Physical inactivity is measured and understood in different ways. For example the mid-decade progress report on national objectives for physical fitness shows zero progress made in the percentage of adults who lead sedentary lifestyles. When

these goals were set in 1990, it was estimated that more than half of the U.S. population was considered sedentary. That is, half the population reported physical activity less than three times a week and/or less than 20 minutes per session. The most active states in the United States are in the west and southwest; the least active extend throughout the southeast and central United States. In Canada, it has been documented that 35 percent of Canadians are essentially sedentary or only somewhat active. Other measures of physical inactivity use the proportion of people who do

·····················

Figure 10-7

Proportion of people eighteen years and over who do not engage in leisure activity: United States, 1991, and year 2000 target. (*Source:* Centers for Disease Control and Prevention, National Center for Health Statistics, National Health Interview Survey.)

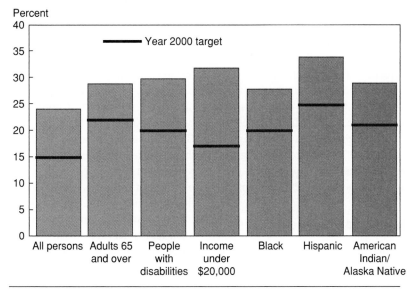

	1991	Year 2000 targets
All persons...................................	24	15
People 65 years and over	29	22
People with disabilities	30	20
Income less than $20,000	32	17
Black...	28	20
Hispanic......................................	34	25
American Indian/Alaska Native....	29	21

not engage in leisure-time physical activity. Nearly a quarter of all U.S. adults fall in this category (figure 10-7).

Physical activity varies by population. Black women, the less educated, overweight individuals, those with low incomes, and the elderly are most consistently reported as inactive groups in terms of overall physical activity. One study found a significant drop-off in exercise for men and women after marriage. For women reduced exercise was linked to pregnancy and feelings of overload; for men it was a gradual decrease. Black men were found to exercise most, then white men, white women, and black women.

Physical Inactivity Among Youth

About one-half of U.S. youth between 12 and 21 years of age regularly participate in vigorous physical activity and about a quarter of young people engage in light to moderate activity nearly every day. About 14 percent of youth report no recent vigorous or light to moderate physical activity. The trend of reduced physical activity is also found in Canada where the Ontario Medical Association reports that Canadian children are up to 40 percent less active than they were 30 years ago. In part this inactivity comes from watching more than 26 hours of television every week and spending up to 30 hours sitting in school.

Participation in all types of physical activity decreases with increases in age and grade in school. In 1995, 59.6 percent of U.S. students in grades 9 through 12 were enrolled in physical education. Enrollment did not vary by sex or race/ethnicity, but did decrease by grade. Although enrollment in physical education programs did not change significantly between 1991 and 1995, there was a significant decrease in daily attendance in physical education classes from 41.6 percent to 25.4 percent.

RECREATION AS HEALTH PROMOTION

Recreation can contribute to mental, social, and physical health. By breaking the commonplace routine of existence, recreation contributes to a greater realization of the individual's potential for living. Recreation alone cannot produce a high level of health, but combined with other factors affecting health it can elevate health for normal individuals. For some people the contribution of recreation to mental health is its greatest value. For others the physical health values or the social values are recreation's most important attribute. For the individual with a disorder or chronic disability, recreation frequently proves important in restoring health. The rehabilitation value of recreation is universally acknowledged.

Mental Health

Many individuals are able to find self-gratification and self-esteem in their regular vocations, but others derive little gratification from the services they give and will seek some other source of emotional satisfaction. Through recreation an individual can achieve a high level of personal performance, experience mastery, and obtain attention, approval,

and praise, all of which arouse emotions of pleasure and elation. Self-esteem, so essential to a high level of mental health, can be enhanced by recreation, which gives the individual an experience in which the self is of importance.

Preventive Benefits   Recreation offers many emotional and intellectual benefits. Competitive games can serve as a healthy outlet for aggression, and research links physical fitness to high motivation, persistence, learning, achievement, self-confidence, and social acceptance. Cooperative activities can provide a sense of belonging and community. Benefits can be attained through creative, aesthetic, social, communicative, and educational activities and through physical activities and performance. For example, relaxation may be achieved through more passive interests such as reading, listening to music, attending lectures, visiting museums, and otherwise serving more the role of the spectator than that of the active participant. Creative urges can be satisfied through programs in crafts, painting, dramatics, music, writing, and other arts.

Therapeutic Benefits   As part of the therapeutic procedure in mental health counseling and psychiatric treatment, specific types of recreation may be prescribed for each patient. Dance therapy and music therapy have become professional subspecialties.

The National Therapeutic Recreation Society, formed in 1982 as a branch of the National Recreation and Park Association, describes the purpose of therapeutic recreation to be the development, maintenance, and expression of an appropriate leisure lifestyle for individuals with physical, mental, emotional, or social limitations. Therapeutic recreation professionals seek to enhance clients' leisure ability in recognition of the importance and value of leisure in the human experience. Therapy services are applied in various settings, including hospitals and residential and community-based health and human service agencies for people of all ages. Halfway houses, community mental health centers, nursing homes, rehabilitation centers, sheltered workshops, vocational training centers, burn centers, and children's hospitals use therapeutic recreation specialists.

Social Health

Human interaction should promote a feeling of worth, a feeling of security from group acceptance, approval, and recognition. Social drives include the desire for new experiences, adventure, and identity with others.

Recreation can elevate the feeling of personal worth in those who already enjoy a high level of social health and in those whose social adjustment has been adequate but unsatisfying. It can be a means by which asocial individuals join in social situations. It also can be a means for preventing or correcting antisocial tendencies. Children and adolescents vulnerable to delinquency can find release and wholesome alternatives to drugs, alcohol, and tobacco in recreational participation. Family recreation in particular can be an aid in preventing delinquency. A Detroit study of over 2,000 court cases showed that 60 percent of the juveniles had little or no recreation within the family group, 32 percent experienced occasional family recreation, and only 8 percent participated regularly in family recreation. A common recreational interest can bring together a diversity of people and promote a general understanding and appreciation of other human beings, which in turn will improve the individual's ability to adjust socially.

Physical Health

The evidence is mounting that the physically fit live longer, perform better, and participate more fully in life than do those who are not fit. Regular, moderate, or vigorous exercise adds to vibrant good health and enhances the capacity for enjoying life and functional health.

Preventive Benefits   The physical exertion inherent in many physical activities creates organic vigor and physiological well-being and increases **physiological efficiency.** Physical activity develops skills, dexterity, coordination, and stamina. If pursued with enough frequency and intensity, a fitness program will provide sufficient physical exertion to stimulate the body to a higher level of efficiency in its functioning.

The actual amount of exercise that recreation or fitness programs should provide should be determined by the individual's general condition and the exercise he or she gets on the job and from other day-to-day living practices. An individual who adjusts activities to capacity and needs can gain certain established benefits. Metabolism will improve, circulation and respiration will function more efficiently, muscle tone and coordination will improve, greater flexibility may be achieved, and general body **efficiency** will increase (figure 10-8).

Therapeutic Benefits   Physical rehabilitation programs employ recreational activities as a large part of their occupational therapy. The motivation that a particular activity can give to a rehabilitation patient often makes the difference between inadequate and adequate recovery. Indeed, the mental and physical stimulation that a recreational or fitness activity can give to a normal individual can be even greater for the individual recovering from extended illness or a disability. More than one-fourth of the hospitals in the United States have organized recreational programs.

SCOPE OF RECREATION AND FITNESS

A wide range of activities provide moderate amounts of physical activity (figure 10-9). Depending on the intent in which they are engaged, these activities can be classified variously, for example, as sports and competition, intellectual pursuits, creative and aesthetic activities, or social events. A specific activity may be considered as being in all of these categories. For example, race walking can be a competitive activity, a brisk walk with a friend

....

Figure 10-8

Cycling laboratories allow exercise physiologists to test physical responses to precise levels of energy expended. (*Source:* University of British Columbia Community Relations Office and Dr. David Sanderson.)

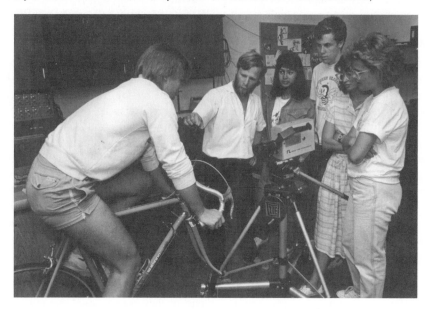

can be a social activity, an active walk in new areas can be a creative activity, or walking from home to work can be a functional activity. For purposes of delineation and convenience, each classification described will include activities whose primary function is in that particular category, although other functions may be served as well.

Physical Activities

Activities with a primary purpose to provide physical exertion, weight control, and exercise include team and individual events.

The number of calories per minute that might be expended by an individual pursuing a physical activity depends on many variables, such as the activity itself, physical build, age, skill at the activity, and adverse circumstances—for example, a strong wind while running, waves while swimming, or an awkward partner while dancing. Table 10-1 is a comparative guide to the relative benefits of vari-

ous physical activities in terms of fitness, weight loss, and general well-being and conditioning.

Intellectual Activities

Many recreational activities that are largely intellectual or educational have other values, although their primary attraction is in the intellectual stimulation or the opportunity for learning they provide. Such activities and interests include astronomy, chess, collecting of scientific materials, computer programming, debates, discussion groups, educational games, educational television, exhibits, fairs, first-aid courses, forums, interest groups and classes, language study, museum visits, ornithology, reading, scouting, stamp collecting, and tours.

Creative and Aesthetic Activities

Most creative and aesthetic activities will have some aspects of a learning experience and will depend on intellectual application. Certain activities

· · · · · · · · · · · · · · · · · · · ·

Figure 10-9

A wide range of moderate physical activities can be incorporated into daily life providing health benefits for people of all ages. (*Source:* At-A-Glance companion document to *Physical Activity and Health: A Report of the Surgeon General.* Centers for Disease Control and the President's Council on Physical Fitness and Sports.)

Examples of moderate amounts of activity

Washing and waxing a car for 45–60 minutes

Washing windows or floors for 45–60 minutes

Playing volleyball for 45 minutes

Playing touch football for 30–45 minutes

Gardening for 30–45 minutes

Wheeling self in wheelchair for 30–40 minutes

Walking 1¾ miles in 35 minutes (20 min/mile)

Basketball (shooting baskets) for 30 minutes

Bicycling 5 miles in 30 minutes

Dancing fast (social) for 30 minutes

Pushing a stroller 1½ miles in 30 minutes

Raking leaves for 30 minutes

Walking 2 miles in 30 minutes (15 min/mile)

Water aerobics for 30 minutes

Swimming laps for 20 minutes

Wheelchair basketball for 20 minutes

Basketball (playing a game) for 15–20 minutes

Bicycling 4 miles in 15 minutes

Jumping rope for 15 minutes

Running 1½ miles in 15 minutes (10 min/mile)

Shoveling snow for 15 minutes

Stairwalking for 15 minutes

Less vigorous, more time

⬆

⬇

More vigorous, less time

---

satisfy the creative urge of people and provide special opportunities for exercise or aesthetic experiences; among these are aerobic and ballet dancing, clay modeling, dramatics, drawing and painting, group singing, instrumental music, jewelry making, leather craft, metal craft, needlework, photography, pottery, puppetry, sculpting, weaving, and woodworking.

Social Activities

Nearly all recreation includes some social aspects. Activities planned primarily for their social value

Table 10-1
Summary of How Seven Experts Rated Fourteen Sports and Exercises

	Jogging	Bicycling	Swimming	Skating (Ice or Roller)	Handball/squash	Skiing-nordic	Skiing-alpine	Basketball	Tennis	Calisthenics	Walking	Golf*	Softball	Bowling
Physical fitness														
Cardiorespiratory endurance (stamina)	21	19	21	18	19	19	16	19	16	10	13	8	6	5
Muscular endurance	20	18	20	17	18	19	18	17	16	13	14	8	8	5
Muscular strength	17	16	14	15	15	15	15	15	14	16	11	9	7	5
Flexibility	9	9	15	13	16	14	14	13	14	19	7	8	9	7
Balance	17	18	12	20	17	16	21	16	16	15	8	8	7	6
General well-being														
Weight control	21	20	15	17	19	17	15	19	16	12	13	6	7	5
Muscle definition	14	15	14	14	11	12	14	13	13	18	11	6	5	5
Digestion	13	12	13	11	13	12	9	10	12	11	11	7	8	7
Sleep	16	15	16	15	12	15	12	12	11	12	14	6	7	6
TOTAL	148	142	140	140	140	139	134	134	128	126	102	66*	64	51

Adapted from President's Council on Physical Fitness and Sports, Public Health Service, U.S. Department of Health and Human Services. Ratings are on a scale of 0 to 3; thus a rating of 21 indicates maximum benefit (a score of 3 by all seven panelists). Ratings were made on the basis of regular (minimum of four times per week), vigorous (duration of 30 minutes to 1 hour per session) participation in each activity.

*Ratings for golf are based on the fact that many North Americans use a golf cart and/or caddy. If one walks the links, the physical fitness value moves up appreciably.

include board games, card games, carnivals, church nights, circuses, concerts, dancing, hobby clubs, holiday parties, and games to teach young children social skills (figure 10-10).

The array of recreational activities suggests that a person who could not find one interest would be destitute. Individuals may need help in understanding the broad array of activities possible and in choosing activities that are suitable to their needs, interests, and resources. It is not surprising to find many people with several recreational interests who benefit physically, intellectually, creatively, aesthetically, and socially from these pursuits.

VALUES IN RECREATION AND FITNESS

Many people associate fitness with good physical performance rather than with good health, improved appearance, or better performance on the job and in the classroom. This has been especially true among the poor, the elderly, and the less educated. Fortunately, perceptions and values are changing in the appreciation of the wider benefits of physical activity and fitness.

Vocational and other interests and activities seem to be adequate to provide some people with the necessary motivation for gratification in living. If recreation merely serves to fill time, its value as

· · · · · · · · · · · · · · · · · · · ·

Figure 10-10

Children learn social skills, ethics, and manners through social games and organized activities under adult supervision. (Photo courtesy M. Jane Ford, Health Director, Lincoln-Lancaster County Health Department, Lincoln, NE.)

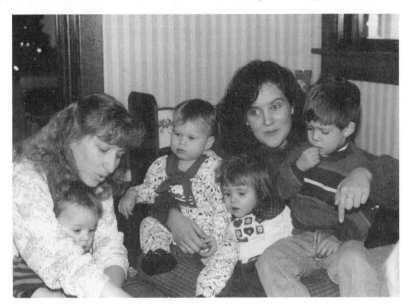

a positive force and profitable investment of time is lost for the individual, the family, the group, and the community.

According to a Louis Harris survey, Americans gave up an average of eight hours of leisure time each week in the 1990s, devoting seven of those hours to work in response to economic pressures. Meanwhile the respondents reported seeing television programs, movies, art exhibits, concerts, and dance performances more often than in the previous decade. Three of every four respondents said the arts give them "pure pleasure." Despite the increase in the United States in the total number of hours worked from 1970 to 1989, participation in the arts has increased. It is estimated that 78 percent of Americans attended movies, 67 percent watch some kind of theater, and 58 percent visit an art museum annually. The shifts appear to be toward more sedentary, spectator forms of leisure.

Bertrand Russell noted how deeply rooted the value attached to exercise is in American tradition: "Unhappy businessmen, I am convinced, would increase their happiness more by walking six miles every day than by any conceivable change of philosophy. This, incidentally, was the opinion of Jefferson, who on this ground deplored the horse. Language would have failed him if he could have foreseen the motor car" (Russell, 1946). The valuing of exercise can be traced at least to Athenian culture, in which the Greek athletic emphasis on health gave rise to the Olympics. The ancient Greek concept of mind and body also gave Western civilization a broader notion of health than mere physical prowess. In his old age, Socrates found time to take lessons in dancing and the playing of musical instruments, and considered it time well spent. Today's lessons on recreation and physical fitness teach us the need to incorporate such activities throughout the life span.

Keeping Fitness in Perspective

A light-hearted but provocative reminder that fitness should not become an end in itself, pursued single-mindedly without connection to deeper or more socially relevant values, is offered by William H. Carlyon's poem "The Healthiest Couple," reprinted with the author's permission:

They brush and they floss
with care every day,
But not before breakfast
of both curds and whey.

He jogs for his heart
she bikes for her nerves;
They assert themselves daily
with appropriate verve.

He is loving and tender
and caring and kind,
Not one chauvinist thought
is allowed in his mind.

They are slim and attractive
well-dressed and just fun.
They are strong and well
immunized
against everything under the sun.

They are sparkling and lively
and having a ball.
Their diet? High fiber
and low cholesterol.

Cocktails are avoided
in favor of juice;
Cigarettes are shunned
as one would the noose.

They drive their car safely
with belts well in place;
at home not one hazard
ever will they face.

1.2 children they raise,
both sharing the job.
One is named Betty,
.2 is named Bob.

And when at the age of
two hundred and three
they jog from this life
to one still more free.

They'll pass through those portals
to claim their reward
and St. Peter will stop them
"just for a word."

"What Ho" he will say,
"You cannot go in.
This place is reserved
for those without sin."

"But we've followed the rules"
she'll say with a fright.
"We're healthy—
"Near perfect—
"And incredibly bright."

"But that's it" will say Peter,
drawing himself tall.
"You've missed the point of living
By thinking so small."

"Life is more than health habits,
Though useful they be,
It is purpose and meaning,
the grand mystery."

"You've discovered a part
of what makes humans whole
and mistaken that part
for the shape of the soul."

"You are fitter than fiddles
and sound as a bell,
Self-righteous, intolerant
and boring as hell."

- What values, besides fitness as an end in itself, might families or couples respond to in participating in community fitness programs?
- By placing fitness in the broader context of recreation and health, how does the community give families and couples broader meaning for their participation?
- By encouraging joint participation of family members in recreational and fitness programs designed for groups, how does the community support values other than fitness as an end in itself?

Individual Benefits

Recreation and fitness activities can offer the individual adventure, physical activity, skill development, release of tension, relaxation, participation and a feeling of belonging, challenges, mastery, success, creativity, stimulation, diversion from boring routines, elation, and a fuller life. Doubtless, these benefits can be acquired from pursuits other than recreation, but for people living in a highly organized and mechanized world, it becomes increasingly necessary to satisfy many personal needs through initiatives outside work and normal living habits.

The benefits of physical or athletic pursuits are felt more intensely by those who engage them at higher levels, than at minimum levels. One study asked reasons for participation in physical recreation; answers included feel better; pleasure; improve flexibility; control weight; reduce stress; be with people; learn new things; challenge personal abilities; and respond to advice by others, including a physician.

One of the barriers for many to overcome is the perception of physical activity as an extra activity to be squeezed into an already busy schedule. Instead, physical activity can be incorporated into daily activities, such as taking the stairs rather than the elevator or taking the farthest parking spot as an opportunity to walk.

Family Benefits

Recreation can serve to integrate family action through joint interest. Social changes and new understandings of what constitutes a family have made the promotion of family recreation more complex. The growing tendency has been to disperse the family rather than to consolidate family living. Women, who once devoted their early marriage years to childbearing, had a different set of recreational and fitness needs than those today who seek careers. Neighborhood cohesiveness has been largely supplanted by friendships based on special interests; social groups are not so often formed on a neighborhood basis today. The increasing complexity and over organization of social services and social structure has had the effect of disrupting the family; children and parents tend not to participate in common events. The child has his or her separate interests and recreational outlets in daycare centers, sports groups, music, art, scouting, and various teenage activities.

Family-centered fun is inclined toward commercialized amusements and sedentary viewing of television. However, there are many other activities in which children and adults have potential mutual interest and can participate. Some degree of promotion may be necessary ("The family that plays together stays together"), but frequently a common interest already exists that merely needs to be realized. Camping, music, painting, badminton, photography, crafts, picnics, hiking, bicycling, volleyball, motor trips, boating, swimming, fishing, folk dancing, skating, skiing, bowling, tennis, golf, gardening, church activities, walking, jogging, and special family nights suggest the variety of activities that lend themselves to total family participation.

To participate as a group, to enjoy common experiences, to share the gratifications of accomplishment, and to pioneer together in new ventures will promote the physical, mental, emotional, and social well-being of the members of the family. The sense of belonging that recreation cements is important in family integration (and group integration). With each member being an individual in his or her own right, joint recreation gives each participant valuable experience in respecting the other members, adjusting to their needs and opinions, and caring about the well-being of the rest of the family.

Surveys show that many adults want their children to be concerned and involved with physical fitness. The growing involvement of women in sports has influenced parental attitudes. With the exception of certain competitive or contact sports, parents are almost as eager for their daughters to be involved in athletics as they are for their sons. Collaborative activities for youth and adults are gaining in popularity.

Group Benefits

Recreation is one means by which the gregariousness of the human species is expressed. Association with others who have the same interests and special needs can be made possible through recreation; in fact, recreational and fitness activities often present the best opportunity for such association and group participation. Engaging in common recreational or fitness pursuits rewards members of the group with a richer experience in group participation, in social adjustment, and in understanding people of like interests and needs.

Children, adolescents, adults, and the aging have different recreational and fitness interests and needs (figure 10-11). Age grouping, however, is not always the pattern on which group recreational or fitness programs are based. The physically challenged and those with impaired vision or hearing often need special group recreational and fitness opportunities. Similarly, the mentally retarded can benefit from special opportunities for group activities. The Special Olympics has demonstrated the

· ·

Figure 10-11

The benefits derived from increasing physical activity from a minimal (sedentary) level to a moderate level are great for young mothers. (*Source:* Photo by Marsha Burkes, courtesy The University of Texas Health Center at Houston.)

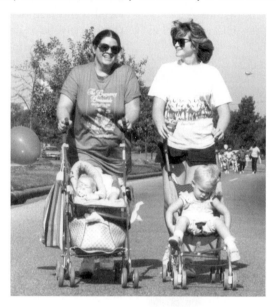

value and need for such activities. Intergenerational grouping has benefits for young and old.

Formal groups find recreation an ideal vehicle for the promotion of group solidarity, morale, motivation, and attainment. Informal groups, which retain more individuality, find recreational activities that will permit individual development within group participation. Organized groups, characterized by individual sharing, and unorganized groups, characterized by a lack of cohesiveness, have equal need for recreational activities. Recreation provides both opportunities for cooperative service and a common interest that can hold a group together.

Whether it serves as a primary or ancillary activity of a group, recreation, like mutual self-help in health and fitness, raises the general value and significance of the group to its members. In this respect, recreation is a means to an end rather than an end in itself.

Community Benefits

The happiness, physical health, character development, and morale of a community are but an expression of these qualities on a composite basis in its residents. Through its social processes, a community can do much to establish the general standard or pattern of community living. In this highly industrial age, a community that provides opportunities for recreation and fitness makes an investment in community stability and integration (figure 10-12).

Economic Benefits

In the United States the amount of personal income available for and spent on recreation has continued to increase from $91 billion in 1970 to over $250 billion in 1990s. The largest amounts were spent on video and audio products ($53 billion); toys and sport supplies ($28.3 billion); wheel goods, sports, and photographic equipment

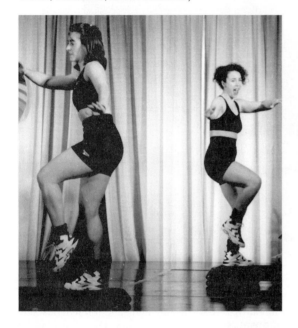

· ·

Figure 10-12

Regular classes with favorite instructors in accessible community centers makes physical fitness fun, as well as conducive to a sense of community. (*Source:* Sandra Wilson, Vancouver, British Columbia.)

($27.7 billion); and books ($19 billion). Substantial sums were spent on attendance at major league sports including $55.5 million at baseball games, $17.6 million at football games, and $12.6 million at hockey games.

The stimulus of recreation and fitness affects all levels of the economy. In the United States jobs in the service sector of recreation in particular have been growing at a faster rate than jobs in all other industries, including other service industries. Another significant impact of recreation on the U.S. economy is the generation of federal, state, and local revenues through sales, income, property, amusement, and gasoline taxes. For example, depending on its proximity to private property, parkland can have a positive or negative impact on property values. Generally, however, recreational improvements enhance the monetary value of nearby properties.

Employers and businesses also gain important economic advantages from investments in exercise facilities and recreation for their employees. The assumed benefits include reduced absenteeism, fewer serious health problems, improved worker productivity, reduced insurance premiums or benefits paid, and improved morale, resulting in better recruitment, less turnover, and consequently lower training expenses.

The provision and maintenance of recreational services is a sizable component of local, state, and federal government budgets. Local government spending for recreation tends to be around 2 percent of county and municipal budgets.

SPONSORS OF RECREATIONAL PROGRAMS

In modern communities planned recreation programs must provide the physical activity that everyday life no longer supplies. The government at all levels, employers, voluntary agencies, schools, and families must join together to provide leadership and facilities for recreation. Programs or activities considered recreational may fall under one or more classifications ranging from commercial entertainment to public recreational and fitness programs.

National Programs and Leadership

In the United States the national physical fitness program sponsored by the U.S. Office of Disease Prevention and Health Promotion and by the President's Council on Physical Fitness and Sports (PCPFS) has the following mission:

- A population committed to physical fitness and possessed of the knowledge and skills to achieve it.
- Acceptance by parents, schools, recreational agencies, and sports organizations of their special responsibilities for fitness.
- Recognition by communities and employers that fitness facilities and programs should be a part of the residential and work environments.
- Maximal use of resources—human and material, public and private—for physical fitness.

· ·
Figure 10-13

Local community centers can provide recreational activities that also promote safety goals. (*Source:* Kitsilano Community Center, Vancouver, British Columbia.)

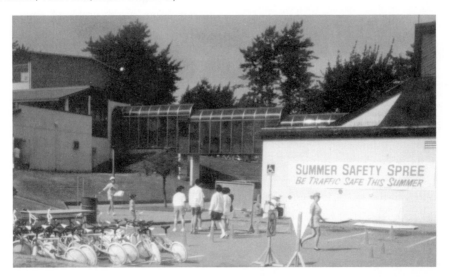

Fitness Canada, the federal lead agency for Canadian programs in physical fitness, has a mission similar to that of the lead U.S. agencies.

The task of the federal government in fitness programs is to educate, advise, and encourage. The U.S. government has developed selected Objectives for the Nation related to physical fitness included in this chapter. The responsibility for action usually rests with parents, school administrators, teachers, coaches, recreation supervisors, civic and business leaders, and others at the community level. One example of a national program is the "Get Moving America" program in which federal agencies joined with twenty-three other major organizations to prevent high blood pressure, including regular physical activity.

National Voluntary Organizations

Hundreds of national organizations in the United States support recreation and fitness activities in local communities. Bikecentennial and the League of American Wheelmen promote the use of bicycles. The American Bowling Congress and the Women's International Bowling Congress standardize rules of play and sanction leagues and tournaments. Aerobics Dancing, Inc., and numerous other vendors of health promotion and fitness programs offer tape recordings, videotapes, scripts, or trained instructors to conduct exercise programs. The National Campers and Hikers Association, the Sierra Club, and the U.S. Forest Service support hiking and camping. Similar organizations for racquetball, running, skating, skiing, swimming, tennis, volleyball, yoga, and even walking (the American Volkssport Association) provide information and guidelines for community organization of programs or events. Directories of these and other resources for **community health events** (figure 10-13) are available through the Office of Disease Prevention and Health Promotion National Health Information Center (P.O. Box 1133, Washington, D.C., 20013-1133) or from Fitness Canada (506-294 Albert Street, Ottawa K1P 6E6).

Commercial Entertainment

Entertainment is a passive type of recreation in which the individual is a spectator or enjoys the activity vicariously. It has become fashionable in some circles to condemn entertainment. The term *couch potato* has been used to disparage the growing popularity of television. The empathy, exhilaration, and enjoyment that come from watching highly skilled athletes and artists perform can have educational, intellectual, and emotional value. Unfortunately, for some, commercial entertainment is a complete substitution for active recreation. Rather than condemn entertainment as damaging to a community's moral fiber, however, the constructive approach is to prepare people for—and provide the means for—physical recreational activities.

Commercial entertainment is big business. It includes professional sports, high school and collegiate athletics, theatricals, concerts, movies, television and radio programs, horse racing, fairs, circuses, and many other activities in which people derive enjoyment from being spectators.

Commercial and Semipublic Recreation

Although certain commercial recreational enterprises actually may be semipublic, the vast majority of them are available to the general public. For example, fitness centers sponsored by hospitals, voluntary health associations, and commercial organizations offer fee-for-service programs in aerobic exercise to individuals and to organizations for their employees.

Semipublic recreation usually is made available through organizations that normally reserve their facilities for their own members, but on occasion make them available to nonmembers. Athletic clubs, golf clubs, tennis clubs, and social clubs may be in this category.

Bowling, roller skating, ice skating, skiing, golf and miniature golf, swimming, canoeing, and horseback riding are examples of commercial and semipublic recreation that can be part of a community's recreational program. Video games are more recent and still dubious entries on the commercial recreation scene, displacing pool halls in many communities.

Private Recreational and Fitness Programs

In providing recreational and fitness opportunities in a community, sports groups and social organizations that limit their facilities and services exclusively to their own members should not be underestimated. Country clubs and private fitness clubs are notable examples of such organizations. It is estimated that as many as 20 million Americans hold a health-club membership. From the standpoint of community recreation, members of these groups are privileged to enjoy recreational opportunities that one might hope everyone could enjoy. Even when formed primarily for recreational purposes, most of these private organizations serve more than one function. Private clubs for golf, swimming, dancing, boating, riding, hunting, skeet shooting, tennis, skiing, weight training, bowling, and other physical activities often include creative, social, and aesthetic activities.

Public Recreational and Fitness Programs

Providing opportunities for recreation and fitness does not mean that all recreation must be planned or in any sense formal. Indeed, it is a justifiable apprehension that, particularly for youngsters, there is too little opportunity for self-created recreational activities. Teen centers have been constructed by some communities to provide for unstructured, but supervised activity.

Urban Areas Recreational services in urban areas are primarily the responsibility of the local government. Communities have the authority to zone and acquire land and to provide public services, including recreation. Political fragmentation too often makes solutions to the problem of providing open space on a regional scale very difficult; it requires a cooperative approach that individual jurisdictions are sometimes reluctant to undertake.

The increasing disparity in wealth of communities—poor core cities surrounded by wealthier suburbs—results in inequitable recreational services. Thus local solutions are sometimes impossible and often inadequate. The assistance of higher levels of government is often needed.

State Government   States and provinces are actively providing, or assisting local governments in providing, urban recreational opportunities. Most provinces and states concentrate their park and recreation efforts on acquiring open space of regional or statewide significance. The potential is great for state and provincial governments to identify urban recreational needs, work with local governments in developing comprehensive strategies to alleviate identified deficiencies, and assign priority to urban recreational projects. States and provinces can encourage localities in metropolitan regions to work together to develop regionwide open space strategies; they can also provide technical assistance to local groups.

Community Actions   Much can be done locally to improve recreational lands and services without any assistance from state, provincial, and federal governments. The following three objectives are suggested for local and state actions. They include actions by public and private (nonprofit and for-profit) providers. In many cases these suggestions are being carried out successfully in communities, states, and provinces in North America, Europe, Australia, and other countries.

1. *Conserve open space for its exercise and recreational value.* Local governments and private organizations must work together at the community level to:
   - Develop procedures for multijurisdictional, public-private conservation of open space through mechanisms such as fee acquisition, purchase of easement, management strategies, or establishment of regional resource conservation and recreation authorities with independent taxing and management roles.
   - Transfer derelict land, tax-delinquent land, surplus highway rights-of-way, and other land not presently in productive use to park agencies through land exchange; purchase; or long- term, no-fee leases.
   - Make maximal use of lands associated with public water supply reservoirs to meet urban recreational needs.
   - Adopt regulations for new residential, business, or industrial development and re-development that require either the dedication of parklands, provision of recreational facilities, or payment of money to a public recreation fund.

2. *Provide financial support for parks and recreation.* Accessible facilities, diverse programs, year-round operation, and good maintenance contribute to citizen satisfaction with community recreation. These elements require substantial numbers of competent staff and a steady source of funds to sustain them. Hiring freezes and staff cutbacks have occurred in a majority of park and recreation departments over the last twelve years in the United States, resulting in reduced program opportunities and facility maintenance.

   Communities and state or provincial governments could address these problems in the following ways:

   - Evaluate user fee policies and identify ways to increase recreation and fitness revenues through user fees and concession royalties.
   - Earmark a portion of local tax revenues for parks and recreational or fitness facilities.
   - Hire grants experts to ensure that local governments are taking advantage of appropriate nonlocal sources of assistance.
   - Adopt legislation giving local governments full authority to set tax rates and to issue bonds.
   - Adopt legislation authorizing localities to deposit revenues earned from specific park and recreational activities (such as

concession stands and golf courses) in accumulated capital outlay funds to be used only for similar park and recreational activities.

- Increase state and local tax incentives for donations of land, easements, and money.
- Create local public trusts and foundations to receive donations that will assist in land preservation or provide programs and services.

3. *Provide close-to-home exercise and recreational opportunities.* Most people, especially in urban areas, want recreational opportunities within walking distance of home. By far the most frequent reason given in most surveys asking people why they are not getting enough exercise is "lack of time" or "inconvenient facilities." For children the problem is often one of transportation.

Many urban neighborhoods lack a variety of year-round programs and facilities that are responsive and available to all residents. About three-fourths of the neighborhoods sampled in field studies reported dissatisfaction with neighborhood recreational opportunities.

Recreation in urban areas includes a wide array of programs provided by many organizations in the community: teen and senior citizen centers; service centers and programs of nonprofit, voluntary agencies; bicycle paths; exercise facilities; parks; and other public and private facilities. Indoor recreational facilities and community centers play a critical role in providing recreational services. General purpose community centers serve as neighborhood meeting places, are usable throughout the year, and often have supervised recreational programs not always available at outdoor sites.

Actions that can be taken by local governments and community groups to assure greater accessibility of recreational resources include the following:

- Establish priorities that recognize the location of potential users when considering acquisition of new recreation land.

- Use streets closed to traffic, rooftops, parking lots, utility rights-of-way, water supply reservoirs, and so on, to provide nearby places for exercise and recreation in heavily developed and densely populated areas.
- Use mobile recreation units where appropriate.
- Coordinate park planning and public transit planning to ensure that new parks and fitness facilities are accessible by public transit.
- Improve public transit service to parks and fitness facilities during weekends and evenings, times of peak use.
- Plan for maximal pedestrian and bicycle access to new parks as an alternative to automobile access.
- Ensure that transit-dependent people have a real voice in the transportation planning process.
- Develop a comprehensive inventory and plan for parks and physical improvements as a first step toward removing or modifying architectural barriers to the physically handicapped.
- Provide specialized staff and equipment for the handicapped, senior citizens, and young children to help them make better use of exercise and park facilities and programs.

Public resources for recreation will be expanded little in the years immediately ahead, with the exception of snow- and water-based facilities. Particular attention must be given to recreation for adolescents and for the elderly in the urban community.

COMMUNITY RESOURCES AND EDUCATION

Physical activity and recreation are influenced by many variables, such as socioeconomic status, culture, age, and health status. Organizations having facilities and members who are willing to contribute their services can add appreciably to the community's recreational and fitness resources. To do so they need to understand the multiple influences on the adoption of physical activity by various population groups including children, adolescents, adults, the elderly, and minorities. Various intervention strategies might be more or less useful for encouraging individuals to adopt and sustain physical activity. The role of different environments in promoting physical activity needs to be examined, along with issues of cost and availability of adequate resources.

For community organizations, it is not just a matter of accepting those who are willing to volunteer, but of recruiting the individuals who may make a contribution to the program. By enlisting the cooperation and active participation of such people and organizations in the community, it is possible to have an extensive communitywide recreational program without huge expenditures on the part of any individual or group (figure 10-14). Casting this wider net for volunteers also helps meet the physical fitness needs of multiple populations.

Community action can expand the use of existing recreational and physical fitness resources through such methods as:

- Use school buildings that have been closed or are underused because of declining enrollment for recreation and fitness.
- Consider the potential for joint recreational use in the planning stages for new or expanded school and park facilities.
- Develop reciprocal, no-fee policies that encourage park use by school groups and school use by park groups.
- Assist in providing services required to open school facilities to the public for recreational purposes after school hours; this will overcome present constraints on joint use, such as prohibitive custodial and maintenance costs.
- Encourage joint use for recreation, wherever possible, of lands and facilities committed to other private and public purposes, including federal property, utility rights-of-way, and the property of institutions and private corporations.
- Encourage use of local park and recreational facilities for a wider range of human delivery services, such as health information, consumer protection, and nutrition information.

Figure 10-14

A national public service campaign sponsored by the Independent Sector and the Advertising Council encourages the American public to give 5 percent of their income to community charity and 5 percent of their time as volunteers to help meet community needs. (*Source:* Advertising Council, New York.)

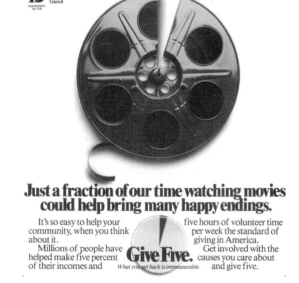

Just a fraction of our time watching movies could help bring many happy endings.

It's so easy to help your community, when you think about it.

Millions of people have helped make five percent of their incomes and

Give Five.

What you get back is immeasurable.

five hours of volunteer time per week the standard of giving in America.

Get involved with the causes you care about and give five.

Relative Strength of the Measures

In the short run, the programs most likely to be successful in recruiting new participants to appropriate physical activity are those that offer services and facilities to individuals and economic incentives to groups and individuals. Programs that can more easily be implemented and are more likely to effect lasting changes include those related to providing public information and education and improving the linkages with other health promotion efforts. The effectiveness of measures is handicapped by the limitation in knowledge about the relationship between recreation and exercise and physical and emotional health; the optimal types of exercises for various groups of people with special needs; and the appropriate way to measure individual levels of physical fitness.

Official Agencies

Tax-supported organizations are regarded as **official agencies.** The state or provincial conservation department providing park, camping, hunting, and fishing facilities is an example of a governmental agency that serves as a valuable resource in recreation. Official agencies on the county and city level include schools, park boards, and public libraries. A city recreation commission, formally organized by the city council with a staff of full-time professional recreational personnel, should be the nucleus of the entire community recreational program. The recreation commission's program can be financed with only 2 percent of the city's annual budget. While various recreational activities do produce some revenue for the city, such income is merely an incidental factor in maintaining the program. Cities accept recreation as a necessary and proper community service and must appropriate funds for its promotion.

Social Groups

People with common interests and needs tend either formally or informally to organize groups to promote their common interests. This is notably true of recreational and fitness interests. These groups usually are limited in their numbers and usually serve only their own members but contribute appreciably to recreation in a community. Dance groups, jogging groups, bridge groups, groups of young married couples, and similar organizations are to be found in most communities. Each group in its own way meets certain recreational needs for its members. Some social groups also undertake to promote recreational activities that will be available to nonmembers. From one social group, many groups may develop to enhance the overall recreational and fitness programs of the community.

Religious Groups

Health and fitness are integral to most religious and philosophical systems. Recreational activities sponsored by religious groups usually are conducted not in competition with official agencies but as supplements to governmental programs. The Young Men's Christian Association (YMCA), the Young Women's Christian Association (YWCA), Boys Clubs of America, B'nai B'rith Hillel Foundations, Jewish Community Centers, Diocesan Youth Councils, the National Catholic Youth Council, and the Methodist Youth Fellowship are examples of religious groups that promote outstanding recreational and fitness programs. Most of these nationally organized groups have local affiliates or facilities in many communities. For example, in the United States there are nearly two thousand YMCA and YWCA facilities. Similar distributions are found in Canada, Europe, Australia, and most other Western countries. Corresponding groups have been established in African, Asian, and Latin American countries, where religious organizations play an even larger role in community life.

Business and Industry

Apart from their commercial interests in health-related products and facilities, employers have many reasons for contributing to the recreation and fitness of their employees, at the worksite and in the community. Although existing programs are too new to yield much statistical data, accumulating evidence from research shows that workers taking part in regular physical activity programs miss fewer workdays when they do get sick, are less vulnerable to accidents, have a higher overall work output, and suffer fewer emotional disorders and physical disabilities.

The most extensive research on employee fitness programs has been carried out in the former Soviet Union, where the tangible economic benefits of regular exercise have been repeatedly documented. Experts found that working people who exercise regularly produce more, visit physicians less, and seem to be more immune to industrial accidents. Japanese companies also routinely provide for exercise breaks.

National Aeronautic and Space Administration employees who participated in a fitness study in Houston, Texas, reported a general

Objective for Physical Activity and Fitness

- By 2000 increase the proportion of worksites offering employer-sponsored physical activity and fitness programs as follows:

Number of Employees	1985	2000 Target
50–99	14%	20%
100–249	23%	35%
250–749	32%	50%
>750	54%	80%

sense of well-being that improved their attitudes about their work and enriched their leisure time. Even more significant was that the results of medical tests bore out the perceived benefits of the program. Those who reported improved stamina, for example, showed marked improvement in cardiovascular performance. Similar results were reported for the employee fitness programs of the New York State Education and Civil Service Department, where risk factors and employee absenteeism were reduced and health problems eased.

The first true fitness program in a U.S. firm began in 1894 at the National Cash Register Company in Dayton, Ohio, where the president authorized morning and afternoon exercise breaks for employees, then built a gymnasium and a 325-acre park for National Cash Register people and their families. Since then, company-sponsored recreational and fitness facilities have become commonplace.

More than half of companies in the United States with 750 or more employees provide fitness programs for their workers. Some companies, IBM for example, subsidize community facilities such as parks or the programs of the YMCA. Others—for example, Tenneco, Conoco, Pepsico, Johnson & Johnson, and Kimberly-Clark—have developed separate facilities at their own sites.

Some companies hesitate to launch fitness programs because they fear they will be liable for injuries to employees. Studies and on-site experi-

ence, however, show that this risk is minimal; where health and fitness programs are properly designed and supervised, the risk of injury is negligible. Anything a company does for its employees— whether a company outing or softball league— involves some liability. A fitness program should be recognized as an integral part of the job, under which the employee is fully protected by worker's compensation or private insurance.

The experiences of Canada and the United States with employee health promotion and fitness programs have been documented and summarized in guidelines available from Fitness Canada and from the U.S. Public Health Service.

Schools

It is recommended that schools provide students at least thirty minutes of vigorous physical education each day. Sending students out to exercise, while teachers and administrative staff retreat to the lounge for a smoke, however, does little to encourage a lifetime of healthful living for students. Physical fitness in schools needs to be part of the overall **school health program.** This includes teachers as role models of physical fitness, incorporating physical activity into other school activities, not using exercise as punishment, and encouraging parents to become educated about active living. Teachers and parents need to be supported by principals who support implementation of physical fitness programs in their schools, by citizen groups interested in physical fitness, and government programs and resources.

Youth-Serving Agencies

Over 250 organizations in the United States work with children and youth under twenty-five years of age. The areas in which these organizations serve are so diverse that it would be difficult to imagine any recreational needs left unprovided. Youth-serving organizations include 4-H groups, Future Farmers of America, Future Homemakers of America, Boys Clubs and Girls Clubs of America, Boy Scouts, Girl Scouts, Camp Fire Girls, Big Brothers/Big Sisters of America, and the Junior

Red Cross. These and other groups in the United States and worldwide indicate the many agencies created to provide the leisure-time and health activities essential for the best development of the children and youth of the community. Use of school facilities after hours by these groups is an ideal way of maximizing resources and addressing the **latchkey syndrome** of unsupervised youth.

Service Groups

Community service groups sometimes sponsor continuing fitness and recreational programs. Equally important is that these service groups are an ever-present resource that can be called on to support any worthwhile recreational program in the community. Rotary Clubs, Lions Clubs, Kiwanis, Junior League, Exchange Clubs, Soroptimists, Grange, Parent-Teacher Associations, and similar organizations provide a diversity of services in their communities, not the least of these being the promotion of recreational and fitness programs.

Neighborhoods

Recreational activities often grow out of group interests, therefore an actual or potential neighborhood interest can serve as a catalyst in initiating and extending recreational activities. Many of these enterprises are self-starting, but others need leadership to crystallize support and to implement the contribution of the group. Interest in building a playground in the neighborhood can be a starting point from which an extensive neighborhood recreational program can be developed. When a playground already exists in the neighborhood, interest can be generated in expanding the facilities and the activities they accommodate.

Special Interest Groups

The typical community has a number of groups with special recreational interests, such as gardening, music, dramatics, computers, chess, stamp collecting, and photography. Through these groups, others can be encouraged to develop new interests or to enjoy an interest they already have. There is something contagious about an intense interest in some fascinating or challenging hobby. As people become exposed to possible recreational outlets, they are more likely to find activities that will appeal to their particular abilities and temperament.

Other Community Resources

Labor unions, industrial firms, retail business houses, chambers of commerce, and fraternal groups promote and support various recreational enterprises. Such organizations find that providing recreation is one of the best public relations services they can contribute to their constituents. In any community it is possible to discover public-spirited organizations that will respond to reasonable requests for support of worthwhile community enterprises. These are the organizations that, with very little fanfare, play an extremely important role in the year-in, year-out promotion of the well-being of the community. They may take an active role and actually administer their own recreational or fitness programs, or their participation may be limited to financial or other support. Resources for the promotion of recreation are rarely more than partially tapped in most communities. To use all possible resources usually requires three things: a worthwhile program, qualified leadership, and an informed community.

Actions that communities can take to strengthen planning, leadership, and public education include:

- Employ professionals to do recreational services planning and fitness program and facility planning, on a continuing basis.
- Improve coordination of planning and implementation efforts to ensure realistic plans and responsive action to meet identified needs.
- Coordinate recreational planning with other health and human service planning; coordinate park and facility planning with overall land use planning and physical fitness planning.
- Develop cooperative programs between resource agencies and local education advisors so that park and recreational resources become an

ISSUES AND CONTROVERSIES
Special Messages for Special Populations

OLDER ADULTS

No one is too old to enjoy the benefits of regular physical activity. Muscle-strengthening exercises can reduce the risk of falling and fracturing bones and can improve the ability to live independently.

PARENTS

Parents can help children maintain a physically active lifestyle by providing encouragement and opportunities for physical activity. Family events can include opportunities for everyone in the family to be active.

TEENAGERS

Regular physical activity improves strength, builds lean muscle, and decreases body fat. It can build stronger bones to last a lifetime.

DIETERS

Regular physical activity burns calories and preserves lean muscle mass. It is the key component of any weight loss effort and is important for controlling weight.

PEOPLE WITH HIGH BLOOD PRESSURE

Regular physical activity helps lower blood pressure.

PEOPLE FEELING ANXIOUS, DEPRESSED, OR MOODY

Regular physical activity improves mood, helps relieve depression, and increases feeling of well-being.

PEOPLE WITH ARTHRITIS

Regular physical activity can help control joint swelling and pain. Physical activity of the type and amount recommended for health has not been shown to cause arthritis.

PEOPLE WITH DISABILITIES

Regular physical activity can help people with chronic, disabling conditions improve their stamina and muscle strength and can improve psychological well-being and quality of life by increasing the ability to perform activities of daily life.

---

instrument for environmental teaching as an extension of school and community health education programs.

- Broaden the scope of interpretive programming to address local environmental issues; sponsor public forums on land use planning, energy conservation, and environmental management programs to involve the public in the decision-making process.
- Encourage residents to assume responsibility for making neighborhood parks safe by giving them a role in park supervision and maintenance.
- Conduct citizen participation and preference surveys to determine recreation deficiencies.
- Publish information on comparative local recreation preferences and needs throughout the state or province.
- Recruit inner city personnel through an office of volunteerism to lead recreational and fitness programs.

Physical fitness through recreation will increase in importance with the increase in leisure time and the extension of life expectancy. Many factors enter into the expansion of community fitness and recreational programs. Understanding by the public must be encouraged, qualified professional leadership must be provided, and adequate resources must be distributed more equitably to serve the needs of special populations.

SUMMARY

This chapter has linked recreation and fitness on the premise that recreation serves a variety of physical, mental, and social health purposes and that a healthful lifestyle can and should be fun and rewarding. For individuals, families, groups, and communities, fitness should not be seen as an end in itself, but as a means to the achievement of other quality-of-life benefits or social goals for different population groups. The reasons people gave in the Canadian Fitness Survey for participating in active physical recreation, for example, reveal that to gain pleasure, fun, and excitement are nearly as important as "to feel better." The desire "to be with people" was given as a reason for participation almost as frequently as "to relax or reduce stress."

When approached as a social issue and a health issue, fitness falls more clearly into place in the development of community programs for recreation and health. The history of recreation and fitness reveals the convergence over the past century of natural allies: the conservation movement, the urban parks movement, the recreation movement, and the fitness movement. New alliances are emerging with physical educators, recreation professionals, health educators, and others working in schools, in community agencies, and at worksites to develop comprehensive fitness programs with recreational and health benefits.

The health benefits of various sports and exercises include those described in table 10-1 as criteria for physical fitness and well-being and various physical, mental, and social health benefits that are less direct.

The scope of recreation and fitness includes physical, intellectual, creative, and social activities. In addition to their health benefits, these activities offer a variety of family, group, and community benefits, including considerable economic value to the community.

Recreational activities can be provided or supported by national programs; commercial entertainment; commercial and semipublic recreation; private recreational and fitness programs; and public recreational programs, including park and open-space programs.

Community resources to support recreational activities include health promotion and educational measures, official agencies, social groups, religious groups, business and industry, service groups, neighborhoods, and special interest groups. Of particular note is the remarkable growth of corporate sponsorship of health and fitness programs for employees at the worksite.

WEB*Links*

http://www.aahperd.org
The American Alliance for Health, Physical Education, Recreation and Dance

http://www.healthandfitness.com/gyms/
Directory of fitness centers in the United States by state.

http://www.hyperlink.com/balance
Monthly newsletter on fitness-related topics.

http://www.activeliving.ca/activeliving/index.html
Active living in Canada—national website for organizations in fitness, recreation, and physical education.

QUESTIONS FOR REVIEW

1. What is the difference between recreation and fitness?
2. To what extent is recreation a vehicle for health promotion?
3. To what extent is recreation a vehicle for the treatment of disabilities?
4. Why are recreation and fitness growing as community enterprises in the United States?
5. What recreational and fitness activities are available in your community?
6. How can recreation promote social health?
7. Why does the public place so much emphasis on physical recreation?
8. Why is an intellectual activity recreational for one person but an unenjoyable task for another person?
9. How can group interests in your community be used to expand the community's recreational and fitness program?
10. What alternatives to the tavern and gambling hall does your community offer its citizens?
11. What role does commercial entertainment play in your community?
12. To what extent does commercial recreation contribute to the total recreational program of your community?
13. What recreational and fitness activities are provided publicly in your community?
14. What recreational areas and facilities are available in your community?
15. What additional areas and facilities should be provided?

READINGS

Blair, S. N., H. W. Kohl, N. F. Gordon, P. S. Paffenbarger. 1992. How much physical activity is good for health? *Annu Rev Public Health* 13:99.

Reviews the epidemiological evidence and historical analyses of energy expenditures and physical activity, concluding that some exercise is essential to good health but showing that moderate physical activity with regularity is just as good for most people as intensive physical activity.

Collette, M., G. Godin, R. Bradet, N. J. Gionet. 1994. Active living in communities: Understanding the intention to take up physical activity as an everyday way of life. *Can J Public Health* 85:418.

A survey of New Brunswick residents age 15–80 applied the Theory of Reasoned Action and discovered strong influence of perceived enabling factors that were more important in predicting exercise than beliefs about physical fitness.

Katz, D. 1994. *Just do it: The Nike Spirit in the corporate world.* New York: Random House

This book is an anthropologist's interpretation of Nike's rise as a multinational corporation. While Nike helped to democratize sports and connect the global village, it created cultural icons, fueled consumer wants, and changed the meaning and importance of footwear.

Kovar, P. A., J. P. Allegrante, R. MacKenzie, M. G. E. Peterson, B. Gutin, M. E. Charlson. 1992. Supervised fitness walking in patients with osteoarthritis of the knee: a randomized, controlled trial. *Annals Intern Med* 116:529.

The positive results presented in this article demonstrate the effectiveness of a program based on a planning process guided by the PRECEDE model (see Allegrante et al. article in Bibliography).

Mills, E. M. 1994. The effect of low-intensity aerobic exercise on muscle strength, flexibility, and balance among sedentary elderly persons. *Nursing Research* 43 (July/August): 207–11.

Elderly persons who participate in low-intensity aerobic exercise may improve their flexibility, balance, and muscle strength, thereby reducing the risk of falls, the leading cause of death for persons seventy-five years and older.

Pate, R. R. 1995. Recent statements and initiatives on physical activity and health. *American Academy of Kinesiology and Physical Education.* 47:304–310.

Official pronouncements from prestigious scientific and medical societies on the health implications of physical activity are reviewed. Pronouncements in the 1970s focused on guidelines for the use of exercise in cardiac rehabilitation and fitness programs. More recent statements addressed the role of physical activity in preventing disease and promoting public health. Emphasis has shifted from endorsement of structured exercise and public health interventions to promoting physical activity through environmental, policy, and personal lifestyle modifications.

BIBLIOGRAPHY

Allegrante, J. P., P. A. Kovar, C. R. MacKenzie, M. G. E. Peterson, and B. Gutlin. 1993. A walking education program for patients with osteoarthritis of the knee: Theory and intervention strategies. *Health Education Quarterly* (spring): 63–81.

American Heart Association. 1995. Exercise standards: A statement for health care professionals from the American Heart Association. *Circulation* 91:580–615.

Astrand, P. O. 1992. Why exercise? J. B. Wolffe memorial lecture. *Med Sci Sports Exerc* 24:153.

Allison, K. R. 1996. Predictors of inactivity: An analysis of the Ontario Health Survey. *Can. J. Public Health* 87:354.

Balcazar, H., and J. A. Cobas. 1993. Overweight among Mexican Americans and its relationship to life style behavioral risk factors. *J Community Health* 18:55.

Bouchard, C., R. Shephard, T. Stephens, eds. 1993. *Physical activity, fitness, and health: consensus statement.* Champaign, IL: Human Kinetics Press.

Boyce, R. W., A. R. Hiatt, and G. R. Jones. 1992. Physical fitness of police officers as they progress from supervised recruit to unsupervised sworn officer fitness programs. *Wellness Perspec* 8:31.

Buchner, D. M., S. A. A. Beresford, E. B. Larson, A. Z. LaCroix, and E. H. Wagner. 1992. Effects of physical activity on health status in older adults. II: Intervention studies. *Annu Rev Public Health* 13:469.

Centers for Disease Control and Prevention. 1997. Guidelines for school and community programs to promote lifelong physical activity among young people. *MMWR* 46 (No. RR-6): 1.

Cardinal, B. J. 1993. Readability of printed materials on exercise. *Wellness Perspec: Theory Prac* 9:48.

Dzwewaltowski, D. A. 1994. Physical activity determinants: a social cognitive approach. *Medicine and Science in Sport and Exercise* 26(11):1395–99.

Eaton, S. B., M. Shostak, and M. Konner. 1988. *The paleolithic prescription: a program of diet and exercise and a design for living.* New York: Harper and Row.

Eichstaedt, C. B., and B. W. Lavay. 1992. *Physical activity for individuals with mental retardation: infancy through adulthood.* Champaign, IL: Human Kinetics Press.

Field, L. K. and M. A. Steinfardt. 1992. The relationship of internally directed behavior to self-reinforcement, self-esteem, and expectancy values for exercise. *Am J Health Prom* 7:21.

Fletcher, G. F., S. N. Blair, J. Blumenthal, C. Caspersen, B. Chaitman, S. Epstein, H. Falls, E. S. Froelicher, V. F. Froelicher, and I. L. Pina. 1992. Statement on exercise: benefits and recommendations for physical activity programs for all Americans, a statement for health professionals by the Committee on Exercise and Cardiac Rehabilitation of the Council on Clinical Cardiology, American Heart Association. *Circulation* 86:340.

Gemberline, C. 1996. Preparticipation sports evaluation: An overview. *Nurse Practitioner* Forum 7(3):125–135.

Godin, G. 1994. Theories of reasoned action and planned behavior: Usefulness for exercise promotion. *Med Sci in Sport and Exercise* 26(11):1391–1394.

Jette, M., J. Quenneville, and K. Sidney. 1992. Fitness testing and counseling in health promotion. *Can J Sport Sci* 17:194.

Johnson, N. A., C. A. Boyle, and R. F. Ketter. 1995. Leisure-time physical activity and other health behaviors. *Aust J Public Health* 19(1):69.

Kusinitz, I., and M. Fine. 1995. *Your guide to getting fit.* 3d ed. Palo Alto: Mayfield.

Laws, A., and G. M. Reaven. 1993. Physical activity, glucose tolerance, and diabetes in older adults. *Ann Behav Med* 13:125.

Lee, C. 1991. Women and aerobic exercise: directions for research development. *Ann Behav Med* 13:133.

Lewis, B. S., and W. D. Lynch. 1993. The effect of physician advice on exercise behavior. *Prev Med* 22:110–21.

Lissau, I., and T. I. A. Sorensen. 1992. Prospective study of the influence of social factors in childhood on risk of overweight in young adulthood. *Int J Obesity* 16:169.

Lock, J. Q., and A. V. Wister. 1992. Intentions and changes in exercise and behaviour: a life-style perspective. *Health Prom Int* 7:195.

Mason, J. O. 1992. Healthy people 2000 goals: How far have we come in physical fitness and activity? *Am Fitness* 10:29.

Mood, D., F. F. Musker, and J. Rink. 1995. *Sports and recreational activities.* 11th ed. St. Louis: Mosby.

Paffenbarger, R. S., Jr., R. T. Hyde, A. L. Wing, I. M. Lee, D. L. Jung, and J. B. Kampert. 1993. The association of changes in physical activity level and other lifestyle characteristics with mortality among men. *New Engl J Med* 328:538–45.

Powell, K. E., and M. Pratt. 1996. Physical activity and health: avoiding the short and miserable life. *The British Medical Journal* 313 (July 20):126–27.

Russell, B. 1946. *History of western philosophy.* London: George Allen & Unwin.

Russell, S. J., C. Hyndford, and A. Beaulieu. 1992. *Active living for Canadian children and youth: a statistical profile.* Ottawa: Canadian Fitness and Lifestyle Research Institute and Active Living Alliance for Children and Youth.

Simoes, E. J., T. Byers, R. J. Coates, 1995. The association between leisure-time physical activity and dietary fat in American adults. *Am J Public Health* 85:240–44.

Singer, J. E., A. Lindsay, and D. M. C. Wilson. 1991. Promoting physical activity in primary care: overcoming the barriers. *Can Fam Phys* 37:2167.

Smith, J. A., and D. L. Scammon. 1987. *A market segment analysis of adult physical activity: exercise beliefs, attitudes, intentions, and behaviors. Advances in nonprofit marketing.* Vol. 2. Greenwich, CT: JAI.

Stewart, G. W. 1995. *Active Living.* Ontario: Human Kinetics.

Verhoef, M. J., and E. J. Love. 1992. Women's exercise participation: the relevance of social roles compared to non-rolerelated determinants. *Can J Public Health* 83:367.

Vertinski, P. 1992. Sport and exercise for old women: images of the elderly in the medical and popular literature at the turn of the century. *Int J Hist Sport* 9:83.

Wagner, E. H., A. Z. LaCroix, D. M. Buchner, E. B. Larson. 1992. Effects of physical activity on health status in older adults: I: Observational studies. *Annu Rev Public Health* 13:451.

World Health Organization. 1990. *Prevention in childhood and youth of adult cardiovascular diseases: time for action.* Geneva: WHO Technical Report Series, No. 792.

YMCA of the U.S.A. 1992. *Programs for special populations.* Champaign, IL: Human Kinetics Press.

Young, M., and T. Schuller. 1991. *Life after work: the arrival of the ageless society.* London: HarperCollins.

Chapter *11*

Communicable Disease Control

*D*isease can never be conquered, can never be quelled by emotion's wailful screaming or faith's cymballic prayer. It can only be conquered by the energy of humanity and the cunning in the mind of man. In the patience of a Curie, in the enlightenment of a Faraday, a Rutherford, a Pasteur, a Nightingale, and all other apostles of light and cleanliness, rather than of a woebegone godliness, we shall find final deliverance from plague, pestilence, and famine.
—Sean O'Casey (1884–1964), Irish dramatist. *Inishfallen, Fare Thee Well,* vol 1., 1949.

*N*ow scientists can identify the key factors responsible for epidemics. We know they're all of our making. They're not some strange thing in nature; it's human intervention all the way. If we're responsible, we can correct it. The message is not go freak out and scream, 'the sky is falling.' Let's look at these amplification factors and come up with policies and behavior changes.
—Laurie Garrett, author of *The Coming Plague,* 1995, interviewed in *USA Today,* Oct. 18, 1995.

Objectives

When you finish this chapter, you should be able to:

- Assess the relative importance of various sources of infection and disease in a community
- Identify the means of transmission of common communicable diseases in a community
- Assess ways to control the spread of an outbreak
- Describe prevention and health promotion methods to reduce the incidence of major communicable diseases by the year 2000

The successful application of immunizations, nutrition, sanitation, and epidemiological principles has caused acute, infectious communicable diseases to give way to chronic diseases as the leading causes of death in the more developed countries. So pervasive are the means of controlling communicable diseases that you probably take most of them for granted in your everyday living.

Much of the remaining infection in the community persists because of lapses in communicable disease control measures, or because poverty, stress, malnutrition, exhaustion, alcohol, or drugs compromise the "host resistance" of individuals. Hence, major defenses against communicable disease include economic development and the promotion of physical and mental health.

Is it necessary to study this aspect of community health if it is so close to being controlled? New communicable diseases seem to emerge to replace the old, eradicated scourges; viral diseases replace bacterial diseases, hepatitis and acquired immunodeficiency syndrome (AIDS) replace gonorrhea, Lyme disease seems to replace Legionnaires' disease, Ebola replaces controlled tropical diseases. These "new" diseases have existed in the past, but their emergence as epidemics seemed to await new social circumstances. This points to a second reason for remaining alert to the communicable diseases—namely, that they are highly sensitive to social conditions; they serve as a barometer of the status and health of a community or population. The third reason is that much of what we know about health, and most of the concepts and epidemiological methods for community and population health, derive from the study and experience of communicable disease control.

CAUSES OF COMMUNICABLE DISEASE

Epidemiology defines **disease** as a harmful departure from normal in individuals or populations. A **communicable disease** is one transmitted from one human being to another or from animals to humans. Communicable diseases result from organisms that are parasitic and **pathogenic,** or disease-producing. Most pathogens of humans are microorganisms, although some, notably the worms, are multicellular forms visible with the unaided eye. **Infectious disease** represents a reaction of the host to the invader. The interaction may destroy the pathogen and produce abnormalities in the host, even to the point of causing the death of the human host.

Infection and Disinfection

Infection is the successful invasion of the body by pathogens under such conditions as will permit them to multiply and harm the host. The mere presence of pathogenic organisms or toxins in the human body does not constitute disease. A person may be harboring millions of pneumococci in his or her lungs or have billions of streptococcus organisms on the skin without having disease. Only when the pathogens cause harm to the body can the condition be classed as a disease.

Disinfection consists of killing or removing organisms capable of causing infection. Disinfection by the use of chemicals is the usual method. Physical disinfection includes the use of such agents as ultraviolet radiation, sound waves, and electron treatment. The two most common means of chemical disinfection are bacteriostasis and antibiosis.

Bacteriostasis is an arrest in the multiplication or metabolism of pathogens. Thus toxin production by the invading organism is reduced or ceases completely. For example, sulfonamides arrest bacterial action by depriving the organism of the material that it must have to carry on normal metabolic processes. The resulting bacteriostasis enables a person's phagocytes to destroy the pathogen.

Antibiosis such as produced by penicillin, means antagonism to specific organisms. The antibiotics have had spectacular effects in combating certain pathogens, but they have not proved to be a panacea. Despite their magnificent contribution to the battle against infection, the antibiotics have limitations. Bacteria develop resistant strains in response to antibiotics. This **mutation,** or adaptability, by the bacteria limits the use of antibiotics. Resistant strains of bacteria are found particularly in hospital-acquired (**nosocomial**) infections. An infection with the same organism acquired outside the hospital will more likely be sensitive to the same antibiotics and respond well to treatment. Indiscriminate use of antibiotics, without proper indication, increases the proportion of organisms that can resist that particular antibiotic.

Contamination and Decontamination

Contamination is the presence of toxins or pathogens of humans on inanimate objects, such as needles (figure 11-1), articles of clothing, furnishings, eating utensils, food, water, or even soil. Certain organisms, such as *Escherichia coli,* live naturally in the intestines of humans, therefore the

· · · · · · · · · · · · · · · · · · · ·
Figure 11-1

Intravenous drug (IVD) users are at particular risk of contracting HIV/AIDS through sharing of contaminated needles. Public service ads in magazines alert IVD users to this contamination risk. (*Source:* National Institute on Drug Abuse, U.S. Department of Health and Human Services.)

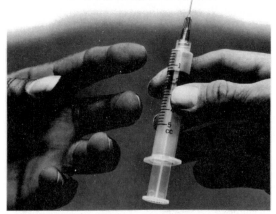

SHARING NEEDLES CAN GET YOU MORE THAN HIGH.

IT CAN GET YOU AIDS.

You can't tell if someone has the AIDS virus just by looking.
You can't tell if needles or works are infected just by looking.
When you shoot drugs and share needles or works you could get AIDS. Even if you think your drug-sharing partners are clean, if the AIDS virus is present, it could be passed to you.
AIDS is not pretty. It's a long, slow, painful way to die. Do the right thing. Get into treatment. It's the best way to make sure you don't shoot up AIDS.

STOP SHOOTING UP AIDS.
GET INTO DRUG TREATMENT.
CALL 1-800 662 HELP.

presence of these organisms in inanimate matter such as water indicates presence of human discharges. Contact with a possibly contaminated object—and therefore with pathogens from the alimentary tract of humans—presents danger. The *E. coli* count serves as a standard measure or index of contaminated water, even though most *E. coli* bacteria are not pathogenic. One variety, however, is highly pathogenic for children and has contaminated food (for example, hamburger and unpasteurized apple juice, see chapter 16).

Table 11-1

Reported Cases of Selected Communicable Diseases, United States, 1900 and 1992

Disease	1900	1992
Diphtheria	147,991	4
Malaria	184,165	1,004
Smallpox	102,128	0
Typhoid fever	35,994	382

Based on data from National Center for Health Statistics (1900 data); and Centers for Disease Control, *MMWR* 41:979, Jan. 8, 1993.

Decontamination means the killing or removing of toxins or pathogens and *E. coli* in or on *inanimate* objects. More drastic measures can apply to inanimate objects than are used in disinfection, including boiling, the use of steam, **pasteurization,** high levels of dry heat, long exposure to the sun, highly concentrated chemicals, and even radiation.

INCIDENCE OF COMMUNICABLE DISEASES

Epidemiology, public health education, socioeconomic improvements in housing, the food supply, and access to vaccines have contributed enormously to the control of infectious diseases. A comparison of reported cases of selected communicable diseases in the United States in 1900 and 1992 indicates the extent of the gain (table 11-1). In appraising the general decline in the number of reported cases of these selected diseases, added weight must be given to the increase in population, now 180 percent greater than it was in 1900.

Gains and setbacks are seen in the comparison of progress in immunization and communicable diseases in the first half of the 1990s relative to the objectives set for the year 2000 (figure 11-2). These figures indicate that the United States has

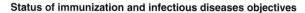

Figure 11-2

Progress toward achieving the immunization and infectious disease objectives and subobjectives for the United States for the year 2000 is shown here as percentage achieved or percentage lost between 1990 and 1995. (*Source: Healthy People 2000: Midcourse review and 1995 revisions,* Boston, 1995, Jones and Bartlett Publishers.)

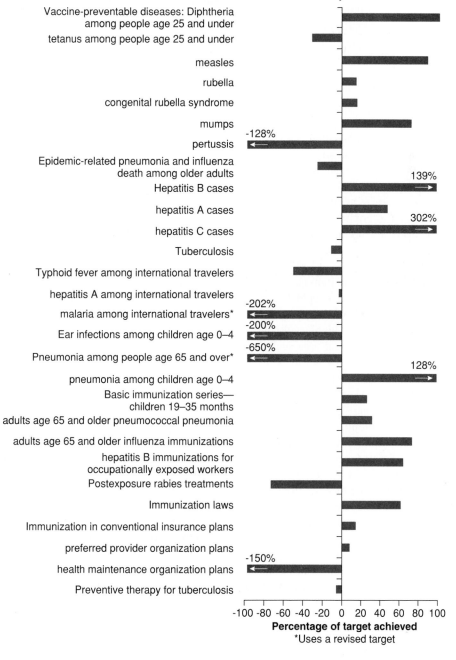

Status of immunization and infectious diseases objectives

Percentage of target achieved

*Uses a revised target

not reached the point where its residents can be complacent about communicable disease. Some of the national objectives for 2000, such as preventing cases of diphtheria and measles, were met by mid-decade, but communicable disease still exists in epidemic proportions for pertussis, malaria, ear infections for children 0 through 4 years of age, and pneumonia among people age 65 and over. In developing countries, endemic malaria continues to lead causes of death, along with other diarrheal and respiratory infections.

Epidemic is from the Greek for *epi,* which means upon, and *demos* for people. It refers to a more than normally expected incidence of cases of a particular disease in a locality such as a city. The number of cases that would classify an outbreak as an epidemic is flexible, depending on the usual frequency of the particular disease, at the same season of the year, and among the specified population and size of the community. In a city of 12,000 people, 10 cases of chickenpox would not be an epidemic, but in a community of 200, that number might well be regarded as epidemic. Ten cases of cholera or paralytic poliomyelitis in a city of 12,000 would be regarded as an epidemic.

Pandemic is from the Greek for *pan,* meaning all. It indicates a considerable number of cases of a disease in a wide geographical area such as an entire nation, a continent, or the world. Thus the outbreak of influenza in 1918 and 1919 was classed as a pandemic. Despite the advance in communicable disease control, no country is completely safe from pandemics. The AIDS and cholera epidemics soon became pandemic for regions of Africa and South America.

Endemic, from the Greek *en,* for in, refers to a steady but limited number of cases consistently present in a geographical area. The term is sometimes limited to diseases peculiar to a particular area.

Infectious diseases in the United States still account for a significant death toll. The increase in some categories such as tuberculosis includes AIDS-related cases.

TYPES OF INFECTIOUS DISEASES

For purposes of community disease control, the most useful classification of infectious diseases is one that incorporates at least a suggestion of how the pathogen escapes from the host or reservoir and how the disease is transmitted. The classification presented in table 11-2 lists some diseases in more than one category. Therefore tuberculosis and smallpox properly can be classed as respiratory diseases and as open lesion diseases. In these infectious conditions, the avenue of spread from the host to a new host can be either from the respiratory tract or from the open sores that these infections produce.

Respiratory Diseases

Respiratory tract diseases are much more common than the other classes of infectious diseases because the respiratory tract is as exposed as the skin but without the defenses of the skin. Diseases of the respiratory tract are particularly prevalent in the temperate zones. Usually acute, they pose a constant threat to the population.

Infectious diseases of the respiratory tract follow a characteristic cycle of periods—incubation, prodrome, fastigium, defervescence, convalescence, and defection, as defined in figure 11-3. An understanding of the typical course of a respiratory disease identifies factors operating at a given stage and where and what control measures should be taken.

Incubation starts with the invasion of the causative agent. Although organisms multiply in the host during the incubation period, no symptoms occur. An infectious respiratory disease normally is not communicable during this period, although chickenpox and measles may be transmitted to other hosts during the last two or three days of the incubation period. Duration of the incubation period varies from disease to disease. Generally the more severe diseases have a short incubation period and the less severe diseases have a longer incubation period, although exceptions to this general tendency do exist.

Table 11-2

Classification of Infectious Diseases by Their Usual Means of Escape from One Host to Reach Another*

Respiratory diseases	Alvine discharge diseases	Vector-borne diseases	Open lesion diseases
Cerebrospinal meningitis	Amebic dysentery	African sleeping sickness	AIDS/HIV
Chickenpox	Cholera	Bilharzia	Anthrax
Coryza	Giardiasis	Encephalitis	Chancroid and chlamydia
Diphtheria	Hookworm	Dracunculiasis	Dracunculiasis
Influenza	Paratyphoid	Hanta virus	Erysipelas
Pertussis (whooping cough)	Poliomyelitis	Lyme disease	Gonorrhea
Pneumonia	Salmonellosis	Malaria	Hepatitis B
Poliomyelitis	Schistosomiasis	Onchocerciasis	Herpes
Rubella (German measles)	Shigellosis (bacillary	Plague	Leprosy
Rubeola (measles)	dysentery)	Psittacosis	Scarlet fever
Scarlet fever	Typhoid fever	Rabies	Smallpox
Smallpox	Viral hepatitis	Relapsing fever	Syphilis
Streptococcal sore throat		Rocky Mountain spotted fever	Tuberculosis
Tuberculosis		Schistosomiasis	Tularemia
		Tularemia	
		Typhus fever	
		Yellow fever	

*In addition to the usual means of transmission, some diseases can be transmitted by hypodermic needles shared by drug users or by blood transfusions.

. . . .

Figure 11-3

The natural history of an infectious respiratory disease typically follows the pattern shown here. The most infectious period is the prodromal period.

Prodromal symptoms: Nasal discharge, headache, mild fever, general aching, irritability, restlessness, digestive disturbances, cough, sore throat.

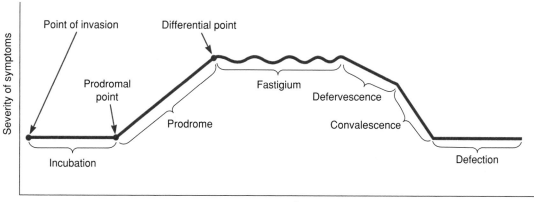

Prodrome begins with the first symptoms in the host and usually lasts about one day. Symptoms during this period are similar for all respiratory infections and resemble those of the common cold; thus, it is difficult to get a definite diagnosis at this stage. From a community health standpoint, there exists a great danger of disease transmission during this highly communicable stage. With the assumption that they "just have a cold," patients continue their normal daily routines and unknowingly expose a considerable number of people.

Fastigium is the period during which the disease is at its height. Differential symptoms and signs appear, making accurate diagnosis possible. Although a highly communicable stage, the fastigium does not represent a serious disease control problem. Patients expose only those who serve their immediate needs because they are at home or in a hospital.

Defervescence indicates that the disease is declining in the severity of symptoms, although a relapse may occur.

Convalescence represents a recovery period. New problems in preventing disease spread arise because patients feel well enough to be up and about and consequently expose those they come in contact with.

Defection is the stage in which the pathogenic organisms are cast off. This occurs through coughing for respiratory diseases and defecating or urinating for most others. It may run concurrently with the period of convalescence. Termination of defection is the sign for the termination of isolation.

Alvine Discharge Diseases

Control of infections of the alimentary canal, or alvine discharge diseases, is essentially a problem in sanitation. Dysentery, typhoid fever, and other *Salmonella* infections are the principal alvine discharge diseases of consequence in North American and European countries. *Salmonella* infections other than typhoid fever are rarely fatal, but the incidence of such diseases is much higher than is recognized. Many cases of digestive disturbances, "intestinal flu," and "summer complaint" technically should be classed as *Salmonella* infections. Environmental control measures for alvine discharge diseases will be covered in chapters 14, 15, and 16.

Vector-borne Diseases

Vector-borne diseases are normally transmitted to humans by intermediate hosts and **vectors,** such as rodents, bats, dogs, cows, snails, birds, fleas, and ticks. The larger animals are usually intermediate hosts for the pathogen, which is then transferred to humans by vectors such as fleas, ticks, or mosquitoes. These diseases pose a far greater problem in the tropics than in Western countries, where only a few exist and then only in endemic form. Intensive campaigns in these affected geographical regions have brought such vector-borne diseases as malaria, rabies, and Rocky Mountain spotted fever under control. Lyme disease, transmitted by ticks from deer, is now endemic in the northeastern states of the United States. Community control measures for vector-borne diseases will be discussed in chapter 16.

Open Lesion Diseases

Syphilis and gonorrhea are the open lesion diseases of primary importance in community health. Infection transfer in this class of disease normally entails direct contact with the open lesion or site of infection. In addition, only certain body tissues, such as the mucous membranes, are specific for the organisms causing these diseases.

Tuberculosis and smallpox, and most venereal diseases producing skin eruptions, technically may be classed as open lesion diseases because the causative agents of these diseases leave their reservoir via the lesions of the infection.

THE CONCEPT OF ERADICATION

The fifteenth through eighteenth centuries saw the New World explored. Transportation and commerce ended the isolation of many remote areas. Smallpox epidemics followed, decimating populations. It is estimated that there were fatalities of 20

. . . .
Figure 11-4

Westward bound on ships, trains, and covered wagons, immigrants and pioneers were interrupted by immigration inspection service doctors for smallpox vaccinations. This scene was sketched on a train in 1883. (*Source: Harper's Weekly* 27:85, Feb. 10, 1883, after drawing by W. A. Rogers, after sketch by R. Davis. Courtesy: National Library of Medicine.)

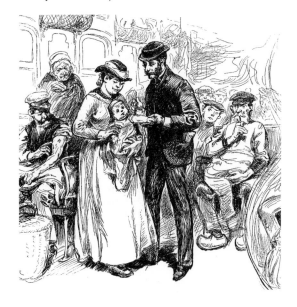

percent to 50 percent among those who contracted smallpox during the epidemics in the seventeenth and eighteenth centuries. By the middle 1700s smallpox was believed to account for 10 percent of deaths in North America and was the leading cause of infant death. Even George Washington bore the scars of smallpox.

Despite the increasingly widespread use of smallpox vaccination in the 1880s (figure 11-4) and early 1900s, the disease remained endemic throughout the world, and those who were not immune still ran a high risk of being stricken sometime during their lifetimes.

Strategy for Smallpox Eradication

The concept of worldwide eradication of smallpox gained new supporters as the disease was suc-

cessfully eliminated from North America, Europe, and a number of other countries following World War II. Travelers without evidence of smallpox vaccination were prohibited from crossing their borders. In 1959 the World Health Assembly passed a resolution directed at smallpox eradication, and the World Health Organization (WHO), UNICEF, and other organizations offered help to those countries willing to undertake mass vaccinations. It was not until 1966, however, that the commitment to worldwide eradication of smallpox was backed up with budget and bilateral agreements sufficient to make feasible the goal of eradication by 1976, accomplished in 1977 (see box on p. 316).

Mass vaccination programs were improved, and costs decreased, with the development of the jet injector gun and the bifurcated needle. Production and quality control of vaccines were also greatly improved. The enlistment of hundreds of thousands of public health workers who educated communities, detected cases, tracked down contacts, and vaccinated entire populations in areas where cases occurred contributed greatly to the success of this effort. A surveillance and containment technique moved these workers rapidly into any area in which a case was detected, sealing off the spread to other areas, isolating and treating the patient, and finding and vaccinating contacts of patients.

Global Victory and New Challenges

The last cases of smallpox in Kenya and Somalia were reported in 1977. A laboratory accident in England in 1978 produced the last verified case of smallpox. The Global Commission for the Certification of Smallpox Eradication required that a two-year period pass without any reported cases before they could declare the disease eliminated. That period ended in 1980, and the smallpox virus is considered extinct.

The expenditures for smallpox eradication from 1967 to 1979 by the international community are estimated at nearly a third of a billion dollars, a small amount in comparison to the annual costs the disease inflicted only fifty years earlier.

Milestones in Disease Eradication

1888	Charles V. Chapin proposes eradication of tuberculosis (TB).
1892	Contagious pleuropneumonia of cattle declared eradicated from United States after five-year campaign costing $5 million, begun in 1884.
1896	Rabies eradicated from England.
1901	Gen. William C. Gorgas eradicates yellow fever from Havana.
1907	Rockefeller Foundation establishes Sanitary Commission for Eradication of Hookworm Disease in the United States; eventually stimulates projects in fifty-two countries.
1915	Rockefeller Foundation establishes Yellow Fever Commission to eradicate that disease, under leadership of Gorgas. Fear of importing yellow fever to Asia via Panama Canal.
1917	Decision to eradicate bovine TB from United States.
1922	Rockefeller Foundation's hookworm campaign begins phasing out after evaluation showed little impact on transmission.
1923	Yellow fever reappears in Brazil after a year's absence.
1928–29	Outbreaks of yellow fever in Brazil, including Rio de Janeiro.
1933	Yellow fever found to be widespread in South American jungles, but absent from coastal cities.
1934	Eradication of *Aedes aegypti* mosquito in Brazil proposed.
1937	Wade Hampton Frost reports human TB was being eradicated in the United States and other countries.

1937–38	Malaria epidemics, widespread and fatal, associated with *Aedes gambiae* mosquito in Brazil.
1939–41	*Aedes gambiae* mosquito eradicated from Brazil.
1943	Bolivia was first country to proclaim eradication of *Aedes aegypti*.
1943–45	Egypt achieves eradication of *Aedes gambiae*.
1947	Pan American Health Organization (PAHO) adopts plan for eradication in the Americas of *Aedes aegypti*.
1950	Pan American Sanitary Conference approves goal of smallpox eradication and yaws eradication.
1951	Malaria eradicated from Sardinia.
1954	Global yaws eradication goal approved by World Health Organization (WHO).
1955	Global eradication of malaria goal approved by World Health Assembly (WHA) of WHO.
1958	Global eradication of smallpox goal approved by WHA.
1966	Intensified global smallpox eradication plan approved with target of 1976.
1969	Admitting impracticability of malaria eradication after spending $1.4 billion from 1955 to 1965, WHO officially changes malaria eradication policy back to malaria control.
1970	Smallpox declared eradicated from the Americas.
1975	Europe free of malaria for first time in history.
1977	Smallpox eradicated worldwide.
1978	Goal of measles eradication by 1982 set by United States.
1980	Smallpox eradication officially declared by WHO. India began

	national dracunculiasis eradication program.
1985	Goal of eradicating poliomyelitis from the Americas by 1990 declared by PAHO; Europe set measles eradication by 2000 goal.
1986	WHA declared global goal of eradicating dracunculiasis.
1988	WHA declared global goal of eradicating poliomyelitis by 2000; African Region of WHO sets 1995 goal of eradicating dracunculiasis in Africa.
1991	WHA declared goal of global dracunculiasis eradication by 1995; last case of indigenous poliomyelitis in the Americas occurred in Peru.
1993	Progress report on measles eradication goal (revised to 2000) for United States showed twenty-one states and District of Columbia had no cases, eight states had ten or more cases. Most cases imported.
1994	WHO reported poliomyelitis eradication strategy on track with only 10,000 cases globally in 1993 and an expected 6,000 to 8,000 cases in 1994. Measles cases increased in United States but still second lowest number in recorded history.
1996	No new polio, no new diphtheria, declines in measles, mumps, and pertussis cases in United States.

Poliomyelitis

Ten years after the eradication of smallpox, enthusiasm began to build about the possibility of achieving the same victory with polio (table 11-3). The World Health Organization has proposed plans for attempting to eliminate polio from the globe by the year 2000. The effort will succeed only if progress is maintained in building immunization levels and other health services around the world. The effort of the Pan American Health Organization to eradicate polio in the Americas by 1990 succeeded in North America and then the following year in Latin America with the final cases reported from Peru in 1991. The feature of polio that will make it more difficult to eradicate is that transmission of polio is far less visible than that of smallpox. Only one in every 100 people who contract the polio virus ever show any major paralytic symptoms. Many people can be spreading the disease without anyone realizing contagion is happening. This means that immunization levels must be much closer to 100 percent. Eradication is technically feasible, but would be greatly facilitated by development of a vaccine that requires fewer doses or is more heat stable. WHO estimates that the costs of eradicating poliomyelitis will be about $1.1 billion (United States dollars).

Measles

Some 1 million persons die annually from measles. Most of them are infants and young children. Hope of wiping out measles was inspired in the 1980s by the near zero level of reported cases in some countries, including Canada and the United States. The disease rebounded in 1990, dashing hopes of eradication. Measles is more visible in most cases than polio, and is harbored only in human hosts, so the isolation and surrounding of cases with a buffer zone of immunized people is technically possible as it was in the smallpox campaign. Measles and polio, and diphtheria and pertussis reduction, will benefit from the global effort to achieve universal childhood immunization in the developing world. Unfortunately, measles has not been eliminated from any large country. The ineffectiveness of the vaccine for infants at birth or soon after and the highly contagious spread of the disease by airborne droplets exhaled by infected persons remain major barriers to eradication.

Tuberculosis

Following several decades of decline in the number and rate of tuberculosis (TB) cases, this ancient scourge of populations rose again in North America in the late 1980s. This was attributed in part to the influx of immigrants from refugee camps in Asia and other refugees from Central America. After declining steadily from over 50 cases per 100,000 in 1950 to less than 10 in 1984, the rate in the United States rose again, especially in Asian-American populations, until 1992 (figure 11-5). Almost 70 percent of TB cases and 86 percent of those among children up to 15 years old occurred among racial and ethnic minorities. Homeless and low-income persons and those with HIV or AIDS are particularly susceptible. Adverse social and economic factors have contributed to the rise, as has the immigration of persons with tuberculosis.

The goal of eradicating tuberculosis is achievable in North America, although it is not achievable on a global level. The strategy should include

- initiating public awareness campaigns to alert communities about the increasing TB problems;
- training and educating public and private health-care providers in the skills needed to relate effectively to the at-risk communities being served, and empowering at-risk populations with knowledge and other resources needed to influence the TB programs directed toward their communities;
- building coalitions to help design and implement intensified community TB prevention and control efforts;
- intensifying the screening of at-risk populations for TB and tuberculous infection (skin tests) and providing appropriate treatment;

Table 11-3

Diseases Considered as Candidates for Global Eradication by the International Task Force for Disease Eradication

Disease	Current annual toll worldwide	Chief obstacles to eradication	Conclusion
Diseases targeted for eradication			
Dracunculiasis (Guinea worm disease)	<2 million persons infected; few deaths	Lack of public and political awareness; inadequate funding	Eradicable
Poliomyelitis	100,000 cases of paralytic disease; 10,000 deaths	No insurmountable technical obstacles; increased national/ international commitment needed	Eradicable
Lymphatic filariasis	80 million cases	Need better tools for monitoring infection	Potentially eradicable
Mumps	Unknown	Lack of data on impact in developing countries; difficult diagnosis	Potentially eradicable
Rubella	Unknown	Lack of data on impact in developing countries; difficult diagnosis	Potentially eradicable
Taeniasis/ cysticercosis (pork tapeworm)	50 million cases; 50,000 deaths	Need simpler diagnostics for humans and pigs	Potentially eradicable
Diseases/conditions of which some aspect could be eliminated			
Hepatitis B	250,000 deaths	Carrier state, infections in utero not preventable; need routine infant vaccination	Not now eradicable, but could eliminate transmission over several decades
Iodine deficiency disorders	Unknown	Inadequate surveillance, lack of environmental sources of iodine	Could eliminate iodine deficiency disorders
Neonatal tetanus	560,000 deaths	Inexhaustible environmental reservoir	Not now eradicable, but could prevent transmission
Onchocerciasis (river blindness)	18 million cases 340,000 blind	High cost of vector control; no therapy to kill adult worms; restrictions in mass use of ivermectin	Could eliminate associated blindness
Rabies	52,000 deaths	No effective way to deliver vaccine to wild animals that carry the disease	Could eliminate urban rabies
Trachoma	500 million cases; 6–8 million blind	Linked to poverty, ubiquitous microbe	Could eliminate blindness
Yaws and other endemic treponematoses	2.5 million cases	Political and financial inertia	Could interrupt transmission*

*Because persons may be infected for decades and the organisms cannot be distinguished from those that cause venereal syphilis, elimination of transmission—not eradication—is the goal.

Source: Recommendations of the International Task Force for Disease Eradication, *MMWR* 42:Suppl.RR-16, Dec. 31, 1993.

· · · · · · · · · · · · · · · · · · · ·

Figure 11-5

The trend since 1950 in tuberculosis rates in the United States showed a steady decline from 50 cases per 100,000 population. The rate began to rise again in 1984. Rates continued to rise to 1992. The year 2000 objective is based on an extrapolation from the earlier trend (regression) line. (*Source:* National Center for Health Statistics: *Healthy People 2000 review, 1995–96,* Hyattsville, MD, 1996, Public Health Service, p. 19.)

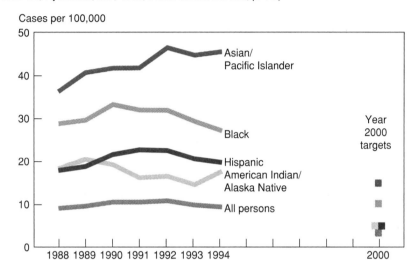

- increasing the speed and completeness of reporting suspected cases to health departments; and
- improving the availability and quality of TB health care services in socioeconomically disadvantaged areas.

Tropical diseases

Table 11-3 lists some of the other candidates on the list for global eradication. Guinea worm disease (dracunculiasis) eradication is feasible if the necessary commitment and resources can be mobilized. Great progress has been made in Africa since WHO declared a goal of eradicating this disease globally, the first such goal since the smallpox campaign. By educating infected villagers who bathe in stream water to keep their open sores out of the water and others to strain the water they drink from infected streams, the

life cycle of the guinea worm can be broken (figure 11-6).

Table 11-4 lists the major criteria in considering whether any disease is potentially eradicable. Four factors that made smallpox eradication possible must be taken into account: (1) No reservoir of the virus existed except in humans. This makes rabies, for example, a poor candidate. (2) Nearly all persons infected with smallpox had an obvious, distinguishable rash. This is what makes TB most difficult to eradicate. (3) Smallpox made people infectious for a relatively short period. (4) The natural infection, even without vaccination, left most people immune for a lifetime. This is not the case with most other diseases. (5) A safe, effective, and inexpensive vaccine was available. It was also highly stable in tropical environments. Many vaccines require refrigeration, which is difficult to arrange in many remote areas.

••••••••••••••••••••

Figure 11-6

The life cycle of *Dracunculus medinensis,* the cause of guinea worm disease, targeted by WHO for eradication by 1995, suggests the points of intervention to interrupt the cycle of infection. (*Source:* Hopkins, D. R., and E. Ruiz-Tiben. 1992. Surveillance for Dracunculiasis, 1981–1991. In CDC Surveillance Summaries, *MMWR* 41:3.)

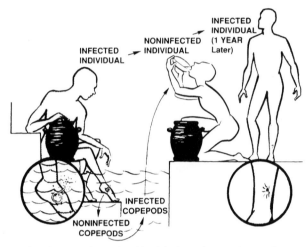

- The mature female worm pierces the skin of the lower leg, causing an ulcer.
- When the ulcer comes in contact with water, the female worm discharges larvae into the water.
- Cyclopoid copepods (small fresh-water crustaceans) become infected by ingesting the larvae.
- Humans drink the water contaminated with the infected copepods.
- The ingested larvae mature in humans in 1 year.

Table 11-4

Criteria for Assessing Eradicability of Diseases and Conditions

Scientific Feasibility
- Epidemiologic vulnerability (e.g., existence of nonhuman reservoir; ease of spread; natural cyclical decline in prevalence; naturally induced immunity; ease of diagnosis; and duration of any relapse potential)
- Effective, practical intervention available (e.g., vaccine or other primary preventive, curative treatment, and means of eliminating vector). Ideally, intervention should be effective, safe, inexpensive, long-lasting, and easily deployed.
- Demonstrated feasibility of elimination (e.g., documented elimination from island or other geographic unit)

Political Will/Popular Support
- Perceived burden of the disease (e.g., extent, deaths, other effects; true burden may not be perceived; the reverse of benefits expected to accrue from eradication; relevance to rich and poor countries).
- Expected cost of eradication (especially in relation to perceived burden from the disease).
- Synergy of eradication efforts with other interventions (e.g., potential for added benefits or savings or spin-off effects)
- Necessity for eradication rather than control

Source: Centers for Disease Control & Prevention. Recommendations of the International Task Force for Disease Eradication. *MMWR* 42:RR-16, 1992.

··················

Figure 11-7

Rates of acquired immunodeficiency syndrome (AIDS) cases for selected countries, 1994 (*Source:* Health Canada, Division of HIV/AIDS Epidemiology, Laboratory Centre for Disease Control, *Quarterly surveillance update: AIDS in Canada,* Jan. 1995.)

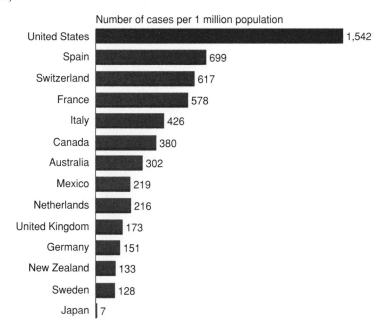

Number of cases per 1 million population

United States	1,542
Spain	699
Switzerland	617
France	578
Italy	426
Canada	380
Australia	302
Mexico	219
Netherlands	216
United Kingdom	173
Germany	151
New Zealand	133
Sweden	128
Japan	7

SEXUALLY TRANSMITTED DISEASES

The major sexually transmitted diseases (STDs)—syphilis, gonorrhea, herpes, chlamydia, and HIV/AIDS—present different clinical and epidemiological patterns. The methodology for syphilis and gonorrhea control has been developed over a long time and has been demonstrated to be effective in reducing the incidence of disease when rigorously applied. Control methods for herpes, chlamydia, and AIDS are still in earlier stages of development.

Acquired Immunodeficiency Syndrome (AIDS)

AIDS brought fear and panic with its sudden appearance and spread in North America, its high mortality rate, and its dramatic debilitation and complications in the few years of life following diagnosis. The death rate for cases discovered in the early 1980s was virtually 100 percent. The full-blown AIDS syndrome includes severe fatigue, persistent cough accompanied often by shortness of breath, persistent diarrhea, persistent white coating or spots inside the mouth or throat, often accompanied by soreness and difficulty of swallowing, purple or brown lumps or spots on the skin. Eventually nervous system impairment occurs, including loss of memory, inability to think clearly, and depression.

The devastating statistics, represented in figure 11-7, are the tip of an iceberg. For every case of AIDS, five to ten times as many people (up to 2.7 million in the United States) have been infected with AIDS-related Complex (ARC). These people suffer some symptoms of AIDS such as enlarged lymph glands, night sweats, and fevers. These may

ISSUES AND CONTROVERSIES
The AIDS Controversy

The pressure on governmental agencies to exercise their police power in matters of health grows intense when the community feels threatened by a new, mysterious, socially stigmatized or frightening disease. Such was the case with the enforced isolation of lepers in the Middle Ages. Such was the case in the 1970s and 1980s with the fear concerning Legionnaires' disease, herpes, and HIV/AIDS. More than 76 percent of the AIDS patients diagnosed before July 1982 had died by mid-1984. Homosexual or bisexual men continue to be, by far, the group at highest risk for the disorder, with 72 percent of the cases occurring in this group. Intravenous drug users make up 17 percent of the cases. The disease evokes more fear and punitive reaction than sympathy, at least in conservative communities.

Even in progressive San Francisco, the controversy over the closing of bathhouses—meeting places for homosexual encounters—led to the resignation of the city and county health officer. In Houston, the city council was forced to place a referendum on the ballot, which allowed the public to vote down a controversial ordinance protecting homosexuals from discrimination in city hiring. An antihomosexual psychologist has suggested that homosexuals be required to stay in their homes until a cure or a vaccine for HIV/AIDS is found. Many states have laws that would empower public health officials to quarantine people who have been exposed to a communicable disease and even to force them to undergo treatment. These laws, however, have seldom been used to quarantine entire groups,

only individuals known to have been exposed. Large-scale quarantines would raise constitutional questions concerning an individual's right to due process and hearings before being placed in custody. Quarantines are more common in institutions such as prisons or boarding schools where many people live in close proximity. The only instances in recent years of entire groups being quarantined have been on ships arriving in port with passengers discovered to have cholera.

If homosexuals were to be quarantined, what about hemophiliacs and other minority groups with higher-than-average rates of HIV/AIDS? Where would you draw the line in evoking the police power of the state in controlling communicable diseases?

---

last for years with a general decline in health, but without developing the full-blown AIDS syndrome.

Deeper still beneath the tip of the iceberg are another 50 to 100 times the number of reported cases, 14 million to 27 million people, who will have been exposed to the AIDS virus and remain healthy carriers of the virus that causes AIDS, the human immunodeficiency virus (HIV). These people may not know they carry the virus unless they have been tested, and so they continue to spread the disease to other people.

In addition to the sexual transmission of HIV/AIDS through virus-infected semen, especially during anal intercourse, AIDS is spreading rapidly among drug users who share needles with partners who infected the needle with virus-infected lymphocytes in their blood (see figure 11-1).

Syphilis and Gonorrhea

Syphilis control involves the reporting of cases, treatment, and follow-up and patient interviews for contact information. Named partners are traced, tested, and treated to interrupt the transmission of disease within the community. The basic technique in syphilis control is contact investigation. Decreases in the rates of syphilis and gonorrhea are attributed in part to changing sexual practices, but also to the aging of the baby boom generation.

The major thrust of gonorrhea control programs is screening by bacteriological culture of all females for asymptomatic gonococcal infection, followed by prompt treatment if they are infected. The examples of syphilis and gonorrhea illustrate the difficulty of prevention and control of sexually transmitted disease, even when the cause is known.

Figure 11-8

Four of the fifteen 10-year Healthy People 2000 objectives for sexually transmitted diseases had been achieved by mid-decade, most of the rest were on track toward being accomplished, but three had gone the wrong direction. Tracking data for 2 of the 15 objectives were unavailable. (*Source: Healthy People 2000 midcourse review and 1995 revisions,* Washington, DC, 1995; U.S. Department of Health and Human Services; Public Health Services.)

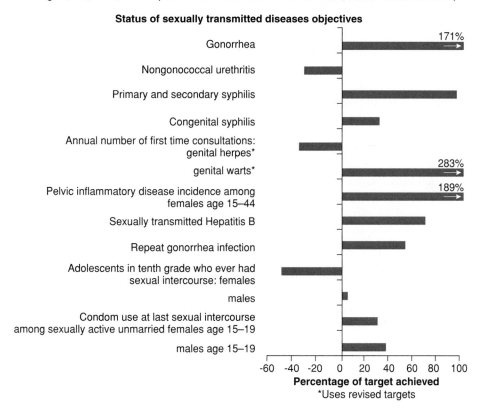

Status of sexually transmitted diseases objectives

The pathogenic organisms are sensitive to drugs, yet behavioral factors are involved that complicate control. Between 1965 and 1975, the number of reported cases of gonorrhea in the United States tripled. Since 1975, however, reported cases have leveled off, with a steady decrease since 1985. The reduction goal for the year 2000 has been exceeded by more than 70 percent (figure 11-8).

Herpes and Genital Warts

Genital herpes infections are very common, with an incidence of one-half to one million new cases an-

nually, with several million recurrences each year. For this painful condition, periodic recurrences are the rule. Herpes-complicated pregnancies often result in spontaneous abortion, stillbirth, or severe neonatal infection; neonatal herpes results in death or permanent disability in two-thirds of the cases.

Hepatitis B

Hepatitis B is caused by a virus transmitted by shared needles, sex, or birth. Homosexual males are at very high risk; nearly 60 percent attending clinics for sexually transmitted disease show evidence of past or present hepatitis B infection. This same population is also at high risk of several other sexually transmitted diseases, including HIV/AIDS, amebiasis, and giardiasis.

Prevention-Promotion Measures

Educational Measures The most fundamental component of a community program to control sexually transmitted diseases is education and training. This includes clinical experience in schools for health professionals; education and information about sexually transmitted diseases for school children before and during the time they are at highest risk; preservice and continuing professional education for health care providers and health educators to deal with sexually transmitted diseases in a confidential, nonjudgmental fashion; and improved public understanding of sexually transmitted disease risks and confidentiality of treatment through effective and continuous campaigns using mass media. Educational measures may be mass directed or may be targeted to special groups such as women, children, homosexual and bisexual men, adolescents, minorities, populations with special language needs, and specific high-risk groups. They may include the counseling of patients being treated for sexually transmitted diseases regarding complications and measures to avoid future infection.

Education is all the more critical to the control of viral STDs because the diseases are not curable. Treatment cannot break the cycle of transmission as it can for syphilis and gonorrhea.

The U.S. Congress, recognizing the importance of education as the "single most effective means available today to slow the spread of the AIDS epidemic," has approved over $1 billion for AIDS research, education, and control each year since 1989. State health agencies also spent increasing amounts with the largest proportion (26 percent) going to education.

Service Measures The second level of community strategy is the provision of diagnostic and treatment services for patients with sexually trans-

mitted diseases and their complications. Also included in secondary prevention and control are detection and referral methods, such as counseling infected patients and tracing and treating their contacts; screening for selected sexually transmitted diseases; and encouraging joint availability of services among related programs such as those for sexually transmitted diseases, family planning, and maternal and child health.

A highly controversial but apparently effective service, implemented in many European and Canadian communities but only in a few U.S. communities, is the provision of new, sterile needles to intravenous drug (IVD) users. This strategy is referred to as a "harm reduction strategy" because its goal is not the elimination of all harm but rather the reduction of the worst harm. The theory behind needle exchange programs is that IVD users will not be easily stopped from using intravenous drugs, so it is better to protect them and others who might share needles with them by providing sterile needles than to do nothing to prevent Hepatitis B or HIV/AIDS in this population.

Technological Measures Properly used, condoms are the best known measure for persons engaging in sexual activity to avoid acquiring or transmitting many of the sexually transmitted diseases, including HIV/AIDS. A vaccine for hepatitis B is being tested for efficacy; vaccines for gonorrhea and genital herpes are at an earlier stage of development. A vaccine for HIV/AIDS is unlikely to be ready for use in the near future.

Legislative and Regulatory Measures Community agencies need to determine the magnitude of the sexually transmitted disease problem and to establish objectives for inclusion in their annual implementation plans. Health planning agencies need to make certain that the health plan for the community addresses gaps in education and service delivery regarding sexually transmitted diseases. Other regulatory activities to support community control might include the examination by certifying agencies or other regulatory boards of health professionals' knowledge of sexually transmitted diseases and competency in dealing with such diseases; the repeal of statutes and ordinances that inhibit the advertising, display, sale, or distribution of condoms; and regulations requiring information about sexually transmitted diseases as part of school health education programs.

Economic Measures The two most needed economic supports for sexually transmitted disease services in the U.S. are (1) prevention-related activities that are exempted from coinsurance or deductible provisions of health insurance, and (2) prepaid health plans with financial incentives for sexually transmitted disease prevention activities, including management of persons who have had sexual contact with the affected person and who are not members of the plan.

THE MICROBIOLOGY OF CAUSATIVE AGENTS

A pathogen is a poor parasite because it arouses the host. It is analogous to a burglar awakening the household on which he is preying. The response of the host is usually a defense reaction, chemical or immunological. Host resistance is the key to preventing disease from those pathogens that cannot be eliminated from the environment.

Infecting Organisms

Most organisms pathogenic to the human species belong to the plant kingdom, specifically to the phylum Thallophyta. Bacteria constitute the greatest number of pathogenic organisms. Rickettsiae are small bacteria, and viruses are ultramicroscopic forms. Certain true funguses, including the molds, are also pathogenic to humans; they may produce infestations (such as athlete's foot) and infections (such as valley fever) in that they live *on* the body and *in* the body. In the animal kingdom certain protozoa and a few metazoa are pathogens of humans. For the purposes of community health, a classification that can be readily applied to existing conditions, such as in table 11-5, is most useful.

Specificity of Infecting Organisms A typhoid bacillus is derived only from a preexisting typhoid bacillus. The virility but not the species may change from generation to generation of a particular type of organism. The severity of the reaction the organism produces in human hosts may rise or subside with subsequent generations of the organism, but the pathogen's action will always be similar in its basic nature. In addition to having specific action, many organisms are harmful only to specific types of human tissue. This basic tendency of pathogens to be specific accounts for the manner in which the organism functions and for the reaction it produces in the host. In some respects the diphtheria bacillus may resemble the typhoid bacillus and in some respects they may produce similar reactions in the host, but the two different organisms have definite identities. This specificity of infecting organisms is a universal phenomenon.

Mode of Action Most pathogens injure human tissue by the toxins they produce; in their normal metabolic processes these pathogens generate substances that happen to be injurious to certain human tissues. Some organisms—for example, the diphtheria bacillus—produce toxins that diffuse through the permeable membrane of the bacterium and for this reason are called exotoxins. Other pathogens—for example, the typhoid bacillus—produce toxins that do not diffuse through the impermeable membrane that encloses the organism and for this reason are called endotoxins. When an organism of this type dies, its enclosing membrane undergoes changes that make it permeable to the toxins.

A small proportion of pathogens invade body tissues directly. Some of the protozoa, such as the malaria plasmodium and the spirochete of syphilis, and some viruses and rickettsiae invade human cells, causing cellular change and sometimes destruction. The AIDS virus (HIV) specifically attacks white blood cells, undermining the body's immune system.

Table 11-5

Examples of Diseases Classified by their Means of Pathogen Transmission

Indirect contact			
Airborne	**Water- and food-borne**	**Vector-borne**	**Direct contact**
Anthrax	Botulism[†]	Dracunculiasis	AIDS*
Cerebrospinal meningitis* ‖	Brucellosis[†]	Glanders[†]§	Anthrax[†]
Chickenpox*	Cholera*	Hanta virus	Brucellosis[†]
Encephalomyelitis, equine[†]	Diphtheria*	Jaundice, infective*	Chlamydia*
Influenza*	Dracunculiasis	Lyme disease	Gonorrhea*
Legionellosis*	Dysentery, bacillary*	Malaria*	Herpes ‖
Measles*	Hoof-and-mouth diseases‡§	Onchocerciasis	Rabies[†]
Mumps*	Poliomyelitis* ‖	Plague*	Smallpox*
Pneumonia[†]	Schistosomiasis	Relapsing fever*	Syphilis*
Psittacosis[†]	Streptococcus*	Rocky Mountain spotted fever*‡	Tetanus*
Tuberculosis[†]	Tuberculosis[†]	Tularemia*	Tuberculosis[†]
Typhus fever*‡	Tularemia*	Typhus fever*§	Tularemia*
	Typhoid fever*	Yellow fever*§	

*Infects humans only.
[†]Infects humans and animals useful to humans.
‡Infects animals or birds only.
§Artificially transmissible by air in laboratory.
‖ Means of transmission unknown.

Reservoirs of Infection

Pathogens are relatively fragile organisms that survive only in a highly selective medium. A reported case of a new host for a particular type of organism means that the organism had been harbored in a medium favorable to the organism's survival, multiplication, and functioning. The medium in which organisms are thus harbored usually must have moisture, a relatively high temperature, nutrients, and an absence of light. Most reservoirs of organisms that affect people are living hosts that provide an excellent medium for harboring these pathogens. However, soil can be the reservoir for some pathogens, such as the tetanus bacillus.

Human Reservoirs   The human body is the greatest reservoir of organisms pathogenic to other human beings (figure 11-9). This is the genesis of the time-tested question asked when a new case of disease is discovered—"Where is the other case?" Thus the human reservoir is the source of the greatest danger of infection. **Frank cases,** or persons obviously ill with a disease, are not of much danger to a community. Although the individual who nurses the ill person may be greatly exposed to the disease and therefore endangered, the community can be effectively protected by isolation of the identified ill person or other means of preventing transfer of infection from the known reservoir to other possible hosts. **Subclinical infections,** variously referred to as missed or ambulatory cases, constitute a reservoir of great danger to the community because the affected individuals usually continue their normal daily routines. An ambulatory patient with diphtheria, scarlet fever, or dysentery could unknowingly infect a considerable number of people before the source of the new cases of the disease was located. **Carriers** are individuals who harbor and disseminate a pathogenic organism without themselves experiencing recognizable symptoms. "Typhoid Mary" was a carrier who became

Figure 11-9

Other human beings represent the reservoir of most pathogens, including the HIV pathogen. Condoms can protect a person from infection from others. This AIDS campaign ad reminds the public of this simple fact. (*Source:* Public Health Service, U.S. Department of Health and Human Services.)

USING IT WON'T KILL YOU. NOT USING IT MIGHT.

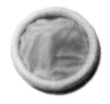

Maybe you don't like using condoms. But if you're going to have sex, a latex condom with a spermicide is your best protection against the AIDS virus.

Use them every time, from start to finish, according to the manufacturers' directions. Because no one has ever been cured of AIDS. More than 40,000 Americans have already died from it.

And even if you don't like condoms, using them is definitely better than that.

HELP STOP AIDS. USE A CONDOM.

infamous because her job as a food handler made her a source of infection for large numbers of people. The longer the duration of the carrier status, the greater the danger to the community. Chronic or permanent carriers pose the most considerable threat; however, once they are identified, control measures can be instituted that will minimize or nearly remove the danger of communicating the disease to others. A convalescent carrier or transient carrier also can be a serious danger to those in the immediate environment. The distribution of AIDS cases shown in figure 11-10 reflects the approximate distribution of human reservoirs for spread of the HIV infection.

Lower Animal Reservoirs   Only a few species of lower animals harbor organisms pathogenic to human beings, and these are principally domestic animals. However, rodents and certain other wild animals also serve as reservoirs of organisms that produce disease in humans. Society has the necessary means to protect the human species against diseases such as anthrax from sheep and cattle; glanders and tetanus from horses; hoof-and-mouth disease from cattle; brucellosis and tapeworm from cattle, swine, and goats; tuberculosis from cattle; trichinosis from swine; psittacosis from parrots and parakeets; rabies from rodents, canines, and bats; toxoplasmosis from cats; Lyme disease from deer; and Rocky Mountain spotted fever, hanta virus, and tularemia from rodents.

Schistosomiasis, the most prevalent of the serious diseases in this category, is an organ-damaging and sometimes fatal disease. It is caused by a parasitic worm whose life cycle takes it from snail to water to human, during which time it grows to be up to one inch long, lays vast numbers of eggs, and has sexual unions that can last thirty years or more. The eggs of the threadlike parasite hatch in humans, are passed through stools and often end up in fresh water where they develop into larvae. This preadult form searches out and infects a snail (the disease is sometimes called snail fever), only to be released again into water where it must burrow into a host within

· ·

Figure 11-10

Reservoirs of HIV as reflected by the distribution of reported adult cases of AIDS, by patient group, Canada, 1994. (*Source:* Health Canada. *Quarterly surveillance: AIDS in Canada,* 1995.)

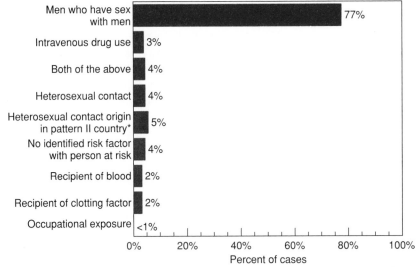

*Countries in which the predominant means of transmission is heterosexual contact

twenty-four hours or die. Damage to human hosts is caused by the great number of eggs produced by the adult worm. The eggs eventually lodge in the liver, causing a nonalcoholic and reversible form of cirrhosis of the liver. Effects also include infection of the bladder and kidney and a slow sapping of energy.

Prevalent in developing countries where water supplies are not adequately treated by modern purification methods and where lifestyles and economics limit hygiene, schistosomiasis is one of the scourges of the Third World. Over 200 million people suffer from this disease, and its devastating effects have been felt throughout the Middle East, Africa, Latin America, the Caribbean, and Asia far more than HIV/AIDS. Health education campaigns to control schistosomiasis have had to struggle against time-honored cultural and agricultural practices that cannot be easily challenged, especially in the face of economic hardships.

Escape of Organisms from Reservoir   That a particular pathogen is harbored in a particular host is important from the standpoint of controlling disease spread, but the organism must escape from the reservoir if other potential hosts are to be endangered. For some diseases, the person harboring the causative agent represents no danger or poses a threat only under most unusual circumstances. For example, a person with trichinosis could endanger only the health of a cannibal, because the causative agent of trichinosis, living in the skeletal muscle of the human, has no avenue of escape. Likewise, under ordinary circumstances a person who has an active case of malaria or who is a carrier does not pose a threat to others, since the causative agent of malaria normally does not escape from the reservoir that harbors it. This pathogen can reach another host only via the female Anopheles mosquito, a blood transfusion, or the sharing of a hypodermic needle by drug users.

The avenues by which pathogens escape from the human body are shown in table 11-4. The avenue of escape depends on the site of infection. The respiratory tract is the most common and most dangerous avenue of escape. While an individual harbors an infection of the respiratory tract, escape of the organism is a continuous process by such means as droplets from coughs and sneezes, eating utensils, or the human hands. Escape via the intestinal tract would be through discharges of the colon and the urinary tract. With HIV/AIDS, other body fluids such as semen and blood have been implicated. Open lesions provide an easy means of escape. With tubercle bacilli this is true whether it is a lesion of lung tissue or of the surface of the body. Tiny, imperceptible tears in the delicate tissues of the rectum provide the open lesion for the spread of HIV/AIDS from the semen of the host into the blood stream of a new host during anal intercourse. Likewise, the open lesions of syphilis, gonorrhea, and common furunculosis (boils) allow the pathogens that produce the lesion to leave the body. Mechanical escape of organisms from the human body is possible by insects or other animals that bite or suck. Here the organism is aided by a specific vector, or intermediate host. This is illustrated by figure 11-11 for schistosomiasis, transmitted by the snail.

Another example is onchocerciasis, carried by the blackfly. It breeds in fast-flowing rivers, hence the name "river blindness." The process begins when the blackfly bites an infected human and picks up the premature form (microfilariae) of the worm *Onchocerca volvulus*. The premature worm develops inside the blackfly, which then infects another person with the larvae. In the new human host, the infective worm matures, becoming an adult that survives for years and reaches over two feet in length while it produces millions of microfilariae. Severely infected people suffer disfiguring skin changes, chronic itching, and various eye lesions that lead eventually to total blindness.

Preventing the organism from escaping from the reservoir obviously provides one means of communicable disease control. Efforts must be based on microbiological knowledge of the nature of the organism and epidemiological knowledge of the specific avenue through which it must escape to spread to a new host.

THE EPIDEMIOLOGY OF INFECTION

Once the organism has escaped from the reservoir it must be transferred to a new host if a new case of the disease is to occur or if the organism is to survive and spread. The normal pathogens of humans do not walk, run, swim, or fly. They must be transported by some vehicle. This transfer can be effected from person to person either directly or indirectly (table 11-4 and figure 11-12).

Direct Transmission

Organisms can be transmitted directly from one person to another without an intermediate object. This usually requires intimate association, but not necessarily physical contact. Therefore coughing and sneezing can be a direct means of transmitting organisms from one person to another without physical contact being involved. This accounts for the high incidence of respiratory diseases in crowded living areas. Proper handwashing can reduce the transfer of most respiratory and intestinal diseases.

Indirect Transmission

When an intermediate object is involved in the transmission of disease from the reservoir to a new host, the mechanism is classed as indirect transmission. Such a transfer can occur with no particular close relationship between the reservoir and the new host. There are, however, two basic requirements for indirect transmission. The first is that the organisms involved must be virile enough to survive a long time outside a living body. Therefore highly resistant organisms such as those causing typhoid, tetanus, and anthrax are most likely to be transmitted by indirect means. On the other hand, highly fragile organisms such as those causing meningitis, syphilis, and gonorrhea are less

····················

Figure 11-11

Life cycle of schistosomes: a complex cycle involving alternate human and water-borne snail hosts. Some 200 million people in 76 countries are affected by schistosomiasis, which can lead to scarring and tissue destruction of internal organs. A patient can be cured for less than $1.00, but the rate of reinfection is high as people return to the same unsanitary streams and ponds. (*Source:* Courtesy National Institutes of Health, U.S. Department of Health and Human Services.)

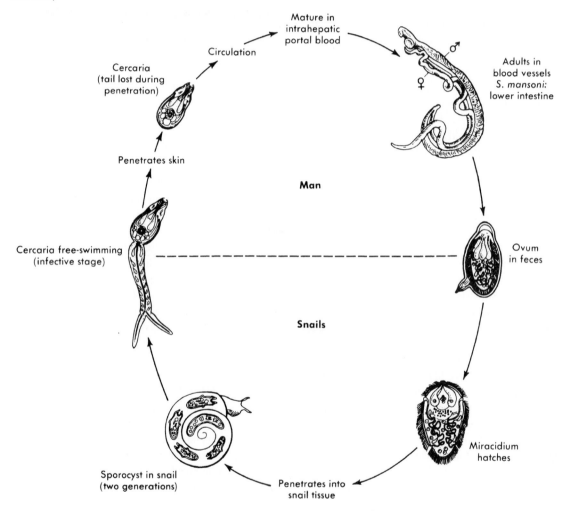

Figure 11-12

Routes over which diseases travel. The blocking of routes prevents pathogens from reaching potential susceptible new hosts.

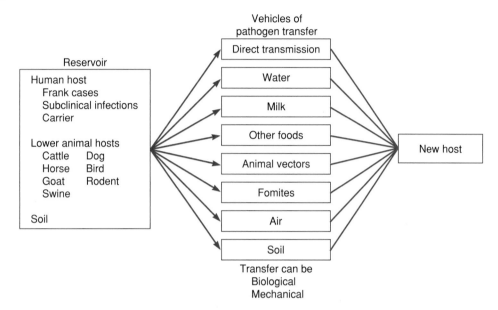

likely to be transmitted by an intermediate object except under very unusual survival circumstances. A second requirement for indirect transfer of infection is a favorable vehicle of transmission. It may be a specific living form of life, such as a mosquito, or a highly favorable substance for growth of the pathogen, such as milk. In a high proportion of diseases that can be transmitted by indirect means, the pathogen involved requires a specific medium for its survival.

Vehicles of Transfer

The expression "vehicles of pathogen transfer" refers to the objects that make the transfer from the reservoir to a new host. They might also be referred to as routes of infection so far as they represent certain pathways by which the organisms are transferred. Vehicles of transfer may be animate or inanimate.

Vectors   Animate vehicles are spoken of as vectors. These intermediate hosts of the organism represent the connecting link between one case of a disease and a susceptible new host. Transfer by vectors can be either biological or mechanical. In a biological transfer the organism spends part of its life cycle in the body of the intermediate host, as illustrated by the Schistosome in figure 11-11. Biological vectors are specific for specific diseases. Malaria is transmitted only by the female *Anopheles* mosquito, yellow fever by the *Aedes aegypti* mosquito, typhus fever by the louse, plague by the flea, schistosomiasis by the snail, river blindness by the blackfly, and Lyme disease and Rocky Mountain spotted fever by the ticks. When a vector makes possible the mechanical transfer of organisms, such species-specific action does not prevail. In this instance the vector comes in contact with infectious agents that mechanically become attached to the vector's body, legs, or other parts as with the transfer of fleas and ticks by a variety of rodents and other mammals.

A vector that normally produces a biological transfer may also effect a mechanical transfer. Normally, the Anopheles mosquito harbors the plasmodium of malaria for about fourteen days while the pathogen goes through a life cycle. The resulting young forms are then introduced into a host. This biological transfer, however, can be short-circuited. The Anopheles mosquito can get some blood from feeding on a human being with malaria, leave this reservoir, and immediately attach to a new host, where the organisms from the original reservoir can be "mechanically" introduced. HIV has not been found to spread by this means.

Theoretically it would be possible to eliminate disease transfer via vectors, but it is not practicable. Epidemiology knows how these vectors operate and how they can be destroyed, but given their almost limitless number, public health has to concentrate on their destruction and control in specific geographical areas or populations with a high incidence of vector-borne diseases.

If an inanimate object is to serve as a vehicle of pathogen transfer it must have certain characteristics; otherwise, the organism will not survive the interval between the time it comes into contact with the object and the time it is transmitted to the new host. If the organism is to survive and remain sufficiently virile to set up a new infection, the time interval during which most organisms are carried by the medium must be relatively short. The medium must be moist, bland, warm (near 100° F, or 38° C), and exist in relative darkness. Water, milk, other foods, air, fomites, and soil are the classes of inanimate vehicles of disease transfer (figure 11-12).

Water Water serves as a medium for the transfer of organisms from the human alimentary tract. Typhoid, paratyphoid, cholera, and bacillary dysentery are examples of diseases spread via water. Although pathogens normally do not multiply in water, an organism such as the typhoid bacillus can live for two or three weeks in relatively cool water. Public health has developed the necessary measures to protect communities against disease transmission via water. Filtration and chlorination of community water supplies have been effective in controlling water-borne diseases.

Milk Milk is an excellent medium for several organisms pathogenic to people. Contamination of milk can come from three sources. The first is infection within the udder from a disease of the cow, such as brucellosis or bovine tuberculosis. The second is infection within the udder by organisms accidentally introduced into the udder by a human being. Septic sore throat and scarlet fever are examples of diseases resulting from this type of contamination. The third type is direct contamination of the milk by a human being after it has left the cow. Thus a milk handler harboring diphtheria, typhoid, or dysentery bacilli may introduce the organism into the milk in the course of milk processing. Through herd testing, dairy sanitation, and pasteurization, public health has been able to prevent the spread of infectious disease via the vehicle of milk.

Other Foods Other foods can be a means of transmitting pathogens but are not offenders as often as the lay public believes. For solid foods to serve as a vehicle of disease transfer, they must be moist, nonacid, not (adequately) cooked, or handled after cooking. Time is also a factor: if a clerk in a bake shop, through handling, should leave dysentery bacilli on baked goods, the likelihood is remote that these few organisms would survive until the pastries were eaten.

There are three common sources of contamination in food. The first is food handlers conveying organisms to food by coughing or by their hands. The second is contamination during growth, as when shellfish develop in a body of water contaminated with typhoid bacilli. The third is when the food comes from infected animals that transmit such diseases as trichinosis and tapeworm. Here, however, proper cooking would destroy pathogens.

Indeed, in most cases, this is the key to protection against transfer via the common foods. Boiling or heating to the boiling point for a time will destroy the usual pathogens that may be transferred via food. HIV/AIDS has never been found to spread by water, milk, or other food vehicles.

Air The dryness, low temperature, and light of the air are highly unfavorable to most pathogenic organisms. Droplets from sneezing and coughing may give pathogens a moist vehicle that will help them survive long enough to set up an infection if they are inhaled into the respiratory passage of a new host. Measles and chickenpox appear to be more readily transmitted by this means than any of the other known respiratory diseases. Generally, however, air is not a principal vehicle of disease transfer. A cubic foot of air may contain a considerable number of pathogens, but they would be so attenuated before being inhaled into a person's respiratory tract that the likelihood that they could cause an infection in the new host is slight.

Fomites Inanimate objects other than water, milk, food, air, and soil that might be vehicles of disease transfer are called **fomites.** The term embraces such things as clothing, bed linen, books, toys, handrails, and similar objects. Fomites are no longer regarded as major vehicles of disease transfer because they do not provide a good medium for pathogens. However, disease spread can occur if a susceptible person handles an object immediately after it has been contaminated and then touches his or her mouth, nose, or eyes. Needle punctures following use by an infected person can transmit pathogens from the blood stream of one person directly to the bloodstream of another. Increasing use of disposable items in medical and nursing care minimizes this vehicle of disease transfer, except for drug abusers.

Soil Soil may harbor the organisms that cause hookworm, tetanus, anthrax, and botulism. Each of these presents a particular type of control problem, but immunization, boiling of food with soil

on it, wearing of shoes and clothing, and other procedures can prevent the transmission of disease by soil. Where an intermediate object is the vehicle for the transmission of disease from a reservoir to a new host, it should be possible to block that route and therefore prevent disease spread. Through proper education of the public and the exercise of community control, it is possible to reduce the transfer of disease via animate and inanimate objects. However, public health officials find that control of the social contact (direct) route is a much more difficult task than control of disease transfer by vectors or inanimate vehicles. Human beings, largely because of carelessness or lack of understanding, often do not take sufficient precautions to prevent the spread of disease.

Entry of Organisms into New Host

Arrival and entry are not synonymous. When the organism arrives at the new host, it still must find its proper port of entry and must overcome certain body barriers. Pathogens producing respiratory diseases must arrive at the mouth or nose to enter the respiratory tract. Likewise, the organism causing an infection of the alimentary canal must find its way to the mouth and into the alimentary canal; even then, acid in the stomach may destroy the organism. Direct infection of mucous membranes such as occurs in gonococcal infection requires that the organism come in contact with those membranes. Although hookworms can go through the unbroken skin and mosquitoes and other animals can penetrate the skin sufficiently to introduce pathogenic organisms, percutaneous infections generally require a cut or an abrasion of the skin for the organism to enter the body.

Defenses of the Host

Even after leaving the reservoir, transferring to the new host, and reaching the right port of entry, the pathogen still encounters a series of defenses by the new host. Indeed, usually a large number of viril organisms must enter the new host if the host's defenses are to be overcome and infection produced.

Host Resistance Resistance is the ability of the host to ward off pathogens. General resistance against infection is nonspecific in that the various human defenses serve as antagonists to all pathogens. The skin serves as a mechanical barrier, and its natural acid state provides a further defense against those pathogens that require a neutral or alkaline medium. The secretion of mucous tissue serves as a defense against pathogens. The ciliated epithelial tissues of certain passages such as the respiratory tract provide an added defense, as the cilia tend to propel organisms to the exterior of the passageway. The acidity of such structures as the stomach, bladder, urethra, and vagina provides additional resistance to infection. Leukocytes, with their phagocytic action, destroy foreign organisms. Lymph nodes filter out infectious organisms and are capable of destroying them. A highly important defense is the ability of the body to produce an elevated temperature, or fever. The optimum temperature for most pathogens is about 100° F (38° C), the approximate normal temperature of the human body. In elevating the temperature by only two degrees, the body is able to inactivate the pathogens so that they are unable to multiply and carry on normal metabolism involving toxin production. During this stasis, the phagocytes of the body are able to engulf and destroy the invading organisms.

From time to time pathogens enter the human body without setting up infections. The human body's general resistance is normally able to provide the necessary defenses to prevent infection. This capacity depends on some of the physical fitness, mental health, and social factors discussed in previous chapters.

Immunity and Susceptibility The host with no specific resistance is termed susceptible and may be converted to immunity status by a variety of mechanisms. Complete resistance is termed immunity and is specific for a particular disease. Immunity is dependent on the presence in the body of specific substances that are most easily identified in the bloodstream but that are present in all tissues. These chemical substances are called antibodies and may be in the form of antitoxin, which neutralizes a particular toxin; agglutinin, which causes organisms to clump together; or precipitin, which produces a disintegration of pathogenic organisms.

Active immunity exists when an individual's own body produces the necessary antibodies. This type of immunity can result either from the actual attack of the disease or from artificial introduction of the necessary antigenic substance into the body by vaccination or immunization (table 11-6). An **antigen** is a substance (for example, toxin) that, when introduced into the body, causes the formation of antibodies.

Passive immunity is "borrowed" immunity; it exists when antibodies produced in some other individual or animal are introduced into a person. The duration of passive immunity is relatively short because the protective substances tend to disappear, not to be replaced by the individual's own antibody production. Passive immunity is employed when a susceptible person has been exposed to a disease and there is insufficient time to produce active immunity. For example, the injection of convalescent serum into a susceptible child exposed to measles would give the child temporary immunity or at least limit the case to very mild symptoms. The infantile immunity that a child experiences during the first six months of life is an example of natural passive immunity; antibodies from the mother's bloodstream diffuse through the membranes of the placenta into the bloodstream of the fetus, but the immunity exists only while the mother's antibodies survive in the child. Infantile immunity is extended during breast-feeding through the antibodies contained in the nursing mother's milk.

Natural immunity exists when a species has a genetic immunity to a particular disease to which some other species is susceptible. For example, mammals are immune to many of the microorganisms that cause infection in birds. Domestic animals are susceptible to some diseases, such as distemper, to which humans are immune. Likewise,

Table 11-6

Adult Immunization Schedules

Disease	Risk group	Primary series	Booster doses	Vaccine
All adults				
Tetanus	All adults	2 doses + 1 dose after 6-12 months	Every 10 years	Combined Td vaccine or combined Td-Polio
Diphtheria	All adults	2 doses + 1 dose after 6-12 months	Every 10 years	
Travel vaccines				
Polio	Travelers to endemic areas, others with occupational risks	2 doses + 1 dose after 6-12 months	Every 10 years*	Salk (IPV) vaccine or combined Td-Polio
Meningococcal	Travelers to epidemic areas	1 dose	Unknown	Meningococcal vaccine
Yellow fever	Travelers to endemic areas	1 dose	Every 10 years	Yellow fever vaccine
Cholera	Where required for foreign travel	2 doses	Every 6 months*	Cholera vaccine
Typhoid	Travelers to endemic areas	3 doses	Every 3 years*	Typhoid vaccine
Japanese encephalitis	Travellers to endemic or epidemic areas	3 doses	Every 4 years*	JEVax
Other adult vaccines				
Influenza	Everyone over 50, others with heart, lung, kidney, or metabolic disorders	1 dose	Every year	Influenza vaccine
Measles	All born after 1956 who are susceptible	1 dose	None	Measles vaccine or combined MMR
Mumps	All young adults with no history of mumps	1 dose	None	Mumps vaccine or combined MMR
Rubella	All susceptible women of childbearing age	1 dose	None	Rubella vaccine or combined MMR
Hepatitis B	Patients on renal dialysis, repeated use of blood or blood products, health care workers exposed to blood, staff and residents of mental institutions, household contacts of carriers, homosexually active males, some travelers	3 doses	Every 5 years*	Hepatitis B vaccine
Rabies	Veterinarians, trappers, animal technicians animal control, zoo keepers, conservation officers, wildlife biologists, travelers to endemic areas, and others at high risk of exposure	3 doses	Every 2 years*	HDC rabies vaccine
Pneumococcal	Everyone over 65, others with medical conditions that increase risk	1 dose	None	Pneumococcal vaccine

*While risk or travel requirement lasts.
Source: National Advisory Committee on Immigration, U.S. Department of Health and Human Services.

domestic animals are immune to diphtheria, small-pox, typhoid fever, and other infectious diseases to which humans are heir. Fortunately, the human species possesses natural immunity to a vast number of microorganisms that could be disease-producing but for the human body's distinctive biochemistry. Communities are able to add to this general protection or defense by offering artificial immunity through vaccination.

Acquired immunity is that particular type of active immunity that comes from having an attack of a disease. In humans second attacks are common with such diseases as influenza, pneumonia, gonorrhea, streptococcal sore throat, and the common cold, but are relatively rare with such diseases as chickenpox, diphtheria, measles, poliomyelitis, scarlet fever, smallpox, typhoid fever, and yellow fever. Vaccines to produce artificial active immunity are available for diphtheria, tetanus, pertussis, smallpox, poliomyelitis, typhoid fever, cholera, Rocky Mountain spotted fever, measles, German measles, mumps, and influenza. Various immunization schedules apply to these vaccines (see chapter 5 and table 11-6).

Smallpox vaccination has been discontinued because there is a greater threat to human health in possible complication from smallpox vaccination than in not being immunized. The spread of an epidemic through a population is determined by the immune/susceptible ratio. When the supply of susceptibles is exhausted, the epidemic ceases. In the case of smallpox, the pathogen was isolated from susceptible populations until the agent-host chain was broken with the isolation of the last case in Somalia.

Agent–Host–Environment

The outcome of disease in the individual is determined by the interaction of agent, host, and environment. The agent may be of high virulence or present in high concentrations. The host's defenses may be compromised by age, exhaustion, or concomitant disease, or the immune system may be affected by drugs or radiation given for chronic disease. The environment may be unfavor-able, as in the case of air pollution. Community action can be applied at any of the three points. Resistance of the host can be enhanced by better nutrition or by vaccination, for example. The agent may be directly attacked by chemicals or antibiotics, and the environment may be altered by sanitation or housing reforms.

This interactive model may also be used to consider conditions other than infectious diseases, such as automobile injuries, where the agent is the automobile, the host is the driver, and the environment is the highway.

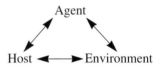

EPIDEMIOLOGICAL PRINCIPLES OF DISEASE CONTROL

Epidemiology is the study of the distribution and determinants of disease in a population. The unit of study is not the individual, as in microbiology and clinical medicine, but the community. Epidemiology compares and contrasts, studying sick and well groups. Variables such as age, sex, race, and occupation are analyzed in an attempt to determine which are found frequently in the sick but rarely in the well. The validity of the conclusions reached is subject to statistical tests.

Disease in the community is first categorized by time, place, and person. By studying the time or place of onset in an epidemic, a shared event, such as a meal, may be identified. It can then be determined if this particular meal was attended by many of the sick persons but by few of a comparison group of well people. Food histories may then be assembled and a suspect vehicle identified. The place of the epidemic may help to identify the offending vehicle, as when there is a density of cases in an area with a common water supply or when the cases are predominantly on the route of a mobile food vendor. The personal characteristics of those afflicted in an epidemic may point to its cause. For example, the sick people might share a common exposure to toxic inhalants in an industrial plant or to asbestos fibers in construction work.

Legal Authority

Communicable diseases are legally controlled through the exercise of police power, the authority or power of the people, represented by government, to protect the well-being of the public. Basically, sovereignty or ultimate authority rests with the people, who vest it in the state or province to exercise for them. The state or province may in turn delegate police power to counties or parishes to exercise disease control measures within their geographical boundaries. Municipalities may be granted a charter that gives broad authority, including police power, to protect the well-being of the people within the political limits of the borough, village, town, or city. Municipalities and counties usually assign some authority to schools to carry out certain control measures.

In practice the state or province enters into communicable disease control practice in a broad advisory capacity to the community governmental units and by direct action when communicable diseases spread beyond a single locality. The state or province usually does not step in and take action unless local authorities request assistance or are unable to cope with the situation.

In the exercise of police power the one governing principle recognized by the courts is that whatever action is taken must be reasonable. Thus it may be reasonable for health authorities to isolate an individual in his home for a period of five days when he suffers from a diagnosed case of a certain communicable disease, but a court might rule that it would not be reasonable to require that patient to be removed to a hospital and isolated there for two weeks. The science of epidemiology has advanced to a point where the action taken is usually reasonable because it is based on sound statistical probability, microbiology, and medical science. People are spared a great deal of the inconvenience suffered by their grandparents because

modern public health science has displaced much of the arbitrary police action based on guesswork once involved in disease control.

Health authorities cannot ignore the personal and religious rights of the individual, but courts have been reluctant to censure official public health action exercised reasonably in the interest of the general population. Courts have ruled that while official health boards cannot require a person to be immunized in opposition to religious beliefs, imposing quarantine on susceptible nonimmunized people when an epidemic threatens the community is just and reasonable. In the present era, however, control measures are so highly effective that if a relatively small percentage of the population is not immunized against a disease, that most of the people are immune nearly eliminates the spread of the particular disease. This is sometimes referred to as "herd immunity." In the final analysis, the exercise of police power often reflects a failure of public health education and other means of communicable disease control.

Segregation of Reservoir

Theoretically, perfect prevention of spread would mean perfect control of communicable diseases. It is possible to establish certain barriers around a reservoir of infection and thus block the spread of the disease.

Isolation   The oldest communicable disease control measure is the segregation of an infected person or lower animal until danger of conveying infection has passed. **Isolation** can be a highly effective control measure, but in practice it occasionally fails because of subclinical cases, variability in the duration of the communicable state, and human failures in observing regulations.

Bacteriological methods can determine the required interval of isolation with precision. Laboratory examination of the secretions of a patient with tuberculosis will establish the presence or absence of the tubercle bacillus and thus determine the continuance or termination of isolation. Likewise, examination of secretions from the nose and throat of a patient with diphtheria will provide an accurate bacteriological determination of whether isolation should be terminated.

The longer the period of isolation, the greater the safety—but also the greater the injustice, because many patients reach a noncommunicable or at least relatively safe state long before the maximum isolation period is reached. No definite rule applies; for this reason, great variation is found from community to community. To set an inflexible isolation period would make no provision for individual variation. For this reason, the usual practice is to set a minimum time that experience has demonstrated will be ample in perhaps 80 percent to 90 percent of the cases, and then leave to the discretion of the attending physician the need for extending the isolation in individual cases. An arbitrary period of isolation can be quite satisfactory for diseases such as measles and chickenpox where no convalescent carriers occur.

Isolation has certain limitations. Hidden cases—those never reported by patients or parents—are not technically under isolation. Carriers of a disease usually do not have overt symptoms and thus are not identified as potential hazards. In addition, during the early or prodrome stage of a respiratory disease, individuals may not be ill enough to remain home, yet they are in a highly communicable state and capable of spreading the disease to others.

Quarantine   The detention of susceptible individuals who have been exposed to a communicable disease is called quarantine. These individuals are often spoken of as "contacts." Nonsusceptible people who have been exposed are not included as contacts. Quarantine is used infrequently in disease control because the individual is rarely in a communicable state during the incubation period of a disease. As a consequence, not until first symptoms appear does the individual present a danger, and, at this point, isolation can be imposed. Measles and chickenpox are exceptions in that they may be communicable during the last two or three days of the incubation period. Even in the case of these two

diseases, however, quarantine is of questionable value in controlling spread.

Quarantine time is based on laboratory findings, the maximum incubation period, or both. Therefore if several laboratory specimens are negative, the person is released from quarantine; or if the usual incubation period for the disease in question is seven days, then after the seventh day following exposure to the disease the subject is released from quarantine if he or she exhibits no symptoms.

Reducing Communicability   Treatment of a patient limits the reservoir and therefore represents an important procedure in communicable disease control. Medical treatment of patients can be highly effective in reducing communicability of certain diseases. For example, through the use of chemotherapy and antibiotics, a case of syphilis can be rendered noncommunicable, although some symptoms may persist in the patient.

Reservoir Eradication

Logically the most permanent and therefore the most desirable measure of communicable disease control would be the complete elimination of the reservoir. This is possible when lower animals serve as reservoirs of organisms pathogenic to humans. Bovine tuberculosis and brucellosis have been eliminated by an orderly, widespread program of testing cattle and then slaughtering those that are reactors.

The principle of reservoir eradication can sometimes be applied to the human organs harboring infectious organisms. This procedure has been directed to the carriers of disease. Some typhoid carriers, for example, have been rendered noncarriers by the removal of the gallbladder.

Environmental Measures

Sanitation measures usually are directed toward the vehicles of disease transfer and are effective in limiting the spread of such diseases of the intestinal tract as hepatitis, typhoid, paratyphoid, dysentery, salmonellosis, staphylococcus infection, and cholera. Application of the principles of sanitation to water supplies, processing of milk and other foods, and sewage disposal has played an important role in reducing the incidence of these alvine discharge diseases since the beginning of the century. Sanitation has been effective also as a measure in controlling vector-borne diseases such as malaria and yellow fever. By destroying the breeding places of the vectors and by using effective insecticides, sanitation programs can effectively control the spread of insect-borne diseases.

Environmental measures are of little value in the control of such respiratory diseases as measles, chickenpox, scarlet fever, streptococcal sore throat, diphtheria, smallpox, and pertussis. Although decontamination measures may be of some value in preventing the spread of respiratory diseases, their effectiveness has never been scientifically established.

Increasing Resistance of New Host

Even when organisms of sufficient number and virility to establish infection invade a new host, measures still may be taken to protect the host and to prevent further spread of the disease.

Passive immunization can give transient emergency protection. Before this procedure is employed, it must be ascertained that the person actually was exposed and is susceptible to the disease. Passive immunization lasts but a few weeks, therefore it provides only a stopgap for a particular situation when no other measures are feasible. Passive immunization has one marked disadvantage in that the serum usually used may sensitize the individual so as to set up the future danger of anaphylaxis—extreme reaction to a second exposure to the foreign serum. For this reason, passive immunization is not regarded as a good community measure to be used on a widespread basis.

Limiting the severity of a disease should be regarded as a control measure. Diseases such as diphtheria and scarlet fever can be modified by treatment, and by this procedure communicability can be reduced. **Immunization** of children and adults has provided the most dramatic examples of epidemiological control of infectious diseases, as in the case of smallpox eradication, which combined immunization with isolation and quarantine. More exclusive use of immunization has accounted for the spectacular drops in poliomyelitis and measles in the past twenty years, as illustrated for measles in the United States in figure 11-13. Measles is now a candidate for possible eradication, at least in some countries.

Personal Hygiene and Health Behavior Individual behavior continues to be a factor in the control of infectious diseases, particularly among those spread by person-to-person contact. Evidence for the continuing importance of proper hygienic measures is illustrated by outbreaks of illness associated with improper food handling in private homes and institutions. Correct use of condoms is an effective measure in the prevention of sexually transmitted diseases. Similarly, simple handwashing techniques will prevent the transmission of many bacterial illnesses in the hospital and the home.

Certain factors such as smoking, alcohol consumption, poor nutrition, drug misuse, and stress place people at increased risk for infectious diseases and subsequent morbidity and mortality. Alcoholics are known to be at higher risk for several infectious diseases, including pneumonia. Smokers are at risk, in particular, for pulmonary diseases such as bronchitis and pneumonia. Intravenous drug users are at risk for HIV/AIDS (see figure 11-1), hepatitis B, and endocarditis (most commonly caused by staphylococcal infection). Poor nutrition, particularly in children, puts the individual at risk for gastroenteritis and respiratory illnesses, secondary to infectious pathogens. Finally, studies indicate that stress can increase people's susceptibility to many kinds of illness, including infectious diseases.

Community Education Measures Community health education and health promotion programs directed at these health practices and lifestyles will contribute to the control of infectious diseases,

Figure 11-13

The decline in reported measles (rubeola) incidence since the measles vaccine was licensed in the United States. The jump in 1989 and 1990 rates was the result of widespread slippage in state and local immunization efforts. (*Source:* Centers for Disease Control: Measles surveillance—United States, 1991, *MMWR* 41(SS-6):1, 1992.)

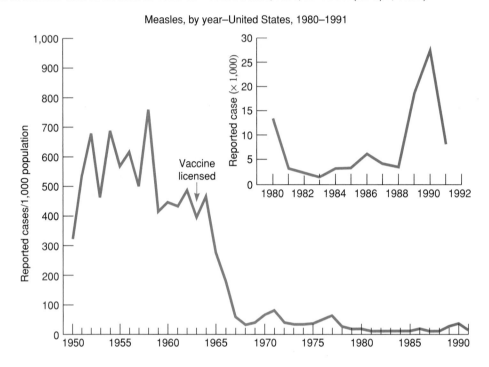

Measles, by year–United States, 1980–1991

even though this may not be the primary objective of such programs. Community health education interventions designed to support behavior conducive to infectious disease control could occur at any of the following five steps when people (1) become more susceptible (lifestyle behavior), (2) become exposed (hygienic behavior), (3) become infected (protective or prophylactic behavior), (4) become symptomatic (appropriate medical care), or (5) suffer complications or relapses (adherence to prescribed medical regimens). The first three points of intervention are primary prevention steps to build host resistance; the last two are secondary and tertiary prevention steps.

In addition, a well-informed public will not be stampeded by scare rumors or fantastic reports such as fatal reactions to immunization. Further, a good community health education program will assist in obtaining funds for the promotion of immunization and other control measures.

Community health education should provide useful immunization information to mothers and new parents through hospitals, physicians, and others; aim educational programs at members of the health care professions; include discussion of immunization and preventive measures in school health curricula; enlist daycare centers, senior citizen centers, and churches to provide immunization information to parents and to older people; use the mass media for immunization activities; and continue the use of volunteers.

Objectives for Immunization

By 2000 at least 95% of children attending licensed day-care centers and kindergarten through twelfth grade should be fully immunized. (In 1988 the immunization level was about 94% for licensed child care, 97% for first school entrants.)

By 1990 all mothers of newborns should receive instruction prior to leaving the hospital on immunization schedules for their babies.

What would you set as corresponding objectives for your community for the year 2000?

Service Measures Community health centers and other medical care settings can contribute to the control of diseases for which vaccines are available by adopting standardized official immunization records; developing and using tickler files and recall systems to ensure that children return for immunizations on schedule; making immunizations available and affordable in all health care settings as a part of comprehensive health services; and using local volunteers who know the population at risk.

Legislative and Regulatory Measures Further organizational supports should include the following legislative and regulatory steps: enforcing existing school immunization requirements and extending them to include children at all grade levels in public and private schools and in organized preschool settings; including coverage of immunization as a health insurance benefit not subject to deductible provisions; requiring carriers under any national health insurance plan to reimburse for immunization services; requiring immunization as a condition of employment (for example, in health care institutions); and including rubella immunization as a service routinely offered in family planning clinics, primary care clinics, hospitals, and Health Maintenance Organizations (HMOs).

Economic Measures Related economic supports for immunization programs include reimbursing for immunizations under public and private health insurance plans; supplying vaccines free to health care providers as long as they do not charge for vaccinations; and offering economic incentives to health care providers and vaccine recipients.

DISEASE CONTROL RESOURCES

Official health agencies require the cooperation and assistance of individuals and other agencies competent to assist in the general problem of disease control. Health education of the public is fundamental to effective communicable disease control measures, and official health agencies recognize that the supplementary health education contributed by other organizations is highly valuable in the general control program. Indeed, education of the public is the primary approach of the official and voluntary health agencies in controlling diseases. In the philosophy of modern community health, a department of health that must rely continually on its legal authority for an effective program would be regarded as an outdated and ineffective agency. Schools, voluntary agencies, hospitals, and medical practitioners should be expected to contribute their resources to the communicable disease control efforts. (See chapters 18 to 21 for descriptions of these resources.)

SUMMARY

The dramatic decline in the relative importance of communicable diseases as causes of death since the beginning of the twentieth century might lead one to believe that little more needs to be done. The inspiring story of the eradication of smallpox might encourage the conclusion that the other communicable diseases are on their way out also. Diphtheria, malaria, poliomyelitis, trichinosis, and typhoid fever seem near extinction, and measles has been targeted for eradication. However if further reduction in any of these diseases is to be accomplished, existing control measures cannot be taken for granted or relaxed. Maintaining high levels of immunization requires persistent effort on the part of community health agencies, schools, and other cooperating institutions. The importance of vigilance was seen in the 1970s and again in 1989 through 1990, when immunization levels in the United States dipped perilously below the 90 percent standard, resulting in the resurgence of measles and certain other diseases.

The distinct modes of transfer for respiratory diseases, alvine-discharge diseases, vector-borne diseases, and open lesion diseases have divided the strategies for control into broad classes of intervention. For respiratory diseases the main control measure has been the strengthening of host resistance, primarily through immunization, but also significantly through improved nutrition and general health promotion. This approach has succeeded where any other hope of controlling airborne transmission would be limited by the realities of social contact and indoor living.

The alvine-discharge diseases are transmitted primarily by water and food contaminated through unsanitary conditions. The major interventions, therefore, have been environmental control measures directed at water purification, sewage disposal and treatment, food protection, and personal hygiene. These means of control also have been aided by more general improvements in housing, urban design, and economic conditions, and by promoting public understanding of disease control.

Vector-borne diseases have been controlled largely through the killing or containment of vectors such as rodents, mosquitoes, flies, ticks, and fleas. Some vectors carry other vectors as part of the life cycle of the pathogenic organism. The vehicles of transfer from reservoir to new host can therefore be mechanical and biological.

The diseases most difficult to control have been those transmitted by direct contact, particularly open lesion diseases. The obstacles here seem to be related to the value-laden, socially and politically controversial aspects and implications of governmental or other third-party intervention in people's intimate relations. The sexually transmit-

ted diseases illustrate the problem most poignantly today, as tuberculosis and leprosy have in the past. For this reason public health education has proved to be the most durable and essential intervention for the ultimate control of these diseases.

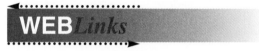

WEB *Links*

http://www.mediconsult.com/noframes/aids/
shareware/aids/index.html
The Virtual Medical Center

http://www.gen.emory/edu/MEDWEB/keyword/pub-
lic_health/infectious_diseases.html
Emory University Health Sciences Center Library - contains links to sites on infectious disease and control, research, immunization programs, and communicable disease prevention.

http://www.nyu.edu/education/health/healthed/taub/
hepr/noframes/index.html
Health Education Professional Resources

http://www.medscape.com
Medscape

http://odphp.oash.dhhs.gov/default.htm
Office of Disease Prevention and Health Promotion

http://www.ams.queensu.ca/sexcntr/links.html
Sexually Transmitted Infections - including HIV/AIDS. Contains a large number of links of interest.

http://hwcweb.hwc.ca/hpb/lcdc/hp_eng.html
English version of the Canadian Laboratory Center for Disease Control

QUESTIONS FOR REVIEW

1. What distinction can be made between infectious disease and communicable disease?
2. If effective methods of immunization were developed for all of the communicable diseases, would humankind eliminate all existing communicable diseases?
3. Of recent outbreaks of communicable disease you have observed or otherwise were acquainted with, do you class these outbreaks as endemic, epidemic, or pandemic?

4. What communicable respiratory diseases are most likely to appear in epidemic form in your community?

5. What disease do you predict will cause the next worldwide pandemic?

6. To what extent is there justification for saying that an epidemic is evidence of an inadequate public health education program?

7. Is pasteurization of the community milk supply less necessary than it was thirty years ago?

8. What services does your health department provide in its communicable disease control program?

9. What organizations or agencies in your community contribute to communicable disease control?

10. What steps should an ordinary citizen take when he or she has evidence that a case of communicable disease may exist in a household where no physician has been called and no precautions are being taken to prevent possible spread of the disease?

11. What is being done and what further should be done in your community to prevent the spread of communicable diseases via foods other than milk or water?

12. From the standpoint of public health education, how would you change this prevailing attitude: "It's just a cold"?

13. Why should passive immunization be rejected as a communitywide procedure?

14. What disadvantages in respect to communicable disease control does a democracy have that a dictatorship does not have?

15. Is there any evidence that new infectious diseases are appearing?

READINGS

Benenson, A. S., ed. 1995. *Control of communicable diseases manual.* 16th ed. Washington, DC: American Public Health Association.

This most widely recognized sourcebook on infectious diseases covers more than 300 communicable diseases. It describes for each disease its infectious agent, occurrence, mode of transmission, incubation period, susceptibility and resistance, and methods of control.

Freudenberg, N., and M. Zimmerman. 1995. *AIDS prevention in the community: lessons from the first decade.* Washington, DC: American Public Health Association.

With descriptions of the experiences of successful and unsuccessful community programs, this book summarizes the experience of the 1980s in educating

people about AIDS, with attention to the social and political forces that shape AIDS educators. Written primarily for practitioners.

Hopkins, D. R., and Ruiz-Tiben, E. 1992. Surveillance for dracunculiasis, 1981–1991. In CDC surveillance summaries, Special focus I: public health surveillance and international health. *MMWR* 41:1.

After successfully eradicating smallpox, WHO designated dracunculiasis (guinea worm disease) as the next disease scheduled to be eradicated (by 1995). This article reports progress on this goal, emphasizing the importance of epidemiological methods of surveillance.

Mann, J., and D. J. M. Tarantola. 1996. *AIDS in the world.* 2d ed. Oxford: Oxford University Press.

This book charts a course into the future based on clear analysis of the global pandemic and response, and lessons learned from the first decade of the prevention efforts.

Smith, L. L., and L. M. Lathrop. 1993. AIDS and human sexuality. *Can J Public Health* 84(suppl 1):14.

Specific strategies for a comprehensive approach to AIDS is outlined using the PRECEDE-PROCEED model introduced in Chapter 4 of this book. This whole issue of the *Canadian Journal of Public Health* is devoted to AIDS.

BIBLIOGRAPHY

Addrein, A., P. Godin, G. Cappon, S. Manson Singer, E. Maticka-Tyndale, and D. Willms. 1996. Overview of the Canadian study on the determinants of ethnoculturally specific behaviours related to HIV/AIDS. *Can J of Public Health* 87:4–9.

Alteneder, R. R., J. H. Price, S. K. Telljohann, J. Didion, and A. Locher. 1992. Using the PRECEDE model to determine junior high school students' knowledge, attitudes, and beliefs about AIDS. *J School Health* 62:464.

Aruffo, J. F., J. H. Coverdale, V. N. Pavlik, 1993. AIDS knowledge in minorities: significance of locus of control. *Am J Prev Med* 9:15.

Barua, D., and W. B. Greenough, III. 1992. *Cholera.* New York: Plenum.

Benenson, A. S., ed. 1990. *Control of communicable diseases in man.* 15th ed. Washington, DC: American Public Health Association.

Centers for Disease Control. 1992. *Health information for international travel, 1992.* Pub. No. (CDC) 92-8280. Washington, DC: U.S. Government Printing Office.

Chen, L. C., J. S. Amor, and S. J. Segal, eds. 1991. *AIDS and women's reproductive health,* New York: Plenum.

Committee for the Study on Malaria Prevention and Control. 1991. *Status review and alternative strategies.* Washington, DC: National Academy Press.

Coyle, S. L., R. F. Boruch, and C. F. Turner, eds. 1991. *Evaluating AIDS prevention programs.* Washington, DC: National Academy Press.

Cutts, F. T., W. A. Orenstein, and R. H. Bernier. 1992. Causes of low preschool immunization coverage in the United States. *Annu Rev Public Health* 13:85.

Dabbagh, L., L W. Green, and G. M. Walker. 1991–1992. Case study: application of PRECEDE and PROCEED as a framework for designing culturally sensitive diarrhea prevention programs and policy in Arab countries. *Int Q Commun Health Educ* 12:293.

Decosas, J., and V. Pedneault. 1992. Women and AIDS in Africa: demographic implications for health promotion. *Health Pol & Planning* 7:227.

Donowitz, L. G., ed. 1991. *Infection control in the child care center and preschool.* Baltimore: Williams & Wilkins.

Evans, A. S. 1991. *Viral infections of humans: epidemiology and control.* 3d ed. New York: Plenum.

Evans, A. S., and P. S. Brachman, eds. 1991. *Bacterial infections of humans: epidemiology and control.* 8th ed. New York: Plenum.

Henig, R. M. 1995. The lessons of syphilis in the age of AIDS. *Civilization* 2(6):36–43.

Hope-Simpson, R. E. 1992. *The transmission of epidemic influenza.* New York: Plenum.

Horowitz, L. G., and L. Kehoe. 1992. Fear and AIDS: educating the public about dental office infection control. *Dent Age of AIDS* Special issue (spring).

Kim-Farley, R. 1992. The Expanded Programme on Immunization Team: Global immunization. *Annu Rev Public Health* 13:223.

Lederberg, J., R. E. Shope, and S. C. Oaks, Jr, eds. 1997. *Emerging infections: microbial threats to health.* Washington, DC: National Academy Press.

Lupton, D. A. 1992. From complacency to panic: AIDS and heterosexuals in the Australian press, July 1986 to June 1988. *Health Educ Res* 7:9.

Manson Singer, S., D. G. Willms, A. Adrian, J. Baxter, C. Brabazon, V. Leanne, G. Godin, E. Maticka-Tyndale, and P. Cappon. 1996. Many voices—sociocultural results of the ethnocultural communities facing AIDS study in Canada. *Can J Public Health* 87:S26.

Murray, C. J. L., and A. D. Lopez, eds. 1996. *The Global Burden of Disease.* Cambridge: Harvard University Press.

National Institute of Allergy and Infectious Diseases. 1992. PID: guidelines for prevention, detection and management. *Clin Courier* 10:1.

National Institute of Allergy and Infectious Diseases. 1992. *Toxoplasmosis.* Bethesda: NIAID, National Institutes of Health.

de Quadros C. A., J. K. Andrus, J. M. Olive, C. G. deMacedo, and D. A. Henderson. 1992. Polio eradication from the Western Hemisphere. *Annu Rev Public Health* 13:239.

Quinn, T. C., A. Ruff, and J. Modlin. 1992. HIV infection and AIDS in children. *Annu Rev Public Health* 13:1.

Richardson, S. 1994. A rash of epidemics. *Discover* 15(1):86–87.

Rhodes, T., and J. Holland. 1992. Outreach as a strategy for HIV prevention: aims and practice. *Health Educ Res* 7:533.

Rozovsky, L. E., and F. A. Rozovsky. 1992. *AIDS and Canadian law.* Ottawa: Canadian Public Health Association.

Skinner, J., L. March, and J. M. Simpson. 1995. Cohort study of childhood immunization in northern Sydney. *Austral J Public Health* 19(2): 58.

Snider, D. E., and W. L. Roper. 1992. The new tuberculosis. *N Engl J Med* 326:703.

U.S. Department of Health and Human Services. 1992. *Healthy people 2000: national health promotion and disease prevention objectives.* Boston: Jones & Bartlett.

World Health Organization. 1995. *National Target: CDD/ARI Programme Management.* World Health Organization, Division of Diarrhoeal and Acute Respiratory Disease Control.

Chapter 12

Lifestyle, Population Health, and Community Health Promotion

*H*ealth promotion is the process of enabling people to increase control over, and to improve, their health . . . Good health is a major resource for social, economic and personal development and an important dimension of quality of life.

—Ottawa Charter for Health Promotion

Objectives

When you finish this chapter, you should be able to:

- Identify the behavioral risk factors that account for more than half of the leading causes of death and disability in populations

- Describe the epidemiological patterns and trends associated with these risk factors

- Propose health promotion strategies combining educational, organizational,

economic, and environmental supports for behavior and conditions of living conducive to health

- Apply the model of community health promotion to the planning of a large-scale program to support lifestyles conducive to health

---

Population health and community health promotion require an understanding of health behavior that goes beyond the specific actions of individuals and includes more than educational approaches alone to changing those behaviors. Lifestyle, a broader concept than behavior, describes value-laden, socially conditioned behavioral patterns. This concept has a rich history of study in anthropology and sociology. Only recently has it taken on special significance in epidemiology, population health, and community health promotion.

The midcentury shift from acute infectious diseases to chronic, degenerative diseases as the leading causes of death in Western societies brought a new perspective in epidemiology. No longer could isolation and suppression of a single germ or agent control the predominant diseases. Now, the causes of most chronic diseases tend to be multiple and elusive. They defy simple environmental control measures because they involve people's pleasures and rewards, their social relationships and physical needs, and ultimately, for some, their habits and addictions.

Table 12-1

The Five Leading Causes of Death in North America and Their Associated Risk Factors or Precursors

Cause of death	Risk factors
Cardiovascular disease	Tobacco use
	Elevated serum cholesterol
	High blood pressure
	Obesity
	Diabetes
	Sedentary lifestyle
Cancer	Tobacco use
	Improper diet
	Alcohol
	Occupational/environmental exposures
Cerebrovascular disease	High blood pressure
	Tobacco use
	Elevated serum cholesterol
Unintentional injuries	Safety belt noncompliance
	Alcohol/substance abuse
	Reckless driving
	Occupational hazards
	Stress/fatigue
Chronic lung disease	Tobacco use
	Occupational/environmental exposures

Source: National Center for Health Statistics, and Health and Welfare Canada.

This chapter examines four kinds of behavior or health-related habits that are or can be harmful: tobacco use, alcohol misuse, drug misuse, and eating patterns. All involve physiological changes and may involve a compulsive or dependency component in behavior. Tobacco, diet (in combination with physical activity), and alcohol use are the three leading causes of the leading types of death in North America (table 12-1). Together they account for 38 percent of premature deaths. With physical activity or exercise, stress management or recreation, and safety practices, these patterns of behavior are termed lifestyle. They are health-related but not necessarily health-directed patterns of behavior.

Figure 12-1

Lifestyle risk factors contribute more than the combination of health care, environment, and human biology to the years of life lost prematurely (before age 75). Nutrition includes overnutrition, obesity, anorexia, bulimia, undernutrition, and control of diabetes. (*Source:* Centers for Disease Control and Prevention, Public Health Service, U.S. Department of Health and Human Services.)

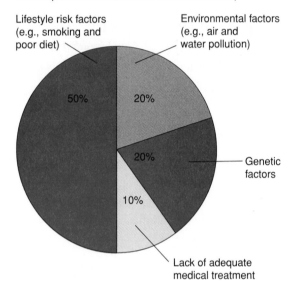

Lifestyle risk factors (e.g., smoking and poor diet) — 50%

Environmental factors (e.g., air and water pollution) — 20%

Genetic factors — 20%

Lack of adequate medical treatment — 10%

EPIDEMIOLOGY OF LIFESTYLE DETERMINANTS OF HEALTH

The health field concept described in chapter 2 has four elements: health services, environment, human biology, and lifestyle. Of these, lifestyle is responsible for most (at least half) of the years of life prematurely lost in the more developed nations (figure 12-1). To put this revealing statistic in more positive terms, the greatest gains in preventing premature death and disability can be achieved through community supports or policies for more healthful lifestyles. Reducing risk means that chances of developing a disease are lowered. It does not guarantee that a disease will be prevented. Several factors are involved in the development of disease, therefore risk reduction usually involves several strategies or approaches.

The entire burden for improved health or reducing risk must not be placed on the individual. The responsibility must be shared between individuals and their families; between families and their communities; and between communities and their state, provincial, and national governments. Each level of organizational influence on behavior must assume some responsibility for setting the economic and environmental conditions that will support healthful lifestyles. Families, for example, must set examples for children. Communities must provide facilities and pass local ordinances to encourage, enable, and reinforce healthful behavior. State and national governments and private organizations must assume responsibility for the production, sale, and advertising of foods and other substances that can be either helpful or harmful to health.

TOBACCO USE

Tobacco use is the single most preventable cause of death in North America (figure 12-2). The use of tobacco can be understood and studied at many levels—from the individual to global markets—and from many perspectives—economic, health, social, legal, agricultural, communication, and political. In 1997 many of these perspectives merged as a cigarette manufacturer, the Liggett Group, admitted publicly for the first time that smoking is addictive and causes cancer. The admission came as part of a lawsuit filed by twenty-two states to recover health care costs attributed to tobacco use. This break in rank among cigarette manufacturers came at a time when they were being investigated for manipulating nicotine levels to increase the addictiveness of their product and marketing cigarettes to youth. While this public admission confirmed what scientists and health advocates have known for many years, it served as a reminder about the importance of studying community health issues from multiple perspectives. Lifestyle is one among many understandings of the use of tobacco and its consequences. Population health provides another perspective looking at the distal

·····················

Figure 12-2

Smoking kills more Americans every year than alcohol, automobile crashes, AIDS, suicides, homicides, fires, and drugs combined. (*Source:* Centers for Disease Control and Prevention, Public Health Service, U.S. Department of Health and Human Services.)

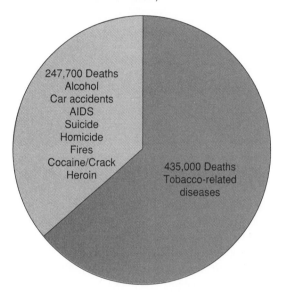

determinants of health. For adolescents, smoking may be less a form of rebellion than submission to well-targeted ads intended to hook them to an addictive product early in life. For middle-aged adults, the difficulties of quitting smoking may be less an issue of being "weak willed" than struggling with the powerful and addictive effect of nicotine. Community approaches to tobacco need to be broad and to impart that broader vision to the public.

Epidemiology of Tobacco and Health

About one-half of regular smokers will eventually die as a result of this addictive behavior. Cigarette smokers suffer the highest **relative risk** with respect to cancer, but the community and population impact of smoking is greatest in cardiovascular disease because the latter is so prevalent. Cigarette

Objectives for Tobacco Control

- By 2000 reduce cigarette smoking to a prevalence of no more than 15% among people aged 20 and older. Baseline: 29% in 1987 - 32% for men and 27% for women.

Special Target Populations	1987	2000
People with high school education	34%	20%
Lower socioeconomic youth	40	18
Military personnel	42	20
Hispanics	33	18
American Indian/Alaska Native	42–70	20
Pregnant women	25	10

- By 2000 reduce smokeless tobacco use by males aged 12 to 24 to a prevalence of not more than 4%. Baseline: 6.6% among males aged 12 to 17 in 1988; 8.9% among males aged 18 to 24 in 1987.

smoking accounts for 21 percent of coronary heart disease deaths and 30 percent of cancer deaths. Selected sites where the **attributable risk** from smoking is high include lung cancer (87 percent) and chronic obstructive pulmonary disease (82 percent). Attributable risk (AR) is the percentage of total cases that can be ascribed to a particular risk factor—in this case, cigarette smoking. The unintentional inhalation of sidestream or environmental smoke is estimated to cause approximately 3,800 lung cancer deaths and 37,000 cardiovascular deaths yearly in the United States alone. An additional 2,500 perinatal deaths were estimated to have been caused by smoking among pregnant women, and another 1,300 deaths resulted from burns related to smoking.

Smoking Trends   The first decline in cigarette consumption in the United States came in 1954 after more than forty years of increases. This was the year that the first American Cancer Society report was published showing that the death rate for cigarette smokers from all causes was much higher than for nonsmokers and that the lung cancer mortality of cigarette smokers was ten times that of nonsmokers. The second decline in consumption came in 1964 when the first Surgeon

General's Report on Smoking and Health was published (see Milestones box). The third reduction in smoking prevalence rates occurred between 1968 and 1970, when the "fairness rule" in broadcasting required television networks to provide airtime for thousands of antismoking messages in response to cigarette advertisements. The more steady decline since 1973 is attributed to the cumulative effects of federal, state, and local action; the growing influence of the nonsmokers' rights movement; and the rising cost of cigarettes, including the U.S. federal excise tax.

The overall prevalence of smoking in the United States has been falling at a rate of approximately 0.5 percent per year. The smoking rate among adults has declined from 40 percent in 1965 to 26 percent in 1994, toward a target of 15% percent by the year 2000. The smoking rate differs between men (28 percent) and women (23–25 percent); see figure 12-3. The smoking rate remains disproportionately high among American Indians/Alaska Natives (40 percent), blue-collar workers (39 percent), and people with a high school education or less (31 percent).

The decline in smoking has been substantially slower among women than among men. By the late 1980s women's death rate from lung cancer

Milestones in the Tobacco Wars

1492   Christopher Columbus observed natives' fondness for chewing an aromatic dried leaf or inhaling its smoke through a pipe called the "tobaca," then found his sailors unable "to refrain from indulging in the habit."

1850   London tobacconist, Phillip Morris, catered to English smokers addicted to smoking during the Crimerian War.

1900   Buck Duke, American Tobacco Company founder, lobbied successfully in U.S. Congress to head off crackdown on cigarettes.

1901   Senator Nelson W. Aldrich of Rhode Island, Senate Finance Committee chair, and three other key members hold tobacco stock worth more than $1 million.

1902   Theodore Roosevelt initiated some forty anti-trust actions against big corporations including Standard Oil, DuPont, Union Pacific Railroad, and American Tobacco.

1903   Buck Duke testified in federal court that his actions were to increase, not decrease, competition.

1906   Congress passed the Pure Food and Drug Act, but tobacco remained the only ingested product subject to processing and containing known toxins and additives not covered by the regulations. The industry continued to argue that tobacco is neither a food nor a drug, therefore properly exempted.

1911   Supreme Court ruled against American Tobacco in the antitrust suit, concluding that "wrongful purpose and illegal combination is overwhelmingly established."

1912   American Tobacco broken up by court ruling to create smaller units, with R. J. Reynolds emerging as the strongest competitor.

1913   Camel introduced the first blended cigarettes in the United States, with instant marketing success.

1916   American Tobacco introduced blended Lucky Strike and the advertising battle ensues with increasingly false claims of health and social benefits from smoking.

1917   Western governments supplied free cigarettes to recruits in World War I, contributing to an epidemic rise in the number of males addicted to smoking during and after the war and to the epidemic rise of cancer deaths in the following decades.

1940s   Government supply of free cigarettes to soldiers during World War II produced another leap in the prevalence in smoking in men.

1950s   Three epidemiological studies demonstrated the multiple risks and vastly higher risks in smokers. Tobacco industry responded with the introduction of filtered cigarettes, setting off another round of exaggerated advertising claims.

1957   Federal Trade Commission hearings in U.S. Congress on cigarette advertising, revealed that the new filtered brands were using stronger tobaccos to yield about the same amount of tar and nicotine as the unfiltered brands.

1958   Surgeon General Leroy Burney declared "The weight of the evidence at present implicates smoking as the principal etiological factor" in the increased incidence of lung cancer. *The Journal of the American Medical Association* published an editorial denying the strength of evidence in Burney's statement. The AMA was believed to have downplayed the tobacco link because it needed congressional support from tobacco states in its fight against Medicare.

1964   First official Surgeon General's report on smoking and health concluded that cigarette smoking was a cause of lung cancer in men and identified many other causal relationships and smoking-disease associations. "Marlboro Country" ads campaign born on Madison Avenue, offsetting health warnings.

1967   As smoking rates declined since the 1964 report, sustained for more than two years the first time since World War I, second Surgeon General's report (SGR) concluded "that smoking can cause death from coronary heart disease" and identified measures of morbidity associated with smoking.

1968   SGR supplement to 1967 report estimated loss of life expectancy among young men as 8 years for "heavy" smokers (over 2 packs per day) and 4 years for "light" smokers (less than 1/2 pack per day).

1969   Confirmed association between maternal smoking and infant low birthweight, and identified associations with prematurity, spontaneous abortion, stillbirth, and neonatal death. U.S. Congress banned cigarette advertising on TV and placed health warnings in other (print) advertising. Concessions to tobacco industry included removal of any mention of cancer from warning labels.

1970   SGR concluded that smoking is associated with cancers of the oral cavity and esophagus and with retarded fetal growth.

1971   SGR concluded that tobacco impairs protective mechanisms of the immune system, and that exposure to tobacco smoke, directly or through air pollution from others smoking, may exacerbate allergic symptoms and the condition of those with chronic lung or heart disease.

1973   SGR found pipe and cigar smokers at greater risk of premature death than nonsmokers, but less than cigarette smokers. Also concluded that cigarette smoking impairs exercise performance in healthy young men.

1974   Surgeon General's tenth Anniversary Report showed strengthened evidence on major hazards of smoking

Milestones in the Tobacco Wars (continued)

previously reported and added evidence on brain infarction and on interaction with asbestos exposure.

1975 SGR noted evidence on involuntary (passive) smoking, especially linking parental smoking to bronchitis and pneumonia in children during their first year of life.

1978 SGR showed smoking increased harmful effects of oral contraceptives on the cardiovascular systems of women. Congressional Speaker "Tip" O'Neill warned Health, Education & Welfare Secretary Joseph Califano that "You're driving the tobacco people crazy. These guys are vicious—they're out to destroy you." President Carter fires Califano the following year.

1979 SGR examined for first time the behavioral and social factors influencing smoking, the role of adult and youth education in promoting nonsmoking, and the health consequences of smokeless tobacco. First Surgeon General's Report on Health Promotion and Disease Prevention placed reduced smoking at the head of the health promotion objectives.

1980 SGR devoted to health consequences of smoking for women, projected that lung cancer would surpass breast cancer as leading cause of cancer deaths in women, and identified a trend toward increased smoking by adolescent females.

1981 SGR reviewed lower tar and nicotine cigarettes, noting reduced risk of lung cancer but no conclusive evidence on reduced risk of other lung, cardiovascular, and fetal damage. Concluded that lower yield cigarettes would produce small benefits compared with stopping smoking.

1982 SGR reviewed evidence of harm to nonsmoking wives of smoking husbands and assessed low-cost smoking cessation interventions. U.S. Congress doubled the excise tax on cigarettes to 16 cents per pack. Cigarette manufacturers used this as a smokescreen to increase their prices swelling their profit margin to well over 20 percent, twice the average return on stocks in corporate America.

1983 SGR concluded that smoking "should be considered the most important of the known modifiable risk factors" for coronary heart disease.

1984 SGR concluded that smoking is the major cause of chronic obstructive lung disease, accounting for 80 percent to 90 percent of deaths and extensive morbidity and extended disability from chronic obstructive lung diseases. Surgeon General C. Everett Koop declares an objective for a smoke-free society by the year 2000. U.S. Congress passes a bill that forces tobacco companies to list their ingredients.

1985 SGR found smoking more important than most workplace hazards for smokers.

1986 SGR concluded that "involuntary smoking is a cause of disease, including lung cancer, in healthy nonsmokers." Reviewed the growth in restrictions on smoking in public places and workplaces, concluding that separation reduces but does not eliminate exposure to environmental tobacco smoke.

1988 Canada adopts a comprehensive bill that bans tobacco advertising. In the United States, a new SGR established nicotine as a highly addictive substance, comparable in its physiological and

psychological properties to other addictive substances of abuse.

1989 SGR reviews twenty-five years of progress on reducing the health consequences of smoking and concludes that smoking, responsible for one of every six deaths in the United States, remains the single most important preventable cause of death in North America.

1994 Canadian federal government slashed taxes on cigarettes to counter the smuggling across the U.S. border that was creating a large black market in cigarettes with 30 percent of cigarettes consumed being imported illegally.

1995 The Supreme Court of Canada struck down the landmark law of 1988 banning tobacco advertising, basing its decision on freedom-of-expression grounds. President Bill Clinton instructed the U.S. Food and Drug Administration to proceed with regulation of tobacco advertising to children and youth, basing his decision on the grounds that nicotine is an addictive drug.

1996 Canadian health minister announced bill to counter the effects of the tax reductions and Supreme Court rulings. The bill would increase taxes, strengthen labeling requirements, reintroduce bans of advertising, and limit sponsorship of sporting and cultural events by the tobacco industry.

1997 The Liggett Group broke rank with the rest of the tobacco industry in conceding that tobacco is addictive and causes cancer and accepting terms that compensate states filing suit against the industry for damages related to health care costs incurred as a result of tobacco promotion.

● ● ● ● ● ● ● ● ● ● ● ● ● ● ● ● ● ● ● ●
Figure 12-3

Current cigarette smokers among persons 18 years of age and over by sex: U.S., 1965 to 1993. (*Source:* Centers for Disease Control and Prevention, National Center for Health Statistics, National Health Interview Survey.)

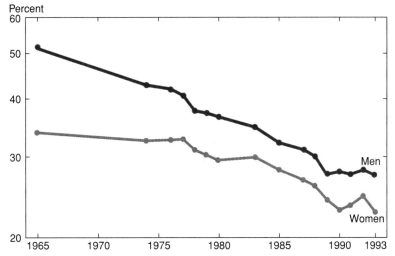

NOTES: Proportions are age adjusted. Data for 1992 and 1993 are not strictly comparable with earlier years or each other due to a change in the definition of current smoker in 1992 and the use of a split sample in 1992. Percents are plotted on a log scale.

surpassed their death rate from breast cancer. The smoking epidemic had caught up with them full force. Although smoking rates for women have fallen again to 23 percent, the rise in the number of women smokers has not escaped the attention of cigarette manufacturers. They have stepped up their promotion of new brands of cigarettes designed expressly for women.

In 1995, 29 percent of Canadians over the age of 12 smoked. This represents approximately 7 million people who smoke an average of 19 cigarettes a day. Although the smoking rates had declined the preceding two decades, by 1990 the smoking rates showed no decline. Some surveys suggest the rate has begun to increase after 1993. Smoking has increased among adolescents age 15 to 19 from 21 percent in 1990 to 29 percent in 1995. Adolescent girls smoke at three times of rate of boys. In 1993, the total direct costs of smoking

in Canada were in excess of $10 billion, which compares with total tobacco tax revenue for the same period of approximately $6 billion. This cost discrepancy can be seen in some antitobacco advertising (figure 12-4).

Smokeless tobacco As smoking decreased in the 1970s, a fourfold increase in chewing tobacco users and a fifteenfold increase in snuff users between 1970 and 1986 prompted new national, state, and community campaigns directed at teenagers. Most smokeless tobacco users begin their use before age 21. Smokeless tobacco use declined among males aged 18 to 24 by 1994, but increased for males ages 12 to 17 to 5.1 percent.

Age and Sex The average age of first use for cigarettes increased to 12.2 years by 1994. Smoking among high school seniors was unchanged

∙∙∙∙∙∙∙∙∙∙∙∙∙∙∙∙∙∙∙∙∙∙

Figure 12-4

Many voluntary agencies provide information and services to help reduce tobacco use or to help the victims of the diseases caused by tobacco. (*Source:* Canadian Cancer Society.)

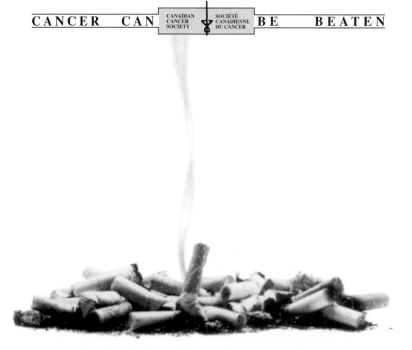

If you won't quit smoking, the least you can do is donate the price of a couple of cartons of cigarettes, so that if you need us, we'll be ready for you.

CANCER CAN | CANADIAN CANCER SOCIETY | SOCIÉTÉ CANADIENNE DU CANCER | BE BEATEN

from the mid-1980s to the early 1990s, but has increased. Tobacco habits established in the teens in the great majority of cases, will persist into adulthood. Teenage girls, who in the past never smoked to the extent that teenage boys did, have caught up. In 1968 only about half as many teenage girls smoked as boys, but by 1979 girls had surpassed boys in teenage smoking. Among lower socioeconomic status youth approximately 40 percent smoke. Smoking declines with age after early adulthood. Smoking parents set the example for children. Studies show that youngsters whose parents smoke are more likely to adopt the habit than are children of nonsmoking parents.

ISSUES AND CONTROVERSIES
Banning Smoking in Public Places, Including Bars?

Toronto passed a bylaw early in 1997, backed by fines of up to $5,000, to stamp out smoking in the city's bars and restaurants. California's statewide law banning smoking in bars went into effect in 1998. Antitobacco groups have applauded these measures, but smokers have challenged the laws with widespread civil disobedience. Many bar owners complain that the laws cost them customers and will put some out of business. Police have not enforced the law with significant surveillance or fines. As the noose tightens around the $170-billion-a-year tobacco industry through court actions to hold the industry responsible for smoking-related deaths, illness, and health-care costs, the beleaguered smokers feel increasingly ostracized. They show signs of flaunting the law, smoking in any part of a restaurant or bar. This is making the air worse than before for non-smokers in those places that previously had segregated smoking areas.

Have the antismoking forces gone too far? Is the tobacco control movement at risk of producing a backlash of the magnitude of the speakeasies and distillers of the prohibition era with alcohol? Will adolescents take this prohibition as one more reason to smoke to defy adult authority? What are the pros and cons of banning smoking in bars? What are the advantages and disadvantages of banning all smoking in restaurants rather than providing segregated, separately ventilated, smoking areas? Is it fair to make the addicted smokers the target of most tobacco control initiatives, rather than the tobacco industry?

International Smoking Rates

Cigarettes are projected to kill one in five people in industrialized countries over the next thirty years. The lag time between smoking prevalence and related morbidity and mortality is seen in different patterns around the globe. Most industrialized countries are experiencing the incongruous combination of declining prevalence and increasing morbidity and mortality from smoking. Less-industrialized countries are entering a period of high prevalence and are beginning to experience some of the disease and disability associated with smoking. The least industrialized countries have low prevalence of smoking and related mortality but have other public health issues to contend with. Eventually, smoking may kill even more in the less industrialized countries. For example, in China, with almost one-third of the world's population, more than 60 percent of the men smoke; in Poland, half of the men who die between the ages of 35 and 69, die of smoking-related causes.

Prevention of Tobacco Use

A national strategy to reduce tobacco use requires multiple types and levels of strategies that are economic, legal, educational, and pharmacological. The six core components of tobacco control programs include: preventing tobacco use, treating nicotine addiction, protecting nonsmokers from environmental tobacco exposure, limiting the effect of tobacco advertising and promotion on young people, increasing the price of tobacco products, and regulating tobacco products. The eventual demise of smoking as a socially acceptable habit will be achieved by persistent action and a variety of concerted approaches. Realistic achievement of goals should be expected in several years, perhaps decades. The U.S. Office of Smoking and Health announced in early 1998 that the nation's objectives for reduction of smoking would not be achieved by the year 2000.

Economics   Tobacco has been a major economic factor in the first 200 years of the development of North America. The profitability of its industry has been legendary and has resulted in lavish promotional efforts. Governments have not been indifferent to this potential source of revenue. The tobacco industry contributes, from the tobacco field to the vending machine, $18 billion to the gross national product of the United States and gives livelihood to a well-publicized segment of the population. These economic activities are protected and fostered by departments of agriculture and the departments of Commerce and add billions of dollars annually to a precarious balance of payments. With billions in U.S. cigarette advertising, the media tend to defend the tobacco industry and resist constraints on advertising on the grounds of First Amendment rights to free press.

The economic revenue from smoking is offset by the compensation for the burden of death, disease, health care, fires, and lost productivity. The U.S. population of civilian, noninstitutionalized persons aged twenty-five years or older who ever smoked cigarettes will incur lifetime excess medical care costs of $501 billion. The estimated average lifetime medical costs for a smoker exceed those for a nonsmoker by over $6,000. The number grows approximately $9 to $10 billion annually because of the additional excess lifetime health care costs of the 1 million teenagers who take up smoking each year.

Legal and Legislative   The tort law in the United States exposes manufacturers to class action suits if they express doubt about the safety of their products. This explains the unprecedented hearings in 1994 where seven top tobacco company executives appeared before Congress to say, under oath, that cigarettes are not addictive and may not even be bad for one's health. The turn around in three years by the Liggett Group to admit the addictiveness of tobacco and their willingness to turn over communications with other companies on this point, portends changes in legal remedies to the tobacco problem.

Traditionally, legislatures have been more sensitive to the immediacy of economic issues and therefore have given only token attention to funding public health needs in smoking. Increasingly, however, local and state legislatures have been passing laws that limit or prohibit smoking in public places such as public buildings, transit, worksites, and restaurants. Forty-one states and the District of Columbia have laws restricting smoking in public places; 38 states and the District have laws and/or executive orders restricting smoking in public workplaces; and 18 states and the District have laws regulating smoking in private worksites. All 50 states and the District have laws prohibiting the sale and distribution of tobacco to youth under the age of 18.

Canada raised federal and provincial per pack cigarette taxes from 46 cents in 1980 to $3.27 in 1991 (figure 12-5). During that time, teen smoking declined by approximately two-thirds and total cigarette consumption fell faster than in any major industrialized nation. Cigarette tax revenue grew from about $1 billion in 1981 to $7 billion in 1991. The subsequent drop in taxes to reduce smuggling across the U.S. border of cheaper cigarettes resulted in a slowing of the decline in smoking rates, but not a reversal of the trend.

Health Education   Communities can mount antismoking campaigns, and local groups can reinforce national leadership on this issue. People must be made aware of the hazards of cigarette smoking (figure 12-6). This awareness results in (1) individuals being motivated not to smoke; and (2) smoking becoming less socially acceptable, which will reinforce decisions not to smoke. Such awareness is important in the young because advertising presently directed at youth depicts smoking as being socially acceptable and desirable.

In the young, it is also necessary to negate peer influence, which often emphasizes risk taking. During the **socialization** process, nonsmoking

Figure 12-5

Annual per capita consumption of cigarettes in Canada went down dramatically after 1981 with the increases in taxes that raised the real price of tobacco (per twenty cigarettes). The large discrepancy in prices between the low U.S. cost for a carton of cigarettes and the high Canadian price resulted in smuggling of cigarettes across the U.S.-Canadian border for illegal profiteering. An adjustment for black market consumption is shown in the last three years before taxes were lowered in Canada. (*Source:* Non-Smokers' Rights Association, Ottawa, Ontario, Canada.)

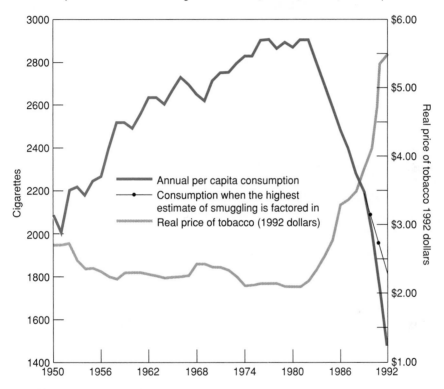

Note: Cigarettes include fine-cut equivalents

must be instilled. Role models—persons teenagers admire—may prove effective. The difficulty is that not smoking is a "nonaction" rather than a dynamic force easy to associate with hero figures. To teenagers, smoking may also be a symbol of independence and rebellion against the norms of the family or group to which they belong.

The educational approach requires identification of, and provision for assistance to, those individuals at an increased risk of tobacco-related dis-

eases (figure 12-7). Epidemiological surveys are conducted to determine the environmental, social, and psychological characteristics of the population at risk. The main thrust in this component of smoking education has been in the development of epidemiological methods for identifying groups at high risk of tobacco-related disease; analysis of smoking patterns and behavior; research in smoking cessation techniques; and evaluation of smoking education programs.

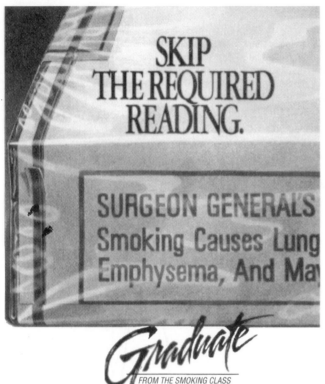

U.S. Department of Health & Human Services

· · · · · · · · · · · · · · · · · · · ·

Figure 12-6

Bold, no nonsense labels on cigarette packages help increase public awareness about the hazards of smoking. (*Source:* U.S. Department of Health and Human Services.)

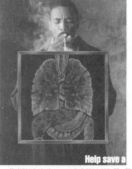
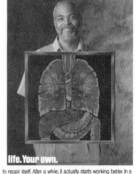

· · · · · · · · · · · · · · · · · · · ·

Figure 12-7

This federal campaign ad targets those who have continued to smoke for long periods of their adulthood, thinking that they have already done irreparable damage and that it is too late to quit. In fact, statistics show that most of those who quit after many years of smoking return to normal cardiovascular and respiratory functioning over a period of two to five years. (*Source:* Centers for Disease Control and Prevention, National Heart, Lung, and Blood Institute; Public Health Service; U.S. Department of Health and Human Services.)

Pharmacological Approaches Cigarette smoking is a form of drug dependence on nicotine. In 1988 the Surgeon General of the U.S. Public Health Service declared tobacco an addictive substance. The Food and Drug Administration is issuing proposals for regulating tobacco as a drug. Nicotine is recognized as a potent drug eliciting pharmacological effects on the central nervous system and playing an important role in controlling smoking behavior. Consequently, pharmacological intervention, such as the nicotine patch, is a possible method for controlling smoking behavior. Such activities are directed at reducing relapse in smoking cessation programs through combined pharmacological, physiological, and psychological approaches; improving and maintaining initial quitting rates; improving people's understanding of the physicochemical properties of nicotine and its metabolites; and identifying substances that taste, smell, or react like nicotine to use as substitutes for cigarette smoking.

Another pharmacological approach is to produce a less hazardous type of cigarette. Average tar and nicotine content of cigarettes sold in the United States have declined by more than 50 percent since 1954 as a result of these efforts, although a truly "safe" cigarette does not exist. Labeling the cigarette package with the amounts of each hazardous substance and with a general health warning has helped remind smokers of the specific risks.

Schools and Worksites The school classroom is frequently regarded as the setting in which antismoking education should take place. Unfortunately, this curriculum focus on schools often ignores the even greater problems and opportunities outside the classroom where children and youth gather, observe, and are exposed to smoking influences. Some of the most promising health education programs in relation to smoking are those addressing the total school environment and "inoculating" pupils against the social pressures they may encounter in that environment. Role playing by rehearsing in the classroom how to de-

Environmental Objectives for Tobacco

- By 2000 establish tobacco-free environments and include tobacco use prevention in the curricula of all elementary, middle, and secondary schools. Baseline: antismoking education was provided by 78% of school districts at the high school level, 81% at the middle school level, and 75% at the elementary school level in 1988.
- By 2000 increase to at least 75% the proportion of worksites with a formal smoking policy that prohibits or severely restricts smoking at the workplace. Baseline: 27% of worksites with 50 or more employees in 1985; 54% of medium and large companies in 1987.
- By 2000 enact and enforce in 50 states laws prohibiting the sale and distribution of tobacco products to youth younger than age 19. Baseline: 44 states had, but rarely enforced, laws regulating the sale and/or distribution of cigarettes or tobacco product to minors in 1990; only 3 set the age of majority at 19, and only 6 prohibited cigarette vending machines accessible to minors.
- By 2000 eliminate or severely restrict all forms of tobacco product advertising to which youth under 18 are exposed.

cline a cigarette offer from a peer has proved effective in delaying the uptake of smoking.

Worksites represent the other environment where people gather, observe, and are influenced by their social and physical surroundings for the greater part of their waking hours. Increasing numbers of businesses in the United States have programs to help their employees stop smoking. Nearly 60 percent of employers with fifty or more employees have policies in place either prohibiting or severely restricting smoking. A significant number have policies to restrict or prohibit smoking in the workplace, most frequently in areas where smoking poses the greatest health hazard. Antismoking programs are the third most common health education program sponsored by companies, after hypertension control and diet-weight management.

ALCOHOL MISUSE

Substance abuse—including alcohol and other drugs—costs the nation almost $240 billion a year, including $100 billion in lost productivity and 13.7 billion in health care. After smoking, alcohol is the most important known cause of mortality and morbidity in most Western countries. The American experience with Prohibition and the longer history of alcohol in civilization indicate that alcohol is a drug that society cannot entirely eradicate. Like most of the lifestyle **risk factors,** the use of alcohol in moderation (with possible exceptions, such as by alcoholics and by women during pregnancy) can be tolerated and even can be beneficial.

Epidemiology of Alcohol Misuse

Alcohol is undoubtedly the most abused drug in North America, Europe, Australia, and New Zealand. Alcohol abuse can lower resistance and increase risk of infectious disease. It contributes to or is associated with ill health, crime, poverty, broken homes, unintended pregnancy, divorce, social conflicts, loss of earning power, loss of productivity, social degradation, and other social pathology. Many social, economic, and political factors influence the role of alcohol in society.

Four to six million Americans have been diagnosed as alcoholics, and 10 percent of the U.S. adult population is believed to have a serious drinking problem. One in four adolescents is at high risk of alcohol and other drug problems, school failure, early unwanted pregnancy, and/or delinquency. The average age of first use of alcohol, 12.9 years, showed little change during the 1990s. This early use of alcohol sets the stage for early and potentially sustained use of alcohol as an indicator of chronic lifelong mental and physical health problems, and social maladjustment.

It is estimated that 50 percent of all traffic fatalities and fatal intentional injuries, such as suicides and homicides, are alcohol-related. Nearly 20,000 people were killed in 1991 in alcohol-related traffic crashes. Overall, such fatalities have declined from 9.8 percent in 1987 to 6.8 percent in 1993; this later figure means that the year 2000 objective was surpassed by middecade. As a result a new year 2000 objective was set of no more than 5.5 alcohol-related motor vehicle crashes per 100,000 people (figure 12-8). Approximately one-third of victims are intoxicated in homicides, drowning, and boating deaths.

Fetal Alcohol Syndrome (FAS), the number one *known* cause of mental retardation and birth defects, results from alcohol consumption by women during pregnancy. The incidence of FAS in Europe and North America is approximately 1 in 300 to 500 live births. FAS can be found in all racial and ethnic groups where women drink a moderate to heavy amount of alcohol during pregnancy. This syndrome is a recognized pattern of malformations, encompassing neurological and behavioral abnormalities, growth retardation, and characteristic physical and facial features. FAS is common, expensive, and preventable.

Cirrhosis of the liver, one of the ten leading causes of death in most Western countries, is caused primarily by alcohol consumption. The cirrhosis death rate has shown a significant decline from 9.1 per 100,000 in 1987 to 7.9 in 1994. Low socioeconomic groups have a higher prevalence of cirrhosis than do high socioeconomic groups.

Costs related to alcohol problems are estimated to exceed $70 billion per year in the United States, with the majority of those costs attributed to low productivity. Over a million people receive alcohol and other drug treatment services annually from publicly funded agencies.

A 1995 survey by Health Canada found that 77.7 percent of Canadians describe themselves as current drinkers, with about 25 percent indicating this means less than one drink a month and 5 percent admitting to daily alcohol consumption. Men are more likely to drink than women and to drink more. Although 80 percent of respondents indicated their alcohol consumption had not harmed others, 73 percent indicated they had been harmed by the drinking of others. The pain caused by others included serious quarrels, being

. . . .

Figure 12-8

Alcohol-related motor vehicle crash deaths: United States 1987 to 1994, and year 2000 targets. (*Source:* U.S. Department of Transportation, Fatal Accident Reporting System.)

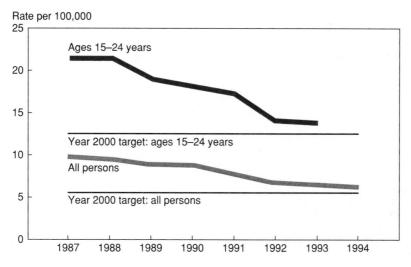

	1987	1988	1989	1990	1991	1992	1993	1994	Year 2000 target
All persons..............	9.8	9.6	9.0	8.9	7.9	6.9	6.8	6.4	5.5
Ages 15–24 years....	21.5	21.5	19.1	18.5	17.2	14.1	13.8	- - -	12.5

- - - Data not available.

shoved or pushed, physical assault, and marital problems. Heavy federal and provincial taxes are placed on alcohol, raising about $4 billion annually in revenue. The costs of abuse, estimated at $5 billion annually, exceed the revenues generated by alcohol.

Prevention of Alcohol Misuse

Like the prevention of tobacco use, the prevention of problems related to alcohol consists of interventions on agent, host, and environment levels.

Agent Alcohol is the agent, an anesthetic that is toxic in overdose. Alcohol has a long history of use across the centuries from medicinal to recre-

ational to spiritual. The revised dietary guidelines issued by the U.S. federal government in 1996, suggest that a glass of wine a day for women and two for men, taken with meals, is healthful. A "drink" is defined as 5 ounces of wine, 12 ounces of beer, or 1.5 ounces of 80-proof distilled spirits. This recommendation is based on data, marshaled in part by wine and liquor manufacturers, that moderate drinking is associated with a lower risk for coronary heart disease.

This dietary recommendation is made in the context of other guidelines that recommend physical exercise; the consumption of less fat; and eating more grain, fruits, and vegetables. The new message is moderation and replaces the 1990

Objectives for Alcohol and Other Drugs

- By 2000 reduce death caused by alcohol-related motor vehicle crashes to no more than 5.5 per 100,000 people. Baseline: 9.8 in 1987.
- By 2000 reduce cirrhosis deaths to no more than 6 per 100,000 people. Baseline: 9.2 in 1987.
- By 2000 reduce drug-related death to no more than 3 per 100,000. Baseline: 3.8 in 1987.
- By 2000 increase by at least 1 year the average age of first use of cigarettes, alcohol, and marijuana by adolescents aged 12-17. Baseline: age 11.6 for cigarettes, age 13.1 for alcohol, and age 13.4 for marijuana in 1988.
- By 2000 reduce the proportion of high school seniors and college students engaging in recent occasions of heavy drinking of alcoholic beverages to no more than 28% of high school seniors and 32% of college students. Baseline: 33% of seniors and 41.7% of college students in 1989.

guidelines, which indicated that alcohol consumption had no health benefit and was not recommended. In fact, the U.S. Department of Health and Human Services and the National Research Council warn that with the consumption of three or more drinks per day, harmful effects such as high blood pressure, cirrhosis of the liver, and even heart attacks begin. There is no known safe level of alcohol consumption during pregnancy.

Alcohol is a readily available drug and, as other drugs, has a reinforcing or anxiety reducing quality, that makes it attractive to use. The use of alcohol, as understood from physical, cultural, legal, and environmental perspectives, may have different meanings. From a physical perspective, the healthy adult liver can oxidize about one-fourth ounce of absolute alcohol per hour. The alcohol content is half the proof, so one-fourth ounce is equal to 0.6 ounce of 86 proof alcohol. The absorption of alcohol into the bloodstream is delayed by food in the stomach, therefore peak blood levels are not reached so quickly after eating. From a

cultural perspective alcohol use can be understood as celebratory by some or immoral by others. From a legal perspective, use may be measured in blood alcohol concentration to determine driving privileges. The decision to consume alcohol or not may be influenced by various factors.

Host   Altering the behavior of the host—in this case the person consuming alcohol—is the most popular intervention. Exhortations to quit drinking, coupled with deprivation, is usually tried. Group therapy and mutual self-help groups using behavioral modification techniques have the best success records. Alcoholics Anonymous is the leading exponent of group approaches. Counselors are frequently former alcoholics, better able to appreciate the difficulties of abstinence than are those who have never overcome such a problem. A nonjudgmental, supportive, understanding relationship must be established. In thinking about the host, it is important to remember that alcohol effects more than the person drinking. Of special importance is the unborn fetus of women consuming excessive alcohol.

Environment   The environment can play a major role in preventing, encouraging, or sustaining alcohol use. Most medical treatment is directed at the alcoholic and merely results in rendering the alcoholic fit enough to resume drinking. Surviving cirrhosis depends on cessation of alcohol consumption. Increasingly, health professionals are engaged in screening and counseling people before alcohol becomes a problem. In hostile environments of poverty, homelessness, unemployment, and racism alcohol may seem an easy escape for some. If people use alcohol abusively to cope with such problems or the alcoholic persists in drinking, medical and surgical measures are to no avail. Worksite and other social networks to help people abstain from alcohol, such as Alcoholics Anonymous, and the help of family and friends, should be supported in the community. Broad based interventions across multiple environmental sections are needed to cope with the diverse causes and consequences of alcohol abuse.

Public Education and Action

The reduction of alcohol-related vehicle deaths is one of the greatest success stories of public health in the 1990s. The communication of effective alcohol-related health messages is particularly challenging and difficult. Few products can match alcohol in the ability to evoke strong sentiments—positive and negative. Most people already have firm opinions concerning the appropriate role of alcoholic beverages in their personal lives, and such beliefs, whether based on accurate information or not, are highly resistant to change.

Perceptions about alcohol use may be acquired through personal experience with alcoholic beverages or through the experiences and influence of associates, friends, and family members. Perceptions may also be acquired vicariously from the depiction of alcohol use in publications and in film, radio, and television dramatizations. Unfortunately, some of these perceptions are incorrect or incomplete. Many people do not know how alcohol is metabolized in the body and have only partial knowledge about the effect that food or time can have on this process; they also assume, incorrectly, that coffee can have a mitigating effect. People are insufficiently aware that consumption of large amounts of alcohol in a short period of time, such as may occur in a drinking contest, can cause death. Often, they are also unaware that drinking can cause or contribute to many health hazards.

Advertising and Counteradvertising An important source of perceptions is alcoholic beverage advertising, particularly for young people. For example, the favorable image alcohol users are given in television advertising and programming creates a barrier to be overcome in alcohol education efforts. The alcoholic beverage industry commits over a billion dollars annually to an extensive array of product advertising in the print and broadcast media.

Considering the pervasiveness of positive images concerning alcohol use, communication

Figure 12-9

The innocent face of this young child serves as a haunting reminder that drinking means more than our own pleasure or escape; it may mean someone else's life. (*Source:* Center for Substance Abuse Prevention.)

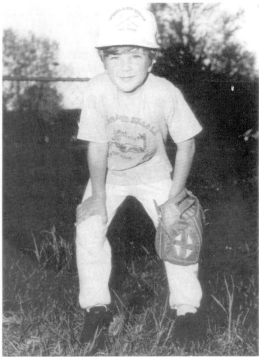

DRUNK DRIVING DOESN'T JUST KILL DRUNK DRIVERS.

Nicholas Esposito, killed Oct. 13, 1989 at 8:25 pm.
Next time your friend insists on driving drunk, do whatever it takes to stop him.
Because if he kills innocent people, how will you live with yourself?

FRIENDS DON'T LET FRIENDS DRIVE DRUNK.

about alcohol must be strategic. It should target current or potential users. It must include mass media campaigns and product labeling to inform, to raise awareness levels, or to reinforce old knowledge, to change potentially harmful responses to social situations in which alcohol use is encouraged, and to understand the consequences of alcohol abuse on self and others (figure 12-9). Education can be used also to raise critical awareness about the methods of advertising alcohol.

Public Policy   In the United States, many different agencies work together at the federal level to combat alcohol and substance abuse, including the Departments of Education, Health and Human Services, Housing and Urban Development, Justice, and Labor. The wide range of services offered through these agencies support programs directly aimed at alcohol prevention and treatment, and programs that deal with problems of homelessness and unemployment that may lead to or sustain substance abuse. In Canada, similar intersectoral cooperation is sought, but the agencies sometimes work at cross-purposes in both countries.

Legal Sanctions   To get intoxicated drivers off the road quickly, thirty-seven states and some Canadian provinces have passed administrative license revocation laws. Drivers who are unable to pass a road-side intoxication test have their licenses revoked immediately. Further, some states have lowered the tolerance levels for blood alcohol concentration from .1 to .08. Enforcement of these laws and education of intoxicated drivers have contributed to reductions in alcohol-related traffic deaths.

Organizational and Environmental Supports Altering the environment is the most effective way of reducing alcoholism in the community. In many instances the social environment of schools, colleges, worksites, and public gathering places creates pressure on the individual to drink. Social ambience must be altered so that alcohol is not regarded as a reward, as a status symbol, or as something that is glamorous.

Economic Supports   The cost of alcohol has increased much less than other beverages. It can be greatly increased by taxation so that a more significant part of discretionary income must be expended to buy alcohol. Mortality from injuries and hepatic disease drops suddenly when alcohol is removed from the community or when supply or demand is restricted by an **excise tax.** This economic approach works best with teenagers, but it penal-izes the poor. It has an effect on overall community consumption, but not necessarily on the most addicted and heaviest drinkers.

Warning Labels   The 100th Congress passed an Omnibus Drug Bill with provisions for a new label on alcoholic beverages that would read: "Government Warning: (1) According to the Surgeon General, women should not drink alcoholic beverages during pregnancy because of the risk of birth defects. (2) Consumption of alcoholic beverages impairs your ability to drive a car or operate machinery and may cause health problems."

Primary Care Providers   Health professionals and other service providers such as social workers, counselors, and teachers can be educated to detect early warning signs of alcohol abuse and other drug abuse. Professionals should be taught to screen and counsel for alcohol and other drug use.

DRUG MISUSE

Drugs have been used throughout the ages for various medicinal, recreational, and religious purposes. As recently as the close of World War II, the term *problem drugs* meant only morphine or its derivative, heroin. This limited concept of problem drugs has expanded to the point where opium and morphine use are the lesser drug problems. As more people become dependent on drugs, there has arisen an alarming misuse of stimulants, depressants, hallucinogens, and narcotics cutting across all social strata. The abuse of illicit drugs drains the U.S. economy of billions of dollars annually. This includes lost productivity, morbidity, and mortality. AIDS resulting from injecting drugs, babies born HIV-positive or exposed to crack cocaine, and drug-related violence are part of the costs of drug use.

Epidemiology of Drug Misuse

Although the use of drugs has declined in some populations, it remains a persistent and increasing problem in others. The mid-decade review of the

....

Figure 12-10

Status of year 2000 substance abuse objectives by mid-decade. (*Source:* Substance Abuse and Mental Health Service Administration.)

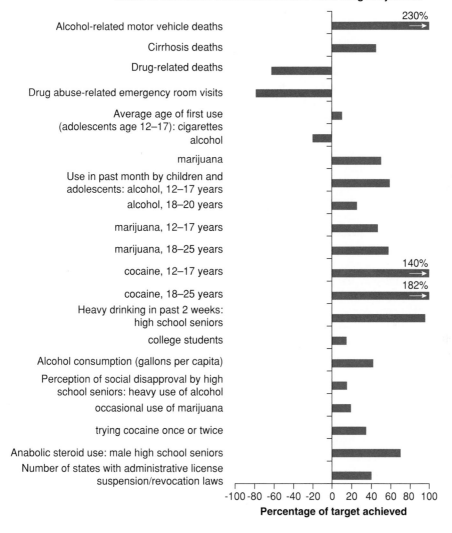

Status of substance abuse: alcohol and other drugs objectives

year 2000 objectives for alcohol and other drugs shows positive movement on a number of indicators, but lack of progress on others, most notably the occasional use of marijuana (figure 12-10).

An estimated 66 million Americans have tried marijuana at least once and 22 million have tried cocaine. The average first age of the use of marijuana is 13.9 years. Marijuana use—as measured by those who reported use in the previous month— remained relatively stable at approximately 5 percent of those 12-years-old and over for the first half of the 1990s. In 1994, the largest age groups of those reporting marijuana in the previous month were 14 to 15 year olds (11 percent) and those 18 to 26 years old (12 percent). Cocaine use—as measured by use in the previous month —remained relatively stable at approximately .6 percent for those 12-years-old and over for the first half of the 1990s. In 1994, the largest age groups of those reporting marijuana in the previous month were 18 to 25 years old (1.0 percent) and 26 to 34 year olds (1.5 percent). Mass media campaigns are one way of reaching these age groups (figure 12-11).

In 1993, 4 percent of adult Canadians reported having used marijuana in the previous year and .3 percent reported use of cocaine or crack in the same time period. A 1995 Health Canada survey, found that women take more medication than men. For example, when asked about the use of tranquilizers, diet pills, antidepressants, painkillers, and sleeping pills, 23.9 percent of women said they had used them as compared with 17.7 percent of men.

Adverse Drug Reactions

In addition to purposeful misuse, the uninformed or misguided mixing of prescription drugs, over-the-counter drugs, alcohol, and certain foods leads to adverse reactions, including hormonal imbalances; digestive disturbances; mood alterations; and other problems that interfere with normal functioning, productivity, and safety. This is problematic at a time when millions of children and adults are on controversial drugs, such as Ritalin or Prozac, to control attention span, mood, or behavior. To say that we are a "pill-happy" society is not an exaggeration, and reliance on pills is the genesis of much drug misuse and abuse.

The Elderly   The elderly, who make up 10 percent of the U.S. population, spend an estimated 20 percent of the national total for drugs. The per capita expenditure by the elderly for prescribed drugs exceeds that for other age groups. The average elderly person spent over $500 in 1990 for prescription and over-the-counter drugs and averaged more than 13 prescriptions (including renewals) a year. It is well recognized that older patients are more likely than younger patients to have adverse drug reactions. Their potential isolation makes such reactions particularly problematic.

Drug Information   There is no readily accessible, single source of information on drugs, their uses, and their monitoring. The most frequently used source is the labeling on each drug approved by the Food and Drug Administration. Education needs to be directed not only at patients taking drugs, but family members, peers, and others who influence them.

Drug misuse is a complex social and health problem. Its solution must come through education and social change, not punishment. Sometimes there is a place for a "crash" program of education, but the problems of drug misuse call for a long-term, continuing program of education and related organizational, economic, and environmental change.

Addiction and Habituation

Drug **addiction** is a state in which an altered state of the body tissue produces a physical dependence that becomes known only after discontinuation of the drug; this dependence is masked while the drug is being taken. The World Health Organization's criteria for addiction are: (1) a compulsion to use and to obtain a substance by any means; (2) a need to increase the dosage to obtain the desired effects; (3) a physiological as well as a psychological dependence on the effects of the substance; and (4) a detrimental effect not only on the individual but also on the community.

Levels of Use   The U.S. National Commission on Marijuana and Drug Abuse has divided the entire spectrum of drug-using behavior into the following five patterns:

1. *Experimental.* The most common type of drug-using behavior—a short, nonpatterned trial of one or more drugs, motivated primarily by the individual's curiosity or desire to experience an altered mood state.

· · · · · · · · · · · · · · · · · · · ·
Figure 12-11

Mass media campaigns are one approach to reaching selected populations to reduce substance abuse. (*Source:* Partnership for a Drug-Free America.)

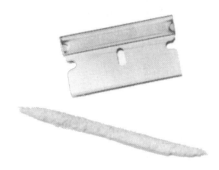

TO MILLIONS OF AMERICAN WORKERS, IT'S CONSIDERED A LUNCH LINE.

If it's not cocaine, it's marijuana or hashish or non-medical use of stimulants, sedatives or tranquilizers. Or any other number of other illicit drugs.

More than eight million employed Americans used an illicit drug at least one time in the last month. Nearly 14 million used one in the past year. And it's not just the users who are paying the cost, it's you, the non-user. Because of accidents, illnesses, absenteeism, thefts, and medical expenses, illicit drug use on the job is costing the nation nearly 60 billion dollars a year.

And while you may not realize it, that loss has a direct effect on your paycheck.

It's enough to make you furious. But after you're finished being angry at what the user is costing you, do something. Speak up. Don't depend on a husband or wife or friend. If you see a problem it's your problem, too. Call 1-800-662-HELP and find out what you can do.

Because the only way to get rid of lunch lines is to help people lose their appetites.

PARTNERSHIP FOR A DRUG-FREE AMERICA

2. *Recreational.* Voluntary or patterned use of a drug, usually in social settings; behavior is not sustained because the user is not dependent on the drug.

3. *Circumstantial.* Behavior generally motivated by the user's perceived need or desire to achieve a new and anticipated effect to cope with a specific problem or situation (for example, amphetamine use by students preparing for examinations or by long-distance truckers).

4. *Intensified drug-using behavior.* Drug use that occurs daily and is motivated by an individual's problem or stressful situation or a desire to maintain a certain self-prescribed level of performance (for example, homemakers regularly using barbiturates or other sedatives, business executives regularly using tranquilizers, youth turning to drugs as sources of excitement or meaning); the salient feature of this group is that the individual still remains integrated within the larger social and economic structure.

5. *Compulsive use.* Patterned behavior at a high frequency and high level of interest, characterized by a high degree of psychological dependence and perhaps physical dependence. This category encompasses the smallest number of drug users. The distinguishing feature of this behavior is that drug use dominates the individual's existence, and preoccupation with drug taking precludes other social functioning (such users include chronic alcoholics and heroin-dependent persons).

Habituation means the customary use of some substance or practice that a person finds pleasurable, either as relaxation or activation. Habituation to a drug differs from addiction in that the drug has not produced a physical or psychological dependence; the individual can terminate the use of the drug without discernible side effects. For example, habituation to coffee, tea, and cola drinks is widespread, but little evidence exists that addiction occurs.

Epidemiological Approach to Drug Misuse

If drug misuse, as other lifestyle issues, is seen as a practice that is transmitted from one person to another, it may be considered for operational purposes a contagious illness. This approach makes it possible to continue to apply the methods and terminology used in the epidemiology of infectious disease (see chapters 3 and 11).

In epidemiological terms, the infectious *agent* is the drug, the *host* and reservoir are the human, the *environment* is the community, and the *vector* is the drug-using peer. The conventional notion of the "pusher" as the vector is effectively dispelled by a careful review of studies in which an effort was made to trace the spread of drug use from person to person. These studies establish that, in the vast majority of instances, the addict or abuser is introduced to the use of the drug by a well-meaning friend, usually in the environment of previously established peer group activity. Beginners must learn snorting or intravenous injection techniques from other addicts or users.

Drug misuse presents the well-known characteristics of epidemics, including rapid spread, clear geographical bounds, and certain age groups and strata of the population being more affected than others.

OBESITY, OVERNUTRITION, AND UNDERNUTRITION

Food intake is a paradox in Canada and the United States. On one hand, nutrition has improved. This is evidenced by the positive dietary changes, such as the consumption of more low fat milk and less red meats (figure 12-12). On the other hand, the mean body weight of Americans has steadily increased leading to increased health problems (figure 12-13). This paradox extends to overnutrition or **obesity** and undernutrition among different population segments. Overnutrition is a major health problem in the United States and in many other Western countries, especially

••••••••••••••••••••••

Figure 12-12

Dietary changes over twelve years for selected foods, 1977 to 1978 and 1989 to 1990. (*Source:* U.S. Department of Agriculture, Human Nutrition Information Service, Nationwide Food Consumption Survey, 1977 to 1978, and Continuing Survey of Food Intakes by Individuals, 1989 to 1990. (Data compiled by National Center for Health Statistics: *Health United States, 1995.* Hyattsville, MD, 1996, Public Health Service.)

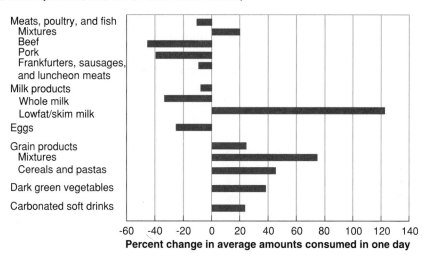

••••••••••••••••••••••

Figure 12-13

Prevalence of overweight among women 20 to 74 years of age by age group: U.S. selected years. (*Source:* Centers for Disease Control and Prevention, National Center for Health Statistics, National Health and Nutrition Examination Survey III.)

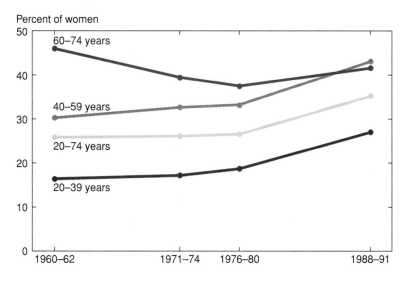

the consumption of dietary fats. One in every three (34 percent) adult Americans and as many as one out of every five adolescents (21 percent) are overweight. Equally problematic is that an estimated one out of eight American children under age twelve suffers from hunger and that many homeless and poor adults experience the same. Overnutrition and undernutrition reflect environmental, cultural, and socioeconomic conditions.

Epidemiology of Nutrition

Status and Trends In the United States, 1976 to 1980 baseline figures indicated that 24 percent of men, 27 percent of women, and 15 percent of adolescents were overweight (that is, at least 120 percent of desirable body weight). Current levels show that 32 percent of men, 34 percent of women, 21 percent of adolescents, and 34 percent of children ages 3 through 17 are overweight. These figures are far from the year 2000 objective that no more than 20 percent of adults and 15 percent of adolescents are overweight.

Women, the poor, and members of certain ethnic groups more often carry the burdens of being overweight. The rates of significant overweight for black men and white men differ very little, but black women are about a third more likely to be obese than are white women. Nearly half of black women and Mexican-American women are estimated to be overweight. Among children, overweight was found in boys more than in girls, lower income children more than higher income, African American and Hispanic children more than white, and older children more than younger.

The economic costs of obesity are reflected in premature morbidity and mortality and reduced productivity. In addition, consumers spend billions of dollars annually on weight loss and exercise programs. The top five diet companies in the United States had, collectively, annual revenues near $4 billion in the early 1990s. The costs of nutrition fraud, which remain unmeasurable and unquantifiable, deserve attention.

North Americans appear to be increasingly concerned not only with the amounts of food they eat, but also with its content. As seen in figure 12-12, Americans increased their consumption of low fat and skim milk; consumed more total grain products; and ate less frankfurters, sausages, and less total dietary fat. Other changes included an increase in the amount of meat and grain mixtures, such as hamburgers. Consumer attention to diet is undoubtedly responsible for average cholesterol levels in the U.S. population declining nearly 10 percent in the past twenty years. Most of this decrease has occurred in higher educational and occupational groups, but it does reflect the potential for change in the populations reachable through community health programs.

Economic factors influenced some of these changes, but most analysts concur that health concerns have motivated much of the shift in diet. Despite some positive changes in eating habits, Americans grew fatter. Other factors need to be considered to explain these seemingly counter trends, including level of physical inactivity and other social and economic factors. For example, consumers are bombarded with contradictory messages to stay fit and eat lean, yet enjoy gourmet ice cream, smell warm cinnamon buns baking at the mall, and return to old-fashioned cooking.

Health Effects Adequate intakes of energy sources and of essential nutrients are necessary for satisfactory rates of growth and development, reproduction, lactation, and maintenance of health. Dietary factors are associated with five of the ten leading causes of death in the United States—coronary heart disease, some types of cancer, stroke, noninsulin-dependent diabetes mellitus, and atherosclerosis. Once prevalent dietary deficiencies have been replaced by excess and imbalance of some food components in the diet, such as the disproportionate consumption of foods high in fat. The consensus of the National Research Council and the Surgeon General's Report on Nutrition and Health is that the U.S. population needs to reduce its percentage of calories derived from fat.

While the "sweet tooth" has gotten most of the publicity, it is the nation's "fat tooth" that has led to an increased consumption of calories and contributed to obesity. Fat is the most calorically dense food at 9 calories per gram and the tastiest in food taste and texture. Americans have one of the fattiest diets in the world: about 37 percent of calories come from fats. This percent is down from 40 percent in 1977, but above the 30 percent recommended by most health organizations and government agencies. Less than 10 percent of calories should come from saturated fat, such as that in cheese, butter, and meat; less than 10 percent should also come from polyunsaturated fats, such as safflower oil, soybean, and sunflower.

Deficiencies of essential nutrients or energy sources can lead to several specific diseases or disabilities and increased susceptibility to others. Excessive or inappropriate consumption of some foods may contribute to adverse conditions, such as obesity, or may increase the risk for certain diseases, such as heart disease, adult-onset diabetes, high blood pressure, gall bladder, osteoarthritis of weight-bearing joints, dental caries, and possibly some types of cancer. Such chronic diseases are clearly of complex cause, with substantial variation in individual susceptibility to the several risk factors. The role of nutrients in some of these diseases is not definitively established, but epidemiological and laboratory studies offer important insights that may help people in making food choices that will enhance their prospects of maintaining health.

Anorexia nervosa and **bulimia** are compulsive disorders with consequences similar to those of malnutrition. Both disorders involve depletion of nutrients, and both are considered epidemic in adolescents and young women in the United States. The fixation on slimness as a necessity causes the anorexic to starve herself or himself or the bulimic to "binge and purge"—eating compulsively, then regurgitating. The bulimic person also suffers from upper intestinal and oral tissue damage from the frequent exposure of the throat and mouth to stomach acids. Dentists are often the first to detect the bulimic, recognizing their pattern of tooth erosion.

Frequent consumption of highly cariogenic (decay-producing) foods (those containing fermentable or orally retentive carbohydrates), especially between meals, can nullify some of the caries-preventive benefits of adequate fluoride intake and can cause rampant caries in children with a fluoride deficiency. No consistent or independent relationship has been shown, however, between sugar consumption and the onset of heart disease or diabetes.

Inadequate nutrition may be associated with poor pregnancy outcome, including low-birthweight deliveries and suboptimum mental and physical development. Excessive sodium intake has been associated with high blood pressure in susceptible individuals. Dietary fat, especially saturated fat and cholesterol, are risk factors for heart disease, along with smoking and high blood pressure. Dietary fat has also been associated epidemiologically with some types of cancer. Indeed, the National Cancer Institute estimates that 35 percent of cancer deaths are attributable to diet. Eating more foods high in fiber may reduce the risk of colon cancer and may alleviate the symptoms of chronic constipation, diverticulosis, and some types of "irritable bowel" in some individuals. Finally, poor nutrition may increase susceptibility to infections, fatigue, and stress.

Overweight infants and children tend to become obese adults. Prevention must begin early, before learned patterns of compulsive overeating are established (figure 12-14). Obesity and overnutrition are associated with increased rates of coronary heart disease, adult-onset diabetes, hypertension, stroke, and accidents, and the combined toll on community health is very large.

Prevention and Nutrition Promotion Measures

Education Nutrition education measures directed at the community should emphasize good nutrition and safe weight control strategies based on energy balance concepts. The public needs to be moved toward setting reasonable and achievable goals in making a lifetime commitment to

· ·

Figure 12-14

These youth are playing a computer nutrition game designed to be culturally appropriate and of interest to this age group. (*Source:* Photo by Marsha Burkes, courtesy The University of Texas Health Science Center, Houston, TX.)

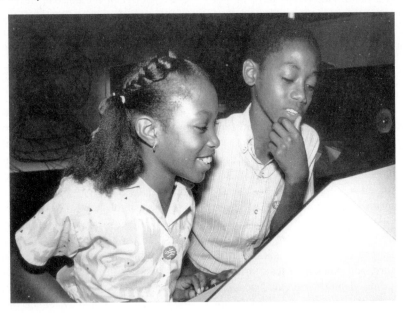

Objectives in Nutrition Health Status

· By 2000 reduce overweight to a prevalence of no more than 20% among people over 20 and no more than 15% among adolescents aged 12 to 19. Baseline: 26% for people aged 20 to 74 in 1976-1980, 24% for men and 27% for women; 15% for adolescents aged 12 to 19 in 1976-80.

Special Target Populations	1976-80	2000
Low income women	37%	25%
Black women	44	30
Hispanic women	37–39	25
American Indians/Alaska natives	29–75	30
People with disabilities	36	25
Women with high blood pressure	50	41
Men with high blood pressure	39	35

dietary and lifestyle changes. For example, the Heart and Stroke Foundation of Canada recommends a "total diet" approach to food selection, meal planning, and eating that stresses the principles of balance, variety, and moderation. To this they add a fourth principle of physical activity. The American Dietary Guidelines were revised in 1995 and offer a similar message of variety, balance, and

1995 Dietary Guidelines for Americans

Eat a variety of foods.

Balance the food you eat with physical activity—maintain or improve your weight.

Choose a diet with plenty of grain products, vegetables and fruits.

Choose a diet low in fat, saturated fat and cholesterol.

Choose a diet moderate in sugars.

Choose a diet moderate in salt and sodium.

If you drink alcoholic beverages, do so in moderation.

Canada's Guidelines for Healthy Eating

- Enjoy a variety of foods.
- Emphasize cereals, breads, other grain products, vegetables, and fruit.
- Choose lower-fat dairy products, leaner meats and foods prepared with little or no fat.
- Achieve and maintain a healthy body weight by enjoying regular physical activity and healthy eating.
- Limit salt, alcohol, and caffeine intake.

moderation. These educational messages focus not just on eating, but selecting foods and planning food consumption. They also balance energy taken in (food eaten) with energy spent (physical activity). Neither message targets "good" or "bad" food; instead they stress balance, variety, and moderation. This is a very different way of thinking about food than that found in most quick fix schemes.

Educational programs can also include awareness of nutrition principles and areas of scientific controversy about the relation of diet to heart disease, high blood pressure, certain cancers, diabetes, dental caries, and other conditions. They can provide information and teach behavioral skills to enable people to select and prepare more healthful diets. More effective means of communicating nutrition information to people in different age and ethnic groups are needed. Nutrition information and education about food choices can be imparted in the home (via the media and outreach services), in schools, at the worksite, by and to health care providers, at the point of purchase (supermarkets and restaurants), as a part of government food service programs (such as the Head Start; school lunch; and Women, Infant, and Child programs in the United States), and by appropriate advertising of food products.

More often than not, women are the family members responsible for meal planning, grocery shopping, and food preparation. These nutrition management responsibilities help establish eating patterns among children, who learn eating habits early in life. What parents eat is still the biggest influence on what children eat and the food habits they develop. Recommendations to parents include: model healthy food choice, know the dietary guidelines, stock the kitchen with food low in saturated fat and cholesterol, teach basic food preparation to children and let them help with grocery shopping and meal planning, and engage in physical activity.

Communication   Consumers rely on the news media for much of their information about nutrition and food safety. The many contrasting news reports related to nutrition are confusing for many consumers. This is especially problematic for consumers who are barraged by the food industry with over $36 billion a year in advertising designed to make people eat more and fashion industry ads that glamorize impossible images. The government expenditures for nutrition are tiny in comparison. For example, the government gives each state $50,000 for such programs. To provide any counterweight to industry marketing, communication messages need to be improved. Ways to improve such coverage is to provide sufficient context in news stories so that consumers can decide the relevance of the story to their own diet. Messages that suggest individual foods are "magic bullets" are less helpful than those that help consumers to see the benefits of a balanced and varied diet. As a rule, information sources should be unbiased and provide all sides in nutrition stories, this includes making the information relevant to various cultural groups and ages.

Service Measures The provision of food and nutrition services in the community should include nutritious breakfast and lunch programs for school children and meals for senior citizens at congregate sites; food stamps for low-income populations; food supplements for low-income women, infants, and children; nutritious food offered in business and institutional settings; dietary counseling routinely offered to high-risk individuals by health care providers, schools, and employers; and psychosocial support groups focused on weight control and weight maintenance.

Technological Measures Most of the technological means of improving nutrition must be exercised at the national or state or provincial level, but some community action is possible in ensuring nutritional quality and content of manufactured foodstuffs, from production through consumption. Communities can support changing livestock practices to produce leaner meat; fortifying certain foodstuffs, such as bread; developing and making readily available new products lower in fat, saturated fat, cholesterol, sodium, and sugar; and positioning products in supermarkets and restaurants so that key information on caloric, cholesterol, fat, sodium, and sugar content is readily apparent. New fat substitutes, such as Olestra, have been introduced on the market as one approach to change eating habits.

Legislative and Regulatory Measures Again, national or state or provincial action is often required to obtain legislation or regulatory changes to maintain or improve the nutritional quality of the food supply; to require nutrition labeling on

> ### Service and Protection Objectives for Nutrition
>
> - By 2000 achieve labeling for virtually all processed foods and at least 40% of fresh meats, poultry, fish, fruits, vegetables, baked goods, and ready-to-eat foods. Baseline: 60% of sales of processed food in 1988.
> - By 2000 increase to at least 90% the proportion of restaurants and institutional food service operations that offer identifiable low-fat, low-calorie food choices, consistent with the Dietary Guidelines for Americans.

foods about which nutrition claims are made or to which nutrients are added; to include information on calories, fat, carbohydrate, protein, cholesterol, sugars, sodium, and other nutrients of public health concern; and to control fortification of foods when this control is of public health significance.

One example of such legislation is the U.S. Nutrition Labeling and Education Act of 1990. It called for activities that educate consumers about the availability of nutrition information on the food label and the importance of using that information to maintain healthful dietary practices. By 1994 food manufacturers were required to comply with the new nutrition labeling. The new nutrition label enabled consumers to make more informed food choices and to understand how a particular food fits into the total daily diet (figure 12-15). The mandatory list of nutrients displayed on the label addresses today's health concerns. The order in which they appear reflects the priority of current dietary recommendations. The regulations included uniform definitions for terms that describe food's nutritional content—such as "light" or "low fat"—to ensure that such terms mean the same for any product on which they appear.

For their part, communities can control food vending practices in schools to reduce or eliminate highly cariogenic foods and snacks; adjust school lunch standards to give greater emphasis to low-fat

. . . .

Figure 12-15

Several consumer studies conducted by the Food and Drug Administration (FDA), and outside groups, enabled FDA and the Food Safety and Inspection Service of the U.S. Department of Agriculture to agree on a new nutrition label. The new label is seen as offering the best opportunity to help consumers make informed food choices and to understand how a particular food fits into the total daily diet. See also the food pyramid in chapter 16. (*Source:* Food and Drug Administration.)

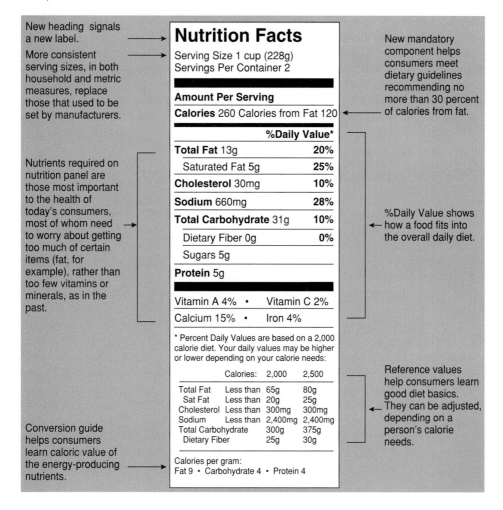

New heading signals a new label.

More consistent serving sizes, in both household and metric measures, replace those that used to be set by manufacturers.

Nutrients required on nutrition panel are those most important to the health of today's consumers, most of whom need to worry about getting too much of certain items (fat, for example), rather than too few vitamins or minerals, as in the past.

Conversion guide helps consumers learn caloric value of the energy-producing nutrients.

New mandatory component helps consumers meet dietary guidelines recommending no more than 30 percent of calories from fat.

%Daily Value shows how a food fits into the overall daily diet.

Reference values help consumers learn good diet basics. They can be adjusted, depending on a person's calorie needs.

Nutrition Facts

Serving Size 1 cup (228g)
Servings Per Container 2

Amount Per Serving

Calories 260   Calories from Fat 120

	%Daily Value*
Total Fat 13g	**20%**
Saturated Fat 5g	**25%**
Cholesterol 30mg	**10%**
Sodium 660mg	**28%**
Total Carbohydrate 31g	**10%**
Dietary Fiber 0g	**0%**
Sugars 5g	
Protein 5g	

Vitamin A 4%   •   Vitamin C 2%

Calcium 15%   •   Iron 4%

* Percent Daily Values are based on a 2,000 calorie diet. Your daily values may be higher or lower depending on your calorie needs:

		Calories:	2,000	2,500
Total Fat	Less than		65g	80g
Sat Fat	Less than		20g	25g
Cholesterol	Less than		300mg	300mg
Sodium	Less than		2,400mg	2,400mg
Total Carbohydrate			300g	375g
Dietary Fiber			25g	30g

Calories per gram:
Fat 9 • Carbohydrate 4 • Protein 4

products; and regulate local televised advertisements directed at young children that promote cariogenic and nonnutritious foods and snacks.

Economic Measures   Possible economic incentives or sanctions include adjusting insurance premiums for corporations offering employee health promotion programs with a nutrition component; assessing feasibility and cost benefits of reimbursement by third-party payers of nutrition counseling services that meet appropriate standards; and decreasing local sales taxes on staple foods.

Appraisal of the Measures   Service programs are likely to be effective in improving the nutritional status of pregnant women and children and in reducing the incidence of low-birthweight infants. Certain segments of the public in the United States have responded to educational messages about fats and cholesterol by reducing intake. Some government messages have been mixed and contradictory, leaving the public confused. Technological measures hold real promise, particularly if governmental policies could be generated in support of such measures and if resultant products are acceptable to consumers. With the exception of food sanitation and labeling, regulation and economic incentives have not been employed and are therefore of uncertain potential.

Changing Diets, World Hunger, and Nutrition

In the global village, food production, population, growth, environmental conditions, and mass marketing are tied. For example, Japanese restaurants are expanding their cuisine to respond to changing food habits that are influenced by international marketing. In the last three decades fat consumption in Japan has increased threefold. Teenagers are bigger than their parents, demand bigger portions, and are eating more protein per capita than well-fed North Americans. The appetites of these Japanese teenagers are directly linked to soybean futures in Brazil and the American midwest. Soybean production, in turn, has suffered from unfavorable weather and possible changes in ultraviolet light, due to a thinning ozone. A change in any one of these sectors influences the others. Improvement in the diet of the world's population is also related to existing food supplies.

Although the developed countries are preoccupied with the problems of obesity and nutritional content, Third World countries and some populations within developed countries have a more compelling problem of malnutrition and hunger. As many as 840 million people are malnourished, yet the world has never produced as much food as it does now. No other factor reveals the commonality and the disparity among the world's population as does food. Developed nations have a special capability and special responsibility to lead the campaign against world hunger. The United States is by far the most powerful member of the world's increasingly interdependent food system. It harvests more than half the grain that crosses international borders, and its grain reserves are the world's largest. The United States automatically exerts a major influence, intended or not, on all aspects of the international food system because of that country's agricultural productivity, its advanced food technology, and its market power. These resources and those of the other developed nations must be deployed to address nutrition and health on a global scale.

The Epidemiology of World Hunger   The major world hunger problem is not periodic famine, but chronic undernutrition, which results when people consume fewer calories and less protein than their bodies require to lead active, healthy lives. It is estimated that 20 percent of the population of the developing countries is constantly hungry. Although chronic or repeated shortages of calories may appear less newsworthy than outright starvation, they steadily take a greater toll in human lives. For example, the much-publicized Ethiopian famine in the mid-1980s and the Somalian famine in the early 1990s are only the tip of a pyramid of some 40,000 deaths monthly from undernutrition in twenty-seven African nations. More than three-quarters of the world's inadequately nourished people live on the Indian subcontinent, in Southeast Asia, and in sub-Saharan Africa. Many also live in parts of Latin America and the Middle East. Pockets of the poorly nourished persist in the United States and other rich countries as well.

In the United States hunger is particularly common among migrant and seasonal farm workers, Native Americans, the elderly, and the 32 million Americans with incomes below the poverty level. Federal programs to alleviate hunger were greatly expanded during the 1960s, and there is evidence

. . . .
Figure 12-16

Educational programs directed at women are one key to changing family nutritional patterns in all countries. (*Source:* UNICEF, World Health Organization.)

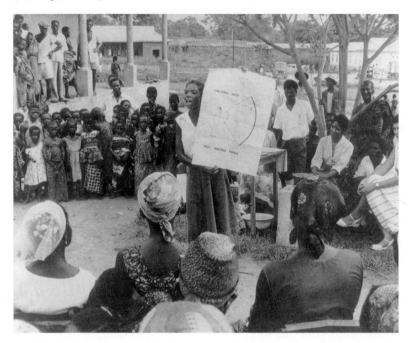

that the nutrition of the American poor participating in the programs improved. Subtler forms of hunger and the malnutrition inevitably associated with poverty persist, exacerbated by economic trends increasing the gap between the haves and the have-nots. Cuts in the federal budget for poverty programs, in general, and food programs, in particular, have strained the resources of church and other private or voluntary relief programs.

Children under the age of 5 years of age make up over half of the world's malnourished population. A survey by the Food Research and Action center found that 5.5 million children in the United States under age 12 are hungry. Overall, 7 in 10 of the world's poor are women and children. Significantly more women are affected by malnutrition than men. Even when there is food, in many countries women feed the men and children first and eat what, if any, is left. Despite its magnitude, moral aspects, and high social and economic costs, world hunger seldom captures widespread public attention except in times of catastrophe. World hunger is at least as much a political, economic, educational, and social challenge as it is a scientific, technical, or logistical one. One solution to this problem by the World Food Summit is to put management and distribution of food aid into the hands of local women. Although women are more likely to get food to their families than other distribution sources, they need to be educated and supported if they are to act in this role (figure 12-16).

Public Education A broad-base plan to eliminate world hunger calls for a major reordering of global and national priorities. For such a marked shift in established policies and practices to occur, public support must be mobilized. The public is only dimly aware of what Western and Third World nations could gain if people in all nations could afford to feed themselves. A successful effort to end hunger will require long-term economic and political support, and this support can exist only if the Australian, North American, and European publics understand the realities of world hunger. Rock concerts such as "We are the World" and local food drives have helped increase public awareness and arouse public concern.

The issue of ending world hunger comes down to a question of political choice—a factor that is no more predictable than the weather, but far more subject to human control. The quantities of food and money needed to eliminate hunger are small in relation to available global resources. Political will is the missing ingredient; it is required in abundance at community and national levels to channel the necessary food resources to those in need.

Nutrition is the foundation on which other aspects of health and lifestyle develop. Without attending first to issues of hunger, community health programs may gain the attention of the affluent at the expense of the poor and disadvantaged populations who have the most to gain from health promotion.

THE COMMUNITY HEALTH PROMOTION MODEL APPLIED TO DRUG ABUSE

Misuse and abuse of drugs, like smoking, alcohol abuse, obesity, and stress management, are intertwined social and health problems. Any program to deal with such complex problems must address the social, environmental, economic, psychological, cultural, and physiological factors encompassed by the lifestyle in question. Communities and health officials recognize the importance of the drug misuse problem, yet only sporadic attempts have been made by communities to deal with it.

Health education traditionally has been called on to alert the public to complex community health problems, but health education by itself can hardly be expected to solve such problems. The lifestyles in question are too embedded in organi-

zational, socioeconomic, and environmental circumstances for people to be able to change their own behavior without concomitant changes in these circumstances. Health promotion combines health education with organizational, economic, and environmental supports for behavior and conditions of living conducive to health.

As this chapter concludes part 3 of this book, the models and concepts introduced in part 1 can be reviewed as they apply to community health promotion and more specifically to the difficult problems of lifestyle exemplified by drug misuse and drug misuse prevention. In chapter 4 the PRECEDE model of health *education* was introduced and applied to problems of maternal and child health. That model will now be expanded to include the additional elements of economic, organizational, and environmental supports for behavior that is conducive to health and applied to health *promotion* for drug misuse prevention. The PROCEED model has been used in health promotion programs at international, national, and local levels.

Drug Misuse Prevention

Health professionals sometimes employ a taxonomy of three levels of prevention: primary, secondary, and tertiary.* Primary prevention is accomplished by activities that promote optimum health and provide specific protection against the onset or incidence of a health problem (for example, proper nutrition, genetic counseling, fluoridation, disease inoculation). In drug misuse prevention, the goal of primary prevention activities is to decrease the rate at which new cases of drug misuse appear in a population by counteracting circumstances conducive to the development of drug misuse before they have a chance to produce drug misuse behavior.

Secondary prevention refers to activities concerned with the early diagnosis and prompt treatment of health problems (for example, the Papanicolaou [Pap] smear, regular physical examination, referral programs for troubled employees, neonatal

---

*The authors thank Dr. Donald Iverson for contributions to this section.

Table 12-2

Examples of Interventional Strategies for Each Level of Prevention of Health Problems, Including Those Associated with Drug Misuse

Type of Strategy	Levels of prevention		
	Primary	Secondary	Tertiary
Educational	Genetic counseling School health education Public education about drugs	Community hypertension screening education programs Teacher training in recognition of drug problems	Drug education programs for patients in coronary care
Automatic-protective	Fluoridation of community drinking water systems Legal control of prescription drugs	Neonatal metabolic screening Requiring medical prescription for drug refills	Referral to community mental health center for counseling following discharge from drug treatment center
Coercive	Immunization requirements for schoolchildren Arrests of drug traffickers	Mandatory classes for persons convicted of drinking while intoxicated or using illicit drugs	Mandatory treatment for persons having an addiction or a sexually transmitted disease

metabolic screening). The goal of secondary drug misuse prevention activities is to reduce the disability rate caused by drug misuse by early treatment of such cases in the community.

Tertiary prevention refers to minimizing the disability from existing illness through treatment and rehabilitation efforts (for example, treatment for persons with lung cancer, alcoholism rehabilitation, treatment of sexually transmitted diseases). The goal of tertiary drug misuse prevention efforts is to reduce the complications and social pathology in the affected population by reducing or eliminating the addiction to drugs. Whereas primary prevention may reduce the *incidence* of drug misuse, secondary and tertiary prevention can reduce its *prevalence* or provide **harm reduction.**

Prevention Strategies Three types of strategies can be used in each of the three prevention levels to accomplish health promotion goals:

- **Educational strategies**—inform and educate the public about issues of concern, such as the

dangers of drug misuse, the benefits of designated drivers, or the relationship of maternal alcohol consumption to fetal alcohol syndrome
- **Automatic-protective strategies**—directed at controlling environmental variables, such as public health measures to track prescriptions, prevent import of drugs, and burn or chemically kill marijuana crops
- **Coercive strategies**—employ legal and other formal sanctions to control individual behavior, such as drug searches for school entry, mandatory drug testing of athletes, compulsory use of automobile breath testing, and arrests for drug possession or use

Table 12-2 gives examples of community health programs and measures classified by level of prevention and category of prevention strategy. The examples illustrate traditional public health strategies and new strategies in community health promotion and drug misuse prevention.

Prevention programs in public health can also be classified by the site where the program occurs.

Although the community has been the primary site for most prevention programs, increasingly such programs can be found in the work, school, and medical care settings. **Employee assistance programs** to detect and refer alcohol and drug misuse problems among workers have become fixtures of most large companies.

Educational Methods in Health Promotion

Regardless of the setting in which the community health promotion program occurs, there are three basic types of educational strategies:

- Direct communications with the target population to *predispose* behavior conducive to health. These include lecture-discussion, individual counseling or instruction, mass media campaigns, audiovisual aids, educational television, and programmed learning.
- Training methods to *enable* or *reinforce* behavior conducive to health. These include skills development, simulations and games, inquiry learning, small group discussion, modeling, and behavior modification.
- Organizational methods to *support* behavior conducive to health. These include community development, social action, social planning, and economic and organizational development. Such methods usually go beyond health education in supporting behavior.

One of the most noticeable changes in prevention and health promotion programs in community health has been the increasing integration of behavioral theory into health education and other phases of program development. So far as health behavior is only partially understood (the level of understanding varies with the complexity of the health behavior), multiple theories have been used in planning for prevention programs. The most successful programs consult relevant theory in their planning to clarify the assumptions about the causes of behavior on the basis of which strategies are selected or developed.

Historical Differences The prevention approach of public health has differed from that frequently found in past drug misuse prevention efforts, but the two fields are converging. Drug misuse programs have differed from traditional public health programs in their educational and behavioral theories and models. The bases of earlier drug misuse programs were drawn primarily from personality, cognitive, and sociological theories. However, taking its cue from the public health field, the drug misuse field is increasingly incorporating principles from developmental and social learning theories.

Another important distinction between the theoretical orientation and underpinning of program development efforts in the two fields is the level of understanding of the target behaviors. Many of the target behaviors of traditional public health programs are relatively simple and easily understood (for example, immunization and proper infant feeding), whereas drug misuse behavior is far more complex.

A third distinction has been in recognizing the role of ethnicity and racial background in influencing health behavior. Public health professionals have always been cognizant of the ethnic and racial influences in health behaviors, such as public use of health practitioners, and have designed prevention programs to account for these influences. People in the drug misuse field have taken increasing notice of ethnicity and racial background as powerful influences on the causes of drug misuse, so major as to alter the nature of the problem and subsequently the prevention techniques that may be effective. For example, the information on drug misuse among black populations has indicated that prevention efforts must focus on social and environmental factors rather than on individual factors, as they often do with white populations.

The drug abuse field and the more traditional public health field are increasingly using similar approaches, as both address social problems involving lifestyle. Strategies for intervention differ; but there are some common elements. They include prevention through education that starts early and extends throughout life; altering the social climate of acceptability; reducing individual and social stress factors; and legal enforcement.

Table 12-3

Priorities for Drug Misuse Prevention Activities Within the Three Spheres of the Health Field Concept

Framework areas from the health field concept	Activities—goals
Lifestyle	Inclusion of drug misuse prevention as a major component of a comprehensive school health education program
	Public and physician education programs to reduce the number of sleeping pill prescriptions, emphasizing problems of cross-addiction
Services	Education of health care providers on the taking of a drug history for adolescents and preadolescents
	Promotion of involvement of national and local youth-serving agencies in drug misuse prevention
	Strengthened drug misuse prevention research
Environment	Encouragement of parent groups to provide supportive networks to help youths resist drug misuse
	Improved enforcement of legal and economic regulations of drug market

The National Institute on Drug Abuse refers to four modalities of prevention: information, education, alternatives, and intervention. Similar to the public health approach, drug misuse prevention programs are targeted at populations (demographically defined groups, families, peer groups) and settings (community, school, workplace) and usually employ multiple educational methods including **community events.**

National Strategies Lengthy and detailed examinations of the public health problems facing the United States, Great Britain, Canada, and Australia were initiated by their respective legislatures and national administrations in the 1970s. A framework similar to the Canadian health field concept described in chapter 2 was useful in devising strategy in the United States and Canada to affect public health problems. The framework included three points of intervention:

1. *Human lifestyle*—recognizing that the choices an individual makes about personal lifestyle behaviors can increase risk of health problems

2. *Human environment*—recognizing that environmental settings and other external sources of hazards can increase health problems and condition health behavior

3. *Human services*—recognizing that preventive services can influence the incidence and effects of preventable diseases and conditions

It is the thesis of the Canadian and the American initiatives in disease prevention and health promotion that programs or interventions in all three areas—lifestyle, environment, and services—are required to combat the leading causes of death and disability. A drug misuse prevention program would include program components, as shown in table 12-3, intended to affect individual behavior (lifestyle), to provide medical treatment of drug misuse and drug dependence as early as possible to prevent permanent damage (human services), and to modify the environmental factors influencing the misuse of drugs (economics and the social environment). The balance of these areas in a community drug misuse prevention program has seldom, if ever, been attained.

Objectives The U.S. initiative in disease prevention and health promotion developed a consensus on specific measurable objectives for each of the high-priority problems related to the goals identified in *Healthy People*. National panels of experts were first convened in 1979 for each of the priorities to formulate measurable objectives.

The U.S. expert panel on drug misuse prevention reviewed information on the status and trends of drug use, the health implications of drug use, and the potential drug-related prevention-promotion measures available, including the strength and feasibility of each measure. The panel then identified two major goals and eleven measurable objectives to be achieved by 1990. These objectives were circulated to more than 3,000 organizations and additional experts for comment and review. This process resulted in the closest that one can expect to come to consensus on U.S. national goals to be achieved in ten years. The objectives for drug misuse were published in the final document *Promoting Health, Preventing Disease: Objectives for the Nation in 1980*. The objectives for the year 2000, published in 1990, followed a similar development process. These objectives were monitored and underwent a mid-decade review in 1995.

Planning Framework Applied to Drug Misuse

Drug misuse prevention efforts have too often been based on fear-arousal strategies. Although such strategies have valid uses, their applicability to community health programs is limited. To maximize the effectiveness of a community drug misuse prevention program, concurrent efforts should be initiated in the three health field categories described in *A New Perspective on the Health of Canadians* and in *Healthy People:* human lifestyle, human environment, and human services. In all three, attention must be given to factors that predispose, enable, and reinforce behavior conducive to health.

Prevention programs, whether they be directed at drug misuse, communicable disease, teenage pregnancy, or some other health problem, have as a base health education activities. Health education is defined in chapter 4 as any combination of learning opportunities designed to facilitate voluntary adaptations of behavior conducive to health. Well-planned drug education programs have been shown to be effective for some people, but they have not demonstrated an ability to resolve a community drug misuse problem. Perhaps no single effort will be able to resolve such problems totally. However drug misuse prevention programs incorporating the integrated health promotion approach of educational, organizational, and economic supports for lifestyle conducive to health have a much greater chance of success than programs directed at only one of these categories.

Health Education Versus Health Promotion

Health promotion has been defined as any combination of educational, organizational, environmental, and economic supports for behavior and conditions of living conducive to health. With health education as an integral part of all health promotion interventions it follows that the interventions should be directed toward voluntary behavior at all levels—individuals, organizations, and communities. At the community, state or provincial, or national level, additional interventions may be legal, regulatory, political, or economic, and therefore potentially coercive. Nevertheless, such interventions to be successful must be supported by an informed and consenting public. Such **informed consent** requires health education. Ideally, the coercive measures are directed at the behavior of those whose actions may affect the health of others, such as the manufacturers, distributors, and advertisers of hazardous products. Even then, public health education is required to ensure the support of an informed public because taxes, prices, availability of services and products, and jobs may be affected by such regulations of health—or of drug-related industries and sources. For example, one part of a health promotion program for drug misuse prevention could target organizational change. Health education could be combined with various incentives (such as free program consultation services) and persuasion techniques (such as program promotion by local public leaders) in an attempt to increase the number of schools offering peer counseling programs for those who misuse drugs. If the program also targeted political change, community organization techniques could be combined with health education activities to develop "concerned parent groups" in neighborhoods and to apply political pressure on local school, law enforcement, and government officials to support drug misuse prevention efforts. If the program directed other efforts toward economic change, health professionals and others could work with representatives of insurance carriers to initiate health insurance reimbursements for counseling and rehabilitation services. The point is simple: when health education activities are combined with appropriate changes in organizations, political systems, and environmental and economic supports for behavior, the end result is more likely to be favorable than is the result achieved by a series of single, uncoordinated changes. Indeed, uncoordinated changes sometimes make things worse by throwing a community system out of balance and forcing an overreaction or overcompensation by the wrong elements in the community.

The relationships of health education and health promotion activities to the three prevention targets and the relationships of these targets to the health or drug misuse objectives set for the community and the nation are depicted in figure 12-17. The three prevention targets are not isolated. Lifestyle is continually affected by the human environment and the organization of services (as seen in chapter 4). Furthermore, a successful program must effectively integrate and coordinate activities in relation to each of these targets. To facilitate the integration of activities within and between the prevention strategies, a planning framework is needed. The planning framework proposed in chapter 4 forces an encompassing and systematic analysis of public health problems in the context of social problems or quality-of-life concerns.

Phases in Planning

The Precede-Procede model applies figure 12-17 to plan community drug prevention programs. One starts with the final consequences—namely, social problems usually defined as community drug-related problems but not necessarily as health concerns. One works back from there to the original causes—that is, the causes of the behavior, which influenced the health problem or community drug-related social problem. The following is an application of the phases, corresponding to those in chapter 4, in this process to prevention of drug misuse.

Phase 1: Social Diagnosis The first phase involves a consideration of the quality of life in a community by assessing the social problems of concern to the various segments of the population. This has the effect of forcing planners to consider the desirable social outcomes of a program before setting priorities on health or selecting program approaches. It also helps justify a program to the community. This is especially important in the planning of community drug prevention programs because of the relationship between drug-related health problems and the social problems of a community. For example, when a community has a large number of drug-dependent persons, it is likely that there will be high rates of crime, school truancy, early dropouts from school, juvenile delinquency, and unemployment (all social problems). Conversely, when a community is experiencing such social problems as high unemployment, inadequate housing, inadequate private and public school programs, or discrimination, a serious drug dependence problem will be present, because the use of drugs for some will be a method of coping with the social problems. By identifying the major social problems of concern to the community, one can select potential outcome evaluation measures and gain an understanding of the community's concerns as they relate to the particular health problem that is the target of the prevention program.

A community's social problems can be diagnosed from analyses of existing records, files,

••••••••••••••••••••
Figure 12-17

The structure of the objectives for the nation in health promotion are seen here as applied to drug abuse prevention. The relationship of community health education and health promotion also is shown as part of the prevention strategies box to the left. Health promotion, however, can serve community development needs other than the prevention of specific diseases or lifestyle problems.

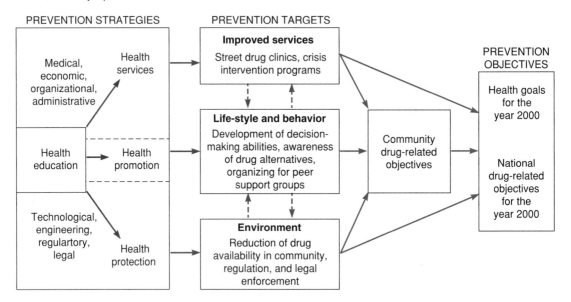

publications, and informal interviews and discussions with leaders, key informants, and representatives of various community populations. This is an important first step that should not be undertaken too hastily, because its outcome may well affect program scope and quality and the extent of community support.

Phase 2: Epidemiological Diagnosis The objective of the epidemiological diagnostic phase is to identify the specific health problems that appear to be contributing to the social problems noted in phase 1. By using data from community surveys, hospital admissions, city and county health departments, health systems agencies, and selected state or provincial and national data, the drug-related morbidity, mortality, and disability trends can be identified. The incidence, prevalence, distribution, intensity, and duration of each identified health problem should be described (see chapter 3). These data can be analyzed to determine the populations most affected by the health problem. This process will often reveal and locate a variety of existing health problems such as drug dependence, drug-related psychoses, drug-related depression or anxiety, injuries, and other drug-related problems such as HIV/AIDS, serum hepatitis, and endocarditis. The use of spatial maps to depict the distribution of the identified health problems within the city or county is an effective way of presenting data if there is reason to believe that the problems vary by geographical location.

By use of the results of epidemiological analyses, program objectives should be developed. The objectives should be stated in epidemiological terms and answer the following: Who will be the recipients of the program? What benefit should they receive? How much of that benefit should they receive? By when or for how long? For example, it has been estimated that in a six-month period, approximately 1,000 persons died of drug overdose in New York City. Therefore, a program objective for a drug prevention program in New York City might have been as follows: "To reduce the number of drug overdose deaths in New York City by 25 percent within one year and an additional 25 percent within the next year, until the national average is reached." The major drug-related health problem for most communities would not be death or drug overdose; rather, it would be physiological or psychological dependence.

Phase 3: Behavioral and Environmental Diagnosis The behavioral diagnosis phase requires the systematic identification of health behaviors that appear to be causally linked to each of the health problems identified in the epidemiological diagnosis. The outcome of the behavioral diagnosis is the generation of a ranked list of specific behaviors to be used as the basis for specifying the behavioral objectives of the program.

The process of identifying the health behaviors linked to the health problems usually relies on the professional literature. The review of the literature can be combined with structured and unstructured interviews of persons familiar with the health problem (such as drug treatment personnel), data from observations, and intuition based on personal experiences. In the case of drug dependence, the behavioral *causes* leading to the health problem are drug use and drug misuse. These should be perceived not as distinct behaviors but, rather, as a continuum of drug use to drug misuse with varying types and amounts of drugs used. Distinct behaviors within the continuum could be specified, such as misuse of prescription medications, use of illicit drugs such as marijuana and cocaine, and use of illicit drugs in a manner that predisposes the user to health problems. To take another example, if the identified health problem was cardiovascular disease, the behavioral problems would include smoking, high intake of saturated fats, heavy alcohol consumption, and a sedentary lifestyle.

A second part of this phase is the identification of environmental factors that contribute to the health problem. These are the organizational and environmental conditions that influence the health problem and the behavior but that are not controlled directly by the behavior of the target population. Nonbehavioral causes of drug dependence include such factors as the housing situation in the community, the school environment, and the law enforcement activity in the community. Identification of these factors is important, because it provides the planners with direction for health promotion activity other than educational measures, such as organizational and economic interventions directed at the regulation of the environment and the availability of services.

Phase 4: Educational Diagnosis The educational diagnosis phase assesses the relative influence of various predisposing, enabling, and reinforcing factors on each of the identified behavioral causes of the health problem. Figure 12-18 focuses attention on the order of causation of behavior, as indicated by the numbered arrows: (1) an initial motivation to act; (2) a deployment of resources and skills to enable the action; (3) a reaction to the behavior from someone else (or in the case of drug use, the drug effects themselves); (4) the reinforcement and strengthening or the punishment and discouragement of the behavior; (5) the reinforcement or punishment of the behavior as it affects the predisposing factors by strengthening or extinguishing the motivation to act; and finally, (6) the increased ability or confidence to take certain actions, which tends to increase the predisposition or motivation to take such actions.

In the process of identifying and listing factors in the three areas, one may include factors that seem to encourage the behavior and those that seem to discourage the behavior. Consider the data in figure 12-19 and their implications for the relative importance of predisposing factors (perceived risk) and enabling factors (perceived availability) for drug use.

• •

Figure 12-18

The three categories of factors influencing lifestyle are shown here as related to drug use and abuse. The numbered arrows indicate the approximate order of expected cause and effect. Arrows 2, 5 and 6 are explained in Chapter 4.

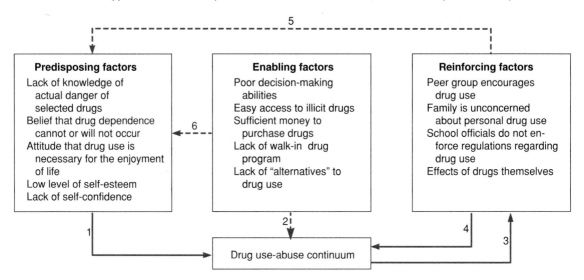

• •

Figure 12-19

Age-adjusted rates for drug-related deaths: United States 1987 to 1993, and year 2000 targets. (*Source:* Centers for Disease Control and Prevention, National Center for Health Statistics.)

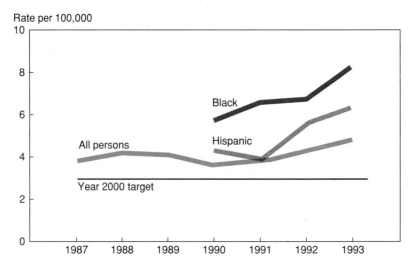

After completing the list, the next step is to select from among the predisposing, enabling, and reinforcing factors those that will be most likely to bring about the behavior desired. The factors that should be selected as targets for the program are those that are most changeable and most important. Importance is determined by answers to the following questions:

- How widespread or frequent is the factor? (For example, low self-esteem, use of drugs by peer group members, easy availability of drugs.)
- How compelling or urgent is the factor? (For example, alternatives to drugs, fear of effects of drugs.)
- How close is the connection between the factor and the behavior? (For example, lack of decision-making skills and drug use, availability of drugs and drug use.)

Changeability is assessed from data or professional judgments addressing the following questions:

- Does the literature suggest that the factor can be changed? (For example, can self-esteem levels be changed? Can decision-making skills be learned? Can school officials be encouraged to enforce regulations?)
- Does the experience of previous programs indicate that the factor can be changed? (For example, have programs been successful in changing parental attitudes and behaviors? Have community organization efforts been successful in stimulating development of drug alternative programs?)

The factors determined to be important and changeable form the basis of the prevention program. This level of specificity helps to use scarce resources in the most appropriate manner and to increase the chances of the program being successful. Difficult choices will be made in this phase of the planning process, but in the decision-making process the level of understanding of the nature of the problem usually increases.

Phase 5: Program Development The program development phase selects the right combination of strategies to affect the selected predisposing, enabling, and reinforcing factors. As a general rule, selected communication methods are effective in altering predisposing factors; organizing resources and training are effective in altering enabling factors; and strategies such as consultation, training, feedback, and group development are effective in altering reinforcing factors. Refer to table 12-2 for an example of considerations in selecting appropriate educational and other strategies according to the level of prevention.

Phase 6: Administrative Diagnosis The administrative diagnosis phase assesses resources available and organizational problems likely to be encountered as the program becomes operational. Factors such as interagency cooperation, staffing patterns, and budgeting should be thoroughly discussed. This phase of planning analyzes the potential problems within programs, within organizations, and between organizations. A well-conceived program is seldom effective without an implementation plan.

SUMMARY

Health-related lifestyle problems such as tobacco use, alcohol misuse, drug misuse, and obesity have no simple solution. Problems as complex as these may defy even well-planned preventive efforts. Nevertheless, the effects of well-planned and systematically implemented preventive efforts are more likely to be successful than the single-focused, uncoordinated efforts that have typified many of the early attempts to address lifestyle, particularly those at the local level.

The Canadian Ministry of Health and Welfare and the U.S. Public Health Service have proposed that their prevention efforts focus on three areas: lifestyle, environment, and services. Specific measurable objectives for the United States were set, which, if met by 2000, will have the effect of substantially reducing the scope and intensity of health problems attributable to lifestyle, the environment, and inadequate health services. These objectives can serve to concentrate the limited resources of communities where they can be most productive. To illustrate community health programs to work toward the objectives, a planning model encompassing the three areas of lifestyle, environment, and services has been presented and illustrated.

Efforts should be directed at individuals and environments, and at organizational, political, and economic systems. Applying the latest findings from the rapidly developing research in designing and evaluating prevention programs and ensuring the necessary quality and quantity of resources for programs will not guarantee success but will increase the probability of reaching the objectives set for a community.

WEB *Links*

QUESTIONS FOR REVIEW

1. What do alcohol misuse, tobacco use, overeating, and drug misuse have in common?
2. Why is alcohol misuse so costly for the community, beyond the direct health effects on the individual?
3. What do population health and lifestyle concepts compare and contrast in understanding alcohol and drug misuse, tobacco use, and overeating.

4. Using the model for drug misuse prevention, how would you design a community program for prevention of alcohol misuse or smoking?
5. How can alcohol misuse, smoking, overeating, anorexia nervosa, bulimia, world hunger, and drug misuse be characterized as epidemics?
6. What should the school teach children about alcohol, smoking, drugs, and nutrition?
7. What does your community have to offer as alternatives to alcohol and drugs for recreation and coping?
8. What can be done in worksites to reduce the prevalence of smoking?
9. Why should women in reproductive ages be singled out as a priority for smoking and alcohol reduction?
10. How does health promotion go beyond health education?
11. When are coercive strategies justified in disease prevention and health promotion?
12. What has public health added to the traditional approach to drug misuse prevention?
13. What are some predisposing, enabling, and reinforcing factors in marijuana use?

READINGS

DeBon, M., and R. D. Klesges. 1996. Adolescents' perceptions about smoking prevention strategies: A comparison of the programmes of the American Lung Association and the Tobacco Institute. *Tobacco Control* 5:19.

This study was done to evaluate components of the teenage smoking prevention programs of the American Lung Association (ALA) and the Tobacco Institute (TI). Although there were moderating effects of gender and race, participants overall strongly favored the ALA program, which consists of seven components: peer pressure/enhanced communications; parents as role models; health consequences of smoking; cost of smoking; smoking as an illegal act; tips for quitting smoking; and responsible decision making.

Glantz, S. A. 1996. *The cigarette papers*. Berkeley: University of California Press.

Dr. Glantz, a noted antitobacco activist, received 4,000 pages of Brown & Williamson tobacco company documents revealing what the tobacco industry knew thirty years earlier but denied consistently. Leaked by a source called "Mr. Butts," the papers can be seen on the Web at http://www.library.ucsf.edu/tobacco.

Green, L. W., and M. W. Kreuter. 1998. *Health promotion planning: an educational and ecological approach,* 3 ed Mountain View, CA: Mayfield.

This book presents the PRECEDE-PROCEED model for planning, implementation, and evaluation of health promotion, with references to some of the more than 700 published applications of the model in various community settings, including schools, workplaces, medical care, and community-wide programs. See updates on http://www.ihpr.ubc.ca.

Mercer, S. L., V. Goel, I. Levy, F. D. Ashbury, D. C. Iverson, and N. A. Iscoe. 1997. Prostate cancer screening in the midst of controversy: Canadian men's knowledge, beliefs, utilization, and future intentions. *Can J Public Health* 88:327.

This application of the PRECEDE-PROCEED model examines how the withering crossfire of public information on a controversial medical procedure affects the target population in responding to that procedure.

BIBLIOGRAPHY

Brown, S. A., A. Gleghorn, M. A. Schuckit, M. G. Myers, and M. A. Mott: 1996. Conduct disorder among adolescent alcohol and drug abusers. *J Studies on Alcohol* 573: 314–324, 1996.

Bulger, R., and S. Reiser S, eds. 1993. *The role of academic health centers in disease prevention and health promotion.* Washington, DC: Association of Academic Health Centers.

Burglehaus, M. J., L. A. Smith, S. B. Sheps, L. W. Green. 1997. Physicians and breastfeeding: beliefs, knowledge, self-efficacy and counselling practices. *Can J Public Health* 88:383.

Carruthe, S., and R. James. 1993. Evaluation of the Western Australian school development in health education project. *J Sch Health* 63:165.

Chapman, S., W. L. Wong, and W. Smith. 1993. Self-exempting beliefs about smoking and health: differences between smokers and ex-smokers. *Am J Public Health* 83:215.

Conrad, K. M., R. T. Campbell, D. W. Edington, H. S. Faust, and D. Vilnius. 1996. The worksite environment as a cue to smoking reduction. *Res in Nursing & Health* 19:21.

Contento, I. R., D. G. Kell, M. K. Keily, and R. D. Corcoran. 1992. A formative evaluation of the American Cancer Society *Changing the Course* nutrition education curriculum. *J Sch Health* 62:411.

Ellickson, P. L., R. M. Bell, and E. R. Harrison. 1993. Changing adolescent propensities to use drugs: results from project ALERT. *Health Educ Q* 20:227.

Environmental Health Directorate, Health Protection Branch. 1993. *Smoking by-laws in Canada—1991.* H46-1-26-1991E. Ottawa: Health and Welfare Canada.

Fawcett, S. B., R. K. Lewis, A. Paine-Andrews, V. T. Francisco, K. P. Richter, E. L. Williams, and B. Copple. 1997. Evaluating community coalitions for prevention of substance abuse: The case of Project Freedom. *Health Educ & Behav* 24:812.

Frankish, C. J., J. L. Johnson, P. A. Ratner, and C. Y. Lovato. 1997. Relationship of organizational characteristics of Canadian workplaces to anti-smoking initiatives. *Prev Med* 26:248.

George, A., L. W. Green, and M. Daniel. 1997. Evaluation and implications of participatory action research for public health. *Prom & Educ* 3(4):6.

Gerstein, D. R., and L. W. Green, eds. 1993. *Preventing drug abuse: what do we know?* Washington, DC: National Academy Press.

Goodman, R.M., A. Steckler, S. Hoover, R. Schwartz, 1992. A critique of contemporary community health promotion approaches based on a qualitative review of six programs in Maine. *Am J Health Prom* 7:208.

Gottlieb, N. H., C. Y. Lovato, R. P. Weinstein, L. W. Green, and M. P. Eriksen. 1992. The implementation of a restrictive worksite smoking policy in a large decentralized organization. *Health Educ Q* 19: 77.

Green, L. W., and M. W. Kreuter. 1992. CDC's planned approach to community health as an application of PRECEDE and an inspiration for PROCEED. *J Health Educ* 23:140.

Health and Welfare Canada Scientific Review Committee. 1990. *Nutrition recommendations.* H49-42-1990E. Ottawa: Health and Welfare Canada.

Herd, D., and J. Grube. Black identity and drinking in the U.S.: A national study. *Addiction* 91:845.

Kaiserman M. J., and B. Rogers. 1992. Forty-year trends in Canadian tobacco sales. *Can J Public Health* 83:404.

Katcher, B. S. 1993. Benjamin Rush's educational campaign against hard drinking. *Am J Public Health* 83:273.

Kok, G. J. 1992. Quality of planning as a decisive determinant of health education effectiveness. *Hygiene* 11:5.

Kluger, R. 1996. *Ashes to ashes: America's hundred-year cigarette war, the public health, and the unabashed triumph of Phillip Morris.* New York: Alfred A. Knopf.

Leukfeld, C. G., and R. R. Clayton. 1996. *Prevention practice in substance abuse.* Binghamton, NY: Haworth Press.

Lewit, E. M., M. Botsko, and S. Shapiro. 1993. Workplace smoking policies in New Jersey businesses. *Am J Public Health* 83:254.

Long, K. A. 1993. The concept of health—rural perspectives. *Nurs Clin North Am* 28:123.

MacCauley, A. C., G. Paradis, L. Potvin, E. J. Cross, C. Saad-Hassan, A. McComber, S. Desrosiers, R. Kirby, L. Montour, D. L. Lamping, N. Leduc, and M. Rivard. 1997. The Kahnawake schools diabetes prevention project: intervention, evaluation, and baseline results of a diabetes prevention program with a native community in Canada. *Prev Med* 26:779.

Mackinnon, D. P., M. A. Pentz, and A. W. Stacy. 1993. The alcohol warning label and adolescents: the first year. *Am J Public Health* 83:585.

Marin, G. 1993. Defining culturally appropriate community interventions: Hispanics as a case study. *J Comm Psych* 21:149.

McGinnis, J. M., and W. H. Foege. 1993. Actual causes of death. *J Am Med Assoc* 270:2207.

McGovern, P. M., L. K. Kochevar, D. Vesley, and R. R. M. Gershon. 1997. Laboratory professionals' compliance with universal precautions. *Lab Med* 28:725.

National Center for Health Statistics. 1996. *Advance report of final mortality statistics, 1993. Monthly Vital Statistics Report* 44(7), suppl. Hyattsville, MD: Public Health Service.

O'Donnell, M., ed. 1993. *Health promotion in the workplace.* 2nd ed. Albany, NY: Delmar.

Palank, C. L. 1991. Determinants of health promotive behavior: a review of current research. *Nurs Clin North Am* 26: 815.

Pasagian-MacCaulay, A., C. E. Basch, P. Zybert, and J. Wylie-Rosett. 1997. Ophthalmic knowledge and beliefs among women with diabetes. *Diabetes Educator* 23:433.

Perez-Rodrigo, C., and J. Aranceta. Nutrition education for schoolchildren living in a low-income urban area in Spain. *J Nutrition Educ* 29:267.

Pill, R., T. J. Peters, and M. R. Robling. 1993. Factors associated with health behavior among mothers of lower socioeconomic status: a British example. *Soc Sci Med* 36:1137.

Pucci, L. G., and B. Haglund. 1994. "Naturally Smoke Free": a support for facilitating worksite smoking control policy implementation in Sweden. *Health Prom Int* 9:177.

Reed, D. B. 1996. Focus groups identify desirable features of nutrition programs for low-income mothers of preschool children. *J Am Dietetic Assoc* 96:501.

Richard, L., L. Potvin, N. Kischuk, H. Prlic, and L. W. Green. 1996. Assessment of the integration of the ecological approach in health promotion programs. *Am J Health Prom* 10:318.

Robbins, A. S. 1993. Pharmacological approaches to smoking cessation. *Am J Prev Med* 9:31.

Rodin, J. 1992. Determinants of body fat localization and its implications for health. *Ann Behav Med* 14:275.

Sharp, P. C., M. B. Dignan, K. Blinson, J. C. Konen, R. McQuellon, R. Michielutte, L. Cummings, L. Hinojosa, and V. Ledford. 1998. Working with lay health educators in a rural cancer-prevention program. *Am J Health Behav* 22:18.

Stimmel, B. 1996. *Drug abuse and social policy in America.* Binghamton, NY: Haworth Press.

Texas Department of Health. 1998. PRECEDE—a powerful planning tool targeting population-based health promotion: linking population risk factors to effective interventions. *Health Prom Interchange* 1(3):1.

Walker, E. A., C. E. Basch, C. J. Zybert, W. N. Kromholz, and H. Shamoon. 1997. Incentives and barriers to retinopathy screening among African-Americans with diabetes. *J Diabetes & its Complications* 11:298.

Warner, K., and G. Fulton. 1995. The importance of tobacco to a country's economy: An appraisal of the tobacco industry's economic argument. *Tobacco Control* 4:180–83.

Wechsler, H. 1996. Alcohol and the American college campus. *Change* (July/August): 20–25.

Weiss, J. R., N. Wallerstein, and T. MacLean. 1995. Organizational development of a university-based interdisciplinary health promotion project. *Am J Health Prom* 10:37.

Wiggers, J. H., and R. Sanson-Fisher. 1994. General practitioners as agents of health risk behaviour change: opportunities for behavioural science in patient smoking cessation. *Behav Change* 11:167.

Part Four
ENVIRONMENTAL HEALTH PROTECTION

We find it convenient in everyday discourse to use the terms *ecology* and *environment,* but they are concepts mainly of theoretical value to the health scientist. They represent bodies of scientific knowledge. They suggest ways of viewing the whole while trying to analyze and solve problems that represent only parts of the whole. Effective community health practice requires the concentration of efforts and actions on specific parts of the environment. Health personnel deal with risk conditions in the environment. Even within categories of environmental conditions, such as water or air pollution, more specific problems or risks must be identified before useful action can be taken. In part 4, you will see how the environment makes up a complementary part of the larger health field concept. You will also delve more deeply into the specific aspects of the environment that must be addressed in community health protection.

Chapter *13*

Community Injury Control

I want to die in my sleep, like my Grandad . . . not yelling and screaming like the passengers in his car.

—Anonymous

Objectives

When you finish this chapter, you should be able to:

- Describe the relative importance of injuries as causes of death in various age groups in a community

- Identify the major causes of injury subject to community intervention

- Propose appropriate combinations of educational, technological, legal, and environmental interventions to prevent injuries and violent deaths

- Propose realistic objectives for the reduction of injuries and violent deaths in a community

As the leading cause of death among environmentally induced and controllable causes of death, injuries and their prevention and control deserve the first chapter in the environmental health protection section of this book. Preventive measures for cardiovascular disease and cancer depend more heavily on behavioral or lifestyle changes such as smoking and diet. Injury prevention also has a large behavioral component, but has made great progress through legislative and regulatory control of the environment, such as with improved automobiles and roads. Control of behavior, as with enforcement of seat belt laws, has also had greater effect than attempts to persuade people to be more vigilant and cautious in self-protection or safety. As with other areas of health promotion covered in the previous section, injury prevention programs require a combination of environmental, social,

and behavioral components. The attention to the physical and regulatory environment has been greater in injury control and other issues in the chapters to follow than in the behavioral and lifestyle areas of community and population health.

Safety professionals often specialize in one aspect, such as occupational, recreational, motor vehicle, school, or fire safety. A community with a well-organized, well-integrated safety program depends on a clear understanding of the epidemiology of injuries and the science of preventing them.

EPIDEMIOLOGY OF INJURIES

The public once considered "accidents" outside the purview of public health. Health promotion and disease prevention professionals and scientists have subjected injuries and traumatic death increasingly to definition, research, and intervention. The term **accident** implies an act of providence or random event over which individuals or communities can exert no control.

Definition

The preferred term is **injury control** rather than accident prevention. This semantic shift was needed for several reasons.

First, an accident is a sudden, unanticipated, unintentional occurrence that may or may not produce a human injury. Many accidents occur with no human involvement at all. Community health is concerned with the prevention of threats to the health of human populations, not primarily with property damage, liability, or other consequences of accidents that are essentially moral, legal, or economic. Thus, human *injury* is the health problem rather than *accidents* per se.

Second, some injuries and deaths have intentional rather than accidental causes, as in the case of homicide, rape, assault, battery, child abuse, and suicide. Community health is concerned with **intentional injury** and **unintentional injury.** Some of the issues surrounding intentional injury have been addressed in chapters 5, 6, and 9.

Third, it is not always necessary to prevent accidents to prevent human injury. Some of the most effective community safety programs limit the impact of accidents rather than prevent them, as in campaigns promoting the use of automobile seat restraints. Some accidents, such as hurricanes and earthquakes, remain unpreventable, but the resulting injuries can be minimized. Planning, organization, public education, training, rescue operations, and preparation can reduce the injuries from natural disasters.

Finally, shifting the focus from accident prevention to injury control has worked to the advantage of public health education. It emphasizes ways in which people can exert control to protect themselves. They can do this partly through direct action in their personal behavior and their personal or family environment. They can also protect themselves and their families through support for legislating or enforcing such measures as safe speed limits, use of child restraints in vehicles, handgun controls, and drunk-driving laws.

The public health approach to injury control emphasizes:

- *training and organization,* such as the first aid and disaster preparedness programs of the Red Cross, to enable families and communities to manage injuries, and swimming instruction and cardiopulmonary resuscitation (CPR) training.
- *legislative measures* such as lowering speed limits or lowering blood-alcohol limits permitted in drivers.
- *law enforcement measures* to improve signs concerning speed limits or penalties for speeding and drinking while driving.
- *product safety,* such as child-proof containers; lowered thermostats on water heaters to prevent scalding; better construction of buildings and highways; fire-safe or self-extinguishing cigarettes; training wheels on bicycles; shatterproof glass; and design of toys, tools, machinery guards, and sports equipment to prevent or minimize injuries.
- *occupational safety* to prevent exposure of workers to dangerous machinery or practices in the workplace.

Injury control indicates not only the prevention of injury but also the control of damage that might result from injury. Communities minimize damage following accidents or injury through 911 telephone systems (figure 13-1), **emergency medical services** (EMS), disaster preparedness organization and training, fire departments, CPR, and rehabilitation training.

A community health definition of **injury** then is an event causing tissue damage, either unintentionally or intentionally, by a rapid transfer (less than minutes) of excessive amounts of energy. The energy may be one of five types: (1) kinetic or mechanical, (2) chemical, (3) thermal, (4) electrical, or (5) radiation. Injuries may result also from the absence of such essentials as heat or oxygen.

WHAT REALLY HURTS IS CALLER MISUSE.

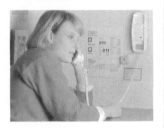

Call EMS in emergencies only.

Some people misuse the EMS system. They call 9-1-1 for reasons other than emergencies. And that really hurts. Because in a *real* emergency—when you think someone is in danger—every second counts.

EMS stands for Emergency Medical Services. Contact EMS for medical help in a serious emergency.

In many communities you can dial 9-1-1 to contact EMS, the police, or the fire department. If you live in an area without 9-1-1, find what the emergency numbers are and keep them by the phone. Know your emergency numbers. And when to use them.

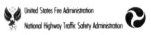

...when life is on the line.

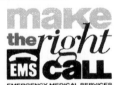
United States Fire Administration
National Highway Traffic Safety Administration

Relative Importance

The priority given injury control by a community depends on its assessment of the mortality and morbidity statistics presented in previous chapters. It also depends on assessment of the various classes and causes of injuries and the fear or other costs associated with them.

Years of Life Lost   As seen in previous chapters, **fatal accidents** are the fourth leading cause of death for all ages combined. Suicides are the eighth leading cause of death. Intentional and un-intentional injuries are higher in the younger groups. Consequently, injuries have greater significance than most other community health concerns when compared on total years of potential life lost (YPLL) from each cause of death (figure 13-2). Unintentional injuries tend to occur at younger ages than deaths from chronic disease, therefore they rank ahead of heart disease and cancer in years of potential life lost. Suicides (in the United States and Canada) and homicides (in the United States) rank fourth ahead of other leading conditions causing death. Alcohol contributes to nearly half of these years of potential life lost from intentional and unintentional injuries.

Classification and Settings   Seven specific causes of injuries—falls, burns, poisonings, vehicle crashes, firearms, sports, and drowning—are preventable. Six settings—highway, home, farm, occupational, school, and recreational environments—are useful areas in which to concentrate preventive efforts.

• •

◀ **F i g u r e   1 3 - 1**

Injury control goes beyond injury prevention to include the community's capacity to limit the damage of injuries through rapid response with 911 telephone systems, disaster preparedness, first aid and CPR training to resuscitate injury victims, ambulance and helicopter transport systems, acute trauma care, and rehabilitation programs. *Source:* United States Fire Administration and National Highway Traffic Safety Administration.

•
Figure 13-2

Potential years of life lost, by cause of death, Canada, 1970–1992. *Source:* Federal, Provincial and Territorial Advisory Committee on Population Health: Report on the Health of Canadians. 1996 Ottawa: Health Canada Communications and Consultation Directorate.

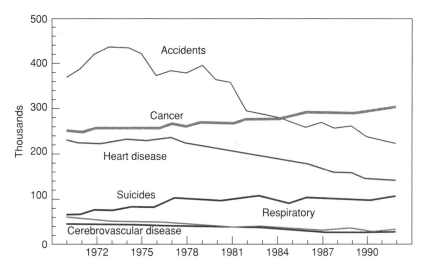

Home, recreational, and farm injuries and violent deaths, and those involving motor vehicles, represent a public health problem of cardinal significance. No strong national preventive focus exists for these in some countries. As with disease control, morbidity and mortality from injuries can be reduced through epidemiological, environmental, and educational approaches. In addition, nations, states and even communities and organizations can reduce injuries through changes in engineering and technology. A community approach to the prevention and control of injuries will focus on those groups at high risk. These are the people most exposed to behavior and environments that increase the risk of injury.

Community programs for injury control should include a surveillance system, epidemiological investigations, standards setting, public education, environmental reforms, and professional training. The primary national role should be one of providing leadership, direction, technical and financial assistance, and information to support injury pre-

vention actions undertaken by state or provincial and local health agencies. The U.S. federal government and some states and provinces have provided this leadership and direction with the formulation and tracking of quantitative goals and targets for injury control (figure 13-3).

State or provincial health agencies can also serve to coordinate the flow of resources and expertise. The local community role is one of innovation and implementation of injury prevention strategies.

Community health priorities based on the relative frequency of fatal injuries would include the following types of unintentional injuries: (1) motor vehicle injuries, (2) falls, (3) industrial injuries, (4) drowning, (5) burns, and (6) poisonings. Injuries disproportionately affect certain age groups, particularly children, adolescents, young adults, and the elderly. Among people aged 1 to 44 years, unintentional injuries are the leading cause of death. Males suffer a much higher death rate from injuries than do females, and the poor

· ·

Figure 13-3

Percentages of the quantitative targets for the year 2000 that had been achieved in unintentional injuries by 1995 at the time of the mid-decade review of national disease prevention and health promotion objectives for the United States.
Source: Healthy People 2000: Midcourse Review and 1995 Revisions. 1996. Boston: Jones and Bartlett Publishers.

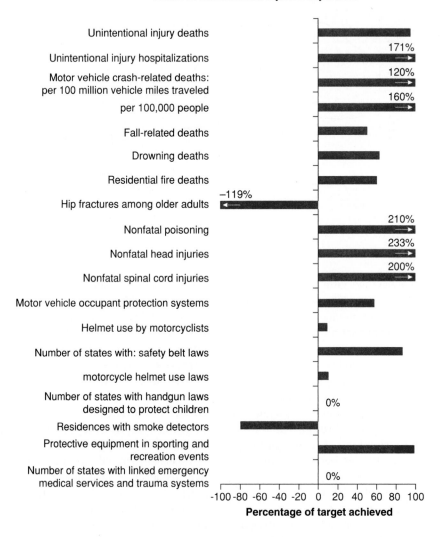

Status of unintentional injuries objectives

• • • • • • • • • • • • • • • • • • •

Figure 13-4

Age-adjusted rates of death caused by unintentional injury have improved, but gaps remain between ethnic groups, especially for males. Progress toward the year 2000 targets was good at mid-decade in the United States. *Source:* National Center for Health Statistics: Healthy People 2000 Review, 1995–96. 1996. Hyattsville, MD: Public Health Service.

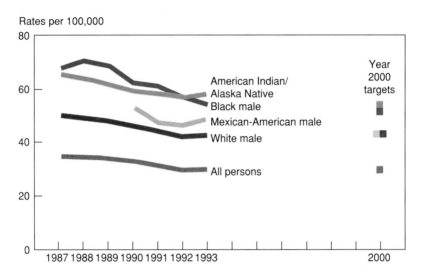

and some ethnic groups suffer a higher proportion of injuries than do other income and ethnic groups (figure 13-4).

Even more relevant as a criterion for community priorities might be the impact of morbidity. Hospital and emergency room (ER) data can measure morbidity better than state or national surveillance systems if the community uses **E-codes** to identify causes. For every death from injury, there are more than forty hospitalizations and more than 1,000 emergency room visits.

Motor Vehicle Injuries

Automobile crashes and motor vehicle mileage have continued to increase, but the death rates have decreased sporadically since 1977. The death rate per vehicle-miles traveled has decreased steadily since 1965. Credit for the reductions accrues generally to increased use of seat belts (see figure 13-5), child restraints, and the re-

newed popularity of larger cars following the emphasis on compact models during the fuel shortages of the 1970s. Nevertheless, automobile crashes still account for thousands of deaths and injuries every year in the United States and Canada. Furthermore, the cost of crashes—including wage loss, **permanent disability** payments, medical expenses, administrative and claims settlement costs, and property damage—amount to billions of dollars.

Age, sex, alcohol consumption, and vehicle size are significant correlates of vehicle injuries. Although psychological factors may also play a role, they are difficult to separate from cultural and social components of behavior.

Age and Sex Male motor vehicle occupants in the 15- to 24-year age group have an exceptionally high death-to-injury ratio. Injuries cause half of the deaths of white males aged 20 to 24 years, and

· · · · · · · · · · · · · · · · · · · ·

Figure 13-5

Motor vehicle death rates per 100,000 population, and percent of motor vehicle occupants who use seat belts, United States, 1987–1994. *Source:* National Highway Traffic Safety Administration, U.S. Department of Transportation, Fatal Accident Reporting System. For seat-belt use: 19 Cities Survey and Population-weighted State surveys. National Center for Health Statistics: Healthy People 2000 Review, 1995–96. 1996. Hyattsville, MD: Public Health Service.

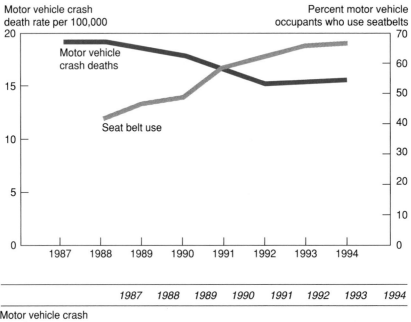

	1987	1988	1989	1990	1991	1992	1993	1994
Motor vehicle crash deaths.............	19.2	19.2	18.4	17.9	16.4	15.4	15.6	15.6
Seat belt use.....	- - -	42	47	49	59	62	66	67

- - - Data not available.

over one-third of all deaths in this age group result from automobile crashes alone. Compare this distribution with that in the 50- to 54-year age group, where only 3 percent of deaths result from automobile crashes.

Age differences in resistance to injury and in the ability to survive a given injury influence the age distribution of injuries and deaths. As a result, decreased ability to survive a crash is a major factor causing older persons to be overrepresented among fatally injured drivers. One must separate the age as it affects the initiation of an event from age as it affects the outcome of the event.

Alcohol Consumption of alcohol is the most important human element known to be causally related to all types of injuries. It is a contributing factor in over half of all fatal injuries (see box p. 397 and figure 13-6). Consumption of alcohol is a factor that tends to increase the severity of the outcome. A drinking driver, for example, will be less capable of escaping from a burning or submerging car. Alcohol impairment makes emergency treatment difficult and can obscure diagnosis.

Size of Vehicle Drivers under age twenty-five run an 87 percent greater risk of being injured in a

························

Figure 13-6

Alcohol use among fatally injured drivers of different ages, 1995, Canada. The proportion of intoxicated drivers has decreased in all age groups, but nearly half of the Canadian 20–45 age groups killed in automobile crashes had blood alcohol levels greater that 80 while driving. *Source:* Mayhew, D. R., S. W. Brown, and H. M. Simpson. 1997. Alcohol use among persons fatally injured in motor vehicle accidents: Canada 1995. Ottawa: Road Safety and Motor Vehicle Regulation, Transport Canada.

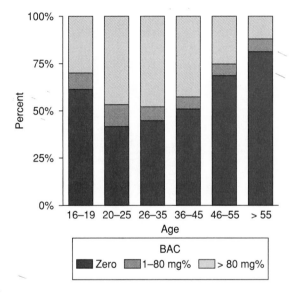

Year 2000 U. S. Safety Objectives Related to Alcohol and Other Drugs

- Reduce deaths caused by alcohol-related motor vehicle crashes to no more than 8.5 per 100,000 people. Baseline: 9.8 per 100,000 people in 1987. Reduce deaths of people aged 15 to 24 years caused by alcohol-related motor vehicle crashes to no more than 18 per 100,000 people. Baseline: 21.5 per 100,000 people in 1987.
- Extend to 50 states administrative driver's license suspension/revocation laws or programs of equal effectiveness for people determined to have been driving under the influence of intoxicants. Baseline: 28 states and Washington, DC, in 1990.

do not provide nearly as much crash protection as heavier vehicles.

Heavy trucks contribute to about one-fourth of fatal motor vehicle crashes. Many of these fatalities result from collisions of large trucks with passenger vehicles. Two-wheeled vehicle and tractor crashes account for the remaining deaths.

Interaction with Other Factors   The interaction of age and alcohol with interpersonal and situational factors predisposes adolescents to injuries on two-wheeled vehicles, including bicycles, motor scooters, motorbikes, and motorcycles. Figure 13-7 shows the interaction of various factors in bicycle injuries. This analytical framework applies the PRECEDE framework introduced in chapter 4. It identifies the psychological, social, and environmental factors amenable to modification through various combinations of educational, legal, and engineering interventions. Such epidemiological and behavioral diagnosis provides the framework for a coordinated community program of safety interventions. A similar analysis and framework could be drawn for each of the following types of injury.

subcompact car than in a full-size one. Nearly two-thirds of the drivers under age twenty-five in the United States drive small cars in the compact and subcompact classes. All age groups suffer increased motor vehicle fatalities with increased use of foreign import cars and as car manufacturers trim automobile weight to meet progressively tougher federal gas mileage requirements and consumer preferences. The population may well pay for these fuel economies with thousands of additional deaths and injuries, unless people drive less often and for shorter distances. Particularly dangerous is the combination of small cars and inexperienced young drivers. Small, lightweight cars

Figure 13-7

This integration of the PRECEDE framework with epidemiological and planning models from the injury prevention field illustrates the interaction of various factors in bicycle-related injuries and the strategies available to address them. *Source:* Gielen, A. C. 1992. Health education and injury control: integrating approaches. *Health Educ Q* 19:203. Reproduced with permission of the author and the Society for Public Health Education.

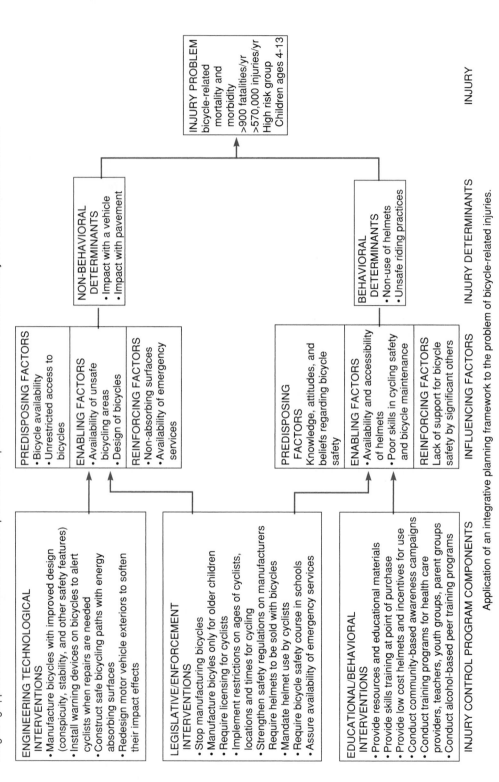

Application of an integrative planning framework to the problem of bicycle-related injuries.

Burn Injuries

Over 1 million Americans and 100,000 Canadians suffer burns each year. About 6 percent of these burns are severe enough to require hospital admission. Of those admitted to a hospital, about 15 percent are likely candidates for intensive burn care. The annual cost of providing intensive burn treatment is about $11,000 per patient. Projection of those figures would place total annual patient costs of specialized burn treatment in the United States at about $100 million and in Canada at $11 million.

Of burn injuries resulting in hospitalization, about two-thirds occur in the home and about one-fifth occur in the workplace. The first decade of life is a period of high risk for injuries and deaths from burns. Other high-risk periods are the early working years and the years after age fifty. Older people are especially susceptible to scalding from bath water because their skin is less sensitive to the heat. Burn injuries occur about twice as frequently in males, and the rate of occurrence for blacks is about three times that for whites.

Each year about 3,500 deaths and 21,275 injuries in the United States result from burns from fires—preponderantly house fires. An additional 1,300 Americans die from other kinds of burns such as scalds and electrical burns. Scalds cause about 40 percent of hospital admissions for burns. A simple environmental intervention effective in reducing scalding is to lower the temperature on hot water heaters to 50° C (120° F) or below. Some communities have put this requirement into their building codes for the installation of new water heaters.

About half of the fatal fires and many of the burn injuries relate to cigarette causes, frequently from people falling asleep while smoking in bed. Painful recovery, permanent disability, and disfigurement can be among the tragic consequences for injured survivors. About 40 percent of the victims of residential fires who have been studied have had blood alcohol concentrations above .10 percent.

Fire incidents and the resulting casualties and income loss per capita for Americans rank among

Figure 13-8

Volcanic fires and mudflows left more than 23,000 persons dead in Armero, Colombia. Earthquakes in other developing countries have caused most of their damage and loss of life through fires. *Source:* Photo by J. Vizcarra, courtesy World Health Organization and Pan American Health Organization.

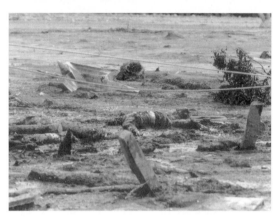

the highest in the industrialized world. Fire burns rank second only to traffic injuries among unintentional fatal injuries when measured as years of potential life lost. The years of life lost from burns in the United States each year approach 225,000. Developing countries suffer greater loss from fires. Their housing stock, building codes, and fire safety enforcement leave more room for fire. This was dramatically illustrated in 1995 and 1997 by fires in department stores, theaters, and hotels that took large tolls in Korea, Thailand, and China. The susceptibility of such countries to natural disasters including earthquakes and volcanic eruptions also produces extensive loss of life in fires (figure 13-8).

Fall Injuries

Falls account for about 12 percent of all deaths related to unintentional injuries. Fortunately, the mortality from falls has been declining, but falls still cause more deaths than any other type of unintentional injury, except motor vehicle crashes.

Objectives for Reduction of Fall Injuries

By 2000 reduced deaths from falls and fall-related injuries to no more than 2.3 per 100,000 (age-adjusted baseline: 2.7 per 100,000 in 1987)

Specific Population Targets

Deaths from falls and fall-related injuries (per 100,000)	1987 Baseline	2000 Target
People age 65–84	18.1	14.4
People age 85+	133.0	105.0
Black men aged 30–69	8.1	5.6
	1990 Baseline	2000 Target
American Indians/Alaska Natives	3.2	2.8

Nearly half of the people treated in emergency rooms with injuries resulting from falls have at least one preexisting health problem (for example, obesity, cardiovascular disease, or arthritis) known to predispose people to falls. Nearly half of children's emergency room visits related to injuries are for those caused by falls, mostly in the home. Alcohol impairment causes many falls.

Over half of fatal falls occur in the home, and 57 percent of fatal falls involve people over seventy-five years of age. Older people who survive falls are more likely to sustain fractures than are younger people. Hip fractures among older adults have increased. They represent one of only two of the U.S. Healthy People 2000 objectives for reduction of unintentional injuries, shown in figure 13-3, in which the mid-1990s trend was in the wrong direction.

Intentional Injury

Intentional injury includes homicide, suicide, rape, and family violence and child abuse. Preventive measures had not yet succeeded in reducing the rates of intentional injuries in the United States before 1995. Reversals in violent crime trends in major cities such as New York and Boston have been encouraging. The U.S. Centers for Disease Control has established a Violence Epidemiology Branch to examine the epidemic character, if not the contagion, of violence.

Homicide   Next to motor vehicle crashes, injuries from firearms cause the greatest number of violent deaths in the United States. The U.S. death rate from firearm injuries is twenty-three times greater than that of England and Wales, eighteen times greater than Canada's. The rates for the U.S. are moving in the opposite direction from the Healthy People 2000 targets (figure 13-9). Gun control laws account for much of the difference between countries, whereas alcohol accounts for much of the difference between these two leading causes of violent death and the others.

Homicides are the fourth leading cause of years of potential life lost in the United States and the second among persons aged 15 to 24 years. Homicide is more common among the poor and among minority groups. Firearm-related death rates increased 13 percent among black persons between 1990 and 1993, almost double the increase for the total population. Young black males remain about five times more likely to become victims of homicide than young white males. Young black females are more than four times as likely to become victims as are young white females. The opposite is true for suicide.

Suicide   White males have a much higher risk of suicide than other males. The suicide rates in most Western countries increase with age and are highest for the oldest men and for northern European and Japanese men. As is true for homicides, females are at consistently lower risk of suicide. The increase in the rate of suicide has also been much greater among young males than among young

Early History of Gun Control

1517   Maximilian I, Roman Emperor, prohibited the manufacture or possession of "self-striking handguns that ignite themselves," in response to early sixteenth century fears that the invention of the handy pistol had served to make firearms suitable for criminal activity in situations where it would have been impossible with the long-barreled musket.

1537   King Henry VIII of England, who had a collection of pistols, attempted to restrict the ownership of guns less than two and half feet in length, stock included.

1563   The Catholic French noble, the duc de Guise, was assassinated with a wheel-lock pistol by one of his Calvinist

enemies. It was possible for the assassin to load this weapon in advance and conceal it.

1575 and 1600   Queen Elizabeth issued proclamations against overly handy firearms, each progressively stronger in wording.

More recently:

1939   A U.S. Supreme Court ruling on the Second Amendment to the Constitution, which protects "the right of the people to keep and bear arms" upheld a law prohibiting private ownership of a sawed-off shotgun.

1968   U.S. federal legislation prohibited the sale of rifles by mail and sale of guns to minors, felons, or addicts.

1986   U.S. Congress eased some of the restrictions in the 1968 law.

1991   Canada passes Bill C-17, the strongest gun-control legislation in North America.

1993   Increasing rates of gun-related crimes precipitated U.S. Congressional passage of the "Brady Bill" named for James Brady, the press secretary wounded in the 1981 assassination attempt on President Ronald Reagan.

1994   U.S. federal crime bill banned the manufacture, sale, and possession of certain assault weapons.

1995   Canadian Parliament introduced Bill C-68, a gun-control bill that includes stiffer penalties for criminals who use firearms and a mandatory registration of all guns. It continued to be debated.

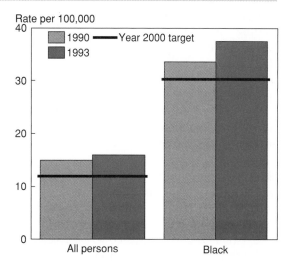

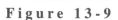

Figure 13-9

Age-adjusted rates for firearm-related deaths, United States, 1990 and 1993, and year 2000 targets for Healthy People 2000 objectives. *Source:* National Center for Health Statistics: Healthy People 2000 Review, 1995–96. 1996. Hyattsville, MD: Public Health Service.

· ·

Figure 13-10

Incidence of injurious suicide attempts among adolescents 14–17 years, United States, 1990–1995, and year 2000 target for suicide reduction objective. *Source:* Centers for Disease Control and Prevention, National Center for Chronic Disease Prevention and Health Promotion, Youth Risk Behavior Survey. National Center for Health Statistics: Healthy People 2000 Review, 1995–96. 1996. Hyattsville, MD: Public Health Service.

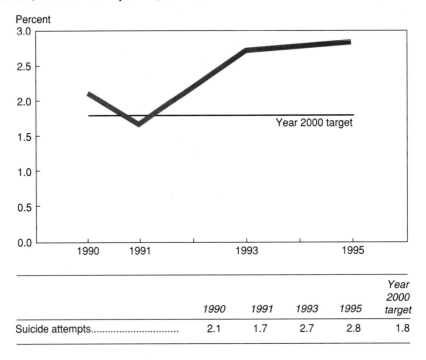

	1990	*1991*	*1993*	*1995*	*Year 2000 target*
Suicide attempts.............................	2.1	1.7	2.7	2.8	1.8

females. Increases in adolescent suicide attempts in the United States follow the trends of homicide (figure 13-10). Firearm use as a method of committing suicide has been increasing at a much faster rate than other means. Over half of the deaths from gunshot wounds in the United States are suicides. The regions where firearms are most prevalent are also the regions with the highest suicide rates. In various countries, high suicide, homicide, and unintentional injury rates occur where highly lethal methods are available.

Rape   Rape had been called the fastest growing violent crime in the United States. After reaching some 90,000 cases per year, reported rape per 100,000 population declined between 1986 and 1992. Criminologists estimate 10 sexual assaults for each one reported. One woman in 10 will be the

victim of attempted or actual rape during her lifetime; in 85 percent of these cases the woman will be beaten or intimidated with life-threatening force. One in four victims is subjected to group rape. Only 50 percent of the accused are brought to trial, and few trials end in the conviction of the assailant.

Three of the more prevalent myths about rape are that it is the result of spontaneous, uncontrollable sex drive in the male; that only young, physically attractive women are targets of rapists; and that women invite rape by going out alone or by provocative attire or seductive behavior. The myth about the "uncontrollability" of the male sex drive is like the attribution of accidents to the uncontrollable fates. Court records indicate that 70 percent of rapes are premeditated, and 50 percent of all rapists have committed violent crimes before. The second myth fell when the incidence of rapes of

······················

Figure 13-11

Incidence of physical abuse directed at women by male partners, United States, 1987–1993. *Source:* Department of Justice, Bureau of Justice Statistics, National Crime Survey. National Center for Health Statistics: Healthy People 2000 Review, 1995–96. 1996. Hyattsville, MD: Public Health Service.

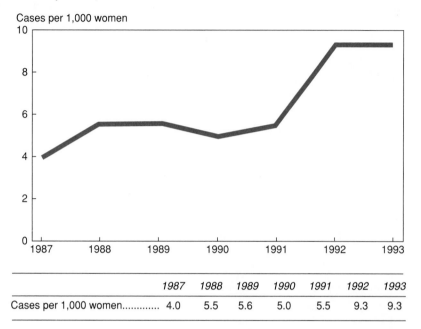

Cases per 1,000 women

	1987	1988	1989	1990	1991	1992	1993
Cases per 1,000 women.............	4.0	5.5	5.6	5.0	5.5	9.3	9.3

women over 60-years-old increased by 800 percent between 1971 and 1981. The myth concerning women inviting rape, especially in strange company or places, is refuted by the fact that only 4.4 percent of rapes are found to have been even partly provoked by the victim's behavior. Furthermore, some 60 percent of rapes occur in the victim's own home. This touches on the subject of family violence.

Family Violence and Child Abuse Although rape decreased, the incidence of physical abuse directed at women by male partners continued to increase from 1987 to 1992 (figure 13-11). **Family violence** affects about 16 million Americans each year, with acts ranging from a sharp slap across the face to murder. In 1985 a federal task force recommended that police should not need formal complaints from victims before pressing charges. Some regard such police intrusion as interference

with family life; others argue that family violence is so prevalent that it must be treated as criminal behavior. Others view family violence as a medical or psychiatric problem to be treated as an illness. The epidemiological or community health approach seeks ways to identify patterns of family violence and to intervene in the antecedent stage to prevent injury (see box for risk factors).

The National Center on Child Abuse and Neglect estimates that some 250,000 children are physically abused each year (figure 13-12). National survey data suggest a rate of 14 child abuse cases out of every 100 children aged 3 to 17 years. This rate would place the number of U.S. cases at 6.5 million per year, possibly 650,000 in Canada. The average number of assaults for these children was 10.5. The only type of family violence to exceed parent-to-child violence is child-to-child violence. The annual incidents of severe violence (kicking, biting, punching, hitting with an object,

Figure 13-12

National campaigns on the prevention of child abuse have assumed the growing problem relates to the growing number of dual earner families with both parents working and having less time and patience with children. *Source:* Courtesy of the Advertising Council and the National Committee for Prevention of Child Abuse.

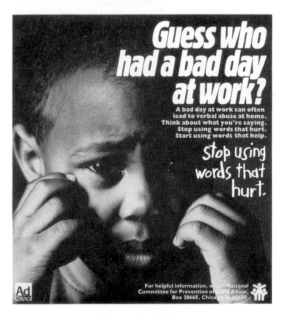

Risk Factors for Intentional Injury

CHILD ABUSE

Family history of abuse (parent or spouse abuse)

Parental mental illness and/or substance abuse

Family dysfunction or disruption (absent parent or inadequate parenting skills)

Socioeconomic stress (poverty, homelessness)

Child characteristics (overactive, difficult, or disabled)

SUICIDE

Psychiatric disorders

Alcohol and other drug abuse by the adolescent or family members

Family history of suicide, violence, and/or disruption

Biochemical (decreased serotonin levels)

Prior attempts

Close relationship with a suicide victim

Incarceration

Ready access to firearms

HOMICIDE

Poverty

Violence in the family and community

Effects of substance abuse

Buying and selling illicit drugs

Ready access to firearms

beating, threatening to use or using a knife or gun) is 14.2 per 100 families for parent-to-child violence. The rate is 53.2 per 100 families for child-to-child violence. The comparable rate for child-to-parent abuse is 9.2 per 100 families, and for spouse abuse only 6.1 per 100 couples.

INTERVENTION TO REDUCE INJURY

Population or community targets for injury control interventions include the agent, host, or environment. Most effort targets the host, for the urge to reform and alter other people's behavior is strong. Although investigation frequently reveals the cause of injury to be human error, this approach to injury control is the least efficient of the three available. Consideration of automobile-related injuries illustrates this point. Three classes of people—young males, alcoholics, and elderly people—are at greatest risk of automobile crashes. These three groups are particularly difficult targets of educational programs.

More efficient intervention modifies the agent so that the product is safer and the potential harm lessened. Manufacturers have done this to some extent with the automobile. Other examples are medication containers designed so that children cannot open them and poison themselves, and children's pajamas made of flameproof fabric. The Consumer Product Safety Commission has required manufacturers to build this into the design of many products. The doctrine of manufacturers' liability for harm resulting from faulty design or operation has done much to accelerate this trend; legal accountability for products used by the public has forced companies to incorporate safety features. Ralph Nader and Joan Claybrook have crusaded effectively on behalf of consumer safety in the United States.

The most effective point of intervention is the environment. Communities can adapt their environments to minimize the incidence of accidents and to minimize harm when they do occur.

Highway Environment

Intervention can make the highway environment substantially safer. Construction of a wide median strip featuring a sturdy guardrail can immediately and permanently reduce fatal accidents. Safe access and exit ramps, clear signs, lighted junctions, and rest areas contribute to safe driving. Other safety methods well known to highway engineers and now available, such as covering frequently struck highway structures with compressible materials and using oil drums filled with sawdust as barriers, also reduce injuries. Communities can make pedestrian areas safe with nonslip surfaces, grading, and lighting. They can modify the environment in industrial areas to increase safety by reducing air and noise pollution and installing guardrails.

The environmental changes necessary for safety frequently involve enforcement of existing regulations (for example, the speed limit). They also require in many cases the enactment of new legislation. Communities proposing such radical changes need to precede them with information campaigns to educate the public about the advantages of the change proposed. Even after enacting a measure, people may not appreciate the ensuing benefit to public health. The public sometimes rescinds such laws. For example, several states rescinded laws requiring the wearing of helmets by motorcyclists because they failed to inform their electorates of the need for these laws (figure 13-13). The public now debates the wisdom of seat belt and air-bag laws (see box on issues and controversies, p. 406).

Seat belts are effective in preventing injury and death, but only about 68 percent of automobile occupants in the United States (see figure 13-5), 90 percent in Canada, use them. This represents a steady increase since 1982. The U.S. Transportation Department requires automobile manufacturers to install shoulder harnesses in the front and back seats of all new cars. Lap-belted drivers have 43 percent fewer serious and fatal injuries than their unbelted counterparts in frontal impact crashes. Provinces in Canada and states in the United States and Australia have reduced crash injuries substantially with the enforcement of mandatory seat belt use (figure 13-14). In 13 cities in states with seat belt laws more than 51 percent of drivers used their belts compared with only 36 percent of the drivers in 6 cities located in states that do not have seat belt laws. Canada and England achieve 90 percent wearing of seat belts; Germany and Australia, 80%; and France, 70%.

The German autobahns have had higher death rates than U.S. interstate highways in all but four years since 1975, despite their greater use of seat belts. They also ban large trucks from using the autobahns on weekends. The Germans limit the driving age to eighteen whereas many states in the United States allow teenagers to drive as early as age 16. The German death rates should be lower than those of the United States for those reasons. The higher German death rates, according to the Insurance Institute for Highway Safety, are because of the unlimited speed laws on the autobahns. Safety epidemiologists expect U.S. federal laws allowing the states to increase their speed limits above the former 55 mph limit (100 km/hr) to result in increased traffic injury and death rates.

Tractor fatalities have declined in those areas where the Occupational Safety and Health Administration (**OSHA**) regulates large farms and requires them to have rollover protective structures on tractors. Most farms do not fall under OSHA's jurisdiction. Tractors account for 40 percent of the work- and non-work-related injuries on farms. More than one-half of these deaths occur when tractors overturn and crush the operator.

....
Figure 13-13

The helmet law experience of several states illustrates the importance of health education to develop an informed electorate as part of the process of legislative action for injury control. Many states allowed their legislators to reverse previously passed laws requiring all motorcyclists to wear helmets because the public never fully understood the rationale for the law. The graphs show how the laws affected motorcycle fatality rates. Proportionate effects on costs to state and community health care systems could be drawn. *Source:* Motorcycle Helmet Laws: Questions and Answers. 1994. Washington, DC: Advocates for Highway and Auto Safety.

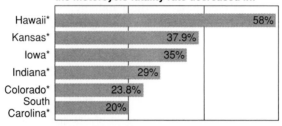

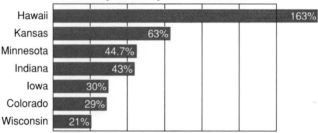

(Motorcycle fatalities/10,000 registered motorcycles)
*All-rider law subsequently repealed

ISSUES AND CONTROVERSIES
Mandatory Use of Seat Belts versus Passive Restraints (Air Bags)
....

Seat belt laws were once resisted by the American automobile industry because they were considered costly and inconvenient. Now the industry favors laws for mandatory use of seat belts to avoid the impending requirement for more costly installation of air bags that inflate automatically on impact and seat belts that lock automatically when the car door closes. Such passive restraints would save an estimated 8,000 lives per year and $2 billion in health care costs, lost wages, and lowered productivity from injuries.

The quandary for community health professionals was whether to work for passage of the seat belt requirements, which could prevent thousands of deaths and disabling injuries, or to hold out for the passive restraints, which would be installed in new cars if the seat belt laws were not passed by enough states. Passive restraints like air bags built into cars would be more effective in the long run only if used with seat belts and shoulder belts, but the experience of some states and other countries has shown that increased use of ordinary seat belts under penalty of law is a guaranteed life-saver in the short run. Which course of action would you have supported, and why?

· ·

F i g u r e   1 3 - 1 4

Safety belt use laws have had greater enforcement and consequently greater impact on public use and reduced crash fatalities. *Source:* National Highway Traffic Safety Administration, U.S. Department of Transportation.

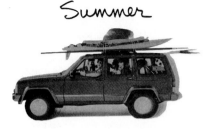

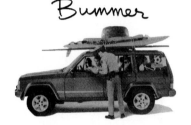

This summer, seatbelt laws are being enforced.
So buckle up. Or you might break more than the law.
And that would be the biggest bummer of all.

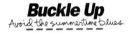

The Chronology of Events Surrounding Seat Belts and Air Bags

December 1991: After Congress mandated that auto manufacturers would install air bags in all cars by 1977, National Highway Traffic Safety Administration (NHTSA) director warned owners of rear-facing infant seats not to use them in the front seats of cars with passenger air bags.

October 1993: U.S. Transportation Secretary warned again about rear-facing car seats but said children in front facing seats and lap/shoulder belts will have added protection from air bag in a crash.

July 1995: First child died in a rear-facing infant seat, but was tenth to be killed by a passenger air bag.

October 1995: NHTSA set up a program to study problems associated with air bags and children.

August 1996: NHTSA proposed new multicolor labels on cars warning that unbelted children are at risk of injury or death from air bags.

October 1996: NHTSA concluded that it is probably safer to use an air bag in conjunction with seat belts, but advised parents not to seat children under the age of thirteen in front seats, and short people to sit as far back from the steering wheel as possible to avoid the impact of the air bag.

November 1996: Transport Canada offered provinces assistance in reaching their own decisions on regulations concerning airbags.

December 1996: NHTSA added to warning labels on air bags new requirements for "smart"

airbags to be phased in beginning in fall 1998 to deploy according to the size of the occupant, a reduction of at least 20 percent in the power with which air bags deploy, permitted manufacturers to install manual cutoff switches on vehicles without a back seat, and allowed dealers to deactivate airbags at request of owners.

April 1997: The Clinton Administration proposed legislation that would reward states for increasing enforcement of seat-belt laws and get more people to wear seat belts, and would later withhold highway funds from states that fail to enact tougher belt laws or to achieve substantial gains in belt use by 2003.

Objective for Home Safety

By 2000 each inhabitable floor of all residential units should have a properly placed and functioning smoke detector. (In 1990 86 percent of inhabited American dwellings and 85 percent of Canadians had systems installed.)

How would you proceed to accomplish this objective in your community?

Home and Childcare Environments

Each year about 22,000 people in the United States and over 2,000 in Canada require medical attention or restricted activity as the result of an injury in the home. Indeed, the home is the leading site for disabling injuries. The most dangerous area for injuries is the bedroom, because it is most often the site of falls, chiefly among older people. The second most dangerous area is the kitchen. These two sites also produce the majority of fires in homes.

Community Home Safety Programs   The combination of residential burns, falls, poisoning, cuts, drowning, and violence means that more injuries occur in the home than in motor vehicle crashes, yet few communities have organized more than fire prevention programs. Such efforts are laudable even though limited to one aspect of home safety. In the United States, for example, Cincinnati has a "Target System" of fire inspections supported by a Tactical Inspection and Educational Unit. Assigned members of each fire company make inspections of structures. They determine the frequency of inspections by the "target" or category of the structure. The inspectors determine the five categories based on the nature of the occupancy and the past inspection record. For buildings in the poorest category, they make inspections as frequently as every two weeks. When persuasion does not result in hazards being corrected, courts may take action to fight noncompliance with fire department orders. In some communities the fire department encourages citizens to request fire inspection by the department staff. They often time this to correspond with Fire Prevention Week.

These fire prevention plans help those who can access them, but such piecemeal home safety programs are not adequate. A communitywide home safety program spanning all aspects of home injury prevention is the goal.

Education is a basic ingredient of home safety promotion, therefore the health education division of the community health department can provide the leadership for a community program to prevent injuries in the home. Health departments spearheading such a program can integrate the safety activities and contributions of organizations (for example, the fire department) and individuals. A communitywide home safety coalition can serve as a sounding board and as a means of access to the public and their homes.

Some combination of improper practices and unsafe conditions cause most home injuries. Promotion of home safety must focus on the correction of these practices and conditions. Efforts to educate the public should precede any legislative or enforcement action directed to improvement of private property. This means the use of all possible communication media and the promotion of special measures for alerting the public to the need for home safety.

Home or Childcare Safety Surveys   Once public awareness and interest have increased, the next step should be a **home safety survey** conducted by householders themselves. Such a survey can identify unsafe conditions and practices and is especially applicable to older homes.

A survey is a means to an end, not an end in itself. Follow-up action to correct unsafe conditions and practices is the logical corollary to the survey. Through the various communication media, sponsors of the survey must place continual emphasis on the importance of corrections if this approach is to yield tangible results. Projects in Denver,

Philadelphia, and San Francisco have demonstrated new approaches to home injury prevention in elderly people and in inner-city black populations.

The injury prevention survey shown in table 13-1 reflects the items that would be important for any home occupied by adults, plus some specific to childcare settings. Additional items that would apply, particularly in homes occupied by older adults, can be obtained from the U.S. Product Safety Commission, Health Canada, or your state or provincial health department or ministry if your local health department does not have them. The additional items for older adults include:

- apply adhesive carpet tape or rubber matting to the backs of rugs and carpet runners (more than 2,000 people sixty-five and over are treated annually in hospital emergency rooms for injuries that resulted from tripping over rugs and runners);
- check smoke detectors, which should be located on every floor, preferably in hallways near bedrooms and away from air vents;
- check bathtubs for installation of at least one, preferably two, grab bars attached to the tile, to structural supports in the wall;
- check setting of water heater at 120° F (49° C) or lower;
- ash trays, smoking materials, or other fire sources (heaters, hot plates, teapots) located away from beds or bedding;
- sturdy handrails on both sides of stairways.

Besides surveys on the home or childcare environment, health or safety agencies can obtain objective data on injuries and how they occur in the home. One method to collect such data is to provide all households with a form for reporting the time, place, and nature of the injury and the factors involved. These collective data can be highly meaningful in pinpointing where emphasis should be placed in the home or childcare safety program.

Fires Some eight out of ten fire deaths happen at home, and more than half of them occur in one- and two-family homes. More than half of the home fires occur between midnight and 6 A.M. Cigarettes, cigars, and pipes are still the major culprits, most often igniting in living rooms and bedrooms. They may smolder for several hours, but it takes only two to four minutes after ignition for combustible materials to go up in roaring flames that release poisonous gases. Unfortunately, this can happen undetected by a sleeping family.

Smoke detectors can often mean the difference between life and death. Technology has produced a ready assortment of low-cost alarms. These devices are particularly effective in detecting fires in their early stages. As their name implies, the design of smoke detectors is to detect the presence of smoke particles in the atmosphere. In the early stages of fires, smoke often develops before there is any appreciable increase in temperature, and smoke inhalation is a major cause of fire deaths. Residences with smoke detectors and fire extinguishers increased in the 1980s in the United States and Canada (figure 13-15), but the U.S. percentage has lost ground in the early 1990s to less than 80 percent.

The distribution of fire locations in houses that have burned shows that the majority of fires start in the three rooms where people spend most of their time. These are living room, bedroom, and kitchen—in that order of frequency. Community agencies can help residents reduce the likelihood of injury residential fires by preparing and practicing home escape plans and fire prevention plans. These should include:

- Plans for at least two escape routes from every room, especially the bedrooms where the most serious injuries result from night fires.
- Obtaining escape ladders for second-story rooms.
- Holding family or resident meetings at least once a year to practice the escape plan.
- Teaching children how to open windows and doors, or to break out glass and screens on windows, and care in breaking off jagged glass.
- Making sure residents know how to exit through all windows and doors and where to meet to be sure all members have escaped.

Table 13-1

This Injury Prevention Survey Was Designed Particularly for Childcare Settings, But Would Apply with Minor Modifications to Any Home Occupied by Adults. Additional Considerations Apply to Home Occupied by Elderly Adults.

Indoor Settings	OK ✓	Action Required Please specify	Assigned to	Date completed
Furnishings: Furniture is in good repair and free of sharp edges, splinters, and pinch or crush points.				
• Rugs are laying flat.				
• Heavy objects are stored on lower shelves.				
Windows: Drapery and blinds cords are out of children's reach.				
Plants: Bulbs and seeds are stored out of children's reach.				
• There are no hazardous or poisonous plants.				
Hazardous Materials: Toxic materials and cleaning products are in original containers and out of children's reach.				
• Ceilings and walls are free of cracked or broken plaster and peeling or chipped paint.				
Hallways • Stairways: These areas are clear of toys, boxes or other items that may limit easy access or cause tripping.				
Gates • Doors: Areas where children are not permitted are protected by secured doors or safety gates.				
Wiring • Electric Plugs • Appliances: Safety covers for electric plug outlets are in place				
• Space heaters are at least 3´ (90cm) away from flammable items.				
• Small electrical appliances are well away from sinks or tubs.				
• Electric fans are out of children's reach.				
• Smoke detectors are tested every month.				
• Batteries in smoke detectors are changed twice a year.				
Toys: Toys are in good repair and free of sharp edges, pinch points, splinters or broken parts.				
Kitchens: Poisonous materials are stored in cupboards with locks or childproof latches.				

continued.

Table 13-1—*Continued.*

Indoor Settings	OK ✓	Action Required Please specify	Assigned to	Date completed
• Scissors, knives, and other sharp items are out of children's reach.				
• Plastic bags are not accessible to children.				
• Highchairs are located away from appliances, windows, and sharp corners.				
Sleeprooms: Cribs are in good condition with no loose or missing slats.				
• Cribs, beds, and mats are located away from windows and blind cords.				
• Cribs have less than 1˝ (2.5cm) gap between mattress and crib side or end.				
• The crib mattress support mechanism is secure.				
• Bumper pads are free of cuts or breaks.				
• Bumper pads and large toys have been removed from cribs of infants who can stand.				
• Toys are not strung over cribs of infants who can sit up.				
• Vinyl covered pads and rail covers for playpens are free of cuts or breaks.				
Gyms • Gross Motor Areas: Equipment is free of loose parts or bolds, protruding nails or splinters.				
• Climbing equipment is located away from windows, walls and other furniture.				
• Structures higher than 2´ (60cm) have resilient mats under and around them.				
Bathrooms: Platforms or stools used at hand basins are stable and slip proof.				
• Toxic materials and cleaning products, skin cream, lotions, and powders are not accessible to children.				
Basements: Paints, insecticides, laundry products, and other toxic items are not accessible to children.				
• Flammable products are stored away from furnace or hot water tank.				
Guns and Rifles: Guns and rifles are unloaded and locked away in an area not accessible to children.				
• Ammunition is stored separate from the firearm and in a locked closet.				
Alcohol: Alcohol is out of children's reach.				

continued.

Table 13-1—*Continued.*

Outdoor Settings	OK ✓	Action Required Please specify	Assigned to	Date completed
Comings and Goings: Fences and gates are stable and free of protruding nails, nuts, or bolts.				
• Walkways are level.				
• Low branches are trimmed from trees and shrubs.				
• Wooden walkways are free of moss and algae and are nonslip.				
• Walkways are swept regularly				
Equipment: Climbing structures, slides, and swings are stable.				
• Rungs, rails, and steps are free of slivers or sharp edges.				
• Swing hangers, chairs, and seats are in good repair and "S" hooks are securely closed.				
• Equipment parts are not broken, worn, cracked, rusted, or missing.				
• Nuts, bolts, and screws are tight, recessed and/or covered with plastic caps.				
• Ropes, chains, and cables are in good condition.				
Resilient Surfaces: Resilient material under and around climbers and swings is between 6–12″ (15–30 cm) deep, depending on equipment height.				
• Loose resilient materials are raked and there are no holes or bare spots.				
• Playground is free of litter, glass, sharp objects and animal droppings.				

Checklist completed by:

Date:

All follow up completed by:

Date:

Source: Community Care Facilities Branch and the Office of Injury Prevention 1994. Preventing Injury in Child Care Settings. Victoria: British Columbia Ministry of Health.

· ·

F i g u r e 1 3 - 1 5

Increases in Canadians age fifteen and over having smoke detectors and fire extinguishers in their homes. More recent declines in the percentage of U.S. homes having smoke detectors suggests a reversal of this trend in the United States. *Source:* Federal, Provincial and Territorial Advisory Committee on Population Health: Report on the Health of Canadians. 1996. Ottawa: Health Canada Communications and Consultation Directorate.

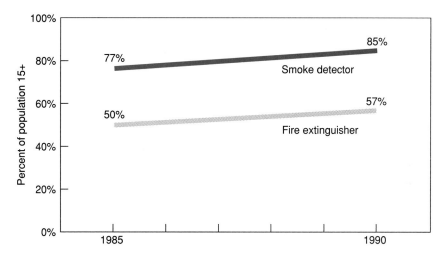

- Inspecting for fire hazards such as frayed wiring, extension cords under rugs, kindling or paper left to close a fireplace or stove, heavy soot buildup in the chimney.
- Maintaining fire department and emergency numbers near the telephone.
- Regular check of smoke detectors and fire extinguishers to insure they are working.

Poisoning Community health would define **poisoning** as a chemical agent ingested, inhaled, injected, or absorbed that results in illness, injury, or death. Poisoning is the fifth leading cause of unintentional injury deaths in the United States. Childhood poisoning deaths declined markedly in the 1990s with the manufacture and enforcement of special child-proof lids on medicine bottles and household chemical containers. The United States had already exceeded its national year 2000 objective for reduction of nonfatal poisonings by 1995.

Homicidal and suicidal poisonings are rare by comparison with unintentional poisoning, though many of the drug-related unintentional poisonings might reflect attempted homicides or suicides. The leading causes of fatal unintentional drug poisonings are opiates and related narcotics and local anesthetics including cocaine. Most of the deaths from other solids and liquids are due to alcohol ingestion. Motor vehicle exhaust (carbon monoxide fumes) accounted for nearly half the deaths attributed to unintentional poisoning by gases and vapors.

The unintentional poisoning mortality rate for males tends to run more than twice as high as that for females. The rates for blacks of both sexes are consistently higher than those for whites in the United States.

The annual observance of National Poison Prevention week in mid-March gives American communities an opportunity to cooperate with over thirty national organizations. These represent industry, consumer groups, poison control centers, health professionals, government, and the media. The community **poison control centers** play a pivotal role in preventing poisonings among children by providing public information, expert consultation, and specialized diagnostic and treatment recommendations within their respective communities.

Other residential or home environment safety issues will be addressed in Chapter 15.

Family Violence Most programs for preventing child abuse and spouse abuse assume that the problem arises from the learning of physical force as a legitimate way to control family members and to express dissatisfaction or frustration. For example, in one survey, nearly 72 percent of the respondents did not consider shaking a child as abusive, yet medical authorities consider shaking an infant or small child to be extremely dangerous. The mass media tend to reinforce attitudes that violence is necessary, legitimate, and effective to maintain family control and to punish transgressions of authority.

Interventions seek to break into this intergenerational cycle. The detection of abusive parents or spouses is a first step. Police have been encouraged to intervene in violent domestic situations without formal complaints from victims. Schools and hospitals previously required to report child abuse should also report abuse of adult partners and the elderly. Broadcasters should voluntarily limit violence on television programs. States that have given police more power in responding to family violence have noted progress in reducing repeat offenses or complaints. Illinois has rules to keep victims from being harassed, and Brooklyn, San Antonio, Los Angeles, and Westchester County, New York, have special units for family violence and sexual abuse cases.

After detection of such cases, group psychotherapy with a heavy emphasis on coping skills can be an effective intervention. Identification of alcohol abuse is often a starting point. Primary prevention strategies include training in parenting skills, emphasis on early bonding between newborns and their mothers (especially important if the baby is born prematurely), and public education to recognize signs of family violence tendencies.

Other Violence Murder, suicide, and rape were the concern primarily of law enforcement agencies, but health organizations have taken increasing responsibility for finding effective interventions. An example is prevention of teenage suicides, which sometimes occur in clusters within communities, suggesting a pattern of contagion. Following an outbreak of teenage suicides, officials may develop a countywide suicide prevention program. Such programs usually include suicide prevention training for teachers, guidance counselors, parents, and students. Telephone hot lines provide a crisis-counseling resource for potential suicide victims who wish to maintain their anonymity.

Rape prevention programs have emphasized public education and security programs for safe transportation for women at night. Other approaches have included the development of more humanitarian, structured assistance for rape victims in the hospital emergency room, at police headquarters, and in the courts. This has required better informed, more sympathetic police officers, physicians, and nurses to interview and treat rape victims. Hospitals have provided standardized kits in emergency rooms for collection of evidence. Other community organizations have provided public education to alter community attitudes toward rape and to gain community support for preventive and control measures.

U.S. data in the 1990s indicated that friends or acquaintances of women committed more than half of rapes and sexual assaults reported. Intimates (partners, lovers) committed 26 percent, while strangers were responsible for only 18 percent. Other violent crimes show men with far more victimization by strangers than women, but much less from intimates (figure 13-16).

Handgun control laws could help reduce several forms of violence and the lethality of resulting injuries. Morton Grove, Illinois, was the first community in the United States to ban the possession of handguns by anyone except law enforcement officers. The citizens of Maryland waged a pitched political battle with the National Rifle Association to pass a statewide gun control measure on the

Figure 13-16

Rate of violent crimes against persons 12 years of age and over committed by a lone offender, by victim-offender relationship and sex of victim, United States, 1992–93. *Source:* Bachman, R., and L. E. Saltzman. 1995. Violence against women: Estimates from the redesigned survey. Washington, DC: U.S. Department of Justice, Office of Justice Programs, Bureau of Justice Statistics, National Crime Victimization Survey.

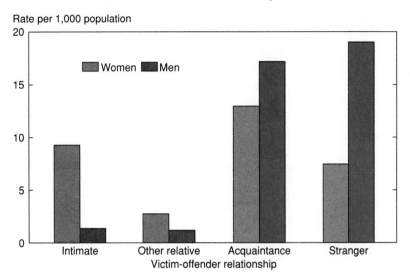

ballot. Polls indicate that most Americans favor stiffer gun control. Most other countries are more restrictive in the possession of handguns than is the United States. Most Western countries have lower rates of violent injuries largely as a result of this difference in gun control.

Farm Environment

Safety on the farm encompasses aspects of occupational, home, motor vehicle, and recreational safety. From the standpoint of occupation, about one-fifth of industrial accident deaths in the United States occur in farming. The rate of accidental deaths in farming, which is higher than that in any other industry, showed the least improvement in the 1990s.

Agricultural work covers a wide variety of jobs depending on the farm's size, its location, its agricultural products, and availability of help. The work is seasonal and often demands long hours, physical strength, and quick execution. Farm workers usually perform multiple job functions, frequently without adequate safety instruction. Many times children, young adults, and uneducated laborers perform urgent work on family farms using a wide variety of heavy equipment, dangerous machinery, and intricate production methods. Farm families and workers are often exposed to the elements and may become vulnerable to sun, heat, and cold. Rural living and farm work also expose these persons to dangerous animals, toxic plants and insects, pesticides, hazardous and volatile chemical compounds, and dangerous equipment (figure 13-17).

Ministries or departments of agriculture and farm extension services hold programs promoting farm safety. Farm organizations such as the Farmers Union and the Grange also have continuing and special farm safety programs. The state department of education usually promotes safety education, including farm safety, in the schools.

....

Figure 13-17

Children on farms encounter hazardous machinery and unregulated use of materials used in building or repairing temporary farm structures. *Source:* Photo courtesy Missouri Department of Health.

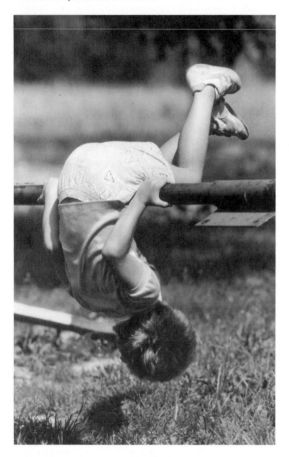

Farm Injuries   Farm life places the agricultural family in a variety of situations with safety problems. Machinery poses a special hazard. Fatal injuries from machines and firearms on farms occur three to five times more frequently than fatal injuries from the same implements in other environments (figure 13-17). Data on farm injuries can identify where to lay the greatest emphasis in safety promotion on the farm. Injuries pose a spe-

cial problem for the farm population, calling for more effective action than has been expended thus far.

Prevention of Farm Injuries   Preventing farm injuries involves the farm families through self-direction as an outgrowth of an extensive program of farm safety education. Correlated with safety education should be a **farm safety survey** that farm families can use profitably.

Combined with the home safety survey (see table 13-1), a farm safety survey can provide the basis for an evaluation of hazards and safety in farm life. Farm families should conduct safety surveys and follow up by correcting any hazardous conditions and practices revealed by the survey.

In some communities a farm safety committee under the aegis of the community safety council coordinates the efforts of organizations and individuals in farm health promotion. More than twenty organizations participate in farm safety on the local level in the United States. These include the Cooperative Extension Service, Grange, Farmers Union, American Farm Bureau Federation, Future Farmers of America, 4-H clubs, and Future Homemakers of America. Meetings, campaigns, contests, demonstrations, and studies are the channels through which these organizations promote safety on the farm.

Occupational Environment

Industrial safety refers to injury control in a branch of trade or production on a wide geographic basis, such as in the steel industry or automobile industry. **Occupational safety** refers to injury control within the confines of a single operational unit, such as the safety program in a specific chemical plant. Industrial safety is of value because of the pooling of experience and knowledge among the various units within an industry. It is on the local operational level where accidents must be prevented and where a safety program will yield the greatest results in **occupational injury** control.

· · · · · · · · · · · · · · · · · · · ·

Figure 13-18

Annual bed days associated with injuries at work by sex, United States, 1982–1994. *Source:* Centers for Disease Control and Prevention, National Center for Health Statistics, National Health Interview Survey.

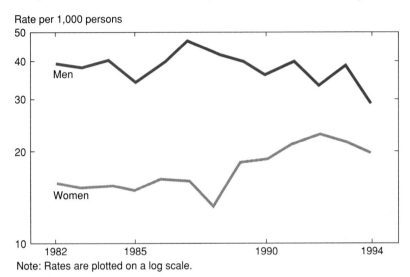

Note: Rates are plotted on a log scale.

Of the major safety programs, occupational safety appears to have made the greatest progress in injury control in the United States. The enactment of Worker's Compensation laws beginning in 1912 made safety economically profitable. Today management and labor have more than a business interest in safety promotion. They have a stake in protecting the lives and health of employees. The drop in the injury frequency rate for companies reporting to the National Safety Council attests to the effectiveness of safety programs. Occupational injury deaths per 100,000 workers dropped 71 percent from 1912 to 1980. Between 1982 and 1994, the number of working women increased by 32 percent. Rates of injuries at work increased during this period for women while rates for men were declining (figure 13-18).

The U.S. Occupational Safety and Health Act mandates the reporting of occupational injuries and illnesses by employers. A new system of uniform reporting and recording has resulted in more complete reporting. Between 1970 and 1980, the number of work-related fatal injuries decreased by 28 percent. However, some of the OSHA standards are not being enforced because of deregulation since 1981.

Industries with the highest injury frequency rates (disabling injuries per 100,000 work hours) also tend to have the highest severity rates (days lost per 1 million work hours). By their very nature, certain industries such as mining, marine transportation, quarrying, and construction tend to be hazardous. Other industries have a minor degree of hazard. Data for a total industry are of value to a local operation, but each plant or place of employment must deal with the hazards in its own operation.

Much as occupational health presents an opportunity for population health promotion and injury prevention, workers suffer more than three times as many accidental deaths off the job than they do on the job. A further consideration is that the probability of an injury incurred at work being fatal is only half that of injuries incurred away from work.

Prevention of Occupational Injuries Organization, a planned program, expert direction, and the enlistment of all personnel are the ingredients of an effective occupational injury control program. Usually such a program consists of the following eight aspects:

1. Leadership by management and labor unions
2. Assignment of responsibility
3. Safe working conditions
4. Safety training of all personnel
5. Accident and injury records
6. Analysis of accidents and research in safety measures
7. Employee and employer acceptance of responsibility for safety
8. First aid and medical services

Industry employs safety experts, sometimes designated safety engineers. Federal and state or provincial regulatory agencies mandate the provision and use of protective equipment or clothing for workers exposed to specific risks (figure 13-19). These environmental approaches to injury prevention and control could apply to other provinces of human activity where injuries are even more prevalent. More will be discussed on occupational health and safety in chapter 16.

School Environment

For school-age youngsters, injuries loom as a greater threat to life and limb than do diseases. In the United States in the 5- to 15-year age group, accidents other than automobile injuries are the leading cause of death.

School Injuries About 43 percent of accidental deaths among school-aged children in the United States are connected with school life. About 6 percent occur on the way to or from school, about 20 percent in school buildings, and about 17 percent on school grounds. Youngsters between the ages of 5 and 14 years have the highest injury rate. Many of the injuries are in sports and recreational activities on school grounds or sponsored by schools. These will be discussed in the next section.

••••••••••••••••••••
Figure 13-19

Federal, state, provincial, and international agencies conduct studies of occupational exposures and risks of injury and have regulatory guidelines or standards for protection of workers in specific industries. *Source:* Photo by P. Larsen, courtesy World Health Organization.

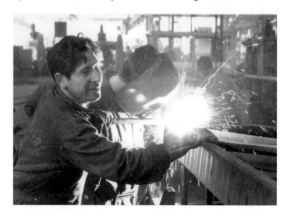

Prevention of School Injuries Schools can prevent accidental deaths and injuries among students and faculty with a systematic, vigorous, and sustained program. Leadership, vision, organization, and teamwork bridging school and community are the ingredients of an effective school safety program, which is one facet of the total community safety program. A school-based driver education training program, for example, can do more harm than good if the community uses it to license youth to drive too early.

A safety council composed of students and faculty supports the school safety program. A school safety patrol can have subdivisions such as a traffic patrol, a building and grounds patrol, and a fire patrol. Student participation under teacher guidance is the working pattern, ideally using school safety checklists as a survey tool and as a safety education opportunity. Involving students actively in the planning and execution of programs helps give the students a sense of ownership and commitment to the programs.

Surveys of conditions and practices affecting safety in the school environment point out hazards and indicate preventive measures that must be taken. These surveys properly include conditions between the school and children's homes and school playgrounds.

A system for reporting accidents and injuries is of legal significance and of preventive value. This is particularly true when a systematic investigation and follow-up is tied in with the reporting system.

Safety education as an integral phase of early health education has been effective in developing good safety attitudes and practices among children. Good safety habits are most readily acquired in the early, formative years of life.

Recreational Environment

Many workers have gained increased vacation time and early retirement as work benefits from business and industry. Others have shifted from employer benefits to self-employment, giving them greater flexibility with their leisure time. Accordingly, the population at risk from various recreational activities has steadily increased. Complete figures on recreational morbidity and mortality have not been compiled, therefore injuries from recreational pursuits have not emerged as a high priority for professional attention except in sports medicine.

It would be unrealistic to restrain recreation for the purpose of preventing injuries. It would be equally unrealistic to think that recreation could be injury-free, but experience has demonstrated that safety promotion can go hand in hand with the expansion of recreation. Clearly, some recreational pursuits carry greater inherent risks than others (figure 13-20).

Injuries in Recreation   Most unintentional injuries and deaths, other than those related to home, noncommercial motor vehicle, and employment accidents, occurred in recreational and leisure settings. Statistics for the age group most affected by recreational injuries show different patterns of sports injuries for males and females in the 5- to 19-year age range (figure 13-21).

Most drownings involve water sports such as swimming and boating. The annual number of

Figure 13-20

Some sports and recreational activities have inherently greater risk than others, but ones that also can be controlled through adequate training, preparation, equipment, regulation, and supervision. *Source:* Photo courtesy World Health Organization.

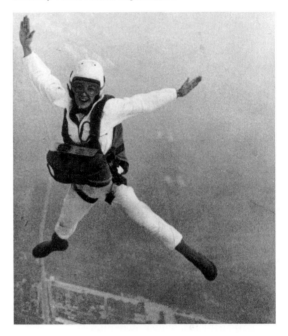

deaths from drowning declined in the 1980s and 1990s despite the increasing numbers of people participating in water sports. About one-third of adults who drown have high levels of alcohol in their blood. Children are at greatest risk.

Approximately 50.5 million boaters use 10 million boats in the waters of the United States. Recreational boating accounts for fewer than 1,000 fatalities each year in the United States. Although few by comparison with the number of motor vehicle deaths, this figure represents a rate of approximately 44 fatalities per 100 million exposure hours compared to the automobile rate of about 55 fatalities per 100 million exposure hours. Hypothermia (exposure) fatalities appear to be increasing with the growing interest in cold weather

· ·

Figure 13-21

Estimates of the most frequent sports injuries, by sport and sex, Canada, 1993. U.S. estimates would be greater for football, less for hockey and soccer. Other estimates are comparable between United States and Canada. The rising popularity of in-line skating produces increasing numbers of injuries not typically classified as sports injuries. *Source:* Canadian Hospitals Injury Reporting and Prevention Program. CHIRRP News, July 1994.

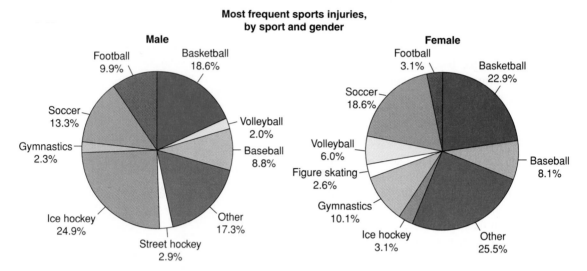

activities and the increasing numbers of individuals participating in winter recreation.

The yearly death toll in recreation has increased. When considered in terms of the increased number of participants in recreation, however, the *rate* of fatal accidents (per 1,000 participants) has declined. Furthermore, not all of these deaths are strictly chargeable to recreation. Flying and railway fatalities can occur in commercial travel and in recreational travel.

Most of the people who lose their lives in recreational injuries are in the prime of life. This is particularly true for injuries in boating and other water sports, with firearms, and in airplane or balloon crashes.

Prevention of Injuries in Recreation   On the community level, organized, supervised recreation is usually safe recreation. Trained personnel, definite responsibilities, enforced codes and regulations, regular supervision, safety surveys, and safety education have produced results. It is in unsupervised recreation that action is most needed, and here the primary approach is safety education. This is not a simple matter because education in one area, such as the safe use of firearms, does not carry over into other areas, such as safe conduct in swimming or boating.

Boating clubs, camping groups, and other sports clubs provide part of the safety education in recreation. The Red Cross, the YMCA, and similar organizations have contributed greatly to the promotion of safe recreation with such activities as swimming instruction and CPR training (figure 13-22). Despite these efforts, an organized community program of safety education in this sphere of activity is a difficult assignment. The efforts of agencies and individuals promoting safety education in other areas make an indirect contribution to recreational safety.

....

Figure 13-22

Training by organizations such as the Red Cross in mouth-to-mouth cardiopulmonary resuscitation (CPR) has been credited with some of the decrease in deaths due to drowning and sudden heart attacks.
Source: Photo courtesy World Health Organization.

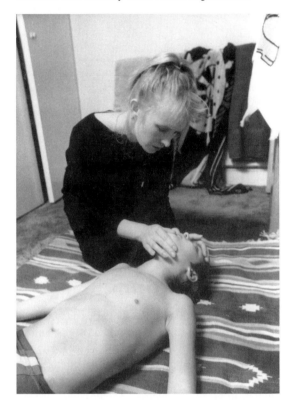

The reductions in drowning deaths during the 1980s could represent an increased number of near-drowning victims saved by CPR and other emergency response capabilities in the community. This has produced an unknown number of near-drowning victims with neurological damage and disabilities.

Regulations governing recreational activities have a considerable effect on the promotion of safety. This is particularly true of regulations designed to prevent the inexperienced from participating in activities for which they are not prepared or qualified. The inexperienced or unskillful participant is most likely to suffer injuries, and the reckless participant is most likely to cause injuries to others.

Each community can survey the recreational safety needs of its people and formulate a program accordingly. The cooperation of all groups sponsoring recreational activities or programs will add assurance for the success of the safety program. Recreational safety promotion should be coordinated with other safety programs in the community.

COMMUNITY SAFETY PROGRAM

The coordination of community safety poses a problem because safety in a community is the province of many organizations and individuals. These include the health department, fire department, police department, recreation department, schools, industry, chamber of commerce, service clubs, Red Cross, civil defense, medical profession, other health and recreation professionals, and news media. One ideal is to integrate the contributions of all agencies into one effective community safety program.

Organization

The community health department is the most logical agency to bring together the various forces influencing injury prevention in the community. While the official health department can be the catalyst, a basic ingredient is a coalition of community groups that have an interest in and a contribution to make to safety. This voluntary, nonofficial body is also a sounding board, a source of information, an expression of community thinking, and a supporter of the various safety programs operating within the community.

Community Safety Promotion

Each agency will continue its ongoing program, expanding as conditions and the council indicate. Unnecessary duplication can be eliminated, but some duplication is highly desirable. Unmet needs will be recognized, and an understanding will be

Elements of Successful Community Injury Control

PLANNING AND PRIORITIZING

A broad-based coalition representing the community of interest; surveillance tools and methods to identify and monitor the number of injuries: the use of E codes to aid in the ascertainment of injury causes; and selection of priority areas for injury control.

COMPREHENSIVE MULTIFACETED APPROACH

Evaluation of prevention strategies to determine effectiveness; dissemination and universal implementation of effective strategies; targeting of high-risk groups, such as low income; and incorporation of prevention messages and efforts into service systems for children and adolescents.

INSTITUTIONALIZATION AND ACCEPTANCE

Coordination of local, state, and federal efforts; institutionalization of injury prevention programming; enforcement of existing legislation protecting children; and development of a societal norm of a "safe childhood and adolescence."

Objectives to Reduce Unintentional Injuries by the Year 2000

Objectives target reducing unintentional injury deaths, nonfatal unintentional injuries, motor vehicle crash deaths, fall-related deaths, drowning deaths, and residential fire deaths; reducing hip fractures among people aged sixty-five years and older; reducing nonfatal poisonings, head injuries, spinal cord injuries, and secondary disabilities associated with head and spinal cord injuries; increasing use of occupant protection systems, and use of motorcycle and bicycle helmets; increasing laws requiring safety belt and motorcycle helmet use; enacting laws on handgun design; increasing installation of fire sprinklers and functional smoke detectors; providing injury prevention instruction in schools; extending the requirement of the use of protective headgear at sporting and recreation events; increasing roadway safety design standards and counseling on safety precautions by primary care providers; and extending emergency medical services and trauma systems.

reached on which agency will deal with a recognized need.

A poison control center is a valuable segment of the community safety program. It is the place where people can call for help in case of unintentional or intentional poisoning. Properly, such a center is open twenty-four hours a day, staffed by a person who knows how to use the standard references on poisons and who can recommend countermeasures. He or she needs to know the physiology and toxicology involved. In small communities a hospital is the logical location for such a center. In larger communities a poison control center may be located elsewhere and staffed with pharmacists.

Safety surveys may be sponsored by health or safety councils or initiated by member organizations. The two essential factors are to discover where injuries occur and where hazards exist in the community. Once hazards are located and the

causes of injuries identified, measures can be initiated within the community to reduce or even eliminate them.

Safety education by various community agencies must be coordinated and integrated to be extensive enough to be fully effective. Safety consciousness in a community can be developed, but it takes a clear focus on specific, attainable objectives.

SUMMARY

In most industrialized countries and increasingly in developing countries, unintentional injuries—once referred to as accidents—account for the first or second largest number of potential years of life lost among all causes of death. Deaths from intentional injuries account for the fourth largest number of potential years of life lost. These facts have turned public health attention to injuries as a health problem subject to epidemiological study and preventive

Objectives to Reduce Violent and Abusive Behavior by the Year 2000

Objectives target reducing homicides, suicides, and weapon-related deaths; reversing the rising incidence of child abuse; reducing physical abuse of women by male partners, assault injuries, rape and attempted rape, and adolescent suicide attempts; reducing physical fighting among youth, weapon-carrying by youth, and inappropriate storage of weapons; improve emergency room protocols to identify, treat, and refer suicide attempters and survivors of sexual assault and of child, partner, and elder abuse; improve child death review systems; improve evaluation and follow-up of abused children; improve emergency housing for battered women and their children; improve school programs for conflict resolution; and increase violence prevention programs and suicide prevention in jails.

still depends on an informed and committed public, which in turn depends on effective health education and the work of community action groups.

The advantages of environmental approaches to injury control lead to intervention strategies aimed at settings where hazards can be analyzed and injuries prevented. These include the home, highway, farm, occupational, recreational, and school environments. Interventions to reduce injuries and deaths from fires, scalds, vehicle crashes, falls, poisonings, drownings, and some types of family violence have gained in effectiveness. Most types of intentional injury, including homicide, suicide, child abuse, and rape, however, have not yielded to comparable interventions. These represent new frontiers for community health. The objectives for intentional injury reductions are summarized in the box regarding reducing violent and abusive behavior.

intervention. The term *accident* has fallen into disfavor because the scientific study of injuries has largely displaced the tendency to think of accidents as uncontrollable events attributable to fate.

Public health leadership has provided a map for community action with national objectives for injury control. The box regarding unintentional injuries summarizes those objectives for the year 2000.

Many injuries can be traced to human error. The frequency of such errors, however, can be reduced most efficiently by structuring the environment or products involved to minimize the need for human decisions or preventive actions. Safety education remains an essential component of community injury control. For those dangerous events that occur most unexpectedly or suddenly, however, the limited opportunity to exercise judgment or take split-second action renders education and training relatively ineffective.

Legal controls on products, structures, and practices that tend to cause injuries help limit the damage that might otherwise result. The passage, retention, and enforcement of such laws, however,

WEB*Links*

http://www.cdc.gov/ncipc/pub-res/prevguide.htm
National Center for Injury Prevention and Control

http://www.nnh.org/Weblinks/isintlk.htm
National Network for Health - intentional injury and safety links

http://www.inj_prev.ab.ca/other.html
Injury Prevention Centre in Canada - list of links to related web sites

QUESTIONS FOR REVIEW

1. To study the epidemiology of injuries in your community, what factors would receive your attention?
2. How would you account for a high injury rate in a community that had a much better safety program than that of another community with a lower injury rate?
3. The death rate from injuries in the United States has declined since the turn of the century, yet injuries rank as the fourth leading cause of death. How do you explain this apparent contradiction?

4. How is your state or provincial highway injury control program organized and administered?

5. In the United States, why are the state industrial safety programs more effective than the state traffic safety or firearm control programs?

6. On the state or provincial level, who has responsibility for the promotion of home safety?

7. What agencies in your locality promote farm injury control?

8. If a car traveling 55 mph crashes into a fixed concrete abutment, with how much force will a person of 160 pounds be thrown forward? Use the equation $MV = Ft$, in which M = mass, V = velocity, F = force, and t = time (1 second).

9. How would you draw an organizational chart for a model motor vehicle safety program for some community?

10. What agencies in your community are engaged in the promotion of poison control?

11. How would you evaluate the safety record and the injury control program of one of the industrial firms in your community or in another community?

12. How effectively have your community's schools taken advantage of their opportunity to promote safety?

13. What obstacles are there to the promotion of recreational safety?

14. If you were to set up a safety council for your community, who would be on the council and what would be the specific provinces of its program?

15. What is the greatest safety need in your community?

READINGS

American Academy of Pediatrics Committee on Injury and Poison Prevention. 1995. *Handbook of Common Poisonings in Children.* Elk Grove Village, IL: American Academy of Pediatrics.

Essential information for the assessment of poisoning exposures in children and the appropriate courses of action to prevent or treat them. Topics include poison prevention and specific poisons such as drugs, chemicals, biological toxins such as spider bites, and poisonous plants.

Female genital mutilation: A joint WHO/UNICEF/ UNFPA statement. 1997. Geneva: World Health Organization.

Societal norms and traditional practices in some areas of the world include female genital mutilation. The United Nations agencies issuing this 20-page statement declare the practice universally unacceptable because it is a form of violence against women. This booklet defines and classifies the practice and practitioners of it, its prevalence and distribution, and its complications.

Farley, C. 1997. Evaluation of a four-year bicycle helmet promotion campaign in Quebec aimed at children ages 8 to 12: Impact on attitudes, norms and behaviours. *Can J Public Health* 88:62.

This long-term study of a program to increase helmet use in young children was designed using the PRECEDE-PROCEED Model outlined in chapter 4. See also the citations: Clarke et al; Farley et al; Gielen, Jones, & Macrina; National Committee on Injury Control; Parks; Reichelt; Sleet; Stevenson et al; and Wortel et al.

Guterl, F. 1996. Gunslinging in America. *Discover: The World of Sci* 17:84.

A handgun is the most dangerous consumer product around, but do the risks of owning one outweigh the risks of not owning one? This article reviews studies that have sought to answer this question.

Levy, B. S., and V. W. Sidel, eds. *War and Public Health.* 1996. Oxford, New York and Tokyo: Oxford University Press.

Documents the impact of war on public health and describes what health professionals can do to prevent war and to minimize its consequences on health and injury. Examines the direct consequences of the use of conventional weapons and the indirect effects on women, children and refugees.

Wortel, E., H. de Vries, and G. H. deGeus. 1995. Lessons learned from a community campaign on child safety in the Netherlands. *Fam & Community Health* 18:60.

This application of the PRECEDE model and related principles of health promotion planning and implementation describes the program directed at parents of preschool-age children. Failures in the campaign are identified to explain the absence of impact on parents' knowledge, beliefs, or adoption of safety measures.

BIBLIOGRAPHY

Adams, O. 1993. Injury control and safety. *Canada's Health Promotion Survey 1990; Technical Report.* Ottawa: Health Canada.

Alagaratnam, M. 1994. Sport and recreational injuries among 5–19 year olds for 1993 from the CHIRPP database. *CHIRPP News* (July). Ottawa: Canadian

Hospitals Injury Reporting and Prevention Program, Laboratory Centre for Disease Control, Health Canada.

Bachman, R., and L. E. Saltzman. 1995. *Violence against women: Estimates from the redesigned survey.* Washington, DC: U.S. Department of Justice, Office of Justice Programs, Bureau of Justice Statistics, National Crime Victimization Survey.

Clarke, V. A., C. J. Frankish, L. W. Green. 1997. Understanding suicide among indigenous adolescents: a review using the PRECEDE model. *Injury Prev* 3:126.

Dowd, M. D., J. Langley, and F. P. Rivara. 1996. Hospitalizations for injury in New Zealand: Prior injury as a risk factor for assaultive injury. *Am J Public Health* 86:929.

Fanslow, J. L., D. J. Chalmers, and J. D. Langley. 1995. Homicide in New Zealand: an increasing public health problem. *Australian J Public Health* 19:50.

Farley, C., S. Haddad, and B. Brown. 1996. The effects of a 4-year program promoting bicycle helmet use among children in Quebec. *Amer J Public Health* 86:46.

Federal, Provincial and Territorial Advisory Committee on Population Health. 1996. *Report on the Health of Canadians.* Ottawa: Health Canada Communications and Consultation Directorate.

Gielen, A. C. 1992. Health education and injury control: integrating approaches. *Health Educ Q* 19:203.

Healthy People 2000: Midcourse Review and 1995 Revisions. 1996. Boston: Jones and Bartlett Publishers.

Jones, C. S., and D. Macrina. 1993. Using the PRECEDE model to design and implement a bicycle helmet campaign. *Wellness Perspec Res Theory Prac* 9:68.

Kelsh, M. A., and J. D. Sahl. 1996. Sex differences in work-related injury rates among electric utility workers. *Am J Epidem* 143:1050.

Motorcycle Helmet Laws: Questions and Answers. 1994. Washington, DC: Advocates for Highway and Auto Safety.

Langlois, J. A., J. S. Buechner, and G. S. Smith. 1995. Improving the E coding of hospitalizations for injury: Do hospital records contain adequate documentation. *Am J Public Health* 85:1261.

Lau, E. M. C., B. G. Gillespie, and D. O'Connell. 1995. Seasonality of hip fracture and weather conditions in NSW. *Australian J Public Health* 19:76.

Liller, K. D. 1997. Teaching Idea: Teaching Preschoolers Injury Prevention. *J Health Educ* 28:50.

Lytle, V. 1996. After the crash. *Discover* 17:98.

Malliaris, A. C., J. H. DeBlois, and K. H. Diges. 1996. Light vehicle occupant ejections—a comprehensive investigation. *Accid Anal & Prev* 28:1.

Massagli, T. L., L. J. Michaud, F. P. Rivara. 1996. Association between injury indices and outcome after severe traumatic brain injury in children. *Arch Phys Med Rehabil* 77:125.

Mayhew, D. R., S. W. Brown, and H. M. Simpson. 1997. *Alcohol use among persons fatally injured in motor vehicle accidents: Canada 1995.* Ottawa: Road Safety and Motor Vehicle Regulation, Transport Canada.

Motorcycle Helmet Laws: Questions and Answers. 1994. Washington, DC: Advocates for Highway and Auto Safety.

National Center for Health Statistics. 1996. *Healthy People 2000 Review, 1995-96.* Hyattsville, MD: Public Health Service.

National Committee for Injury Prevention and Control. 1989. *Injury prevention: meeting the challenge.* New York: Oxford University Press, as a supplement to the *Am J Prev Med* 5(3) (whole issue).

Ontario Public Health Association. 1992. *Report of the Injury Prevention Priorities Consultation.* Toronto: Ontario Ministry of Health.

Parks, C. P. 1995. Gang behavior in the schools: reality or myth? *Educ Psychol Rev* 7:41.

Reichelt, P. A. 1995. Musculoskeletal injury: ergonomics and physical fitness in firefighters. *Occup Med* 10:735.

Scheidt, P. C., Y. Harel, and P. E. Bijur. 1995. The epidemiology of nonfatal injuries among U.S. Children and Youth. *Am J Public Health* 85:932.

Schnitzer, P. G., and C. W. Runyan. 1995. Injuries to women in the United States: an overview. *Women & Health* 23:9.

Sleet, D. A. 1987. Health education approaches to motor vehicle injury prevention. *Pub Health Rep* 102: 606.

Stevenson, M., S. Jones, D. Cross, P. Howat, and M. Hall. 1996. The child pedestrian injury prevention project. *Health Prom J Australia* 6:32.

Tellez, M. G., R. C. Mackersie, D. Morabito. 1995. Risks, costs, and the expected complication of reinjury. *Am J Surg* 170:660.

Wortel, E., G. H. deGeus, G. Kok, and C. van Woerkum. 1994. Injury control in pre-school children: a review of parental safety measures and the behavioural determinants. *Health Educ Res* 9: 201.

Chapter *14*

Community Water and Waste Control

*I*n the world there is nothing more submissive and weak than water. Yet for attacking that which is hard and strong nothing can surpass it.
—Lao-Tzu (sixth century B.C.)

Objectives

When you finish this chapter, you should be able to:

- Identify the sources and contaminants of community water supplies

- Describe the major procedures for sewage and solid waste disposal, including toxic agent controls

- Plan for the improvement and enforcement of environmental protection measures directed at water and waste control

---

Community and population health strategies fall under three broad headings: health promotion, health protection, and health services. Health protection measures consist primarily of environmental controls, including those directed at safety, water, waste, food supplies, vectors, housing, work environments, air, noise, and radiation. Among these, water and waste management have had the most direct, pervasive, and continuous relationship to health. Most of the other factors have much to do with esthetics, comfort, and quality of life but usually threaten health less directly, less immediately, or less frequently. This could change in the future, with growing pollution of the atmosphere and of food supplies. These issues will be addressed in subsequent chapters in this section. This chapter will address water supply and liquid and solid waste control.

SOCIAL AND ECONOMIC IMPORTANCE OF WATER TO COMMUNITIES

The life and the economy of nearly every community depend on water supply and quality. With 80 percent of water consumption going for irrigation, an average of 7 percent is left for municipal use, and the remainder is divided almost equally among manufacturing, mining, livestock watering, and hydroelectric generation. Greater congestion of people in urban areas, concentration of industry, population mobility, and sheer increases in numbers have made control and distribution of the water supply more efficient but more vulnerable to crises and unintended pollution (figure 14-1).

Metropolitan centers, which have usually developed near waterways or lakes (**surface water**) for historical and economic reasons, actually have fewer problems in maintaining an adequate, safe

· · · · · · · · · · · · · · · · · · · ·
Figure 14-1

The hydrologic cycle refers to the recycling and purification of water through the air and soil. It also includes the contamination of streams and groundwater sources in the water table aquifers and the lower artesian aquifer. *Source:* U.S. Environmental Protection Agency.

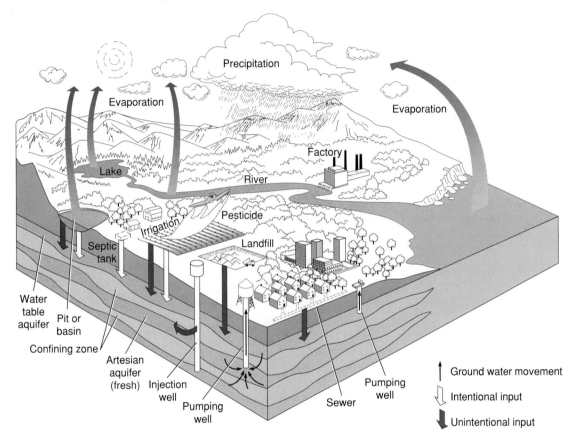

water supply than do rural areas with dispersed populations, individualized wells and septic tanks, irrigation runoff and insecticide use. On the other hand, the urban planting of trees, each of which consumes 300 gallons of water per day, and the paving of surfaces that once absorbed water have caused the reservoirs and water tables of some cities to subside. Cities also depend more on water for industries, extinguishing fires, street cleaning, carrying wastes to treatment facilities, and many other purposes. Therefore, there are many trade-offs between quality of life (as determined by such things as trees, paved streets, manufactured goods, irrigated and fertilized foods) and the resulting depletion and pollution of the water supply.

Public concerns with the factors influencing health clearly center on the two main determinants—lifestyle and the environment—as shown in figure 14-2. The public recognition of these two factors as important also implies a possible understanding of the interdependency of lifestyle and environment, the role of populations in pollution

· ·

Figure 14-2

Opinions of the Canadian public concerning the relative importance of various health risks indicated that North American populations inherently understand that our lifestyles and our environments are intertwined. *Source:* The Environmental Monitor, 1994, in Federal, Provincial and Territorial Advisory Committee on Population Health, *Report on the Health of Canadians, Technical Appendix,* Health Canada Communications and Consultation Directorate, September 1996.

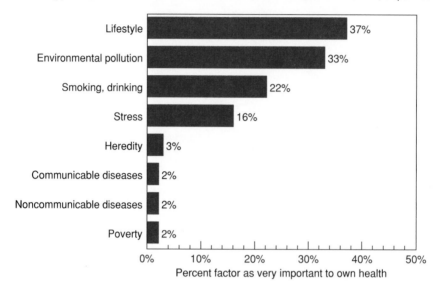

of the environment, and the role of the deteriorating environment in compromising lifestyle or quality of life. The fundamental ecological understanding is that our protection and management of the environment and the health problems or improvements that may result from environmental determinants depends on managing lifestyles of populations. We do not manage environments, we manage our interaction with them.

Fortunately, most of society's uses of water allow it to be used over and over—recycled through soil, retrieved as surface water from lakes, streams, rivers, and as **groundwater** from **aquifers,** then redistributed through evaporation and rain or snow (see figure 14-1). The growing populations and the runoff conditions of some regions, however, place an increasing burden on communities, states or provinces, and national governments to negotiate the control and distribution of water supplies.

EPIDEMIOLOGY OF WATERBORNE DISEASES

Health problems attributed to infectious and toxic agents in water include acute and chronic effects. Acute effects are from infection and poisoning, or **teratogenesis** (abnormality produced in the fetus during pregnancy). Chronic effects include developmental abnormalities; **mutagenesis** (damage to genes); **oncogenesis** (including cancer); neurological and behavioral impairment; immunological damage; and chronic degenerative diseases involving the lungs, joints, digestive and vascular systems, kidneys, liver, and endocrine organs. These effects may be caused variously by contamination of water supplies by organic and inorganic chemicals, radioactive material, and pathogenic microorganisms.

Distribution and Trends

Infectious and toxic agents affect people differently, depending on their sex, age, history of past

Water Rationing as a Way of Life

You rise for breakfast on a Saturday morning in the year 2010. Since the turn of the century (year 2000) you have been warned that your community's water supply was drying up. You draw exactly 8 ounces of water for your morning cup of coffee and boil the measured amount in a microwave oven. Your shower is from a metered, low-pressure valve. You save this water to fill the toilet, which has been disconnected, like most private toilets, from the water main. Your yard has been planted mostly with desert plants requiring no water, but the city ordinances allow you a 5-square-meter area in which to grow a garden or lawn. You attach your garden hose to a 200-liter barrel of partially treated wastewater, because this is much less expensive than water from the metered outdoor spigot and you need to conserve your household allotment for essential washing and domestic uses.

This scenario is a matter of history for some communities, a threat to others in the near future, and a high probability for many more if water resources are not better protected. How might you contribute to community action to prevent the need for future rationing of water to this degree?

Objectives for Regulation of Water Contaminants by the Year 2000

- Reduce human exposure to toxic agents by confining total pounds of toxic agents released into the air, water, and soil to no more than 0.24 billion pounds of those toxic agents included on the Department of Health and Human Services list of carcinogens. Baseline: 0.32 billion pounds in 1988.
- Reduce human exposure to solid waste-related water, air, and soil contamination, as measured by a reduction in average pounds of municipal solid waste produced per person each day to no more than 3.6 pounds. Baseline: 4 pounds per person each day in 1988.
- Increase to at least 85% the proportion of people who receive a supply of drinking water that meets the safe drinking water standards established by the EPA. Baseline: 74% of 58,099 community water systems serving approximately 80% of the U.S. population in 1988.

See figure 14-3 for mid-decade progress on these and other goals for water and waste control in the United States.

exposures, and possible predisposing genetic conditions. Similarly, the genetic and chronic disease effects of infectious and toxic agents may be manifested in varying ways in future years or future generations. For these reasons, the incidence and prevalence rates of diseases associated with waterborne agents do not accurately measure either the true potency of some of these agents or the effectiveness of control and protection measures.

Such uncertainties make the tasks of risk identification and risk reduction enormously difficult. With hundreds of new compounds appearing on the market each year and more than 13,000 substances identified as being toxic, complete control is impossible. Many of these toxic substances and microorganisms find their way into water systems. Most of the infectious agents of greatest concern were mentioned in chapter 11 (for example, see

table 11-2, p. 313 for the list of alvine discharge diseases). This chapter will address the control of infectious and toxic agents in the water supply.

Control Measures

Current evidence builds a convincing case for the carcinogenicity in humans of twenty chemicals and compounds; over 2,300 specific chemicals are suspected carcinogens. Also, more than twenty agents are known to be associated with birth defects in humans, and many times this number are associated with birth defects in animals.

Regulation and Surveillance   Serious contamination of drinking water supplies in North America average from 1 percent to 2 percent each year. This may expose as much as 10 percent of the population. The U.S. Environmental Protection Agency (**EPA**) and the Health Protection Branch

· · · · · · · · · · · · · · · · · · · ·
Figure 14-3

Progress at mid-decade on the ten-year objectives for water and waste control for the year 2000, United States, 1995. The objectives for safe water supplies and surface water pollution have seen the least progress with conditions worsening on some of the objectives. *Source:* U.S. Department of Health and Human Services, Public Health Service. 1996. *Healthy people 2000: midcourse review and 1995 revisions.* Boston: Jones and Bartlett Publishers.

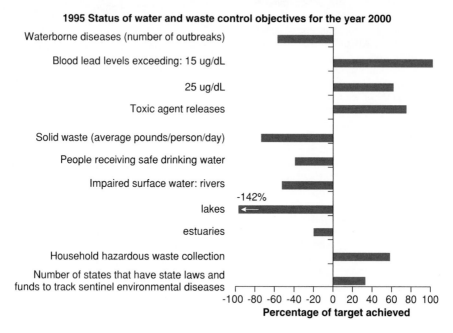

1995 Status of water and waste control objectives for the year 2000

of Health Canada operate programs to prevent new contamination. If EPA guidelines are followed, there should be almost no preventable contamination of water associated with wastewater management. A related goal is to develop a plan to protect communities from the consequences of toxic agents in existing sites of toxic solid waste disposal, as from the Love Canal in upstate New York. Approximately thirty thousand solid waste disposal sites may be involved.

As yet no country has a comprehensive surveillance system to monitor new or continuing environmental threats to health. The development of such a system to assess and reduce the risks from infectious and toxic agent exposures is a particularly important objective for communities and populations (figure 14-3).

Health Education   Access to information and education about hazardous exposures is an essential goal. Objectives include informing managers of industrial firms; increasing the ability of consumers and health professionals to detect, control, and deal with the effects of hazardous exposures; and increasing the capabilities of community health agencies and hospitals to respond appropriately.

Water Uses

Populations need water for recreation, irrigation, industry, esthetics, and domestic use. The population increases, industry expands, and other water uses multiply, yet the quantity of water remains fixed. Water must be reused because the supply is finite. Society's ingenuity is economically and technically challenged by the task of maintaining the quality of water.

A century ago communities used water that people assumed was safe for household purposes as long as it was clear. Not until residents recognized that water was a vehicle for disease transmission was preventive action taken. It took years of community education before citizens understood what had to be done to safeguard the water supply. In some communities officials took the lead in providing the people with a safe and adequate water supply, whereas in other communities the people had to push the officials to take necessary action.

Concern is as much with toxic agents in the water as with infectious agents. Contamination by chemicals and nuclear wastes threatens community water supplies in ways that worry citizens as much as organic pollution ever worried their parents and grandparents. It is not known what the additive effects of these chemicals will be on the total incidence of cancer. As water resources become in shorter supply, more and more surface water used for drinking water will be recycled or reprocessed, continuing the recycling of chemical pollutants.

Water is the most important commodity humans consume, and the consumption of water has increased steadily, so that in the United States the average daily use for domestic purposes is 150 gallons per person. Communities with industries requiring vast amounts of water may have a total use that reaches 2,000 gallons per person per day. Many areas will experience an increasing shortage unless low-cost desalinization of sea water is employed or the harnessing of runoff from glaciers is successful. The cost of water may double or triple in the future, especially if desalinization remains an expensive procedure. The Arab Gulf States and the Canary Islands of Spain have made extensive use of desalination, drawing up to 99 percent of their water from the sea, but poorer countries have not been able to avail themselves of this technology.

Of the 500 million people living in sub-Saharan Africa in 1990, the World Health Organization estimates that 265 million—more than half—lacked safe drinking water. Progress achieved in water supplies since then has been largely offset by population growth. In some of the worst drought-affected regions, renewable fresh water per person has dropped by more than 65 percent since the 1950s.

Etiology and Effects of Toxic Agents

Substances found naturally in water or occurring as industrial pollutants can be harmful when they reach concentrations above levels established by regulatory bodies. Regulatory guidelines include the Safe Drinking Water Act in the United States, the Federal-Provincial Advisory Committee on Environmental and Occupational Health of Canada, and the guidelines of the World Health Organization.

The primary drinking water contaminants and the sources and possible health effects of each contaminant are shown in table 14-1. All chemicals are poisonous in some quantity, so it is the dose or concentration of the chemical in the water that makes it a threat to human populations. Maximum levels permitted are usually stated in milligrams per liter of water (or picocuries in the case of radionuclides). The significance of selected chemical elements and compounds in water are discussed in the following sections.

Pesticides Various insecticides, fungicides, rodenticides, and herbicides, present in water primarily as a result of vector control efforts, crop spraying, and agricultural runoff and spills, pose increasing problems because they are environmentally persistent and cumulative in the water and food chains (figure 14-4). These chlorinated hydrocarbons are neuropoisons that can cause symptoms ranging from dizziness to convulsions and even to death by either cardiac or respiratory arrest. Some pesticides may be teratogenic or mutagenic (causing species abnormalities or species alterations). Endrin and Lindane, pesticides commonly used on field crops, are the most toxic and must be limited in their concentration in the

TABLE 14-1

Major Pollutants of Water, Their Sources and the Threats to Human Health They Pose.

Substance	Main source	Health risk
Chlorinated solvents	Industrial pollution. Used for chemical degreasing, machine maintenance, and as intermediaries in the manufacture of other chemicals	Cancer
Trihalomethanes	Produced by chemical reactions in water that has been disinfected with chlorine	Liver and kidney damage, possibly cancer
Lead	Old piping and solder in public water distribution systems, homes, and other buildings	Nerve problems, learning disabilities in children, birth defects, possibly cancer
PCBs	Wastes from many outmoded manufacturing operations	Liver damage, possibly cancer
Pathogenic bacteria and viruses	Leaking septic tanks, overflowing sewer lines (see table 14-2)	Acute gastrointestinal illness, more serious diseases such as meningitis

Source: U.S. Environmental Protection Agency.

•••••••••••••••••••••

F i g u r e   1 4 - 4

Spraying of larvicides, insecticides, and herbicides on or near waterways produces an ecological chain of events that can harm human populations directly through the water supply or indirectly through the food chain. *Source:* Photo by R. Witlin, courtesy World Health Organization.

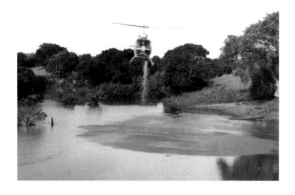

water supply. Herbicides used in weed control may cause muscular tenseness, paralysis, and coma and may trigger mutations and teratogenic effects.

Radionuclides   Uranium, radon, and radium occur naturally in groundwater and to a lesser degree in surface water, as a result of leaching from rock deposits. These radiochemicals are proven carcinogens. The standard limits in drinking water are somewhat arbitrary.

Selenium   A chemical element obtained as a by-product of copper mining, selenium (Se) is normally found in groundwater and occasionally in surface water as a natural occurrence. Selenium attacks the central nervous system and can be fatal in extreme cases. Minor amounts, however, may be beneficial to health. There is some evidence of lower cancer rates in areas where the level of selenium in the water supply exceeds the 0.01 mg/L standard.

Other Standards   Most other chemical agents in water are not toxic but need to be restricted in drinking water resources for other reasons. **Turbidity** refers to cloudiness of water caused by a variety of suspended materials, sometimes organic, but usually inorganic. Turbidity makes disinfection and proper bacteriological analysis more difficult, so a standard limit has been established as 1 turbidity unit (tu). Turbidity can also harbor viruses and cause tastes and odors.

Corrosivity is the tendency of water to corrode metals. It is related to pH, alkalinity, hardness, and dissolved oxygen. Chloride (Cl) in drinking water produces a salty taste when combined with sodium (Na) and may cause corrosiveness, so a limit has been set. Salinity might indicate contamination with seawater in groundwater near seacoasts. The presence of color makes water objectionable primarily for visual reasons but may also indicate organic contamination from decaying vegetation.

Waterborne Infectious Diseases

Pathogens of humans do not normally multiply in water, yet they can survive in water and remain virulent enough to set up an infection in a new host. Water serves as a vehicle of transfer of diseases of the alimentary canal and of transfer of certain worms, notably the schistosomes. Evidence is conclusive that five infectious diseases—typhoid, paratyphoid, giardiasis, cholera, and bacillary dysentery—are transmitted by water. The contention that HIV/AIDS, viral hepatitis, amebic dysentery, and poliomyelitis are transmitted by water is not substantiated. Likewise, no evidence exists that respiratory diseases of humans are conveyed via water.

Since 1975, *Giardia lamblia* has been the most commonly identified pathogen in waterborne disease outbreaks in the United States and Canada (table 14-2). Giardiasis, an intestinal infestation by a single-celled protozoan, is transmitted more frequently in daycare centers where frequent diaper changes carry the organism, than in drinking water. Most water outbreaks occur where sewers and people pollute surface water and backpackers, hikers, and others drink untreated water from lakes and streams. Upstream human and animal feces deposited in or near waterways can infect public water supplies.

Less than 2 percent of reported cases of typhoid fever, salmonellosis, shigellosis, or infectious hepatitis since 1951 have been traced to water. In contrast, more than one-fourth of reported cases of

TABLE 14-2

Pathogenic Microorganisms in North American Waters, and Their Sources of the Water Contamination.

Disease organism	Source
Giardia (parasite)	Most animals, especially aquatic mammals such as beavers and muskrats
Cryptosporidium (parasite)	Most animals
Campylobacter (bacteria)	Mammals, including livestock, domestic pets, humans
Salmonella (bacteria)	Most animals, birds, waterfowl
Hepatitis (virus), Shigella (bacteria), fecal streptococcus (bacteria)	Humans

Source: British Columbia Ministry of Health and Ministry Responsible for Seniors, 1995. *Safe water supply: vital to your health.* Victoria, BC: BC Ministry of Health, Health Protection and Safety Branch.

giardiasis were attributable to water. One reason *Giardia* slip by community water systems is that in small communities, especially recreational communities, the treatment of water is limited to disinfection with chlorine. Standard chlorine treatment may kill coliform bacteria, but *Giardia* cysts survive, especially when the water is unfiltered so that other turbid matter absorbs much of the chlorine. Filtration is the key to stopping *Giardia* cysts from surviving chemical treatment of water.

SOURCES OF WATER

For community and population health purposes, water must be in sufficient supply and free from contamination and pollution. For economic and esthetic purposes, it must be relatively free of

TABLE 14-3

The Two Main Water Sources for Human Populations, their Advantages and Disadvantages.

Water source	Advantages	Disadvantages
Surface water (lakes, ponds, rivers and streams)	Often abundant Easily found	Easily contaminated by sewage/animal feces, car accidents Needs disinfection Not always accessible Commonly cloudy (turbid) Usually only recommended when groundwater is unavailable
Groundwater (aquifers, springs and underground streams)	Often abundant Naturally protected from contamination Usually accessible Water quality is usually stable	Sometimes hard to find May be costly to draw Shallow groundwater may need disinfecting May be contaminated with natural or humanmade chemicals If contamination does occur it may persist for a long time Requires power supply

Larger, deeper lakes have more stable water quality than smaller lakes and streams.
Groundwater is usually safer than surface water.
Deep groundwater is usually safer than shallow groundwater and is less susceptible to contamination.

Source: British Columbia Ministry of Health and Ministry Responsible for Seniors. 1995. *Safe water supply: vital to your health.* Victoria, BC: BC Ministry of Health, Health Protection and Safety.

corrosivity and turbidity. Water that may be suitable for household purposes may not be satisfactory for individual use if it is high in mineral content.

Rainfall is the primary source of water, whether it is surface water in a river, lake, pond, or reservoir created by a dam, or whether it is groundwater that has percolated through the ground to a stratum of gravel (see figure 14-1 and table 14-3). In nature there is no pure water. All untreated water contains dissolved gases, minerals, and organic matter from the decay of algae, funguses, and other life forms. The challenge for community and population health, usually managed by public health agencies, is to ensure the minimal concentration of contaminants and to monitor outbreaks with specific intervention on the source of any outbreak.

Hardness of water is caused by the presence of calcium and magnesium salts. Water with a hardness of 100 parts per million (ppm) or less of cal-cium carbonate is soft enough for household use. Drinking water containing too much sulfate (2,000 ppm), chloride (1,000 ppm), or calcium carbonate (300 ppm) will cause digestive disturbances in most people. Too much fluoride may cause mottling of teeth, but the benefits of chlorination and fluoridation have been well established as public health measures (figure 14-5).

Groundwater Supplies

Groundwater from shallow wells and deep wells is usually the preferred source for communities with populations of under 50,000. Rarely will a larger city locate sufficient groundwater for its needs, although San Antonio, Texas, the tenth largest city in the United States with more than 1 million people, depends on a groundwater supply. Groundwater has certain merits. It is relatively free from contamination, pollution, turbidity, and color. Its disadvantages are its scarcity, its high mineral

Figure 14-5

Adding fluoride to community water supplies has long served population health with dramatic reductions in dental caries. *Source:* National Institute of Dental Research, National Institutes of Health, U.S. Department of Health and Human Services.

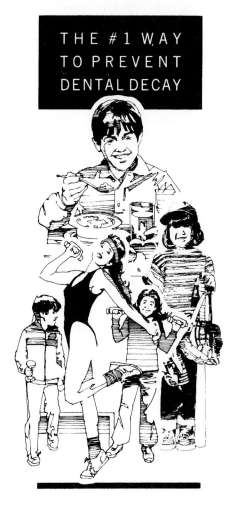

content, and the threat of sinking property when groundwater levels are lowered by overuse. It also requires a power supply to pump water from deep levels (table 14-3).

Underground Source   As a community supply, groundwater is usually safe, and the low capital funds and operating costs involved make groundwater an economical source. The first requirement is to find an adequate supply. This means locating a gravel bed that serves as a natural reservoir. Test wells are drilled to outline the reservoir. The object is to locate a yard-thick gravel bed below an impervious layer 60 feet or more beneath the surface.

Wells   Wells are cased with pipe that has a brass intake screen where the pipe is embedded in the gravel. Spacing of wells depends on the underground flow and community needs. Electrically operated centrifugal pumps raise the water into a concrete receiving reservoir. A second pump forces the water up into a large storage or pressure tank.

Bacteria attach to sand grains and secrete a sticky covering that causes other bacteria to adhere to this biological film. As water percolates into the ground, the sticky film filters out bacteria. This natural process purifies groundwater. Groundwater may be contaminated by seepage along the well casing, limestone, other previous material above the groundwater supply that does not intercept bacteria, sea water near the seacoast, and direct surface contamination into the groundwater stratum (see figure 14-1).

Well water is normally free from turbidity and can be chlorinated without filtration. Frequently, it is unnecessary to chlorinate groundwater, although it may be done as an extra precaution. Some communities do not chlorinate their groundwater but have a chlorination unit on hand in case the water should become contaminated.

Surface Water Supplies

New York City requires more than 1 billion gallons (4.224 billion liters) of water a day. Multiply this by 365 for an idea of the annual tasks that city has in supplying its population with water. New York gets only 10 percent of its water from wells; the remainder comes from surface water and necessitates a number of protected storage reservoirs and flumes. Cities such as Chicago and Milwaukee are fortunate in having Lake Michigan as an excellent water source. The Mississippi River serves as a water source and a sewage disposal receptacle for a long string of cities, including Minneapolis, St. Louis, Memphis, and New Orleans. Surface water has certain merits. It is more abundant, more easily measured, and softer than groundwater. It is frequently polluted, however, by shore wash, transportation waste, industrial waste, and human waste. It is usually contaminated, highly colored, and often turbid.

Treatment   With the increasing population and the high mobility of people today, nearly all surface water must be treated before it is safe for human consumption. Some lakes and streams have clear water, so no filtration is necessary; however, chlorination may be required. Most surface water is so turbid, polluted, and contaminated that filtration and chlorination are necessary.

Rapid sand filtration is designed to filter out particles and bacteria. If the water contains considerable **sediment,** a preliminary settling chamber may be used to precede the treatment process. Otherwise, the water is pumped directly from the intake in the river or lake into the series of tanks comprising the treatment plant. These tanks are usually of concrete construction; frequently, surplus tanks will be constructed so that some tanks may be shut off and cleaned or repaired while the rest of the tanks carry on the treatment process. The treatment usually consists of five steps: **flash mix, flocculation, sedimentation, filtration,** and **chlorination,** as shown in figure 14-6.

Flash mix is done in a relatively small tank. Aluminum sulfate is fed into the incoming water. It combines with solids to form a flaky hydrate, or floc. At the same time, chlorine is added.

Flocculation consists of trapping particles by the mechanical process of adsorption of suspended solids. Flocculation causes an increase in the density and size of coagulated particles, therefore floc particles settle at a fast rate. Flocculation tanks are fitted with slowly rotating wooden paddles to ensure an even and continuous water-chemical mixture.

Sedimentation is the settling of the floc and is carried out in sedimentation tanks connected directly to the flocculation tanks (figure 14-7). Water is retained here for about two hours to allow the floc to settle to the bottom of the tanks where it will be scraped into troughs. Other troughs around the top of the tanks collect the upper layer of water, which is relatively free of floc.

If the water has an odor, activated carbon may be added to the water in the sedimentation tank or may be added at another stage of treatment. The activated carbon is effective in removing odor and objectionable taste.

Filtration removes whatever turbidity may remain after the flocculation and settling. At the bottom of a filtration tank is a layer of gravel, topped by either sand or anthracite coal. Water percolates through this medium and goes out via drains at the bottom of the tank. To clean floc that accumulates on the anthracite coal or sand, the water level is lowered to the top of the troughs just above the coal level. The water flow is then reversed so that the accumulated floc is flushed into the troughs and carried off as waste.

Chlorination, the final step, decontaminates the water and is a simple, effective method for destroying bacteria. Postchlorination is designed to bring the residual chlorine to a level between 0.25 and 0.7 ppm. The chlorine residual level is determined for water in the distribution system and at the plant of origin. Two samples a day at the plant and one from the system are recommended. At standard concentrations, neither taste nor smell can detect the chlorine. In emergencies a chlorine residual of 0.7 ppm may be maintained. Although chlorine can be detected at this concentration, it is not harmful to humans.

· · · · · · · · · · · · · · · · · · · ·

Figure 14-6

Flow diagram of water treatment, beginning with the introduction of the floc material, then through flocculation, sedimentation, and filtering. The clear water is then ready for final chlorination to assure potability.

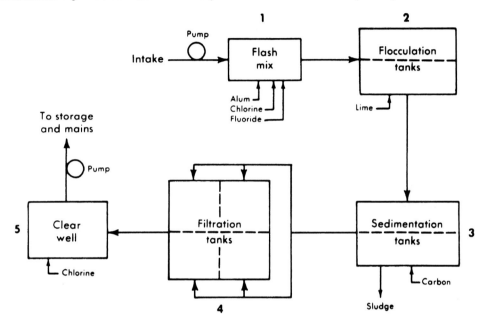

· · · · · · · · · · · · · · · · · · · ·

Figure 14-7

Flocculation tanks in a series. The separation of tanks allows for cleaning and repairing some tanks while others remain in use. *Source:* Texas Department of Health.

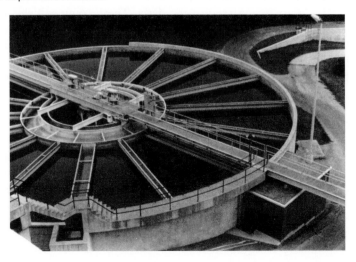

The *slow sand* (European) method of filtration uses a film produced by bacteria as the interceptive medium. The rapid sand method is forty times faster and generally more reliable; therefore, it is preferred in most communities establishing new water systems.

Addition of Fluorides

Based on available knowledge, the most effective, inexpensive, and simple method of preventing dental caries is the fluoridation of the public water supply. By studying local areas where people had a low incidence of dental caries, scientists discovered that these areas had water that naturally contained about 1 ppm of fluorides. Where the fluoride content of water was much lower than this, the incidence of caries was high (see figure 14-5).

Distribution   On the recommendation of dentists and public health scientists, U.S. municipalities began adding fluorides to water supplies as a preventive measure against dental caries. Most water supplies contain a small amount of fluorides; this is to add enough fluorides to bring the concentration up to 1 ppm. Northern cities in the United States raise the fluoride content slightly above this level, and southern cities hold the fluoride content slightly below 1 ppm. This is an adjustment to the difference in water consumption and average water temperatures.

One national health objective for the year 2000 is to increase to at least 75 percent the proportion of persons served by community water systems providing optimal levels of fluoride—a goal already achieved by twenty states and the District of Columbia. To achieve this objective nationally, an additional 30 million persons must receive optimally fluoridated water from public water systems. People in more than 5,860 communities have public water supplies containing an adequate concentration of fluorides.

It has been the history of public health that the small communities are the last to adopt new health measures, and this has held true for fluoridation.

Only about 40 percent of U.S. cities with populations between 2,500 and 10,000 have adopted fluoridation, and less than 20 percent of communities under 2,500 fluoridate their water supplies. Canada, Sweden, the Netherlands, West Germany, Japan, and many other nations are making fluoridation available to their populations.

Controversy   Health innovations for whole populations have usually been opposed. Vaccination, pasteurization of milk, chlorination of water supplies, and even indoor plumbing were initially opposed by the misinformed, the uninformed, and those who resisted change. Fluoridation has been debated in many communities and where it has been placed on ballots for public voting it often has been defeated. It gradually gained acceptance, but the proportion of the U.S. population covered by community fluoridated water supplies has not increased in the past ten years. Courts in the United States have ruled that fluoridation is a reasonable legal exercise of the local police power in the interest of the public health and is not a violation of individual rights.

Some communities have water supplies with a high natural fluoride content of 8 ppm. This concentration prevents caries but causes mottling (discoloration) of the teeth. The only other suspected harm to the human body from such a high fluoride content is possible orthopedic problems for the elderly. These communities add phosphate to the water to reduce fluorides to a level of 1 ppm. In communities having a water supply with a natural fluoride content of 2 ppm, people have health histories showing no deviation from that of the population at large.

Alternatives   In communities that do not fluoridate their municipal water supply, some citizens have their family dentist or physician brush their children's teeth with a covering of fluoride at each visit. As a similar preventive measure, some elementary schools have their children "rinse" or retain fluoridated water in their mouths for about 40 to 60 seconds.

TESTING OF WATER

As a community health measure, bacteriological and chemical examination of a municipal water supply can be of great importance to industry and to the general public. Radiological examination of water is of more recent vintage and not usually a concern, but in specific instances the possibility of radioactive contaminants in water can be significant. **Bioassays** are necessary to evaluate toxicity in fish (figure 14-8), and biological examinations are used to determine the extent of plankton and other life forms in the water.

The Coliform Test

For seventy years the standard test of drinking water safety was the **Coliform** determination. Coliform organisms are not pathogenic, but because they are always present in the human intestinal tract their presence in water is a sure indicator of fecal contamination. Unfortunately, the test for Coliform bacteria *(E. coli)* is tedious and time-consuming, providing results too late to prevent the ingestion of water from the supply being checked. For quality control purposes, the quicker chlorine test is used.

The Chlorine Test

The chlorine residual determination is a simple test to ensure that a sufficient level of chlorine is being maintained, given the temperature and pH of the water, to destroy organisms of the Coliform group and organisms pathogenic to human populations. Turbidity may interfere with the effectiveness of chlorine, therefore the turbidity limit was lowered in the EPA standards. Water purveyors are still required to take bacteriologic samples at regular intervals. The number of samples required ranges from one sample per month for communities with fewer than 2,500 residents to 3,000 samples per month for communities with populations greater than 1 million.

Other Tests

Virological techniques have barely advanced to the point that efficient tests can be used for routine

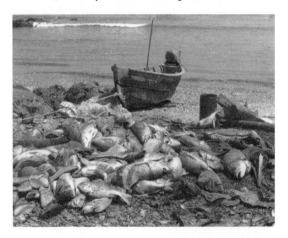

Figure 14-8
Pollution of coastal waters is a serious source of fish poisoning and often represents an important loss of income for fishers of the region. *Source:* Photo by T. Farkas, courtesy World Health Organization.

monitoring of water quality. Viral agents of human infection correlate with Coliform organisms, suggesting that it should be possible to estimate the presence of enteric viruses by using the Coliform test. Unfortunately, viruses are more resistant than are Coliform organisms to water treatments, including chlorination; therefore the ratio of viruses to Coliform organisms might be much higher during an outbreak of a viral disease, such as hepatitis type A.

Chemical examination of water varies, depending on the specific chemical one wishes to detect. Tests for hardness are most frequent. A test for chlorine residual is used to determine the decontamination effect of chlorination.

REGULATION OF WATER SUPPLIES

Providing water to a community is a recognized function of local government in most countries (figure 14-9). The city government usually constructs and manages the water system as a corporate function. This is not a responsibility of the

··················

Figure 14-9

Roman aqueducts were an early example of government assuming responsibility for delivery of water to populations. These Roman aqueducts still transport water in Mediterranean countries. *Source:* Photo by D. Keckemet, courtesy World Health Organization.

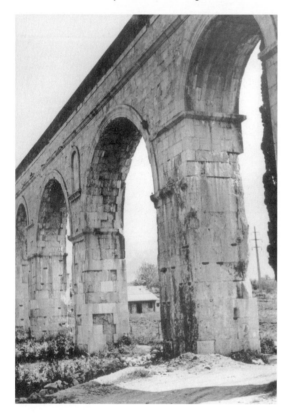

health department. In most communities a special water department or the department of public works operates the water system. A few communities grant a franchise to a private corporation to sell water as a commodity to the public.

Although providing water to the community is a local government function, the regulation of public water supplies is the legal responsibility of the state, which usually delegates this authority to the state or provincial department of health. A public water system is one that provides piped water for human consumption and has at least

fifteen service connections or regularly serves at least twenty-five people. If a city wishes to build a water plant, engineers from the state department of health must approve the plans. In practice, these engineers serve as advisors for the city in developing the plans. This advisory service is without cost to the city. Even though the city pays to have plans drawn and the water system constructed, it is the state that ensures the adequacy of the plans and the construction.

Once the plant is in operation, the state continues its supervisory authority. Plant operators must be certified by the state. Regular reports on water analysis must be submitted to the state as the state department of health decrees. The state representative serves as a consultant should the community encounter a problem in the operation of its water system. This service is free of charge to the community.

Safe Drinking Water Legislation

A 1970 national community water supply study in the United States revealed that the quality of household water was declining. Part of this decline was attributed to the careless use of various chemical substances and other toxic wastes. As an outgrowth of this study by the EPA and growing public concern, Congress enacted the Water Pollution Act of 1971 and the Safe Drinking Water Act of 1974. This provided for the periodic updating of water standards. Congress also authorized the EPA to support state and local community drinking water programs by providing financial and technical assistance. The federal government, through the EPA in the United States and through Environment Canada under the Canadian Environmental Protection Act (CEPA) in Canada, has the authority and responsibility for setting and enforcing standards and otherwise supervising public water systems. The following paragraphs illustrate for the United States how EPA's authority applies to drinking water safety.

Standards   The EPA establishes standards for drinking water quality in the United States. For

Canada, the *Guidelines for Canadian Drinking Water Quality* set maximum levels of chemicals and microorganisms appearing in drinking water. The EPA and Canadian standards represent the Maximum Contaminant Levels (MCLs) allowable and consist of numerical criteria for specified contaminants.

Treatment and Monitoring   Local water supply systems are required to monitor their drinking water periodically for contaminants with MCLs and for a broad range of other contaminants as specified by EPA. Additionally, to protect underground sources of drinking water, the EPA requires periodic monitoring of wells used for underground injection of hazardous waste, including monitoring of the ground water above the wells.

Enforcement   States have the primary responsibility for the enforcement of drinking water standards, monitoring, and reporting requirements. States also determine requirements for environmentally sound underground injection of wastes.

Grants   The Safe Drinking Water Act authorizes the EPA to award grants to states for developing and implementing programs to protect drinking water at the tap and groundwater resources. These several grant programs may be for supporting state public water supply; wellhead protection; and underground injection programs, including compliance and enforcement.

Therefore a vigorous, organized program was authorized by Congress to ensure the nation's people safe drinking water. A state can continue to enforce its own laws and regulations governing drinking water supplies if it complies with certain requirements such as the following:

1. Adoption of regulations at least equal to federal regulations
2. Adoption and implementation of adequate enforcement procedures
3. Provision for emergency circumstances
4. Keeping adequate records and providing reports for the EPA

Controversies   The Clean Water Act, as the Water Pollution Act of 1971 came to be known, must be reauthorized every five years. The debates on attempts to reauthorize the act set the stage for struggles over enforcement and administration of this legislation in the years ahead. According to national surveys, public support for clean water has increased. The Chemical Manufacturers Association emphasizes deregulation, however, countering this public support. They have suggested amendments to the act that would (1) delay or abandon the act's cleanup goals for toxic waste sites; (2) roll back deadlines for industries to clean up their own toxic wastes; (3) weaken or eliminate the national standards for limiting toxic agents in drinking water (described earlier in this chapter); (4) curtail the EPA's budget, strength, and authority; and (5) revert to regulatory policies that Congress rejected as unworkable in 1972.

One of the central strategies in the nationwide cleanup of water would control "nonpoint" sources of water pollution; these involve toxic agents that do not come out of a specific drainpipe but run off from fields. Although these nonpoint sources of water pollution have been given less attention than the industrial-point sources, they account for over half of all water pollution (table 14-4). Other new provisions in updates of the safe drinking water law would require public water utilities to report to their customers regularly—and in plain English—what is in their drinking water and what health problems could result from exposure to contaminants. This "right-to-know" provision is accompanied by authorization of EPA to make grants to rural, disadvantaged communities to address their wastewater treatment needs.

DRINKING WATER IN DEVELOPING COUNTRIES

The World Health Organization (WHO) declared 1981 to 1990 the International Drinking Water Supply and Sanitation Decade. This represented an essential first stage in the global strategy of "Health for All by the Year 2000." Only 43 percent

ISSUES AND CONTROVERSIES
Why Are Waterborne Infectious Diseases a Growing Problem?

- Rapid population growth in many cities is straining municipal water treatment facilities.
- Funding for water treatment and testing has decreased.
- Many city sewer systems do not adequately remove protozoa from sewage before it is discharged into rivers or lakes. Some cities still discharge raw sewage into ocean waters.
- Many city water treatment plants and the pipes that distribute water to houses are old, outdated, or in need of repair.

- Implementation of new water treatment technology has not kept pace with contaminants. Water treatment plants have long used chlorine to kill bacteria and viruses. Chlorine is not effective against Cryptosporidium and is only slightly effective against Giardia, two protozoan cysts in North American water supplies.
- With the growing popularity of outdoor recreation, more people are at risk for illness caused by hepatitis A, Shigella, and Cryp-

tosporidium, which are common in lakes and rivers used for water sports and recreation.
- More North Americans—the very young, the very old, those with weakened immune systems—are more likely to develop severe illness when they become infected with many of the waterborne disease agents.
- How safe is the water supply in your community?

Source: World Health Day, 1997. Washington DC, 1997, American Association for World Health.

TABLE 14-4
Water Pollutants and Their Sources

	BOD	Bacteria	Nutrients	Ammonia	Turbidity	TDS	Acids	Toxics
Common pollutant categories								
Point sources								
Municipal sewage treatment plants	•	•	•	•				•
Industrial facilities	•							•
Combined sewer overflows	•	•	•	•	•	•		•
Nonpoint sources								
Agricultural runoff	•	•	•		•	•		•
Urban runoff	•	•	•		•	•		•
Construction runoff			•		•			•
Mining runoff					•		•	•
Septic systems	•	•	•					•
Landfills/Spills	•							•
Silviculture runoff	•		•		•			•

Source: U.S. Environmental Protection Agency.
Abbreviations: BOD, Biochemical Oxygen Demand; TDS, Total Dissolved Solids.

Figure 14-10

Bringing water from streams and wells has been the burden of women in many developing countries, as in this typical community pump in the Ivory Coast. *Source:* Photo by R. Massey, courtesy World Health Organization.

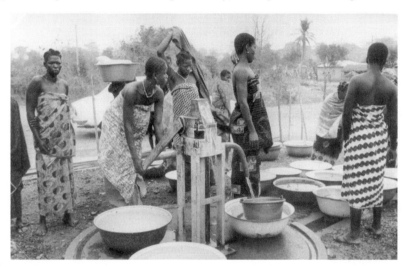

of the people in developing countries had access to safe drinking water. In rural areas of these countries only 29 percent had such access. By increasing the quantity and quality of water supplied to these 3 million people, WHO's "Decade" program helped reduce the incidence of many diseases among the people most at risk. The estimates are that one-half billion rural residents and several hundred million city dwellers in the developing world lack safe drinking water (figure 14-10).

New technologies are sought to provide higher standards of service at lower unit cost to large numbers of relatively dispersed and isolated villages and towns. Local community and external resources must be increased to provide for the construction and maintenance of public and private water supplies. A Japanese citizens' movement has provided a model of such a technology, in which fresh water and sanitation systems are being provided inexpensively to poorer neighborhoods through a combination of simple technology, decentralized systems, and community orga-

nization. The Jishu-Koza Citizen's Movement has helped communities build backyard ponds to recycle sewage and has installed waste disposal systems that require little water, unlike the large, centralized public systems of urban communities in developing and industrialized countries.

COMMUNITY WASTES

Household, commercial, recreational, and industrial wastes are the general sources of community wastes. These are in the form of garbage; refuse; street cleanings; human and animal discharges; kitchen, scavenger, and commercial wastes; and wastes from manufacturing and processing plants. The sheer volume in a year would run into millions of tons and would make a mountainous stockpile. If each year's wastes accumulated, in a period of twenty years a community would be buried by its own waste products. Fortunately, the lowly bacteria, by decomposing animal proteins, not only reduce the great mass of wastes to

· ·

Figure 14-11

The nitrogen cycle explains the decomposition of organic material in the soil, which goes on continuously thanks to four varieties of bacteria that save communities from burying themselves in their own waste.

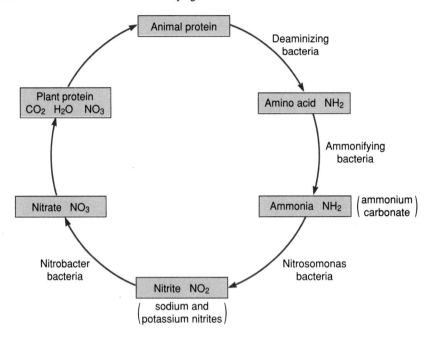

a negligible volume but also make invaluable nitrogen available for reuse. This process is customarily referred to as the **nitrogen cycle,** as shown in figure 14-11.

Nitrogen Cycle

Animal proteins begin decomposing by the action of bacteria that convert the proteins to amino acids. Another set of bacteria next converts the amino acids to ammonia. The ammonia combines with carbon dioxide to form ammonium carbonate, which in turn is converted to nitrites by a third type of bacteria. Nitrites combine with sodium and potassium, and the resulting nitrites are converted into nitrates by yet another group of bacteria—*Nitrobacter* organisms. Nitrates dissolved in soil water diffuse into the root hairs of plants, where they combine with carbon dioxide and water to form plant proteins. The plant proteins are consumed by animals and converted into animal proteins, thus completing the nitrogen cycle.

Communities aid nature in this process of waste disposal by providing the beneficial bacteria with a favorable environment and by the dilution, chemical treatment, burning, and recycling of wastes. The task of disposing of wastes is a continual one that is important and costly. Processes involved in getting rid of human wastes are also processes for destroying or removing pathogens that can cause disease and death. Perhaps the most important of these processes is sewage disposal.

SEWAGE DISPOSAL

Sewage consists of the liquid wastes from household effluents, commercial effluents, and industrial liquid wastes. It is carried in a system of pipes and other means of conveyance called a

· · · · · · · · · · · · · · · · · · · ·
Figure 14-12

In the absence of sewerage systems and even pipes to discharge household and other effluents, they typically mix with rainwater in open drainage systems in the streets, as in this refugee camp in Central America. *Source:* Photo by C. Gaggero, courtesy World Health Organization, Pan American Health Organization.

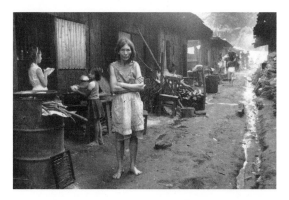

sewage system. In some communities storm water also is carried in the *sewerage system;* in other communities a separate system of pipes carries off storm water, saving the wastewater treatment plant from having to treat large volumes of rain water (figure 14-12).

Community sewage consists of about 99 percent water, which contains animal, plant, and mineral matter in solution and in suspension. Bacteria of many types, mostly nonpathogenic, are always present. Paper, sticks, grease, and other materials are in suspension.

Biochemical oxygen demand (**BOD**) measures sewage strength. BOD is the quantity of oxygen required in a given time to satisfy the chemical and biological oxidation demands of the sewage. A high BOD means that an excessive quantity of oxygen is being used by the biochemical action in the sewage, indicating a high sewage concentration.

The primary purpose of sewage treatment is to prevent the spread of disease among human beings. For additional reasons the proper disposal of sewage is imperative in any community or nation,

particularly one with a high population concentration. Sewage treatment protects water supplies, fish and other aquatic life, food (by preventing soil pollution), livestock, and renders water fit for industrial use. Therefore, in addition to preventing disease spread, sewage treatment returns water to a condition such that it can be reused with safety and with its general condition unimpaired.

Sewage Treatment

Treatment of community sewage addresses five factors: solids in suspension, organic matter in suspension, inorganic matter in suspension, organic matter in solution, and bacteria. A properly designed and efficiently operated sewage disposal plant will eliminate all five of these undesirable factors and leave an end product of clear, uncontaminated water that can be safely consumed.

Before discharging wastewater, industries may be required to provide for *pretreatment* to remove some pollutants from their wastewater (figure 14-13).

A community sewage disposal plant that does the complete job of treatment involves the following six steps: preliminary treatment, primary treatment, secondary treatment, tertiary treatment, chlorination, and final disposal.

Preliminary Treatment   A series of parallel screens set at an angle permit sewage to flow through but intercept large, suspended objects (figure 14-14). Mechanically or manually operated rakes clean the debris and dump it into receptacles, where it is burned. Some community sewage plants use shredders which cut coarse material into fine enough particles to pass through with the effluent for further treatment. Grit chambers for preliminary treatment cause gravel, sand, and other heavy materials to settle to the bottom.

Primary Treatment   The effluent flows into the center of the circular sedimentation or clarifier tanks through a pipe coming up from the bottom. This prevents agitation of the effluent in the tank and ensures that particles will settle to the bottom. To aid this sedimentation, chemicals are added to

· ·

Figure 14-13

Problems that may occur when industries discharge their wastewater into sewage treatment systems can be controlled through pretreatment of pollutants by the industry source before discharging its wastes. *Source:* U.S. Environmental Protection Agency.

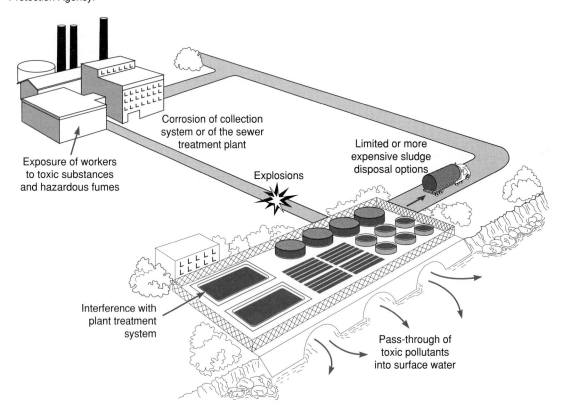

form a gelatinous floc that settles, carries suspended solids to the bottom, and forms sludge.

Anaerobic bacteria or chemicals digest the sludge in the sedimentation tank or in separate sludge tanks. Undigested sludge is hauled away to be dehydrated and used as fertilizer because it is rich in nitrogen.

Secondary Treatment To reduce the oxygen demand (BOD) of the sewage, the secondary treatment requires aeration so that organisms can convert the organic matter in the effluent into stable nitrogenous products. Trickling filters are

constructed of concrete with a bed of gravel, crushed stone, or similar material that provides good ventilation of the bed.

The trickling filter system uses an aeration tank and gently stirs the wastewater to further separate the solids. At that point, air is bubbled through the wastewater, which is piped back through the clarifying tanks one more time, resulting in a cleaner end product.

Tertiary Treatment Most community sewage treatment plants use a third process to remove or reduce certain chemicals such as phosphates, nitrogen,

....
Figure 14-14

A flow diagram for a sewage treatment plant proceeds from preliminary treatment through primary (anaerobic) treatment, to secondary (aerobic) treatment, to final chlorination before returning the safe water back to a large body of water.

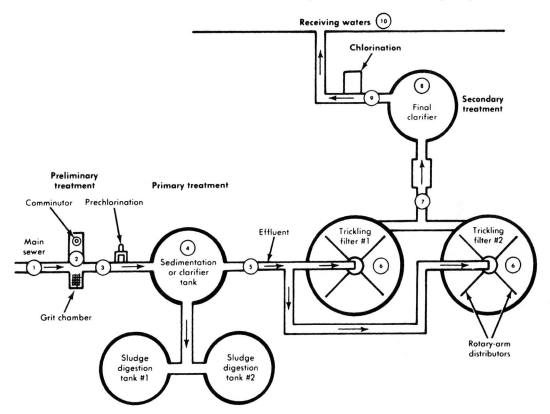

and carbon. Removal of these chemicals is desirable and even necessary because they can lead to eutrophication, a process that occurs naturally in bodies of water but normally takes thousands of years. The process is accelerated dramatically when excessive nutrients (such as nitrates and phosphates) stimulate marked growth of algae and other aquatic plants. The flourishing plants consume elements essential to marine life and to the natural purification of wastes. This essentially was the condition in Lake Erie for several years.

Phosphorus compounds that contaminate streams, lakes, and other bodies of water derive from synthetic detergents, domestic wastes, and runoff from farms and other land. Detergents are not the major source of phosphorus in the effluent of sewage treatment plants, and this phosphorus is no more difficult to remove than that from other sources. In community sewage more than 50 percent of the total phosphorus comes from domestic wastes, detergents account for about 35 percent, and the remainder comes from fertilizers used in farming and lawn care.

Removal of phosphorus involves conversion of soluble phosphorus into insoluble forms and then precipitation of the insoluble forms, which is usually done by adding metal salts—for example, aluminum sulfate or ferrous chloride. When settled, the phosphorus compounds are removed with the sludge, which is disposed of where it will not enter a body of water.

Nitrogen removal is not so simple. One method for removing nitrogen uses a stripping tower from twenty-five to fifty feet high. The inside of the tower is laced with wooden slats. Effluent is pumped to the top of the tower and is distributed uniformly from a horizontal tray across the top of the latticework. As the falling water strikes the slats, droplets are formed. Droplet surface films are of minimum thinness, which favors the escape of ammonia gas from the droplets. Air in the tower enters through side louvers and, by completely surrounding the droplets, promotes a maximum transfer of ammonia from the water to the air. The process of water falling and forming new droplets is repeated at least 200 times. This tertiary treatment vastly improves the efficiency of chlorination.

Tertiary treatment of most community sewage is imperative if the United States is to save its streams, lakes, and ponds. Ecology makes clear that all life on earth (human life included) depends on good quality water. Complete sewage treatment will be expensive, but essential to sustainable life on this planet. An informed public is necessary for this to occur.

Chlorination Primary treatment of sewage may be all that is necessary when the effluent from community sewage is emptied into receiving waters (such as lakes or rivers) that provide extreme dilution. In some instances, the dilution is great and after secondary treatment it is safe to empty the effluent into the final disposal lake, river, or sea. When the population concentration is great and available bodies of water are not adequate, however, a good safety measure is to chlorinate the effluent coming from the primary or secondary treatment unit. In some instances chlorination is necessary only during the summer months when available stream flow is low. Two-stage chlorination, in which chlorine is added to the grit chamber at the beginning of treatment and again to the final effluent, provides added safety.

Besides destroying organisms, chlorine reduces the BOD and odor of effluents. The chlorine injection mechanism is similar to that used in water treatment plants.

Final Disposal The receiving waters into which the final effluent is emptied are usually public waters and, as such, are under the jurisdiction and supervision of a federal, provincial, or state agency. Other communities and citizens have a claim to the use of the waters. The larger the body of receiving water, the greater the safety factor. Although the supervising state agency recognizes practical considerations, no community has the right to jeopardize the public health. If a community is to be granted the privilege of disposing of its wastes, it must take reasonable precautions to ensure that its sewage effluent is not a threat to human life and welfare.

Lagoon Treatment

Cost of a typical sewage treatment plant can be beyond the financial means of a small community. Fortunately, raw sewage lagoons can provide economical and satisfactory treatment of community sewage. A lagoon is a shallow pond in which natural processes produce an acceptable purification.

A lagoon is usually located at least a quarter of a mile from residential areas, where seepage will not pollute groundwater that may be used for domestic purposes. A lagoon is a rectangular excavation, at least half an acre in area and from three to five feet in depth (figure 14-15). The soil at the bottom of the lagoon should be relatively impervious to prevent excess loss of effluent by seepage. Embankments prevent outside surface drainage from entering the lagoon. The inlet from the community's sewerage system should be near the center of the lagoon.

Organic material that settles to the bottom of the lagoon is decomposed by bacteria and is converted into ammonia, carbon dioxide, and water. Algae feed on these soluble nutrients and, in the presence of sunlight, produce oxygen and therefore maintain aerobic conditions and help prevent

· ·

Figure 14-15

Lagoons serve as an alternative for sewage treatment in small communities that cannot afford a full-scale sewage treatment plant. *Source:* Photo by K. Mott, courtesy World Health Organization.

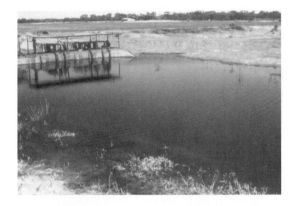

odor. If the lagoon freezes, the ice shuts out sunlight and interferes with the treatment process.

Decontamination of sewage effluents may be necessary if they are being discharged into public waters, especially during the summer months. Raw sewage lagoon effluents are generally not discharged into public waters in quantities that would result in greater than 1 part effluent per 20 parts dilution. Lagoon treatment is not the equivalent of the standard methods of treatment, but it can be acceptable. It serves when the community concerned is not able to finance the more costly, more elaborate primary and secondary treatment plants.

Financing Sewage Treatment

Sewage treatment plants are costly but are a necessary community investment in protecting health, in maintaining an esthetic environment, and in disposing of community wastes. No fully equitable method has been developed for paying the costs of treatment plant construction and maintenance. Nearly all payment methods are based on the volume of water citizens use from the community's water supply.

In view of the investment it represents for future generations, most communities in the United States and Canada find it necessary and appropriate to issue bonds for the construction of a treatment plant. The security for the bonds is the community's ability to collect future fees and to levy taxes to redeem the bonds when due. All establishments connected to the public sewerage system are charged a monthly sewer fee based on the amount of water the establishment used during the month. The practice is based on the assumption that the amount of water a household uses is a reasonable index of the extent to which the household uses the sewer service. The sewer fee is usually higher during winter months than during summer, when the sewer rate is lowered to compensate for the fact that much of the water going through the meter is used for lawn sprinkling and does not go into the sewer lines.

Regulation of Sewage Disposal

In North America construction and operation of sewage treatment facilities and disposal of the final effluent are the responsibility of the community, but the regulation of the sewage treatment plants and disposal of final effluents are the responsibility of the province or state. This authority may be vested in the sanitary engineering division of the provincial Ministry of Health, state department of health, or in a special state sanitation authority. There are advantages in having a special authority to regulate sewage disposal, largely because water pollution is an increasing problem. In addition, a separate authority can deal with air pollution and other problems in the total environment.

The state or province can order a community to treat its sewage before emptying the final effluent into public waters. Courts have held this to be a proper function of the state and have ordered communities to raise the necessary funds to provide for proper sewage disposal. Plans for a community sewage treatment plant must be approved by state engineers, who also work with communities in an advisory role. Sewage disposal plant operators should pass state certification examinations, and the operation of the sewage plant must meet state sanitation requirements.

Septic Tanks

A serious community health problem may exist when sewers do not serve a residential area. A septic tank for each domicile is the means used for sewage disposal in such areas, which are usually the fringes of a city or the outlying districts just beyond the city limits.

A septic tank can be satisfactory for the disposal of household liquid wastes if the tank, drain tile, and seepage pit are properly constructed. When improperly installed, however, a septic tank can constitute a hazard to health and, esthetically, can be a severe nuisance. Sewage sporadically coming to the surface or, during flooding, washing over a neighborhood can constitute a hazard to the well being of everyone in the vicinity. Such situations generally produce a certain pattern of citizen response: first, a long-time toleration of the situation; next, protests to the health officials or others; then, perhaps, court action. The final solution is usually the installation of sewers as a part of the community sewerage system. When at all feasible, even at considerable cost, sewer lines rather than septic tanks should be the choice.

Pit Latrines

The outhouse or pit latrine still does service in industrialized countries as a temporary facility on construction sites or at outside concerts, tent fairs, and picnic or park areas. In developing countries it is the primary means of shifting rural populations from unsanitary conditions of waste disposal to safe disposal. Pit latrine technology is simple, but the acceptability of designs is highly dependent on local toilet customs, cultural taboos, and environmental and economic conditions (figure 14-16).

Cities without Sewage Systems

Cities with inadequate sewage systems pose possible danger to health and life. As a consequence, pressures are exerted on officials and on voters to provide the necessary finances and planning for an

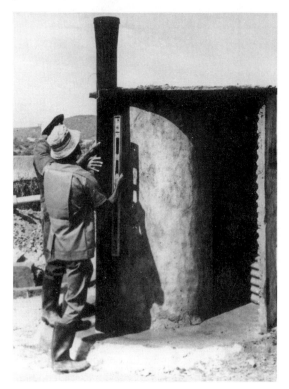

Figure 14-16

The Blair Research Laboratory in Harare, part of the Zimbabwe Ministry of Health, developed the Blair latrine. It can be seen all over southern Africa, appreciated for its control of infectious diseases and its esthetic improvements over the latrines and open pits that preceded it.

adequate sewage system for their community. Federal and state funding adds to the incentive to provide the community with an approved, safe means for water disposal.

One can find cities of more than 1 million inhabitants without a sewage system. Tokyo, with more than 10 million people, has one of the largest populations of any city in the world, yet it depends on collection tanks and tanker trucks to collect and dispose of sewage.

Hiroshima was leveled by a nuclear bomb, which necessitated a complete rebuilding of the city. Environmentalists assumed that Hiroshima would begin by putting in a complete sewage system before erecting structures above the ground. The situation was ideal for this sequence. However, no such system was built. The tank system apparently is preferred in Japan. This choice could cause Western countries to ask themselves whether they have overemphasized the necessity for all of the sewage systems they have built.

STREAM POLLUTION

Although stream pollution is thought of only in terms of a threat to human health, it actually affects many factors of economic and other significance. For example, it can render water unsuitable for industrial use. It affects agriculture by altering the taste of milk from cows drinking polluted water. Polluted irrigation water represents possible dangers. Waterfowl and other animals are exposed to botulism and cyanide poisoning. Turbidity and thermal pollution can destroy fish and other marine life. Decomposition of nitrogen wastes forms nitrates and, because all of the oxygen is consumed, green plants die and anaerobic bacteria (for example, botulism) survive. Farther down the stream where little pollution exists, green plant life may be profuse and give off oxygen. Pollution with acids may cause dock deterioration, and pollution from such industries as mining and quarrying may interfere with navigation and thus necessitate dredging.

Criteria of Stream Pollution

Organic Criteria   In the final analysis, the most reliable single index of stream pollution can be the BOD, expressed as the quantity of oxygen required for oxidation of organic matter (expressed in pounds). The capacity of any body of water to oxidize organic wastes depends on its oxygen content, including oxygen resulting from photosynthesis in algae and other green plants. If oxygen use exceeds oxygen production, a negative oxygen balance occurs and an anaerobic condition results that produces undesirable bacterial action. A stream need not be in a state of negative oxygen balance to be badly polluted, however.

Chemical Criteria   Trace metals polluting many rivers and streams include iron, manganese, copper, zinc, lead, chromium, nickel, tin, cobalt, cadmium, and mercury. These metals settle in the river sediment and can be transported to humans, along with organic pollutants, by any of the routes shown in figure 14-17.

Acid Rain   Sunlight triggers the photochemical conversion of pollutants in the air to acidic substances. These combine with water vapor and return to the earth's surface as acid rain or snow. Sulfur dioxide emissions from coal-fired power plants are the main cause of acid rain, which contaminates surface waters and damages humanmade structures in eastern North America and Europe. The most acidic rain ever recorded fell on Wheeling, West Virginia; it was 5,000 times as acidic as unpolluted rain. Although not a direct health threat for humans, acid rain is believed to account for a decline in fish populations in high-altitude lakes in the northeastern United States and Canada. The two countries are negotiating for a solution to the problem of acid rain. The acid rain falling on Canada is largely caused by pollution produced in the United States. Much of the damage to forests and crops once blamed on acid rain is now attributed to ozone. Like the EPA "Superfund" for cleanup of toxic dumps and the regulation of water pollution by industry, created by the Clean Water Act, the regulation of air pollution by industry has become a political and economic issue of greater proportion because of the problems of international trade balances. Some Western industries say the trade balances are tilted in favor of the countries with less costly controls on pollution. More on acid rain and ozone will be addressed in chapter 17.

Standards   In the United States classification of streams was established by the first state stream regulating agency, the Pennsylvania Sanitary

· · · · · · · · · · · · · · · · · · · ·

Figure 14-17

Several pathways are shown by which pollutants can work their way from the sediment at the bottom of a stream or river to human hosts. *Source:* Courtesy Regional Office for Europe, World Health Organization.

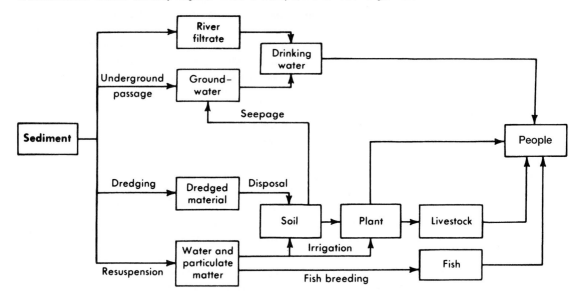

Water Board, created in 1923. This board established standards for three classes of streams. Class A streams are those in their natural state, probably subject to chance contamination by human beings but unpolluted or uncontaminated from any artificial source. They are fit for domestic water supply after chlorination, will support fish life, and may be safely used for recreational purposes. Class B streams are those that are more or less polluted. The extent of regulation, control, or elimination of pollution from these streams will be determined by a consideration of

- the present and probable future use and condition of the stream;
- the practicability of remedial measures for abatement; and
- the general interest of the public through the protection of the public health, the health of animals, fish, and other aquatic life, and the use of the stream for recreational purposes.

Class C streams are so polluted that they cannot be used as sources of public water supplies, will not support fish life, and are not used for recreational purposes. From the standpoint of the public interest and practicability, it is not necessary, economical, or advisable to attempt to restore them to a clean condition.

Stream pollution control boards have established other standards. Some boards also zone rivers. The 1985 amendments for reauthorization of the Clean Water Act set the new timetables and standards for controlling the discharge of hazardous chemicals into lakes and streams and for industry to comply with the standards.

Control of Stream Pollution

The long-established principle of Riparian rights holds that landowners have the right to have a stream come down to their property with its quality unimpaired and its quantity undiminished (figure 14-18). Most people agree that there should be

······················
Figure 14-18

Violations of Riparian rights to clean water downstream are illustrated in this wood engraving of the "The Water Supply of New York" with nineteen vignettes of dams, watersheds, pollution, and pastoral scenes on the water making its way from the mountains through farms to the city. *Source:* Wood engraving after photographs and sketches by J. O. Davidson, in *Harper's Weekly* 25 (May 28, 1881):348–49, courtesy National Library of Medicine.

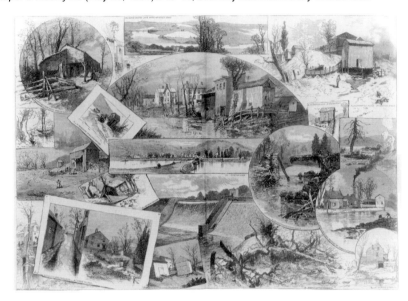

an equitable distribution of water, particularly between states and between communities. Obtaining some degree of equitable distribution while protecting natural waters is a formidable assignment.

A series of Canadian laws protecting the waters of Canada are shown in the box at the end of this chapter. U.S. laws are discussed here. The Federal Water Pollution Control Law went into effect in 1948. This legislation declared the pollution of *interstate* waters to be a public nuisance that must be abated. It protected the rights of the states in controlling water pollution. It also provided funds for surveys, investigations, and research. The essence of the law was the cooperation and coordination of all federal, state, and community agencies engaged in efforts to reduce or eliminate pollution of interstate waters and tributaries. Funds were made available for the construction of community sewage treatment facilities.

The 1965 Water Pollution Act passed by the U.S. Congress provided that each state determines the uses of its lakes and rivers. This water quality approach has much to recommend it, but it proved to be difficult to administer. After ten years, many states had not established water quality standards, and other states were unable to reconcile the relationship between pollutants and water use.

In 1971 the Federal Water Pollution Control Act went into effect. It shifted the emphasis from water quality standards to direct effluent limits, with the theoretical goal to be zero discharge. This act requires polluters to apply for a discharge permit from the EPA. The first phase of this program ended in 1976, by which time all firms and agencies were obligated to use the best available means to control water pollution. The goal of the second phase, achieved in 1981, was to achieve water clean enough for swimming and fish propagation.

Progress on reduction of stream pollution appears to have been steady from 1975 through 1981, but deregulation in the federal administrative policies of the early 1980s resulted in some reversals and slowing of the improvements. Communities and industries have found the costs of effluent elimination to be the main hurdle. The National Council on Environmental Quality acknowledges that costs rise exponentially with the degree of cleanliness sought, so that the last 1 percent of treatment could cost as much as the previous 99 percent. Zero discharge may be an unattainable and perhaps unnecessary goal because costs may be prohibitive even with federal subsidies. Something less may be satisfactory.

Some communities have developed land disposal systems in which wastes are routed through a simple treatment, then stored in lagoons, and finally sprayed over a wide acreage of land. Ecologists favor such an approach, because it returns invaluable nutrients to the soil. This type of simple technology may provide an acceptable, if not completely satisfactory, answer to the problem of effluent discharge.

Two or more states set up compacts when a stream adjoins more than one state. Some of these agreements are formal, others informal, some even cross national borders as between a province in Canada and a state in the United States. Usually, an interstate commission or water control council is created. Cooperation is the purpose for and the key to these joint programs for pollution control.

Within a state or province, responsibility for pollution control may be vested in the state department of health; or some other agency will be responsible for general environmental health problems, including water pollution. The state agency may set up districts or drainage areas to provide control measures best suited to particular problems in specific sections of the state. The state sanitation authority may establish standards of pollution, conduct surveys, and take action to abate a pollution nuisance. Only after all cooperative measures have failed will the state agency resort to legal measures. There is a need for waste

disposal and a need for water protection. To reconcile the two is the task that faces every community and every country.

SOLID WASTES

Solid waste may serve as one link in the transmission of infectious disease or toxic chemical exposures. Community solid wastes consist of garbage, ashes, rubbish (boxes, papers, other scraps), street sweepings, trade wastes, and occasionally dead animals. Leaves, grass, and shrub cuttings will often be considered wastes that must be disposed of. Industrial wastes are normally not a community problem, because industries are expected to dispose of their own wastes.

Of the solid wastes of a community, garbage poses the most significant health menace, because it provides feed for stray dogs, rats, and insects. In some regions this may be a minor factor in health, but in other geographical areas dogs, rats, and mosquitoes are hosts of serious diseases and therefore constitute a significant threat to health. Rubbish can also harbor rats and insects, but the removal of rubbish usually is more a matter of esthetics and convenience than of health (figure 14-19).

Collection

The collection and the disposal of garbage and refuse are accepted government functions in most countries. Some communities collect household and commercial garbage and rubbish without charge, the cost being met through general tax funds; others charge for garbage and rubbish collections. The responsibility for collection usually rests with the department of public works or some other comparable department, and responsibility for proper sanitation relating to garbage and rubbish usually rests with the health authorities of the community.

Some communities contract with private firms to collect garbage and rubbish. Specifications for collections are set up by the city council, and bids are called for. The successful bidder is then

Figure 14-19

Community participation in the Philippines: Residents of a Manila suburb help the garbage collectors clean up their neighborhood. *Source:* Photo by E. Ouano, courtesy World Health Organization, Western Pacific Regional Office.

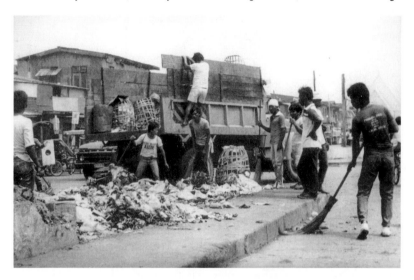

granted a franchise for a period of about five years, when bids are again called for. The city council specifies what the charges will be and stipulates the frequency of collections. Each householder pays the disposal company for hauling garbage and refuse. Garbage is usually collected at regular intervals, whereas rubbish is hauled away only on the special request of the householder. Some cities have a can exchange arrangement, in which the city provides a can, picks up the filled can, and leaves a clean, empty one at each collection location. The frequency of garbage collections in residential areas varies from weekly to every other day. When ashes are kept separate, a weekly collection of ashes is frequently the pattern. Collections from commercial districts are usually made six times a week.

A 30-gallon container for garbage or two large plastic bags per week is usually adequate for a typical family, especially if recycling is handled separately. Community regulations specify that the containers must be of plastic, metal, rubber, or other special composition. The containers must be watertight, fly-tight, and easily cleaned or disposable. A tightly fitting lid is required. The householder is responsible for cleaning out the container and occasionally decontaminating it with some strong germicide such as Lysol. Some communities require that garbage and ashes be separated when incineration is the method of disposal. This may also be required when reduction (garbage disposals in sinks or compactors) or hog feeding is the method of disposal.

Most communities require that garbage be wrapped in wet-strength plastic bags. Enclosed trucks with hydraulic hoists for loading, compressing, and unloading are sanitary and economical (figure 14-20). At least once a week the trucks are steamed and cleaned with detergents.

Disposal

Open dumps, sanitary landfills, incineration, hog feeding, reduction, and grinding are the recognized methods of garbage disposal. Most communities

. . . .

Figure 14-20

Raw refuse is collected by truck, shredded, and put through a series of procedures to recover reusable material and energy. The residual refuse then can be buried more safely in landfills, and the community benefits from the salvage of materials and energy. *Source:* Texas Department of Health.

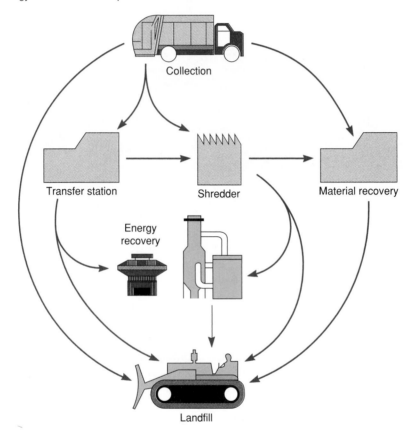

use dumps for the disposal of garbage and refuse, but this choice is less than desirable. Burning at the dump creates a fire hazard and obnoxious smoke and odor. In addition, dumps are breeding grounds for rats and vermin. Only when the dump is in an isolated area and properly supervised can it be an acceptable method of disposal.

Sanitary landfills require a land depression or excavated trench into which garbage and refuse is dumped and then covered with dirt. This method serves to reclaim wastelands, does not require sep-

aration of ashes and garbage, can be virtually odorless, and can be free of rats and vermin. Availability of an acceptable area may be a problem, however.

Incineration is an expensive and controversial disposal method but is regarded as the most acceptable, especially in combination with a recycling program for plastic, glass, aluminum cans and other metals, and paper. Garbage and rubbish need not be separated. Ashes are excluded and usually magnetic separators are used to remove cans and other metal objects. Incinerators are composed of a receiving bin from which refuse is carried by conveyor to a hopper that feeds the refuse into a furnace. Oil, coal, or gas may be used as supplementary fuel for maximum combustion in the furnace. The final ash is removed from the bottom of the furnace and hauled to a dump or a landfill. When air pollution laws were enacted in the 1970s, they made incinerators less economical. Many facilities had to be closed. Shortages of landfill space has reversed this trend. Combined with energy generation from incinerators for some communities, incinerators have made a comeback, but remain controversial.

Hog feeding is an old method of garbage disposal still in use but not approved by health authorities. It requires a separation of garbage from other wastes and a sorting of the garbage. An area of 2 acres and a ton of garbage per day for 100 hogs is the usual standard. Even if the hog farm is well operated and is far removed from the community, feeding garbage to hogs is objectionable. Spreading garbage, raw and cooked, creates an unsanitary and malodorous environment where flies and rats proliferate. As a source of human trichinosis, garbage-fed hogs must always be regarded as a primary threat, even when an informed public cooks pork adequately before serving it.

Grinding of garbage and disposal of it in the community sewage is effective and practical. A large grinding plant receives garbage from the collection trucks and empties the ground garbage into the trunk sewer. This task has been made easier with the widespread installation of home garbage disposals. Experience indicates that ground garbage causes no serious interference with sewage treatment. Oxygen demand of the sewage is increased, but not to a degree that would have an adverse effect on the treatment of the effluent or on the terminal waters into which the sewage effluent is emptied.

Domestic garbage grinders attached to kitchen sinks are highly satisfactory, although some objects must be separated out. The individual householder can purchase his or her own grinder from a commercial firm, the city may install home grinder units on a citywide basis and resell to the householder on an installment plan, or the city may retain ownership and charge a monthly rental fee. The municipal sewage treatment plant can handle the ground garbage if the biochemical oxygen demand is within a controllable range. To take care of household garbage in this manner, the community rightfully makes a regular monthly sewage charge. Controversy continues around the question of ground food wastes contributing to the amount of wastewater contaminants discharged into nearby streams, lakes, and ocean waters. This problem arises most where sewage treatment is inadequate.

Recycling

Recycling certain combustible and noncombustible solid wastes is receiving increased attention by research agencies and community officials. Over 75 percent of municipal solid waste in the United States is recyclable. Only 30 percent of these materials are being recycled because of deficiencies in technology, public cooperation, and markets. Community programs to increase this rate of recycling have included educational campaigns, and incentives such as cash prizes, refundable deposits, and surcharges on garbage bags for nonrecyclable wastes. Mandatory programs obtain greater participation but also result sometimes in public antagonism and illegal private dumping on roadsides.

Successful community programs have emphasized colored containers in which residents can sort their recyclable materials and set them out with their trash cans. Garbage trucks are equipped with separate bins for the color-coded bags for glass, aluminum, plastic, and paper. The high visibility of the colored bags makes the recycling act a more public act that builds a neighborhood norm. Some communities have achieved 80 percent participation rates with such voluntary programs (figure 14-21).

Wilton, New Hampshire, collects glass, metals, paper, and hazardous household wastes in separate

. . . .

Figure 14-21

Community recycling programs have been supported by national media campaigns to educate and encourage the public to sort and recycle its household wastes. *Source:* Environmental Defense Fund and Advertising Council.

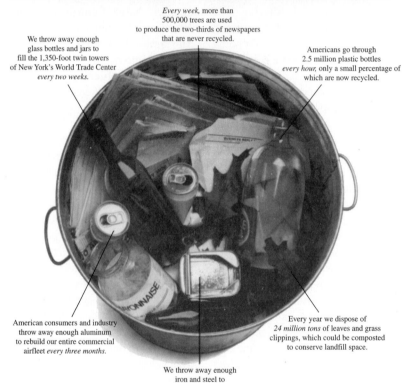

TAKE A FEW MINUTES TO GO THROUGH YOUR GARBAGE.

Every week, more than 500,000 trees are used to produce the two-thirds of newspapers that are never recycled.

We throw away enough glass bottles and jars to fill the 1,350-foot twin towers of New York's World Trade Center *every two weeks.*

Americans go through 2.5 million plastic bottles *every hour,* only a small percentage of which are now recycled.

American consumers and industry throw away enough aluminum to rebuild our entire commercial airfleet *every three months.*

Every year we dispose of *24 million tons* of leaves and grass clippings, which could be composted to conserve landfill space.

We throw away enough iron and steel to *continuously* supply all the nation's automakers.

The ordinary bag of trash you throw away is slowly becoming a serious problem for everybody.

Because the fact is, not only are we running out of resources to make the products we need, we're running out of places to put what's left over.

Write the Environmental Defense Fund at: 257 Park Avenue South, New York, NY 10010, for a free brochure that will tell you virtually everything

you'll need to know about recycling.

One thing's for certain, the few minutes you take to learn how to recycle will spare us all a lot of garbage later.

IF YOU'RE NOT RECYCLING YOU'RE THROWING IT ALL AWAY.

® 1988 EDF

Canadian Federal Legislation Applying to Water and Liquid or Solid Waste Control

Canadian Environmental Assessment Act (CEAA) Establishes a federal environmental assessment process for projects conducted at, on or affecting federal lands.

Canadian Environmental Protection Act (CEPA) Provides for the identification, assessment, and management of toxic substances and authorizes regulations controlling their discharge into the environment, including ocean dumping.

Canadian Water Act Provides for the management of the water resources of Canada, including research, planning, and implementation of programs for conservation, development, and use of water resources.

Fisheries Act Provides for control and prosecution of any deposit of a deleterious substance into waters frequented by fish or in an area where such a substance may enter any such water; offenses include $1 million fines and three years' imprisonment.

Fertilizers Act Controls and regulates agricultural fertilizers.

Provincial Acts parallel the federal acts. In addition, they include acts for waste management prohibiting the discharge of *all* wastes to the environment unless the discharge is specifically exempt or is made to conform to a system of permits or approvals. Fines up to $1 million per day of discharge, or $3 million if bodily harm is done to people, and three years imprisonment apply to companies or individuals violating these acts.

containers with a mandatory program. This program has saved the town about $50,000 in waste-disposal costs per year and has brought in about $25,000 per year in revenue from the sale of recycled materials. Such programs do not necessarily pay for themselves, but for communities with dwindling landfill space and with air quality problems prohibiting incineration, recycling becomes increasingly attractive. Some states and communities are giving tax incentives to businesses that in-

corporate recycled materials into their manufacturing process. Recycled plastic is relatively inexpensive at $0.40 per pound compared with $0.60 per pound for pure plastic. Recycling appears to be a winning strategy for waste management on the supply side and the demand side.

Reducing Litter

Litter serves as a signal of a blight on the community that disregards the common good. It would be difficult to establish a relationship between litter and physical health, but the effect of litter on mental health certainly could be appraised.

Litter reduction, to be effective, must be based on organization of resources and voluntary leadership. In the United States principal voluntary organizations for the prevention of litter are Keep America Beautiful, Inc. and the Sierra Club.

Some states and provinces have passed "bottle bill" legislation making mandatory a deposit for the return of certain containers and responsibility for preventing and controlling litter. Total litter in Oregon and Vermont was reduced by more than 10 percent.

SUMMARY

This chapter began with an examination of how water can be protected, derived, and treated for safe consumption. It ended with a discussion of ways in which that same water can be recycled back into the environment after domestic and other uses by treating wastewater and by handling other toxic wastes so that they do not contaminate the water supply beyond recovery.

The entire process of consumption and disposal of water is analogous to digestion on a community scale. The water must be protected, like other parts of the environment, if it is to remain usable without health risks. Protection includes treatment and testing of water supplies, disposal and treatment of wastes, control of pollution, and the maintenance of standards for these several processes.

Organic pollution of water has been controlled primarily with the use of chlorine. Inorganic pollution by trace metals and other toxic chemicals cannot be so easily neutralized with a single substance. The only hope for control of the thousands of possibly toxic chemicals that pollute water is control of the disposal of toxic wastes. In addition to efforts to prevent the continuing pollution by industry and restrictions on agricultural use of pesticides, a "Superfund" had to be created in the United States for cleanup of the major sites where large quantities of toxic substances had been dumped in the past. For a summary of Canadian legislative acts pertaining to water, liquid wastes and solid wastes, see the box on page 459.

Disposal of human and industrial wastes has become a spiraling problem demanding greater investments and control. There is no other choice, for safe water and soil are essential to survival.

WEB Links

http://www.epa.gov/
U.S. Environmental Protection Agency

http://www.doe.ca/envhome.html
Environment Canada

http://www.lycos.com/wguide/wire/wire_144531_
47234_0_5.html
Lycos links to waste management sites

QUESTIONS FOR REVIEW

1. How does treating water for consumption differ from treating wastewater for release back into the environment?
2. If water is more important to a human being's health than any drug, why does water cost less than any drug?
3. If the total water supply in the world remains the same, why is water management important?
4. Who has the safer water, urban dwellers or rural dwellers?
5. What is the source of your community's water supply, and what are its merits and hazards?
6. How is it possible for water to be contaminated and still be safe?
7. Why is the bacteriological examination not directed at finding the typhoid bacillus?
8. Why are chemical wastes in water more difficult to test for and to neutralize than organic wastes?
9. What problems of waste disposal have been created by the development of suburban areas?
10. How would you initiate a program to make your community more conscious of its water protection needs?
11. What is the most equitable and efficient method of charging for sewage services?
12. If communities are responsible for the construction and operation of their own sewage treatment plants, why should the state be the regulating agency?
13. Industrial stream pollution has existed for more than ninety years; why is there so much concern about it now?
14. Why are toxic waste dumps in dry fields a threat to the water supply?
15. How can chemical or trace-metal sediment at the bottom of a stream reach people to do any harm?

READINGS

Blumenthal, D. S., and J. Ruttenber. 1993. *Introduction to environmental health.* 2d ed. New York: Springer Publishing Co.
This book is written specifically for students of the health sciences and focuses primarily on the relationship between the environment and human health.

Greenberg, A. W., L. S. Clesceri, and A. D. Eaton, eds. 1995. *Standard methods for the examination of water and wastewater.* 19th ed. Washington, DC: American Public Health Association.
The all-inclusive reference tool covering all aspects of 340 water analysis techniques for assessment of chemical constituents, sanitary quality, and physical and biological characteristics.

The Presidential/Congressional Commission on Risk Assessment and Risk Management. 1997. *Framework for environmental health risk management.* Final Report. Vol. 1. Washington, DC: The Commission
This Commission's framework defines a clear, six-stage process for risk management that can be scaled up or down in its complexity depending on the public health and ecological importance of a particular threat. (WWW: http://www.riskworld.com)

Sloan, W. M. 1992. *Site selection for new hazardous waste management facilities.* Geneva: World Health Organization, WHO Regional Publications, European Series, No. 46.

Guide to the selection of new sites where hazardous wastes can be collected, treated, stored, and disposed of in a safe manner acceptable to the general public. Gives particular attention to the measures to protect health, preserve environmental quality, and respect the social values and economic well-being of the host community.

BIBLIOGRAPHY

Albert, R. E. 1994. Carcinogen risk assessment in the U.S. Environmental Protection Agency. *Critical Reviews in Toxicology* 24:74.

British Columbia Ministry of Health and Ministry Responsible for Seniors. 1995. *Safe water supply: vital to your health.* Victoria, BC: BC Ministry of Health, Health Protection and Safety Branch.

Burke, T. A., N. M. Shalauta, and N. L. Tran. 1995. Strengthening the role of public health in environmental policy. *Policy Studies* 23:76.

Cairncross, S., and P. J. Kolsky. 1997. Water, waste, and well-being: a multicountry study. *Am J Epidemiology* 146:359.

Carr, P. A., J. R. Hoey, and P. Moccio. 1996. Evaluation of tax bill inserts as a public health strategy to influence septic tank pumping practice. *Canadian J Public Health* 87:343.

Chen, A. T. L., J. A. Reidy, and L. E. Sever. 1996. Public drinking water contamination and birth outcomes. *Am J Epidem* 143:1179.

Chess, S., K. L. Salomone, B. J. Hance, and A. Saville. 1995. Results of a national symposium on risk communication: next steps for government agencies. *Risk Analysis* 15:115.

Doyle, T. J., W. Zheng, and A. R. Folsom. 1997. The association of drinking water source and chlorination by-products with cancer incidence among postmenopausal women in Iowa: a prospective cohort study. *Am J Public Health* 87:1168.

Faustman, E. M., and G. S. Omenn. 1995. Risk assessment. Chap 4 in Casarett and Doull's *Toxicology: The basic science of poisons.* 5th ed. New York: McGraw-Hill.

Federal-Provincial Working Group on Recreational Water Quality. 1992. *Guidelines for Canadian recreational water quality.* Ottawa: Canada Communica-tions Group for the Federal-Provincial Advisory Committee on Environmental and Occupational Health.

Fewtrell, L., D. Kay, and G. O'Neill. 1997. An investigation into the possible links between shigellosis and hepatitis A and public water supply disconnections. *Public Health* 111:179.

Forbes, W. F., J. F. Gentleman, and C. A. McAiney. 1997. Geochemical risk factors for mental functioning, based on the Ontario Longitudinal Study of Aging. *Can J Aging* 16:142.

Freeman, M., ed. 1995. *The letters of Rachel Carson and Dorothy Freeman, 1952–1964.* Boston: Beacon Press.

Goldstein, B. D., and M. R. Greenberg. 1997. Toxicology and environmental health. In *Oxford textbook of public health,* edited by R. Detels, W. W. Holland, J. McEwen, and G. S. Omenn. 2d ed. Vol. 2. New York, Oxford, Tokyo: Oxford University Press.

Grainger, C. R. 1996. Radon in surface water on Jersey. *J Royal Soc Health* 116:237.

Griffiths, R., and P. Saunders. 1997. Reducing environmental risk. In *Oxford textbook of public health,* edited by R. Detels, W. W. Holland, J. McEwen, and G. S. Omenn. 2d ed. Vol. 3. New York, Oxford, Tokyo: Oxford University Press.

Health and Welfare Canada. 1990. *Guidelines for Canadian drinking water quality.* 4th ed. Ottawa: Canada Communication Group.

Hellard, M. W., M. I. Sinclair, and C. K. Fairley. Commentary: drinking water and microbiological pathogens—issues and challenges for the year 2000. *Public Health Med* 19:129.

Hoque, B. A., and M. M. Hoque. 1994. Partnership in rural water supply and sanitation: a case study from Bangladesh. *Health Policy and Planning* 9:288.

Hoxie, N. J., J. P. Davis, and K. A. Blair. 1997. Crytosporidiosis—associated mortality following a massive waterborne outbreak in Milwaukee, Wisconsin. *Am J Public Health* 87:2032.

Jasanoff, S. 1996. The dilemma of environmental democracy. *Issues in Science and Technol* (fall):63.

Jones I. G., and M. Roworth. 1996. An outbreak of *Escherichia coli 0157* and *Campybacteriosis* associated with contamination of a drinking water supply. *Public Health* 110:269.

Lioy, P. J. 1997. The analysis of human exposures to contaminants in the environment. In *Oxford textbook of public health,* edited by R. Detels, W. W. Holland,

J. McEwen, and G. S. Omenn. 3d ed. Vol. 2. New York, Oxford, Tokyo: Oxford University Press.

Monto, A., and C. Marrs. 1997. Infectious agents. In *Oxford textbook of public health,* edited by R. Detels, W. W. Holland, J. McEwen, and G. S. Omenn. 3d ed. Vol. 1. New York, Oxford, Tokyo: Oxford University Press.

National Academy of Public Administration. 1995. *Setting priorities, getting results: a new direction for EPA.* Washington, DC: National Academy of Public Administration.

National Research Council. 1996. *Understanding risk: informing decisions in a democratic society.* Washington, DC: National Academy Press.

Noah, N. 1997. Microbiology. In *Oxford textbook of public health,* edited by R. Detels, W. W. Holland, J. McEwen, and G. S. Omenn. 3d ed. Vol. 2. New York, Oxford, Tokyo: Oxford University Press.

Omenn, G. S., and E. M. Faustman. Risk assessment, risk communication, and risk management. 1997. In *Oxford textbook of public health,* edited by R. Detels,

W. W. Holland, J. McEwen, and G. S. Omenn. 3d ed. Vol. 2. New York, Oxford, Tokyo: Oxford University Press.

Pilotto, L. S. 1995. Disinfection of drinking water, by-products, and cancer. *Australian J Public Health* 19:89.

Reiff, F. M., M. Roses, V. M. Witt. 1996. Low-cost safe water for the world: a practical interim solution. *J Public Health Policy* 17:389.

Sharma, V., A. Sharma, and H. Tiwari. 1995. A medico-social profile of adolescent rag-pickers handling hospital wastes. *J Adolescent Health* 17:66.

St. John, R. 1996. Emerging infectious disease: repeat of an old challenge. *Can J Public Health* 87:365.

Taylor, G. A., A. J. Newens, and D. P. Forster. 1995. Alzheimer's disease and the relationship between silicon and aluminum in water supplies in northern England. *J Epidem & Community Health* 49:323.

Zmirou, D., S. Rey, and R. Mounir. 1995. Residual microbiological risk after simple chlorine treatment of drinking ground water in small community systems. *European J Public Health* 5:75.

Chapter *15*

Community Food and Vector Control

Objectives

When you finish this chapter, you should be able to:

- Describe the modes of transmission of disease by food and other vehicles and vectors
- Identify the major food protection and vector control strategies for communities and sources of their authority
- Develop objectives for a community food and vector control program

Hamburgers and mosquitos have something in common—the potential to transmit diseases to humans. While North American headlines carry stories about *E. coli* fatalities from contaminated hamburgers, concern in other parts of the world is about malaria carried by mosquitos. This chapter focuses on how food and vectors transmit diseases to humans and the kinds of regulatory and educational measures needed to address these threats to public health.

The development of systems to protect consumers from the dangers of unapproved food contaminants and vectors that transmit disease have been a major public health accomplishment. It is a longer stretch from farm to table, however, than in the days of Charles Warner. There are multiple links in the food production, processing, and packaging chain in which contamination can occur. Food safety requires vigilance against special interests, training and technology to keep abreast of advances in science, and oversight responsibility (figure 15-1).

Despite effective procedures, outbreaks of foodborne diseases leading to illness and death still occur. For example, in 1997 headlines were made when one of the largest fast-food chains temporarily pulled hamburgers off its menu. The decision was made following a massive recall of over 25 million pounds of tainted beef produced by a food processor in the Midwest. Consumers, who often take the safety of their food for granted, have been confronted with other headline stories about contamination that affected food safety: contaminated fruit juice ingested by children, *E. coli* deaths from undercooked hamburgers, and "mad cow" disease in England. Together these various headlines remind us that food safety matters, not only in the global chain of food production, but in our homes.

463

Figure 15-1

Popular wisdom suggests that "an apple a day keeps the doctor away," but one covered with pesticide may produce the opposite effect. Keeping apples and other food safe takes cooperation among regulatory agencies, food producers, researchers, and an educated public. *Source:* photo by Zafar, courtesy World Health Organization.

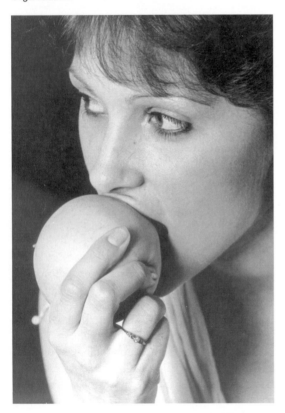

EPIDEMIOLOGY OF FOODBORNE DISEASE

Milestones in food protection have lead to our current level of safety. However, foodborne illness continues to be a major public health problem in the United States and Canada. Foodborne diseases sometimes result from failure in protective systems, but are more often the result of improper food handling. Annual estimates of foodborne cost and illness are estimated to be in the billions of dollars, with estimates of foodborne disease cases varying from 6–81 million in the United States. This wide range in estimates of disease cases is evidence of the difficulties in gathering accurate information in this area. The Centers for Disease Control and Prevention estimate that between 4,000 and 9,000 Americans die each year from food-borne illnesses. It is estimated that 30 percent of foodborne illness results from unsafe handling of food at home.

Common Pathogens

The prime causes of food-borne illness are a collection of bacteria: *Campylobacter jejuni, Salmonella, Staphylococcus aureus, Clostridium perfringens, Vibrio vulnificus,* and *Shigella.* Other causes are the protozoa *Giardia lamblia* and *Entamoeba histolytica* and hepatitis A virus. They are found in a wide range of foods, including meat, milk and other dairy products, coconut, fresh pasta, spices, chocolate, seafood, and even water (figure 15-2). Egg products, tuna, potato and macaroni salads, and cream-filled pastries may contain these pathogens, along with vegetables grown in soil fertilized with contaminated manure. Poultry is the food most often contaminated with disease-causing organisms.

These pathogens pose increased risk for children, the very old, and people with immunological deficiencies. For example, of the estimated 200–225 yearly *E. coli* deaths, most are in children. Common symptoms of foodborne illness include diarrhea, abdominal cramping, fever, sometimes blood or pus in the stools, headache, vomiting, and severe exhaustion. Symptoms vary according to the type of bacteria and the amount of contaminants eaten.

Sources of Contamination People are the most common source of food contamination. Bacteria have no mobility, but are transported into food by various means **(vehicles),** including on parts of the human body, unclean utensils, and working surfaces. Hands are a chief carrier of bacteria because they come into contact with so many different

Milestones in Food Protection

1203   England's King John promulgated the first Assize of Bread, the foundation of food regulation in the English-speaking world.

1785   Massachusetts passed the first comprehensive food adulteration law in the United States.

1820   Friedrich Accum published *Treatise on Adulteration of Food and Culinary Poisons.*

1850   Lemuel Shattuck's report for Massachusetts recommended control of adulterated food.

1862   Congress established the U.S. Department of Agriculture.

1880   The National Board of Trade conducted a competition for a draft of a national food law, which ultimately lead to the Pure Food and Drug Act of 1906.

1884   Bureau of Animal Industry was created to prevent interstate shipment of diseased cattle.

1890   Congress passed a law to prohibit the importation of adulterated food.

1906   The Pure Food and Drug (Wiley) Act prohibited interstate commerce in misbranded and adulterated foods, drinks, and drugs. Federal Meat Inspection Act passed.

1916   USDA published *Food for Young Children,* first dietary guidance pamphlet.

1917   U.S. Food Administration established to supervise World War I food supply. USDA's first dietary recommendations—Five Food Groups.

1924   Addition of iodine to salt to prevent goiter, first U.S. food fortification program.

1927   Food, Drug, and Insecticide Administration established. Name is changed to Food and Drug Administration (FDA) in 1932.

1933   Agricultural Act amendments permitted purchase of surplus commodities for donation to child nutrition and school lunch program.

1938   The Food, Drug & Cosmetic Act included provisions for food standards. FDA nutrition research program established. Social Security Act supported role of nutrition in health.

1941   President Roosevelt's National Nutrition Conference and first Recommended Dietary Allowances by the Food and Nutrition Board. FDA promulgated standards for enrichment of flour and bread with B-complex vitamins and iron.

1946   National School Lunch Program established.

1958   Food Additives Amendment Act prohibited use of a food additive until safety established by manufacturer. Delaney Clause prohibited carcinogenic additives. GRAS (Generally Recognized as Safe) list established.

1965   Food Stamp Act passed by Congress. Nationwide Food Consumption Survey collected first data on dietary intake of individuals.

1967   U.S. Congress passed first major meat inspection law since 1906, requiring states to have inspection requirements at least equal to federal requirements.

1972   Special Supplementary Food Program established for Women, Infants, and Children (WIC). Agriculture and Consumer Protection Act provided price support to farmers. Amendments to Older Americans Act of 1965 established a congregate and home-delivered meals program.

1980   USDA and USDHHS jointly issued *Nutrition and Your Health Dietary Guidelines for Americans:* DHHS issued *Promoting Health/Preventing Disease: Objectives for the Nation,* with seventeen nutrition objectives for the year 1990.

1984   The U.S. Surgeon General's Workshop on Breastfeeding and Human Lactation developed strategies for promoting breastfeeding.

1988   DHHS published *The Surgeon General's Report on Nutrition and Health.*

1989   National Academy of Sciences released *Diet and Health* and the role of pesticides in agriculture and food safety.

1990   The U.S. *Healthy People 2000* included four objectives for reduction of foodborne illnesses.

1991   FDA completed the Total Diet Study on Americans' dietary intake of pesticide residues.

1992   Food Guide Pyramid published. The use of irradiation as an adjunct to other food safety technologies and procedures federally endorsed.

1993   Federal policy on pesticides reversed. Now endorsed the use of "integrated pest management" with beneficial insects and crop rotation for some pesticides.

1994   New food labels required on U.S. canned and packaged foods to enable consumers to make informed nutritional choices.

1995   New federal rules and HACCP regulatory programs to required food industries to design and implement preventive measures making them more responsible for control of their safety assurance actions.

1996   Food Quality Protection Act streamlined regulation of pesticides by FDA and EPA and puts new public health protections in place, especially for children.

1997   President Clinton announced new Early-Warning System to gather critical scientific data to help stop foodborne disease outbreaks and a $43 million program, "Food Safety from Farm to Table," including greater FDA surveillance over imported foods.

· · · · · · · · · · · · · · · · · · · ·

Figure 15-2

Food needs to be not only wholesome but safe. The high fat and cholesterol content of these foods can lead to obesity and heart disease as discussed in earlier chapters. Unless safely produced and handled on its way to market, food can do further harm if contaminated with foodborne pathogens. *Source:* Photo by J. Vizcarra, courtesy World Health Organization, PAHO.

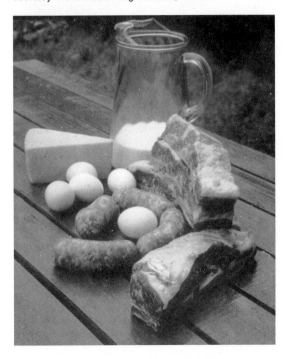

surfaces. Food preparation and eating utensils may cross contaminate food when a clean product comes into contact with a contaminated one. Insects and rodents transfer filth to food through their waste products, mouth, feet, and other body parts.

Modes of Transmission

Food can transfer disease by five different means: (1) inherently harmful characteristics, (2) allergy, (3) ptomaine poisoning, (4) toxin transfer, and (5) infection transfer. Other harmful effects of food consumption behavior have been addressed in the chapter on health promotion in terms of excess consumption of dietary fats, cholesterol and alcohol and insufficient consumption of nutrients and fiber. The focus in this chapter is on the environmental aspects of food protection and the related behavioral aspects of gathering, processing, transporting, storing, and preparing food.

Inherently Harmful Characteristics **Food poisoning** is a term used so generally that it encompasses a spectrum of digestive disorders. Distinction should be made between a food that is itself poisonous and a food that merely serves as a vehicle for the transmission of pathogens to humans. For example, some 70 to 80 species of mushrooms are inherently poisonous to people. These poisonous plants are not a serious community health problem because the public is informed in this regard and many do not have access to the wide variety of such potentially poisonous plants. Commercial producers of foods such as mushrooms have the knowledge and the legal responsibility to provide the market with safe foods.

Allergies A food may also be classed as poisonous for a person who is allergic to it. An allergy is a condition of altered tissue reaction, in which reexposure to a substance produces disturbing effects. About 30 percent of Americans and Canadians have food allergies. Rarely does a person have an allergy to a single food. Community health strives through public health education to assure that the public knows that food allergy may cause **rhinitis,** asthma, gastrointestinal disturbances, cardiovascular disturbances, and various skin disorders. Informed citizens can then seek medical services to determine whether they have allergies that would account for having one or more of these symptoms.

Ptomaine Poisoning A ptomaine is a toxin formed in the decomposition of protein through bacterial action. Meat that is sufficiently decomposed to possess ptomaines would be totally unpalatable. Even if meat is this badly decomposed, there would be no harmful results if it were well

Botulism Case Studies

Case 1

A twenty-two-year-old California man awoke at 2:00 A.M. with vomiting, blurred vision, and a "thick tongue." Symptoms progressed to total quadriplegia, then respiratory failure requiring mechanical ventilation. Two days earlier the patient had eaten stew prepared by his roommate from fresh ingredients (including meat and unpeeled potatoes and carrots) then left overnight at room temperature. The roommate ate it hot on the first night with no subsequent illness. The patient tasted it without reheating 16 hours later and complained of a bad taste. The roommate confirmed a sour taste, immediately spit it out, rinsed his mouth, and remained well. The patient was treated with antitoxin and recovered after extended hospitalization.

Case 2

A man of Egyptian descent, age thirty-two years, was admitted to the hospital after a series of emergency visits because of rapidly progressive problems including dizziness, facial drooping, dry mouth, weakness, and respiratory failure requiring mechanical ventilation. Three family members developed similar symptoms the next day. The New Jersey Department of Health traced the source of botulism to an ethnic preparation of fish known as moloha, an uneviscerated, salt-cured fish product. The family consumed the moloha without cooking or heating it the day before the man appeared with symptoms. The fish market from which the family bought the fish denied selling moloha or similar fish products, and none could be found on the premises. The public was alerted through the new media to avoid eating moloha. No additional cases were reported.

Why did these incidents occur even though the food was not home canned and had been cooked in one case?

Cases summarized from reports in *MMWR* 34:146, 1985; and 41:521, 1992.

---

cooked before being eaten because the heat would break up the protein chains that compose the ptomaines. It is doubtful that anyone in the United States or Canada dies of ptomaine poisoning.

Toxin Transfer   Food occasionally serves as the vehicle for transferring toxins to the digestive system of humans. Normal cooking processes usually disintegrate toxins, but because of a lack of understanding people may fail to take precautions necessary to protect themselves against poisoning by foodborne toxins.

Botulism is caused by a neurotoxin produced by the spore-forming organism *Clostridium botulinum,* found in alkaline and neutral soils. Raw vegetables have vast numbers of the organism on them but are not a threat to health because the organism is **anaerobic,** meaning that it does not produce toxin in free air. A person eating raw beans, peas, beets, or other vegetables would not be affected. However, if these vegetables are subjected in the canning process to an ordinary boiling temperature of 212° F (100°C), the spores withstand that temperature and the organism survives. Placed in the anaerobic conditions of a can or jar, the organism produces toxin. If the vegetables are well cooked before they are eaten, the toxin is destroyed. If the vegetables are eaten without being brought to a boil, however, the toxin can be fatal, as it is one of the most potent of known poisons. Commercial canners eliminate the possibility of botulism poisoning by using pressure cooking at 248° F (120° C).

The community health problem is that of educating the public about the need either to use pressure cookers for canning or to use tyndallization, which means bringing the food to a boil (212° F) on three consecutive days before canning. The public should know that, in any case, the best preventive measure is always to bring previously cooked vegetables or meat to a boil before serving.

Infection Transfer   A food cannot transfer pathogens unless the following favorable conditions exist:

1. The organism must be virile and exist in large numbers.
2. The time interval from reservoir to a new host must be short.
3. The temperature must be favorable (in the neighborhood of 100° F; 38° C, optimum for pathogens of humans).
4. Moisture must be available.
5. Very little light can be present.

Except for a few respiratory diseases transferred via milk, nearly all infectious diseases transferred by food are those of the digestive system—amebic dysentery, salmonellosis, tapeworm, trichinosis, typhoid fever, and viral hepatitis. Cow's milk can be an excellent medium for pathogens affecting the respiratory and other human systems, therefore a few other diseases also transferred by milk must be mentioned—bovine tuberculosis, brucellosis, diphtheria, human tuberculosis, Q fever, and streptococcal infections. Protection of food primarily seeks to prevent food becoming a vehicle of pathogen transmission, a task that can be accomplished by preventing pathogens from reaching food and by destroying the organisms that have reached food.

FOOD PROTECTION OBJECTIVES

The overall goal of food safety is to protect the community from foodborne illness. Specific objectives for a given community should be adapted from the national food safety objectives shown in the box "Food Safety Objectives for the Year 2000." Food Safety was designated as a priority area for the year 2000 national objectives in the United States in recognition of the importance that food plays in reducing the risks to public health associated with contaminated foods and foodborne pathogens.

Food Safety Objectives for the Year 2000

HEALTH STATUS OBJECTIVES

- Reduce infections caused by key foodborne pathogens to incidences of no more than (See table):

Disease (per 100,000)	1987 Baseline*	2000 Target
Salmonella species	18	16
Campylobacter jejuni	50	25
Escherichia coli 0157:H7	8	4
Listeria monocytogenes	0.7	0.5

- Reduce outbreaks of infections due to *Salmonella enteritidis* to fewer than 25 outbreaks yearly. (Baseline: 77 outbreaks in 1989.)*

RISK REDUCTION OBJECTIVES

Increase to at least 75% the proportion of households in which principal food preparers routinely refrain from leaving perishable food out of the refrigerator for over 2 hours and wash cutting boards and utensils with soap after contact with raw meat and poultry. (Baseline: For refrigeration of perishable foods, 70%; for washing cutting boards with soap, 66%; and for washing utensils with soap, 55%, 1988.)**

SERVICES AND PROTECTION OBJECTIVES

Extend to at least 70% the proportion of states and territories that have implemented model food codes for institutional food operations and to at least 70% the proportion that have adopted the new uniform food protection code ("Unicode") that sets recommended standards for regulation of all food operations. (Baseline: For institutional food operations currently using FDA's recommended model codes, 20%; for the new Unicode released in 1991, 0% in 1990.)***

Baseline data source: Center for Infectious Diseases.
**Baseline data source:* FDA Food Safety Survey, USDA Diet-Health Knowledge Survey.
***Baseline data source:* Center for Food Safety and Applied Nutrition.

Figure 15-3

Status of food and drug safety objectives in the 1995–1996 Healthy People 2000 Review. *Source:* U.S. Department of Health and Human Services, PHS/CDC/NCHS.

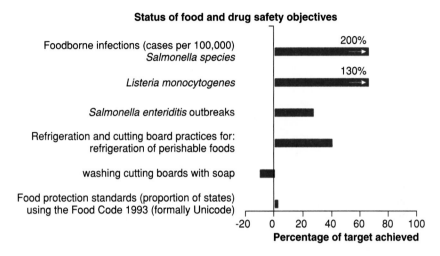

The 1995 mid-decade review of national objectives shows progress on food safety objectives (figure 15-3). The majority of states report the rate of *Salmonella* infections below the year 2000 target number of 16 per 100,000 people although 12 states and the District of Columbia still exceed the target. The practice of refrigerating perishable foods is slowly increasing, while that of washing cutting boards with soap showed little change. There was a reduction in the observed incidence of *listeriosis*—one of the four most common pathogens—largely as a result of industry, regulatory, and educational efforts conducted by public and private sector organizations working together. Replication of this success may not be possible with other pathogens because of changing epidemiology of foodborne diseases, increased consumer demand for fresh foods year-round, and the appearance of emerging pathogens in new products.

Some of the successes in food safety are found in targeted prevention efforts. For example, safe food preparation practices and the use of pasteur-

ized eggs in nursing homes have been encouraged because of the increased susceptibility to *Salmonellosis* by the elderly and those with compromised immune systems. There has also been an 81 percent decline in the incidence of gastrointestinal illnesses since 1974 among American Indians and Alaska Natives reflecting the success of educational efforts directed at food handlers.

CONTROL OVER FOOD PRODUCTION

In the United States the Food and Drug Administration (FDA) has the main responsibility to protect the safety and quality of foods. One of its concerns is to ensure the safety of the food supply by reducing and eliminating the health risks posed by contaminated foods, foodborne infections, and improper handling of food, by commercial food handlers and consumers. The closer the implementation of this control is to the consumer, the more effective the control. On the state or provincial level, the departments or ministries of agriculture

· · · · · · · · · · · · · · · · · · · ·
Figure 15-4

New regulations in the United States require industry to identify critical points in the food chain from farm to table where contamination can occur and to take preventive action. What are some of these critical points? *Source:* Photos by P. Almasy, courtesy World Health Organization/FAO.

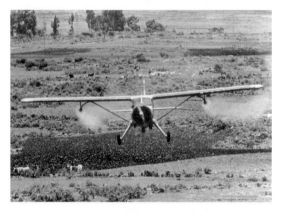

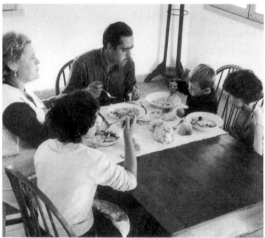

and of health have responsibility for controlling foods. On the community level, the county, district, or city health department usually has this responsibility.

Major changes are in place in the way the food supply is protected in the United States. Underlying these changes are two major themes. The first

is a shift toward greater industry responsibility for producing safe, not just wholesome, products. This means industry no longer can rely on government to determine "safe" production. Instead, industry is legally responsible for analyzing food production processes and identifying critical control points where contamination might occur and take preventive action. The principles of Hazard Analysis Critical Control Points (**HACCP**) will help identify hazards from farm, feed lot, or lake to the table (see figures 15-4).

The second shift in food protection incorporates the best science available into decisions about food safety. Rather than inspecting meat with reliance only on senses of sight, touch, and smell, new protocols aim to make food-safety regulation more science-based (see figure 15-5). While the old system focused on animal health and food quality issues, the new system focuses on preventing risks to people.

In the global economy, however, external pressures are brought on countries about issues such as food safety. For example, the United States and the European Union have had extensive negotiations about meat safety. The Europeans claim the U.S slaughterhouses have lazy hygiene, while the United States claims the European standards are protectionist. In the balance are not only public health concerns, but over $700 million annually in dairy, egg, and fish products.

Control of Milk and Dairy Products

Pathogens can enter milk from many sources, but there will likely be only two reservoirs: the cow and human beings who handle the milk. Accordingly, cows should be tested for tuberculosis, brucellosis, and mastitis, and those who test positive should be culled from the dairy herd. Even though pasteurization would destroy the organisms causing these diseases, it would be foolhardy not to take the extra precaution of preventing pathogens from entering milk to be consumed by humans. Clinical examination of dairy personnel is of questionable value except where there is a history of tuberculosis or typhoid fever.

•••••••••••••••••••

Figure 15-5

New food regulations will give meat inspectors more scientifically based tests to determine contamination rather than relying solely on sight, smell, and touch. *Source:* Photo by P. Almasy, courtesy World Health Organization.

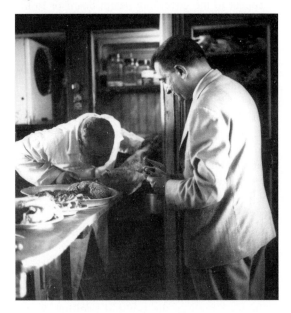

Milk Processing   With the use of modern equipment, milk can go from the cow's udder to the bottle without ever being exposed to light. However even with the finest equipment, milk processing still requires training of the operating personnel, well-constructed stables with cement gutters, ample light, well-maintained ventilation, and fly control. A separate milking room has merit from the standpoint of sanitation. Whether hand milking or machine milking is used, objects that might contaminate the milk should be decontaminated or removed from the milk house. Producing farms should filter or strain milk and cool it to 50° F (10° C) immediately after milking.

Pasteurization   As the best available safeguard against transmission of disease via milk, **pasteurization** consists of heating to a temperature for a period of time that will destroy pathogens but will not appreciably affect the quality of the product. The "holding" method of pasteurization heats the milk to 143° F (62° C) and holds it at this level for 30 minutes. This method destroys pathogens but does not affect taste, proteins, fats, sugars, or salts. It does reduce the level of vitamin C, but milk is not relied on as a source of this nutrient anyway, since the vitamin C content of milk is normally low. The "flash" method of pasteurization does the same job by heating the milk to 161° F (72° C) for 15 seconds.

Cooling and bottling should be done immediately after the pasteurizing. A temperature of 50° F (10° C) should be maintained. Paper containers have some advantages over bottles.

Salmonellosis Outbreaks   The largest recorded outbreak of **Salmonella** poisoning in the United States occurred in 1985 in Illinois. The Illinois Department of Public Health confirmed 5,770 cases of Salmonellosis. The pathogen was isolated from unopened containers of two lots of 2% milk processed at the same dairy plant in Illinois. The milk must have been inadequately pasteurized or contaminated after pasteurization. The contaminated milk was sold in three supermarket chains in Illinois, Indiana, Iowa, and Michigan. After the source of the outbreak had been identified, the dairy plant was closed immediately and all milk produced by the plant was removed from store shelves. In addition to the Illinois cases of Salmonellosis, 289 cases were reported in Indiana, 43 in Michigan, and 28 in Iowa. Three other states reported 19 cases among persons returning from one of those states.

The rate of Salmonellosis cases, excluding typhoid fever, increased in the United States from 1955 when the rate was only 3 per 100,000 to 77 per 100,000 in 1989. Figure 15-6 shows a downward trend starting in the early 1990s.

Regulation of Milk Supplies   In some countries, state or provincial agricultural departments regulate milk supplies. In others the agricultural

••••••••••••••••••

Figure 15-6

The year 2000 objective to reduce outbreaks of infections due to *Salmonella enteritidis* to fewer than twenty-five reported outbreaks per year will be difficult to achieve if trends after 1985 continue. *Source:* U.S. Department of Agriculture, Centers for Disease Control and Prevention, and the Food and Drug Administration.

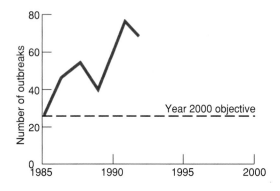

department regulates economic factors and the health department regulates sanitation of milk supplies. Some states have a milk control board. State regulations set standards, but the most effective control exists on the local level. Accordingly, on the recommendation of the city health department, cities pass ordinances regulating the sale of milk in the community. A county, through its health department, also can regulate the sale of milk within its jurisdiction. These regulations can exceed state standards but cannot be lower than state standards.

The U.S. Public Health Service has developed a model ordinance governing the marketing of milk. Communities adopt ordinances adapted from this model. The model ordinance recognizes two grades of milk to be sold to the public. In addition to specifications dealing with farm facilities, processing methods, and other essentials, the ordinance sets up laboratory examination criteria of grades of milk.

Regulations are enforced by the issuance of a permit to sell milk following approval of the farm, the processing facilities, and other factors. Peri-

odic inspections by sanitarians will apprise the dairy farmer of the sanitary quality of his or her operation. A health department, after reasonable warnings, may order a dairy farmer or milk plant to discontinue the sale of milk or refuse to renew the permit when it expires. The seller has the right to appeal to the governing health board or to the courts.

Milk Products   Manufacture of milk products has become big business, with processes controlled through state or provincial regulation, supplemented by local supervision, protecting the community against epidemics.

Ice cream mixes are pasteurized and stored at 10° F (minus 12° C). Contamination would come from containers, dippers, and dispensers. Processing of frozen desserts comes under the same official scrutiny as does processing of other dairy products.

Butter requires pasteurization at higher levels than market milk. The fat is promptly cooled and then held in vats for churning. Cheese, because its curing process kills most pathogens, is relatively safe. "Green" cheese (not time-cured) can transmit pathogens such as the typhoid bacillus. Some cheese manufacturers take the precaution of pasteurizing the milk they use, but most do not deem this necessary. Cottage cheese, unless pasteurized and stored at 40° F (4° C), could easily transmit pathogens to human populations.

The managers of most processing plants take pride in their business and can be relied on to produce a safe product. The relationship between processors and inspectors is usually harmonious. Inspectors serve in an advisory capacity on sanitation and in a regulating role. Legal measures to enforce sanitary standards for dairy products are usually employed only after all other means have failed.

Control of Meat, Fish, and Poultry

The public rebels against eating the meat from diseased animals. In 1996, "mad cow" disease in England caused an international uproar in the beef industry. Even though cooking or curing kills

ISSUES AND CONTROVERSIES
Mad Cows? Mad Response?

In 1996 a panic over "mad-cow disease" in England attracted worldwide attention. The panic heightened when the British government acknowledged a likely link between mad-cow disease (Bovine spongiform encephalopathy—BSE) and a rare neurological disorder in humans (Creutzfeldt-Jakob disease). While a pathogen such as *E. coli* 0157:H7 can be destroyed with proper cooking, the infectious protein involved in these diseases seem difficult to kill with heat. Despite the small number of cases, both diseases were given much ink by the tabloid press. As a result, many countries banned British beef causing huge economic losses and a political uproar. Consumers across the world boycotted beef over fears of mad cow disease, sending beef sales slumping and threatening meat industry jobs. Plans were made in Britain to destroy up to 30,000 cattle a week. Beef is used in a wide variety of products, such as gelatin used in jellies, biscuits, and pies; keratin used in shampoo, and oleic oil in margarine, therefore concerns about beef safety spread to other industries. Charges were made that early research on the effects of these diseases were ignored, while questions about liability for destroying animals and compensating ill humans remain to be resolved.

How is it that rare diseases such as BSE and Creutzfeldt-Jakob disease can cause such an international stir when common food pathogens such as *Campylobacter jejuni* and *listeriosis* are unheard of tongue twisters to the public? What are the contributory roles of the media, regulatory agencies, politicians, researchers, health professionals, talk show hosts, and business to such a global event?

pathogens, biochemical changes in the animal can give the meat a foul taste and even produce human illness. In addition, how meat is processed after slaughter affects its palatability and nutritional qualities. Improper canning can also be a danger to humans in that pathogens conveyed to the meat can survive and cause disease. The public also expects to be protected against the adding of cornmeal or other grains to ground meat or processed meats.

Control Measures   Training of personnel, health education, demonstrations, and conferences have supported proper meat processing. Nevertheless, there remains a need for governmental inspection of meat on the national, state or provincial, and local levels.

The Meat Inspection Act of 1906 created the Meat Inspection Division of the U.S. Department of Agriculture. The act sought to safeguard the public by eliminating diseased or other bad meat from distribution, to supervise the sanitary preparation of meat and meat products, and to prevent the use of false or misleading names or statements on labels. Technically, the authority of the federal agency extends only over meats and meat products shipped in interstate or international commerce. However, courts have interpreted "interstate" so broadly that nearly all transported meat is being so classed. This has caused some conflict between federal and state inspection functions, particularly in those states with decidedly inadequate meat inspection programs. In general, the large meat plants have fallen under federal regulation and the small local plants have been left to state or community inspection.

In 1967 Congress passed the first substantive legislation on meat inspection since the original act of 1906. The new act provided that the states had to have inspection requirements at least equal to those of the federal government. The act authorized the U.S. Secretary of Agriculture to take over interstate meat inspection in states falling below the federal standards. Title I of the act greatly broadened the scope of inspection, so that more than five-hundred additional plants were subject to federal regulation.

In 1992 the U.S. Public Health Service and the U.S. Department of Agriculture endorsed the use of **irradiation** as a safe and effective means to control *salmonella* and other foodborne bacteria in raw chicken, turkey, and other poultry. Up to 60 percent of poultry sold in North America is contaminated with *salmonella,* and studies suggest that all chicken may be contaminated with the *Campylobacter* organism. Consumer apprehension of irradiation has been a drawback to implementing the procedure, even though irradiation does not make food radioactive or increase human exposure to radiation. Some states either banned or issued a moratorium on the sale of irradiated foods in response to public fears. The World Health Organization concluded that irradiation can substantially reduce food poisoning, although it should not be used as a substitute for careful handling, storage, and cooking of food. Irradiated poultry can become recontaminated.

One other control measure not yet adopted in North America, but developed in Japan and widely used there and gradually in Europe, is **high-pressure food processing.** Not to be confused with home pressure cooking, this commercial process uses water pressure instead of heat. In conventional pasteurizing of packaged liquid products, food makers typically boil the food in batches to kill bacteria, but this destroys some taste and up to 30 percent of vitamins and minerals. High-pressure food processing preserves the fresh taste and nutritional quality of the food. It is most widely used with jams and other fruit products but is increasingly applied to meat, fish, and poultry processing.

Fresh Meats   Some slaughterhouses limit their activities to slaughtering and the necessary cold storage, but many meatpacking plants combine slaughtering, cold storage, freezing, smoking, and pickling operations. In the United States most states supplement the federal meat inspection program by having their own inspection services for most slaughterhouses and all packing plants not under federal inspection.

Inspection of animals before slaughter serves to detect any disease or other adverse conditions. Killing, bleeding, and postmortem inspections of the hides, carcasses, and organs will detect gross pathology, and tissue examination will further detect disease conditions. Questionable carcasses are condemned, although the meat may be used for some purposes. A "grade" stamp on meat designates the grade quality of the meat, while the "inspection" stamp indicates that the meat has been passed as being safe.

Beef is placed immediately after slaughter in a cooler at 34° F (1° C), where it will be stored from 4 to 6 weeks. This storage improves flavor and texture because of the autolysis that occurs. Beef frozen at minus 15° F (minus 26° C) can be stored for more than a year. Pork, veal, and mutton are usually held for 3 days before being cut (see table 15-1).

Cured and Processed Meats   Curing of such products as bacon, ham, and frankfurters calls for chilled meat that is moderately moist, pickling solution and brine, and a covered vat to prevent contamination. Cured meats are not necessarily completely protected against spoilage or deterioration. Proper storage is always necessary.

Processed meats pose the greatest danger of meats and meat products. The usual processing of luncheon meats does not assure the destruction of all pathogens. Packaging and storage under inadequate refrigeration can provide a medium in which pathogens of humans can readily multiply; once the package is opened and the food handled, the remaining meat is often left at room temperature for some time, and then, in many instances, placed in refrigerators with temperatures considerably above 50° F (10° C).

Canned Meats   Canned meats are first cooked. High temperatures and pressures are used without seriously affecting the quality of the product. Bacterial contamination can occur, with C. botulinum being one of the pathogens that might survive. Modern methods of meat canning minimize this risk.

Table 15-1

Guidelines for Market and Home Storage of Fresh Meats and Dairy Products Underscore the Importance of "Use by" Dating of Products to Indicate How Long a Product Will Retain Optimum Quality before Consumption.

These SHORT but safe time limits will help keep refrigerated food from spoiling or becoming dangerous to eat. These time limits will keep frozen food at top quality.

Product	Refrigerator (40° F)	Freezer (0° F)
Eggs		
Fresh, in shell	3 weeks	Don't freeze
Raw yolks, whites	2–4 days	1 year
Hardcooked	1 week	Don't freeze well
Liquid pasteurized egg or egg substitutes, opened	3 days	Don't freeze
unopened	10 days	1 year
Mayonnaise, commercial		
Refrigerate after opening	2 months	Don't freeze
TV Dinners, Frozen Casseroles		
Keep frozen until ready to serve		3–4 months
Deli & Vacuum-Packed Products		
Store-prepared (or homemade) egg, chicken, tuna, ham, macaroni salads	3–5 days	These products don't freeze well.
Pre-stuffed pork & lamb chops, chicken breasts stuffed with dressing	1 day	
Store-cooked convenience meals	1–2 days	
Commercial brand vacuum-packed dinners with USDA seal	2 weeks, unopened	
Soups & Stews		
Vegetable or meat-added	3–4 days	2–3 months
Hamburger, Ground & Stew Meats		
Hamburger & stew meats	1–2 days	3–4 months
Ground turkey, veal, pork, lamb & mixtures of them	1–2 days	3–4 months
Hotdogs & Lunch Meats		
Hotdogs, opened package	1 week	
unopened package	2 weeks	In freezer wrap,
Lunch meats, opened	3–5 days	1–2 months
unopened	2 weeks	
Bacon & Sausage		
Bacon	7 days	1 month
Sausage, raw from pork, beef, turkey	1–2 days	1–2 months
Smoked breakfast links, patties	7 days	1–2 months
Hard sausage—pepperoni, jerky sticks	2–3 weeks	1–2 months

continued.

Table 15-1—*Continued.*

Product	Refrigerator (40° F)	Freezer (0° F)
Ham, Corned Beef		
Corned beef		Drained, wrapped
In pouch with pickling juices	5–7 days	1 month
Ham, canned		
Label says keep refrigerated	6–9 months	Don't freeze
Ham, fully cooked—whole	7 days	1–2 months
Ham, fully cooked—half	3–5 days	1–2 months
Ham, fully cooked—slices	3–4 days	1–2 months
Fresh Meat		
Steaks, beef	3–5 days	6–12 months
Chops, pork	3–5 days	4–6 months
Chops, lamb	3–5 days	6–9 months
Roasts, beef	3–5 days	6–12 months
Roasts, lamb	3–5 days	6–9 months
Roasts, pork & veal	3–5 days	4–6 months
Variety meats—Tongue, brain, kidneys, liver, heart, chitterlings	1–2 days	3–4 months
Meat Leftovers		
Cooked meat and meat dishes	3–4 days	2–3 months
Gravy and meat broth	1–2 days	2–3 months
Fresh Poultry		
Chicken or turkey, whole	1–2 days	1 year
Chicken or turkey pieces	1–2 days	9 months
Giblets	1–2 days	3–4 months
Cooked Poultry, Leftover		
Fried chicken	3–4 days	4 months
Cooked poultry dishes	3–4 days	4–6 months
Pieces, plain	3–4 days	4 months
Pieces covered with broth, gravy	1–2 days	6 months
Chicken nuggets, patties	1–2 days	1–3 months

Source: U.S. Department of Agriculture, Food Safety and Inspection Service, 1990.

Fish and Shellfish   Fish is processed much like beef products. Fish can be held at a temperature of 40° F (4° C) for two weeks and be in excellent condition. Quick-freezing of fish, followed by a dip into clean water, produces an airtight coat of ice around each fish. All equipment used in processing fish should be decontaminated daily.

Other seafood, especially raw shellfish and fish harvested in unfavorable environments, pose a greater risk of foodborne illness. Ranking highest in risk of transmitting seafood-borne illness are raw or undercooked molluscan shellfish (oysters, clams, and mussels). Clams and oysters live by filtering 15 to 20 gallons of water per day, so they become concentrated storehouses of bacteria and viruses if they live in polluted waters. The human risk is 1 illness per 250 servings of raw shellfish, whereas the risk from other seafood is 1 illness per 5 million servings. The comparative risk for poultry is 10 times less—1 in 25,000 servings. Raw shellfish account for 85 percent of the illnesses caused by eating seafood. Thorough cooking (internal temperature 140° F) will kill nearly all bacteria and viruses.

Waters polluted with human sewage and chemical contamination are major sources of problems. The most effective ways of protecting the safety of this food supply is preventing human wastes from getting into the waters and improving the monitoring of estuaries to prevent illegal harvesting of shellfish from polluted waters. Sixty percent of health warnings against fish consumption are related to mercury contamination, mainly because of air pollution from coal-burning power plants, industrial sites, and incinerators. Other contaminants include PCBs (a banned electrical insulator), the pesticide chlordane, dioxins, and the banned pesticide DDT. Fish advisories are issued by states to limit consumption of certain species of fish taken from waters where these chemical contaminants are present. Most of these advisories apply to non-commercial fishing.

Various measures help protect against these contaminates. Proper cooking, once again, is the best self-protective measure individuals, families, and other food preparers can take. In the 1997 recall of millions of pounds of tainted beef, some policymakers expressed concern that such a massive recall gave the public a false sense of security that their food supply is safe. The only safe courses are cooking ground beef to at least 160° F or industry irradiation of food. On-site inspection methods (sight and smell) between these two ends of the food protection chain cannot detect the viruses that cause hepatitis and the several types of bacteria that cause gastroenteritis from contaminated shellfish (figure 15-7). Unlike meat and poultry, seafood is not subject to comprehensive mandatory inspections in North America. The FDA inspects only a tiny fraction of the 2.9 billion pounds of seafood imported each year, despite that 50 percent of all seafood consumed in the United States is imported.

Canada has become increasingly concerned with the growing presence of toxins found in its fish. This is becoming a greater problem in

Figure 15-7

As North Americans become more concerned with high fat foods, they are turning more to fish and experiencing more seafood-borne illnesses. Japan has long depended more on fish and has developed a wider range of inspection and testing methods, especially with those varieties used in sushi and other raw fish preparations. *Source:* World Health Organization.

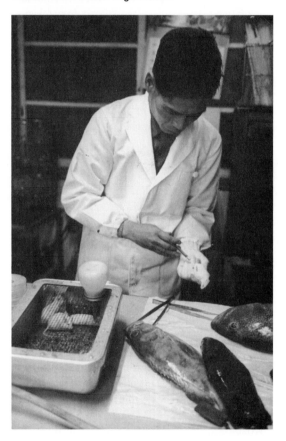

Canada than the problems of bacteria or virus in seafood, especially for Native Indian and Inuit populations that depend heavily on fish for sustenance and for the regions in which heavy runoff of pesticides in agricultural areas are finding their way up the food chain to fish. The Great Lakes produce fish with high levels of industrial chemicals, and these are harvested as game fish.

Poultry Poultry should be observed for a few days before killing. Poultry is quick-frozen at minus 30° F (minus 34° C) and stored at minus 10° F (minus 23° C). Canned poultry is processed under steam pressure of about fifteen pounds per square inch, which should kill the salmonella organism that fowl may harbor. If cold turkey or chicken is eaten without having been refrigerated since being served hot, salmonellosis transmission might occur.

Modern refrigeration and cooking facilities leave no excuse to transmit disease via meat. Unfortunately, handling of cold meats by a person who has an active case of or is a carrier of one of the food-borne diseases remains a likely mode of disease transmission via meat.

EATING ESTABLISHMENT REGULATIONS

No overwhelming evidence exists that dust or other dirt or a person coughing on food will transfer disease to the person who eats the food. However the public is entitled to sanitary and safe food when it eats in a public eating establishment. Cases of salmonellosis and viral hepatitis acquired in public eating places are more common than is realized. Amebic dysentery and typhoid fever can also result from eating in restaurants, schools, company cafeterias, and other institutions.

Citizens patronizing a public eating establishment may be neither qualified nor in a position to judge its sanitation. They must depend on the expertise and vigilance of the community health staff. However a better informed public could be a positive aid to the health staff by looking for restaurant ratings and by insisting that public eating places practice sanitation standards set forth by the health department. Children and the elderly deserve special protection because they are more vulnerable.

Control Measures

Licensing of public eating places provides the instrument of control. To qualify for a license, the establishment must satisfy the equipment and operating requirements of the health department (see figure 15-8). Once the license has been issued, health department sanitarians make periodic inspections. Frequency and timing of inspections will depend on the known conditions of the restaurant and the number of available sanitarians.

Inspections

Rating of the restaurant usually follows the first inspection. Sanitarians find precise numerical rating to be difficult. Some health departments give A, B, or C ratings. Other departments give a rating of "approved." A restaurant disapproved following an inspection will be given a probationary period in which to correct the deficiencies shown on the inspection form. Renewal of the operating permit will be denied if the establishment has failed to correct its faults. The owner may appeal to the community board of health and, in the event of an adverse decision, may appeal to the courts.

Personnel Clinical examinations of new employees, even if accompanied by laboratory tests, are of limited value as a means for preventing disease spread via the restaurant. A more effective measure is to have employees well informed on the nature of disease spread and to enlist their active support in control. Above all, they should not come to work when they may have a communicable disease. Workshops for food handlers are held periodically by health departments to protect the patrons of eating establishments against infectious disease.

Facilities Another key in the protection of the public is a safe water supply, a proper toilet and lavatory facilities, and approved methods of waste disposal. Proper refrigeration and storage of food is highly important. Corrosion-proof utensils and equipment should be properly sanitized with detergents, decontaminants, and hot rinse water. All other safety factors are significant but perhaps not as vital as those mentioned. Many sanitarians contend that rodent control is particularly important.

· ·

Figure 15-8

Inspectors for a local health department, wearing identification badges and using a check list and testing equipment, examine the sanitary conditions at a local restaurant. *Source:* Missouri Department of Health.

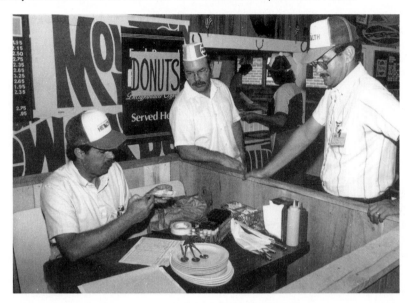

A meaningful overview of a full inspection can be garnered from the items in eating and drinking establishments that most local departments of health require their sanitarians to inspect. These items are listed not by order of importance, but for inspection convenience in the box on page 480.

The integrity of the management and the training and supervision of the employees produce restaurant personnel who are aware of their responsibility to the public and who know how to prepare and serve food properly.

Bakeries and Confectionaries Safeguards in producing bakery and confectionary products are similar to those essential to restaurant operations but are somewhat less demanding. Employee exclusion when necessary as a communicable disease control measure, safe water supply, proper waste disposal, protection against rodents and insects, proper refrigeration, and sanitizing of utensils are all important. The use of sanitary ingredients and the exercise of sanitary precautions during manufacture are also significant. Wrapping and other sanitary provisions are essential in handling and storing the finished product. Although sanitary inspections should be made at intervals, these establishments are rarely a cause of disease transmission.

Retail Food Stores In retail food stores, safety of food is a first consideration in protecting the public. Refrigeration and storage are of primary importance. Elimination of spoiled foods should be prompt and complete. Employees convalescing from an infection of the digestive tract should not handle uncovered foods. It would be difficult for organisms they might transfer to lettuce, tomatoes, or other produce to survive the customer's journey home, but the risk should not be ignored.

Cleanliness is an important consideration. The customer is usually assured of clean food because of modern packaging. Self-service gives customers

A Food Inspector's Checklist

Floors
    Cleanable, good repair; smooth, nonabsorbent; cleaned properly.

Walls and Ceilings
    Clean, good repair; finished, light color; washable to level of splash.

Lighting
    Adequate light; working surfaces; storage rooms, preparation areas; fixtures clean.

Ventilation
    Adequate ventilation; free from odors, condensate; stove hoods and ventilators, adequate design.

Toilet Facilities
    Clean, ventilated; convenient, ample number; proper construction, good repair.

Water Supply
    Adequate supply and pressure; approved construction; safe, complies with state standards.

Lavatory Facilities
    Adequate, convenient to kitchen; hot and cold water; soap, sanitary towels, or air dryer; clean; good repair.

Construction of Utensils, Equipment
    Cleanable construction; self-draining, no corrosion; free from cracks, chips; no open seams; no toxic utensils.

Cleaning of Equipment
    Clean cases, counters, shelves, tables, meat blocks, refrigerators, stoves, hoods, can openers, freezers, and so on; clean cloths used.

Cleaning of Utensils
    Single service used only once; dishwasher, sinks, drainboards approved and maintained; kitchenware, tableware clean; dishwashing procedures approved.

Bacterial Treatment of Utensils
    Approved sanitization, time, temperature, chemical concentration; machine properly operated; kitchenware adequately treated; dishtowels not being used.

Storage and Handling of Utensils
    Protected from contamination; no handling of contact surfaces; single serviceware properly handled; dippers kept in running water.

Disposal of Wastes
    Approved liquid waste disposal; plumbing complies with state code; approved garbage cans; covered, pending removal; clean and in good repair; garbage storage and removal approved.

Food Temperatures
    Cold perishable food below 45° F (7° C); hot perishable food above 140° F (60° C); ice storing, handling approved; thermometer in each refrigerator; refrigerators maintained.

Wholesomeness of Food
    Clean, no spoilage, safe; approved sources.

Wholesomeness of Milk Products
    Milk, milk products approved; milk dispensed properly.

Wholesomeness of Shellfish
    Approved sources; stored in original containers.

Preparation and Storage of Food
    No contamination by immersion, leaking, or condensation; neat storage, off floor.

Display and Serving of Food, Drink
    Minimum manual contact; food wrapped or covered; cafeteria front protected.

Vector Control
    Fly control approved; roaches, insects controlled; rodents under control; structure rat-proof; no animals or fowls; all poisonous compounds stored away from food, proper use.

Cleanliness of Employees
    Clean outer garments; clean hands and nails; no spitting, no tobacco used in rooms where food is prepared.

Housekeeping
    Site, premises neat and clean; no operations in private quarters; adequate clothing lockers and dressing rooms kept clean; storage of soiled clothing, linens, mops, and so on.

Control
    No person at work with any communicable disease, sores, or infected wounds; washing sign posted in all toilet facilities.

an opportunity to do some inspecting themselves. However the cleanliness of the whole store is desirable, and store managers know they will not be in business long if their store is not clean. Safe water should be used for all store purposes.

Community health departments do not find retail food stores a great problem. Occasionally the health department will have complaints against a market. For example, failure to dispose of discarded produce does pose a problem when employees are lax. A written warning by the health department sanitarian usually produces the necessary remedy.

FOOD SAFETY EDUCATION FOR THE HOME

Despite the many technical advances in safeguarding the food the public eats, the need for individuals to contribute to their own protection is ever present. Recent research, however, shows a decline in consumer knowledge about safe food handling. In addition, consumers do not appear to be acting on food safety messages that have been used for years by government and industry. This is not good news when the estimates are that up to a third of foodborne illness results from unsafe handling of food at home.

Cases of home-based food-borne illness may become a bigger problem partly because today's busy family may not be as familiar with food safety issues as more home-focused families of past generations. Knowledge about food safety varies by gender and age. One study found that men tended to be less safe about food practices than women and that those younger than forty years tended to be less safe than those over forty years. The increased use of convenience foods, which are specially preserved, gives the consumer the false idea that equivalent home-cooked foods, without such preservatives, are equally safe. Different technologies, such as the microwave, require consumers to be informed about safe cooking containers so that packaging components such

as paper and adhesives do not migrate into food at excessive heat levels.

To bring issues of food safety to the public's attention a new public/private partnership is planned among several federal agencies and consumer and food industry groups. This new consumer education campaign is sponsored under the Partnership for Food Safety Education. Education from farm-to-table is considered a top priority. The partnership plans to develop accurate, science-based, and consumer-oriented messages to promote safe handling behaviors by the public. Such public education programs aim at not only providing information about food safety, but suggest cooperative strategies that food handlers and the public can use to put such information to work.

Prevention of foodborne illnesses for the home starts with food choices at the local supermarket. Public messages can increase awareness of the hazards of out-of-date products, torn packages, or loose and bulging lids on jars and cans. In the home, food safety concerns revolve around three main functions: food storage, handling, and cooking. Careless food handling sets the stage for the growth of disease-causing pathogens. For example, hot or cold foods left standing too long at room temperature provide an ideal climate for bacteria to grow. Improper cooking also plays role in foodborne illness whether eating at home or eating out (see table 15-2). Foods may be cross-contaminated when cutting boards and kitchen tools that have been used to prepare a contaminated food, such as raw chicken, are not cleaned before being used for another food, such as vegetables.

These possible sources of food contamination lead to identification of essentials in home food safety. The year 2000 objectives for food safety includes refrigeration and cutting board practices for perishable foods. These are practices that apply not only to public eating establishments, but the home kitchen.

Educational messages need to be timely, culturally appropriate, geographically relevant, and economically feasible. For example, figure 15-9

Table 15-2

Guidelines for Cooking Temperature of Egg and Meat Products.

Product	Fahrenheit
Eggs & Egg Dishes	
Eggs	Cook until yolk & white are firm
Egg dishes	160
Ground Meat & Meat Mixture	
Turkey, chicken	170
Veal, beef, lamb, pork	160
Fresh Beef	
Rare (some bacterial risk)	140
Medium	160
Well Done	170
Fresh Veal	
Medium	160
Well Done	170
Fresh Lamb	
Medium	160
Well Done	170
Fresh Pork	
Medium	160
Well Done	170
Poultry	
Chicken, whole	180
Turkey, whole	180
Poultry breasts, roasts	170
Poultry thighs, wings	Cook until juices run clear
Stuffing (cooked alone or in bird)	165
Duck & Goose	180
Ham	
Fresh (raw)	160
Pre-cooked (to reheat)	140

Source: U.S. Department of Agriculture, Food Safety and Inspection Service, 1990.

Home Food Safety Musts

- Get perishable foods into the refrigerator as quickly as possible after buying them.
- Wash raw vegetables thoroughly
- Keep your kitchen or food preparation areas clean.
- Wash your hands before preparing food.
- Keep hot foods hot and cold foods cold after they are prepared.

Source: DHHS publication no. (FDA) 91-2244

APPRAISAL OF FOOD CONTROL MEASURES

Constant vigilance by health officials is essential to protect the public against foodborne diseases. Customers cannot make their own inspections of restaurants, dairies, slaughterhouses, or canneries, and they cannot see what goes on in the back room of retail stores and bakeries. They must depend on the technical expertise of officials paid from taxes. Customers can aid their own cause by being knowledgeable and by cooperating with public officials who are protecting them.

Many technical fields have provided communities with methods and procedures for protection against the transmission of disease and poisons. Freezing as an alternative to canning is convenient and safe. Chemical additives lend protection and danger. Legislation protects consumers against the indiscriminate use of ingredients such as soybeans in hamburgers. Legislation also protects the public by requiring sanitation and proper food handling in the retail business. This has become increasingly important with the growth of food chains and franchise marketing. The "natural food" fads have required some degree of official supervision, though largely in the area of fair trade rather than as vehicles of disease spread.

New foodborne diseases, such as *Campylobacter,* are emerging and previously common but

shows that illness from four of the most common foodborne pathogens increase during the summer months. Figure 15-10 shows how these data can be transformed into a timely summer message to the public about safe cooking outdoors.

· · · · · · · · · · · · · · · · · · · ·

Figure 15-9

Cases of illness from foodborne pathogens vary throughout the year. Such data can be used to produce timely messages to the public about food safety. *Source:* Data from report to Congress. Food Safety and Inspection Service/CDC/FDA.

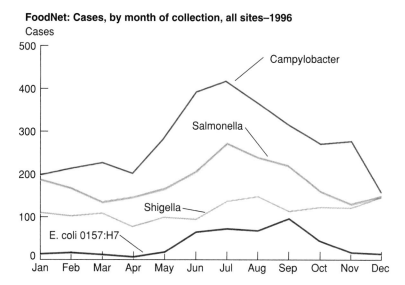

· · · · · · · · · · · · · · · · · · · ·

Figure 15-10

This summertime message states the problem, provides strategies to deal with the problem, and offers a hotline number for more information.

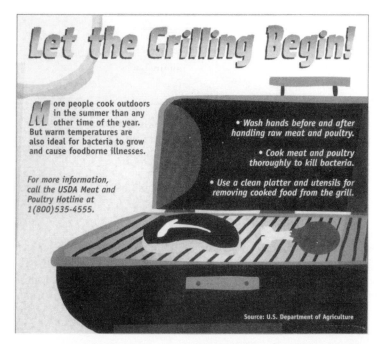

....

Figure 15-11

Many factors or combinations of factors are making it easier for infectious diseases to become bigger problems now and in the future. *Source:* American Association for World Health.

Why some infectious diseases are making deadly comebacks

Changing lifestyles ─────────────────────────────

Changes in food processing . . . . *E. coli* O157:H7
handling, and consumption
                                      Hepatitis A
                                      Listeriosis
                                      Salmonellosis

Increased use of childcare facilities . . . . Cryptosporidiosis
                                      Giardiasis
                                      Hepatitis A
                                      Meningitis
                                      Shigellosis

Substance abuse and . . . . Chlamydia
unsafe sexual practices
                                      Hepatitis B
                                      HIV infection

Increased air travel
                                      All infectious diseases

Growing global population and movement ────────────

Changes in land use . . . . Hantavirus pulmonary syndrome
                                      Lyme disease
                                      Rabies

Increased urbanization . . . . Dengue hemorrhagic fever
in the tropics
                                      Yellow fever

Changing public policies ──────────────────────────

Breakdown in public health . . . . Cryptosporidiosis
prevention programs
                                      Dengue hemorrhagic fever
                                      Measles
                                      Rabies
                                      Tuberculosis

---

usually benign organisms, such as *E. coli* and *salmonella,* are increasingly sources of outbreaks, even as scourges of the past, such as botulism and trichinosis, are declining. Several factors account for the rise in foodborne illnesses (see figure 15-11). Ironically, the health interests of large numbers of people seeking lower-fat alternatives in poultry and fish are one contributing factor. Per capita consumption of chicken in the United States rose from 40 pounds in 1970 to 70 pounds in 1990. Other causes lie in new food processing technologies introducing new risks, the aging of the population, and growing numbers of immunosuppressed people with HIV infections who are more susceptible to foodborne illness and more vulnerable to severe outcomes. Food control measures become more important as new technologies allow transport and prolonged storage of foods produced in large, centralized plants. This means that a single contaminated product can infect more people in a larger geographic area. Similarly, the global marketplace makes the variations in regulations between countries more problematic.

Community control mechanisms provide a critical link in the food safety chain, but individuals must still exercise caution and hygienic practices to protect themselves. Consumers cook less, use more rapid cooking methods such as microwaves, rely on prepared foods, and often have less training and experience in food handling than in times past. The federal governments of the United States and Canada encourage communities to develop tailored educational materials to increase consumer and food handler awareness of methods to prevent foodborne diseases. Farm management strategies and fishery practices to reduce pathogens in poultry, fish, and shellfish, and to reduce pesticide residues in fruits, vegetables, and fish are of growing importance.

VECTOR AND ZOONOSES CONTROL

In the preceding section the focus was on food as a carrier of foodborne pathogens that threaten the public's health. This section focuses on other kinds of transmitters—*vectors*—of pathogenic organisms. A vector is a person, animal, or plant that carries a pathogenic agent and acts as a potential source of infection for members of another species. Commonly known vectors include flies and mosquitos. In community health practice the term vector is not limited strictly to forms of the class Insecta, but includes allied arthropods, such

Figure 15-12

A close-up vividly shows the wings, feet, and body of a fly that can transmit pathogens from one site to another. This particular fly is the Black Fly whose bite transmits onchocerciasis, or river blindness. *Source:* Drawings by Jacqueline Bradshaw-Price, courtesy World Health Organization.

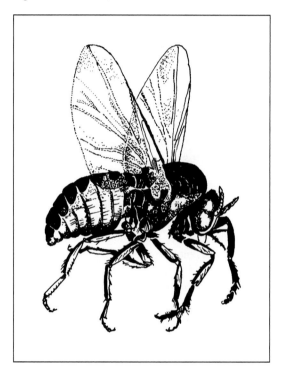

as ticks and mites. The health interest in these forms is in their role in harboring and transferring pathogenic organisms. Nearly all of these are *biological vectors* in that the pathogen passes through part of its life cycle inside the vector or intermediate invertebrate host. The common housefly, however, is strictly a *mechanical vector* that transfers pathogens on its wings, feet, or body (see figure 15-12). Some biological vectors, under certain circumstances, can also function as mechanical vectors.

Zoonoses are the infections or infectious diseases transmissible under natural conditions from vertebrate animals to human beings.

Epidemiology of Vectors

The tick and the common housefly may transfer pathogens even in the northern climates. Communities everywhere have to contend with the nuisance of mosquitoes, flies, lice, and other arthropods, but the significant health problem is their role as vectors of disease.

Transmission of disease by vectors can be described by three patterns or routes over which a disease is transmitted:

Humans—vector—humans

Humans—vector—lower vertebrate—vector—humans (zoonoses)

Lower vertebrate—vector—humans (zoonoses)

Vector—Disease Relationships   Known vector–disease relationships indicate that a *specific* pathogen is transmitted via a *specific* vector. For example, to say that the mosquito transmits yellow fever is not a completely accurate statement. It is only the *Aedes aegypti* mosquito that serves as the intermediate host for the pathogen causing yellow fever. For present purposes, however, the following list identifies the general type of vector with the disease(s) it transmits to humans:

General Vector	**Disease(s) Transmitted**
Mosquitoes:	yellow fever, malaria, encephalitis, filariasis
Fleas:	bubonic plague, murine typhus
Ticks and mites:	Rocky Mountain spotted fever, tularemia, Lyme disease
Biting flies:	tularemia
Lice:	epidemic typhus, relapsing fever
House flies:	salmonellosis

In addition, roaches are suspected of transmitting intestinal diseases, and bedbugs are suspected of conveying relapsing fever. HIV/AIDS cannot be transferred by food or animal vectors (see figure 15-13).

Control Measures   The first principle of vector control is to identify the specific vector and to plan control measures accordingly. When the tick

Figure 15-13

Communication campaigns need to dispel inaccurate beliefs and provide accurate information. This campaign addresses misinformation about how AIDS is spread and provides a hotline number to call for more information. *Source:* America Responds to AIDS.

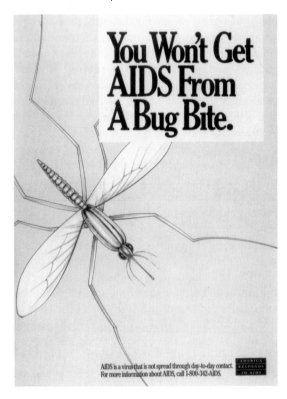

is the known vector, for example, control measures will differ from measures taken when a mosquito is the intermediate host. However three factors must always be considered in vector control: elimination of breeding places, destruction of the insect or its larva, and protection of possible human hosts by preventing the vector from reaching humans. Mosquito control is representative of the classic techniques of insect control, whether the particular species is a vector or simply a general annoyance. Minor variations to the classic approach applies for ticks, flies, lice, and mites.

- Eliminate breeding places
  - —Destroy or empty containers holding water
  - —Fill water holes
  - —Drain ponds, marshes, and swamps
  - —Render bodies of water unsuitable for breeding by using larvicides, releasing water at high velocities, and fluctuating the water level
  - —Divert stream flow
  - —Trim the banks of ponds, lakes, and streams to prevent swamps
  - —Introduce natural antagonists of mosquito larvae, such as fish (Gambusia)
- Destroy adult insects
  - —Spray insecticide in areas populated by mosquitoes
  - —Spread insecticide-impregnated sawdust on surface of flowing streams
  - —Put oil-solution insecticide over rain barrels and other water containers
- Protect humans against contact by mosquito
  - —Screening
  - —Clothing
  - —Nets
  - —Repellents

Insecticides

Like most technologies, insecticides can have harmful and beneficial effects. People, lower vertebrates (wildlife especially), and vegetation (including crops) can be harmed if the insecticide solution is too highly concentrated. Controlling the use of insecticides is imperative. Overuse of insecticides is destroying wildlife. Air and water pollution can be created by insecticides. Unfortunately, because the effects of insecticides on vector populations are only temporary, it is necessary to spray or otherwise apply the insecticide weekly.

The community has a responsibility to reduce vector populations in its area. In North America this is usually a function of the community health department and is carried out in cooperation with state or provincial agencies. Community authorities

Figure 15-14

Chemicals can serve a role in vector control. However national and international collaboration is needed to minimize potential health risks to humans, animals, and the ecology. *Source:* World Health Organization/Documeria.

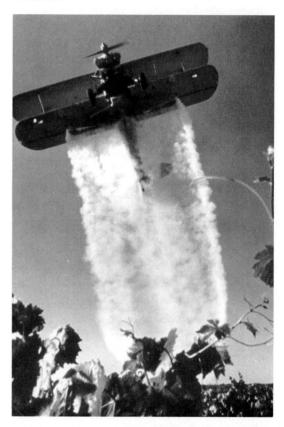

also have a responsibility in regulating the use of insecticides by private citizens. This is primarily a problem of public education directed to specific groups or individuals. Research on insecticides is being carried on by governmental agencies and by scientists in universities and colleges. Identifying permissible concentrations of insecticides is the immediate problem, but the long-range objective is that of developing insecticides that destroy insect vectors but are harmless to people, other animals, and vegetation (see figure 15-14).

Rodent and Zoonoses Control

The term *rodent* encompasses all animals belonging to the order Rodentia. It includes squirrels, rats, mice, and other animals. The ground squirrel can harbor the pathogens that cause Rocky Mountain spotted fever and tularemia in humans and can transmit rabies directly. A vector must transmit most pathogens from rodent to human—for example, the tick for Rocky Mountain spotted fever and the horsefly for tularemia. In the United States control of squirrels is essentially a state and federal problem, and the federal and state governments have extensive programs to eliminate ground squirrels. Field teams using guns, traps, and poisons carry on a constant campaign to eliminate ground squirrels in regions with endemic Rocky Mountain spotted fever and tularemia.

In communities the rodent problem is essentially confined to rats and mice. These rodents cause economic loss, create esthetic problems, and transmit disease. Rats and mice destroy and eat poultry and eggs, grains and sprouts, and corn. They also destroy merchandise. Despite the enormity of this economic loss, it is as carriers of disease that rodents pose the greatest threat to communities.

Rat-Borne Diseases   Rats harbor several pathogens. In many instances the rat dies of the disease. In other instances it remains a carrier of the disease over a considerable time. Although many misconceptions exist regarding the relationship of rats to human disease, at least six diseases of humans are definitely known in which the rat (or house mouse) serves as a reservoir of infection.

Murine typhus:	rat—rat fleas—humans
Bubonic plague:	rat—rat fleas—humans
Weil's disease (infectious jaundice):	urine of rat
Salmonellosis:	feces of rat and house mouse
Rat-bite fever:	bacteria via bite
Rickettsialpox:	house mouse—mite—humans
Leptospirosis	rodents, such as rats

Obviously, not all rats harbor pathogens of humans, but the greater the rat population, the greater the potential reservoir.

Varieties of Rats   Three types of rats are of health concern. The black rat lives in walls and between floors. It has a pointed muzzle, slender body, long tail, and a sooty color. The roof rat is more brown, but otherwise resembles the black rat and usually lives off the ground. The brown rat is also called the sewer rat, wharf rat, and Norway rat. It is a large rodent with a blunt head, short ears, and short tail. It burrows and nests in the ground. Also of concern is the house mouse, which lives in walls, furniture, and other protective places.

Control Measures   A community rodent control program must begin with a well-thought-out plan based on surveys and participation by residents. Education of the public is essential to ensure the type of cooperation on which a successful program must be based. When all residents make their premises rat-free, the task of community officials is not a difficult one. A community program has five aspects: survey likely areas to determine the extent of the problem, elimination of food sources, elimination of nesting and breeding places, rat-proofing, and killing of rats. Each aspect involves certain measures.

1. Surveys
   a. Poor sanitation areas
   b. Substandard housing
   c. Tenements
   d. Railroad areas
   e. Areas near dumps
2. Elimination of food sources
   a. Placing all food in rat-proof containers
   b. Covering garbage cans
   c. Prohibiting dumping of food wastes in open areas
3. Elimination of nesting and breeding places
   a. Disposing of debris
   b. Burning trash and rubbish
   c. Prohibiting piles of building materials

4. Rat-proofing
  a. Closing external openings
  b. Placing screens and metal over cracks and openings
  c. Eliminating all possible passages
5. Killing of rats
  a. Trapping
  b. Using approved rodenticides with all possible safeguards
  c. Fumigating with warning signs and other safeguards

Droppings of infected rats and mice on food consumed by humans transmit disease. Keeping all food where rats and mice cannot reach it is of primary importance. Of secondary importance is the practice of all possible safety measures when using rodenticides and fumigation to kill rats. Eliminating mice by trapping is relatively simple.

SUMMARY

Food is essential to life and health, yet it can transmit disease and can be a poison itself. Much of our food supply comes from animals. Insects facilitate the pollination of food-producing plants. Much of the grain grown as food is shared with animals. However these animals can become vehicles of disease transmission to humans, and food can become contaminated by animals, including rodents and insects acting as vectors. The food chains and cycles inherent in the relations between people and other animals are countless in their variety, their potential benefits, and their potential hazards. This chapter has emphasized those relationships controlled by health agencies in the interests of community food protection and community health. It has noted the kind of community health education that needs to accompany control measures.

The essential features of these relationships can be summarized in the flow chart in figure 15-15. This figure ties this chapter's content with the concepts introduced in earlier chapters on communicable disease control and epidemiology. In figure 15-15 the control of disease-transmitting vehicles, including animals and food itself, is divided into four broad strategies. Among these, food hygiene is divided into the phases of food production and distribution. Each of these phases has specific objectives and activities associated with it, as seen on the right side of the figure.

http://www.aces.uiuc.edu/~food-lab/lectures/twelve/sld001.htm
Slide show on foodborne diseases

http://www.cdc.gov/ncidod/diseases/foodborn/foodborn.htm
National Center for Infectious Diseases—list of links to more information about foodborne diseases

http://www.usda.gov/
U.S. Department of Agriculture

QUESTIONS FOR REVIEW

1. How might lifestyle changes toward healthier eating contribute to increases in foodborne illnesses?
2. What factors would contribute to a decline in recent years about consumer knowledge in safe food handling?
3. Why are most cases of foodborne infections to be found in the lowest economic, social, and educational groups?
4. In your community and state or province, is there overregulation of the food industry or underregulation? Why?
5. To what extent is the prevention of foodborne disease a matter of community health education? To what extent is it a matter or regulation?
6. In home canning, botulism occurs from improper procedures in preparation. How can this be corrected?
7. Why are respiratory diseases not transmitted via solid foods such as vegetables, fruits, and baked goods?
8. If pathogens are destroyed by pasteurization, why are cows with brucellosis, tuberculosis, or mastitis culled out as producers?

· ·

Figure 15-15

Summary of methods of control of food and other vehicles of disease transfer. *Source:* Extracted and modified from various Expert Committees on Bacterial and Viral Zoonoses of the World Health Organization.

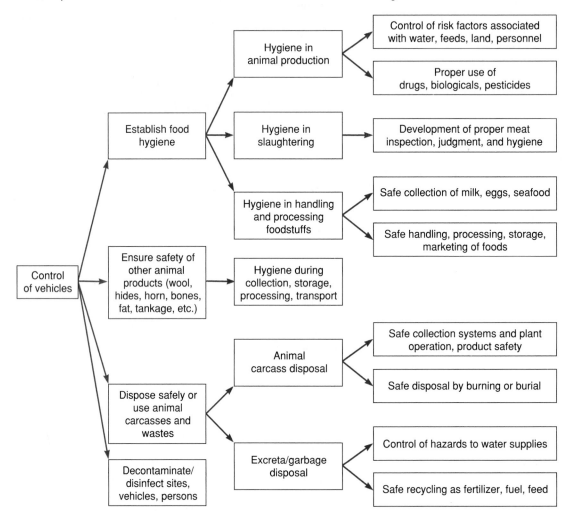

9. What are some of the critical points in the food production chain at which prevention measures might be introduced for the following: dairy products, ground beef, or vegetables? How are the critical points the same or different among these?

10. Why is more attention given to underpasteurization than to overpasteurization of milk?

11. When some cases of disease, such as salmonellosis, are traced to pasteurized milk, what are some possible breakdowns in the milk processing operation that could account for the disease transmission?

12. Should governmental officials prohibit adding ingredients to meats or permit adding ingredients under governmental inspection and control?

13. Which is more important in restaurant sanitation: what is done in the dining area or what is done in the food preparation area? Why?
14. In restaurant rating, which system do you prefer, an A, B, or C rating or an "approved" or "not approved" rating? Why?
15. How does the control of vectors such as flies and rodents protect the community food supply?

READINGS

American Public Health Association and Model Standards Work Group. 1991. *Healthy communities 2000 model standards: guidelines for community attainment of the year 2000 national health objectives.* 3d ed. Washington, DC: American Public Health Association. As for each of the other sets of national objectives shown in previous chapters, this volume provides community-level elaborations of the year 2000 objectives for the nation in food safety and vector control.

Rhodes, R. 1997. *Deadly feasts: Tracking the secrets of a terrifying new plague.* New York: Simon and Schuster. This book gives a comprehensive and compelling understanding of conditions surrounding the 1996 outbreak of "Mad Cow" disease in England and its economic and health consequences. In addition to explaining the animal and human neurological diseases involved, the author details related regulatory practices and lack of response to research outcomes.

U.S. Food and Drug Administration, PHS, DHHS. 1995. *Food Code.* National Technical Information Service, Technology Administration, U.S. Department of Commerce. The code gives the latest advice for protecting food where it is received by the consumer. It provides guidance for preventing foodborne illness in food establishments, such as institutions, grocery stores, restaurants, and food vending locations. It is available in handbook or diskettes formats.

Vanderzant, C., and D. Splittstoesser, eds. 1992. *Compendium of methods for the microbiological examination of foods.* 2d ed. Washington, DC: American Public Health Association. Presents a comprehensive selection of proven methods for processing and testing the safety and quality of foods. Chapters on microorganisms involved in processing and spoilage of foods, pathogenic organisms, foodborne illnesses, and rapid and automated methods of food processing.

World Health Organization. 1992. WHO Expert Committee on Rabies, eighth report, Tech Rep Ser No 824. Geneva: World Health Organization. Reviews new knowledge from basic and applied research on rabies and the prevention of this zoonotic disease. Prospects for controlling the spread of rabies in wild animal populations with new oral vaccines are discussed.

BIBLIOGRAPHY

Auld, M. E., and D. A. Weinreich. 1990. Foundations of American food safety. *Top Clin Nutr* 6:32.

Barnes, A., D. Vilaineurn, and C. Apiwathnasorn. 1994. Evaluation of the safety of domestic food preparation in Malaysia. *Bull World Health Org* 72:877.

Benson, W. 1995. Strategies and willingness of rural restauranteurs to promote healthy foods. *Can J Public Health* 86:181.

Blaser, M. J. 1996. How safe is our food? Lessons form an outbreak of salmonellosis. *N Eng J Med* 334:1324.

Blumenthal, D. 1991. *Food irradiation: toxic to bacteria, safe for humans.* DHHS Publ No (FDA) 91-2241. Washington, DC: Food and Drug Administration. (Reprinted from FDA Consumer Mag Nov 1990).

Centers for Disease Control and Prevention. 1993. Preliminary report: foodborne outbreak of *Escherichia coli* 0157:H7 infections from hamburgers—Western United States. *MMWR* 42:85.

Coulson, N., J. R. Eiser, and C. Eiser. 1996. Children's awareness of additives in food. *H Educ J* 55:375.

de Casas, S. I C., and R. U. Carcavallo. 1995. Climate change and vector-borne diseases distribution. *Soc Sci & Med* 40: 1437.

FAO Panel of Experts on Pesticide Residues in Food and the Environment and the WHO Expert Group on Pesticide Residues. 1992. *Pesticide residues in food— 1991.* Geneva: World Health Organization.

Gordon, L. J. 1994. Food protection: The mission may be hazardous to your health. *J Public Health Policy* 15:393.

Hubalik, Z., J. Halouzka, and Z. Juncova. 1996. A simple method of transmission risk assessment in enzootic foci of Lyme borreliosis. *Eur J Epidem* 12:331.

Hedberg, C. W., and N. Hirschhorn. 1996. Annotation: Why foodborne disease surveillance is critical to the safety of our food supply. *Am J Public Health* 86:1076.

Kemp, S. F., R. F. Lockey, and T. L. Glaros. 1996. Peanut anaphylaxis from food cross-contamination. *J Am Med Assoc* 275:1633.

Mathis, R. G., R. Sizto, and W. Cocksedge. 1995. The effects of inspection frequency and food handler education on restaurant inspection violations. *Can J Public Health* 86:46.

Office of Communications, National Institute of Allergy and Infectious Disease. 1992. *Lyme disease: the facts, the challenge.* NIH Publ No 92-3193. Bethesda: U.S. Department of Health and Human Services.

Palmer, S., and K. S. Bakshi. 1992. Chemical contaminants in food. In *Principles and practice of environmental medicine,* edited by A. B. Tarcher. New York: Plenum.

Patlak, M. 1991. Looking ahead to the promises of food science in the future. NRC News Rep 41:13.

Tilden, J., Jr., W. Young, and J. G. Morris, Jr. 1996. A new route of transmission for *Escherichia coli:* infection from dry fermented salami. *Am J Public Health* 86:1142.

Usera, M. A., A. Echeita, and F. Martinez-Navarro. 1996. Interregional foodborne salmonellosis outbreak due to powdered infant formula contaminated with lactose fermenting Salmonella virchow. *Eur J Epidem* 12:377.

Wei, M., B. D. Mitchell, and M. P. Stern. 1996. Entomologic Index for Human Risk of Lyme Disease. *Am J Epidem* 144:1058.

World Health Organization/FNU/FOS. 1997. *Basic principles for the preparation of safe food for infants and young children.* Geneva: World Health Organization.

World Health Organization/FNU/FOS. 1997. *Food safety measures for eggs and foods containing eggs.* Geneva: World Health Organization.

Chapter *16*

Residential, Occupational, and Other Environments

A *house is not a home.*

—Polly Adler

Objectives

When you finish this chapter, you should be able to:

- Describe the major health hazards in residential, occupational, and other environments

- Identify the agencies, standards, and laws regulating these environments

- Recognize strategies to improve or maintain the quality of housing, worksites, and other environments

People in industrial countries spend more than 90 percent of their time indoors. Most of us, however, are more concerned about outside air and other environmental hazards than we are with such hazards indoors. The air we share outdoors provides a point for social action and concern that dissipates in the individual space within our homes. Gone are the days of communal barn raising when people not only built their homes, they knew the materials that went into them. Few of us know what lies beyond the walls in our homes or what materials fill the furniture we sit on or the air we breath. Even when we read the tags on furniture or pillows that we are scolded by law not to remove, we have little idea how these products affect our health. With increases in allergies, headlines about sick buildings, and photographic blow-

ups of the dust mites under our beds, it is hard to avoid the impact of indoor environments. The environments in which people live, work, and play affect their quality of life.

The public health concern with the relationship between health and the environment—indoors and outdoors—is long standing. Housing, worksites, and recreational environments affect and are affected by the demographic, behavioral, economic, organizational, and genetic factors influencing community health. As discussed in chapter 3, human ecology, demography, and epidemiology interact to produce community health problems and influence community health strategies. This chapter focuses on indoor environments and the ways in which they effect health and community strategies for addressing them.

HOUSING: RESIDENTIAL ENVIRONMENTS

The old adage that begins this chapter reminds us of the differences between the social environment and the structural environment in which the family exists. The health impact of housing encompasses important physical, social, and environmental effects. The house provides shelter for the smallest social unit of society, the family, and must provide shelter against the external elements and safety in its internal construction and components. In most countries, housing is a private concern. Housing is also a public health responsibility, a matter of economics, and a measure of personal and family status. The disparity between the rich and the poor is most visible in their housing (figure 16-1). Housing arouses emotion and controversy when threatened by neighborhood change, new zoning ordinances, economic swings, or highway construction. Citizens have gone to court to bar waste disposal sites, mental health clinics, drug abuse and HIV/AIDS treatment centers, and family planning clinics from being constructed in their neighborhoods. Chapter 13 touched on the safety and injury prevention aspects of housing, occupations, and recreation. This chapter will concentrate on the ways in which these environments affect health and the ways in which communities respond.

Epidemiology of Housing and Health

The home is not just where the heart is, it is also the primary site of disabling injuries and the second most frequent site of injury and death in the United States. Over 21,500 fatal injuries and 3 million disabling injuries occur annually in homes or on home premises. The most common residential injuries result from falls, fires, scalding liquids, immersions, poisonings, suffocation/asphyxiation, and firearms. The young and old are disproportionately affected. Some residential injuries vary according to socioeconomic status. The poor are more likely to live in homes that have greater risk for fire, lead exposure, or failure to meet safety codes.

Figure 16-1

The sanitation facilities, solid structures, and spacing of middle-class housing leaves its residents less susceptible to health problems than those who live in the shadows of such structures. *Source:* Photo courtesy World Health Organization.

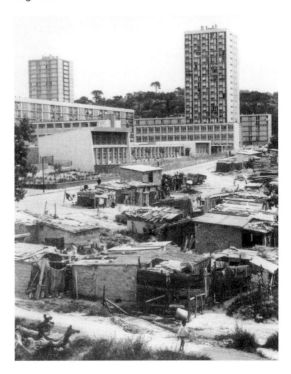

In most societies income plays a large part in narrowing the range of available housing options. Higher income levels correlate with higher levels of education, and these together produce neighborhoods with greater access to medical care facilities, good nutrition, and social standards for childcare and personal health practices, all of which influence health. Other housing influences on health include crowding, indoor air, structural factors, and mental health.

Crowding The transmission of communicable diseases increases with crowding, as studies on the incidence and spread of these diseases have

· · · · · · · · · · · · · · · · · · ·

Figure 16-2

Structures may meet ordinary requirements but fail under severe stress such as this hospital in the 1985 earthquake in Mexico City. *Source:* Photo courtesy World Health Organization.

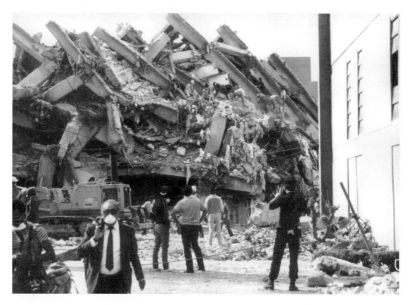

revealed. Incidence rates of the common communicable diseases are higher for residents in densely populated areas than for the general population. At the least, crowding adds to the stresses of daily living; at worst, crowding may contribute to more antisocial behavior.

Indoor Air Insufficient **ventilation,** inadequate artificial lighting, and lack of sunshine can have adverse effects on air quality and health. Chemical emissions from building materials located inside the home, and furnishings, can be a major source of indoor pollution, particularly when new. Other indoor air pollutants include dust, bacteria, and fungus. Even our beloved fireplaces, along with wood stoves, furnaces, and water heaters under the right conditions can backdraft causing indoor pollution. To remain healthy we need a constant source of fresh air and an exhaust system that will effectively remove the moisture, carbon dioxide, and odor we release into our well-sealed environments.

Structural Factors Defective heating units can cause carbon monoxide poisoning and fires. Defective or deteriorated floors, stairs, railings, and other structures account for high rates of injuries. Inadequate plumbing and toilet facilities can be a constant threat to health. When the structures we depend on for protection fail, they can cause injury and death (figure 16-2).

Mental Health Poor housing conditions can be depressing and can lead to a decline in pride and motivation, both essential to optimum mental health. Confusion, noise, and a lack of privacy are not conducive to a feeling of high self-esteem. Graffiti may send racist or obscene messages that discourage and demoralize not only local residents, but discourage customers and residents from the area. There frequently follows carelessness in living practices, in personal grooming, and in self-growth. Social and esthetic decline results from the uncleanliness and disorder often associated with

substandard housing. A person living in substandard housing conditions easily acquire feelings of oppression, powerlessness, and alienation.

Criteria of Substandard Housing

The American Public Health Association Committee on the Hygiene of Housing declared in 1952 that if *any four* of the following criteria existed, the term **slum** applied:

1. Contaminated water
2. Water supply outside
3. Shared toilet or outside toilet
4. Shared bath or outside bath
5. More than 1.5 persons per room
6. Overcrowding of sleeping quarters
7. Less than 40 square feet of sleeping room per person
8. Lack of dual egress
9. Installed heating lacking in three-fourths of the rooms
10. Lack of electricity
11. Lack of windows
12. Deterioration

Substandard Housing   Found particularly in the blighted areas of cities, substandard housing is usually a deteriorating section between the business center and the principal residential sections of the community. This is the area on the fringes of the business section, where people live in retail store buildings that are no longer acceptable for commercial purposes. Many owners put nothing back into the buildings in the way of maintenance. As a consequence, deterioration, rubbish, garbage, flies, vermin, rats, and fire hazards prevail.

Principles of Healthful Housing

In contrast with the preceding discussion of substandard housing, is a set of minimum standards of housing developed by the American Public Health Association. It is based on fundamental human needs and necessary protection against hazards to health and life.

Fundamental Psychological Needs   Healthful housing provides adequate privacy for the individual, and opportunities for normal family and community life. Such facilities that make possible the performance of household tasks without undue physical and mental fatigue and for maintenance of cleanliness of the dwelling and of the individual. Possibilities exist for esthetic satisfaction in the home and its surroundings, and concordance with prevailing social standards of the local community.

Protection Against Communicable Disease   Healthful housing provides for a water supply of safe, sanitary quality, available to the dwelling and protected against pollution within the dwelling. It also provides toilet facilities of such character as to minimize the danger of transmitting disease; protection against sewage contamination of the interior surfaces of the dwelling; avoidance of unsanitary conditions in the vicinity of the dwelling; exclusion from the dwelling of vermin, which may play a part in the transmission of disease; facilities for keeping milk and food from decomposing; and sufficient space in sleeping rooms to minimize the danger of contact infection.

Protection Against Injury   Healthful housing is built with such materials and methods of construction as to minimize danger of injury due to collapse of any part of the structure. It provides for control of conditions likely to cause fires or to promote their spread (figure 16-3); adequate facilities for escape in case of fire; protection against danger of electric shocks and burns, gas poisoning, falls and other mechanical injuries in the home; and protection of the neighborhood against the hazards of automobile traffic.

These basic housing needs may vary from one community to another and even from one section of a community to another. Housing needs in the center of a metropolitan area may best be served

....
Figure 16-3

This home safety checklist from the Consumer Product Safety Commission targets one population—the elderly—who are particularly susceptible to home injuries. *Source:* Consumer Products Safety Commission.

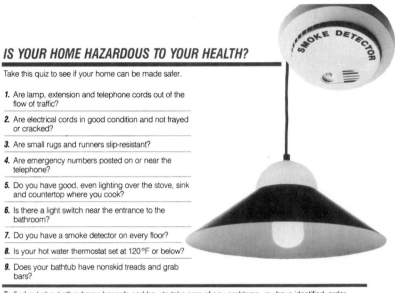

IS YOUR HOME HAZARDOUS TO YOUR HEALTH?

Take this quiz to see if your home can be made safer.

1. Are lamp, extension and telephone cords out of the flow of traffic?

2. Are electrical cords in good condition and not frayed or cracked?

3. Are small rugs and runners slip-resistant?

4. Are emergency numbers posted on or near the telephone?

5. Do you have good, even lighting over the stove, sink and countertop where you cook?

6. Is there a light switch near the entrance to the bathroom?

7. Do you have a smoke detector on every floor?

8. Is your hot water thermostat set at 120°F or below?

9. Does your bathtub have nonskid treads and grab bars?

To find out about other home hazards and how to take care of any problems you have identified, order The Home Safety Checklist for Older Consumers, available free from the Consumer Product Safety Commission, Washington, DC 20207, (800) 638-2772. Write or call for your copy today.

by high-rise apartments; in the periphery by single-unit dwellings. The housing requirements set forth by the American Public Health Association can serve as a guide wherever needed, regardless of the circumstances.

Indoor Air Pollution

Indoor air pollution violates the principles of healthful housing. The concentration of many pollutants is greater indoors than outdoors (see box, p. 498). This is a public health concern because so much of our time is spent indoors, in home, work or recreational environments. Table 16-1 summarizes six sources of indoor air pollution and the various respiratory and other effects they have on health. Although presented in this section on resi-dential environments, many of these pollutants are of concern also in occupational environments.

Environmental Tobacco Smoke   Tobacco smoke is a major source of indoor air contaminants. Environmental tobacco smoke is a dynamic, complex mixture of more than 4,000 chemicals found in vapor and particle phases. Many of these chemicals are known toxic or carcinogenic agents. Research has found it infeasible to totally remove tobacco smoke through general ventilation, therefore more home and business environments are banning it completely. Although many smokers have taken to the outdoors, unless doors and windows are well sealed the smoke is likely to return inside the structure.

Indoor Pollution

An irony of the times is the price we are paying for the energy consciousness of the 1970s. All the caulking and weather-stripping has sealed out atmospheric air but has sealed in household pollutants. Cigarette smoke, paint odors, mildew, insecticide spray, **asbestos,** animal hairs, oven fumes, and **radon** accumulate in unventilated household air. These indoor pollutants have been linked to increased respiratory distress (coughs, asthma, bronchitis, and flu-like symptoms), allergies, and increased risk of lung cancer and emphysema.

The attention given over the past twenty years to pollution in offices and public buildings has turned to air pollution in homes. Research has found indoor atmospheric concentrations of some chemicals much higher than outdoor concentrations. In the early 1970s, the stagnant air inside an average home would have exchanged with outside air once every hour. Now, with improved insulation, the **air exchange rate** in many homes is only once in ten hours.

If improved ventilation and controlled use of selected substances in the home are sufficient remedies for the indoor pollution threat, how would you mount a community program to address this problem? Considering the present consequences of measures taken to control energy expenditures, what community health problems might you expect in the year 2000 as a consequence of today's lifestyle and environmental modifications?

Table 16-1

Environmental Contaminates and Associated Physical Symptoms

Signs and symptoms	Environmental tobacco smoke	Other combustion products	Biological pollutants	Volatile organics	Heavy metals	Sick bldg syndrome
Respiratory						
Rhinitis, nasal congestion	■	■	■	■		■
Epistaxis				■[1]		
Pharyngitis, cough	■	■	■			■
Wheezing, worsening asthma	■	■		■		■
Dyspnea	■[2]		■			■
Severe lung diseases						■[3]
Other						
Conjunctival irritation	■	■	■	■		■
Headache or dizziness	■	■	■	■	■	■
Lethargy, fatigue, malaise		■[4]	■[5]	■	■	■
Nausea, vomiting, anorexia		■[4]	■	■	■	
Cognitive impairment, personality change		■[4]		■	■	■
Rashes			■	■	■	
Fevers, chills			■[6]		■	
Tachycardia		■[4]			■	
Retinal hemorrhage		■[4]				
Myalgia				■[5]		■
Hearing loss				■		

[1]Associated especially with formaldehyde. [2]In asthma. [3]Hypersensitivity pneumonitis, Legionnaires' Disease. [4]Particularly associated with high CO levels. [5]Hypersensitivity pneumonitis, humidifier fever. [6]With marked hypersensitivity reactions and Legionnaires' Disease.

Source: U.S. Environmental Protection Agency.

Combustion Products Stoves, space heaters, furnaces, and fireplaces are another major source of pollutants. Added to these would be vehicle emissions, if houses and garages are close or if loading docks are located near building air intake vents. The gaseous pollutants from combustion sources include carbon monoxide, nitrogen dioxide, and sulfur dioxide. Carbon monoxide (CO) is an odorless, colorless, tasteless, nonirritating gas that is estimated to claim over 1,500 lives annually. CO occurs where there is insufficient oxygen to allow for complete combustion of the fuel in use. High and low levels of CO can prove fatal. In the latter case, it slowly builds in the blood stream and eventually replaces oxygen needed to sustain life. Devices similar in appearance to smoke detectors can be purchased to test for CO. Periodic inspection of equipment can reduce this source of pollution.

Biological Pollutants Animal dander, molds, and dust mites are common pollutants found to some degree in every home, school, and workplace. Environments with high humidity supports the growth of these pollutants. Biological agents indoors are known to cause infections, hypersensitivity diseases, and toxicoses. The transmission of airborne infectious diseases, such as tuberculosis, is increased with poor indoor air quality. Allergic reactions to such pollutants are fairly common. Among the remedies to biological pollutants are adequate outdoor air ventilation, relative humidity under 50 percent, and controlled pet exposure.

Volatile Organic Compounds Formaldehyde, pesticides, solvents, and cleaning agents are common pollutants of this type. Included among these are personal items such as scents and hair sprays. At room temperature, these compounds emit gases from certain solids or liquids. These pollutants are consistently measured at much higher levels indoors than outdoors. Formaldehyde is one of the best known volatile organic compounds and is probably human carcinogen. Although once widely used in construction, Urea-formaldehyde

shows up more often in some finishes, paneling, and particleboard. Increased ventilation when using such products or avoiding their purchase can reduce this source of pollution.

Heavy Metals Airborne lead and mercury vapor are examples of this type of pollutant. Lead poisoning is the foremost preventable disease of children in all socioeconomic and demographic strata. Lead in paint has long been recognized as the major source of high-dose lead exposure and asymptomatic lead poisoning for children in the United States. Since 1977, paint produced for household use must, by regulation, contain no more than 0.06 percent lead. In contrast, some paints manufactured in the 1940s for indoor use contained more than 50 percent lead, and an estimated 27 million households in the United States remain contaminated by **lead paint.** Lead poisoning typically occurs in children under six years old living in deteriorated, pre-World War II housing. It has been found also in children whose parents moved to older housing as "urban homesteaders," exposing the children to paint chips, dust, or fumes as the old lead-based paint was removed during remodeling or renovation.

Sick Building Syndrome The term sick building syndrome was first used in the 1970s to describe situations in which reported symptoms among a population of building occupants can be temporally associated with their presence in that building. Although a variety of specific and nonspecific complaints are associated with this syndrome, the key factor is that the symptoms abate when individuals are no longer in the building. Various causes are suspected including poor building design, maintenance, and/or operation of the structure's ventilation system.

Long-Term Risks Asbestos and radon are among the most publicized indoor air pollutants. Asbestos is a known carcinogen. Once widely used in structural fireproofing, it may still be found in insulation, tiles, and shingles in older

Sources of Lead Exposure and Responsible Regulatory Agencies in the U.S.

The federal agencies—and their areas of responsibility—involved with regulating lead exposure or researching the effects of lead:

FDA has responsibility for regulating lead in: bottled water; calcium supplements; ceramic and other foodware; commercial coffee urns; decorated glassware; food, including ingredients; and packaging lead crystal lead-soldered food cans.

EPA (Environmental Protection Agency) researches and/or monitors lead content in air, water, and soil, and has some involvement monitoring lead-based paints.

NIOSH (National Institute for Occupational Safety and Health) conducts research and surveillance on occupational lead exposure and offers health hazard evaluation

programs on worksites when requested and industrial hygiene training.

OSHA (Occupational Safety and Health Administration) regulates lead exposure at the worksite.

NIEHS (National Institute of Environmental Health Sciences) conducts basic biomedical research on human health effects of lead.

HUD (U.S. Department of Housing and Urban Development) funds public housing authorities to contain or remove lead-based paint in public housing units.

CPSC (Consumer Product Safety Commission) requires warning labels on lead solder for drinking water pipes; monitors lead paint on children's toys to ensure compliance with the federal standard limiting

lead in paint to no more than 0.06 percent; regulates the labeling of artists' materials; and has issued safety warnings about hazards of use of lead-based paint in the home.

ATSDR (Agency for Toxic Substances and Disease Registry) is responsible for health assessment for areas near Superfund sites (toxic waste sites that pose an environmental threat); wrote case study on lead for health professional training; and authored 1988 congressional document about the nature and extent of lead poisoning of American children.

Source: FDA Consumer July–Aug. 1991, Food and Drug Administration.

houses. The risk of disease depends on exposure to airborne asbestos fibers. In 1989, the United States banned new uses of asbestos, but uses before this date are still allowed. Radon is a cancer-causing, radioactive gas (see figure 16-4) It comes from the natural breakdown of uranium in soil, rock, and water and gets into the air. The most likely exposure to radon for most people is in their homes. It gets into homes through cracks in the floors, construction joints, and the water supply. Nearly one out of every fifteen homes in the United States is estimated to have elevated radon levels. Testing for radon is easy and inexpensive.

Building Regulations and Codes

Regulation of housing construction has long been a recognized governmental function in most countries. Such codes can help address some of the indoor air pollution problems previously discussed,

and important structural features of housing. In the community this authority is exercised through ordinances providing for building zones and for codes governing construction.

Zoning   Zoning is designed to control the type of building erected in a given section of a community. One zone may provide only for single-family structures. Another zone may provide for single- or two-family dwellings. In another zone the construction of multiple-dwelling structures may be permitted as well. Some areas may be zoned commercial, and others may be zoned industrial. **Zoning** protects the interests of those owning houses or other structures in an area against having their mode of life jeopardized and the value of their property reduced. It also provides a degree of uniformity in planning. In some communities a special planning commission considers matters of

· · · · · · · · · · · · · · · · · · · ·
Figure 16-4
Relative magnitude of annual deaths from Radon are compared with other fatalities for the United States. *Source:* National Safety Council; Environmental Protection Agency.

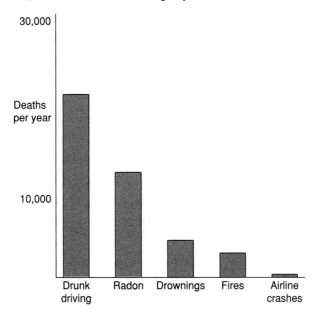

zoning and makes recommendations to the city council, which alone has the legal authority to enact local zoning ordinances.

Building Codes Community **building codes** have their roots in ancient history. As far back as 3500 B.C., regulations applied to the making of bricks and hinges used in the construction of public buildings. Significant events that led to the evolution of the modern building code are shown in the box on page 502. Codes specify the type and quality of materials that may be used, standards of construction, the quality and proper installation of plumbing fixtures, wiring specifications, fire prevention, energy conservation, and accessibility. These and other provisions will give the prospective dweller, the neighborhood, and the community assurance that the building will meet the needs of the inhabitants in terms of safe and secure living.

Communities can enforce building codes by requiring a permit to build. The fee for the permit may be nominal, but in granting the permit the issuing community authority specifies that the permit is issued on the provisions of the building code. Plans for the building must meet zoning and code standards and must be followed in the construction.

Smoke detectors and sprinklers are examples of codes that have contributed to public safety, as discussed in chapter 13. While the percentage of households with smoke detectors has increased from 22 percent in 1977 to 86 percent in 1990, the number of fire deaths per million in the same period decreased from 34 to 21.1. This decrease is in part attributable to the increase in smoke detectors. Although less common, studies have shown that sprinklers would save nearly two-thirds of the people who would not have been saved by smoke detectors alone.

Milestones in the History of Building Codes

1700 B.C. Babylonia's Code of Hammurabi stated that "if a builder has built a house for a man, and his work is not strong, and if the house he has built falls in and kills the householder, that builder should be slain."

1st Century Roman Law regulated building heights, light, ventilation, sanitation, party walls (divisions separating properties) and setbacks.

1189 A.D. England's "Henry Fitz-Elwyne's Assize of Buildings" addressed problems due to dense populations in cities, specifically party wall provisions and criteria for roof materials to decrease risk of fire spreading from building to building.

1625 In New Amsterdam, the first building law on record in America governed the types and locations of roof coverings to prevent fire transmission from sparks emitted from chimneys.

1666 After the "Great Fire of London," the first document resembling a building code was written and led to the passage of the Metropolitan Building Act, which recognized the need for building officials to enforce codes.

1791 At the suggestion of George Washington, the Commissioners of Washington, DC, adopted the first official building regulations, which limited the height of wood frame structures to 12 feet.

1850s The first city building codes in North America were established by New York City.

1896 National Fire Protection Association was established in response to the need to create a standard for the uniform installation of sprinklers.

1915 Building Officials and Code Administrators (BOCA) was established.

By 1920 The first mandatory statewide codes were developed and adopted by Wisconsin.

1922 International Conference of Building Officials (ICBO) was established.

1940 Southern Building Code Congress International (SBCCI) was established.

1972 Council of American Building Officials (CABO) was established.

Source: Trauma Foundation of San Francisco.

Model Codes   The American Public Health Association developed a model housing ordinance regulating construction, maintenance, and occupancy of dwellings and dwelling units. The International Conference of Building Officials also developed a Uniform Housing Code. These instruments represent an intervention mechanism to control many types of injuries, especially those resulting from residential drowning, fires/burns, and falls. They also can serve as excellent guides for health personnel and community authorities in developing local ordinances or codes.

A building erected before a building code was in effect will be bound by the requirements of the code if remodeling is to be done. Requiring a permit to remodel provides community officials with a means for requiring that the completed structure conform to code standards.

Sanction   When health officials judge a particular dwelling to be a threat to the health of the public, they can take necessary steps to abate the condition by consultation and negotiation with the owner or, as a last resort, court action to declare the condition a **public nuisance** (see Chapter 19). The housing problem of greatest general concern to the community—and of particular concern to the health department—is the building that was constructed years before a code existed but that has deteriorated to a substandard condition and will continue to decline. All of the objectionable aspects of deterioration will become progressively more apparent.

In such cases it is doubtful that provisions of the building code can be enforced; thus the avenue for relief may be closed. In this type of situation health departments can play a vital role. Inspections are made, hazards and other unsatisfactory conditions are reported, and a notice is issued to correct the unsatisfactory condition. Diplomacy and reasonable restraint are usually exercised by health officials. Legal measures are taken only as a last resort. Public support, always essential to the health department, is developed by a continuing program of public education and by the health staff's exemplary professional service to the community.

Community Responsibility

People living in substandard housing sometimes become so discouraged that they do not recognize the deterioration going on about them. Those who are homeless may move from shelter to shelter or find themselves on the streets. Tragically, children growing up under these circumstances can become so conditioned that they expect nothing else. Many people in substandard housing would like to find something better, but their economic situation has them enslaved (figure 16-5).

Government Role For centuries housing was left to the individual or to private enterprise, but country after country recognized that this was inadequate. The entry of governmental agencies was a logical development if government was to serve the public in fulfilling its needs, and one of the primary human needs is adequate housing.

In 1937 the U.S. federal government instituted a slum clearance and low-rent housing program by creating local housing authorities committed to slum clearance and to the construction of low-rent housing. Community agencies constructed and operated the housing. Federal funds made up 90 percent of the financing, with the remainder from municipal or private sources. Loans of federal funds at low-interest rates were available. Communities receiving funds were required to eliminate a slum dwelling unit for each new low-cost dwelling unit constructed.

The Housing Act of 1949 further extended federal aid to housing by authorizing financial assistance to communities for the clearing of blighted areas and slums and for redevelopment sites. Federal financial assistance for housing was also given to private enterprise through local agencies. Communities, in turn, could build on the cleared sites or could interest private capital in purchasing the sites from the city and in building approved dwellings or other structures. Certain tax benefits were granted to private purchasers and developers.

Urban Renewal Urban renewal was established by the Housing Act of 1954 as a combination of federal, community, and private resources to replace slum and blighted areas with adequate residential and business facilities. To qualify for federal aid, the community had to agree to certain requisites, such as a comprehensive plan of development including administrative organization, financial adequacy, citizen participation, and responsibility for adequately relocating persons displaced by urban renewal. Not all urban renewal leads to better housing, but the business and other structures that were constructed during this period were in harmony with the concept of urban renewal and contributed to the esthetic improvement of communities.

Urban Decline In the 1960s there was a breakdown of the environment within the semipublic domain—that which falls between the responsibility of the individual household family on one hand (for example, indoor cleanliness, safety) and municipal government on the other (public water supply, public sanitation, sewage disposal, etc.). Most of the problems in this domain are with low-rent apartment or tenement housing. Poor maintenance was the primary problem. Buildings often were structurally sound but poorly maintained. Building superintendents were poorly paid.

Shelter Poverty of the 1970s Soaring interest rates, inflation, and the dramatic appreciation of housing costs in the 1970s and early 1980s put rents and mortgage rates out of reach for many young couples and individuals. In addition, the changing family structure put relatively more single individuals in search of housing. For many

. . . .
Figure 16-5

Wood engraved vignettes of a "tramp's lodging house" in New York City around 1875. Housing improvements in the nineteenth century have been credited with a large proportion of the reduction in communicable diseases in that century, but poor people in cities depended on charity and shared sleeping areas. *Source:* National Library of Medicine.

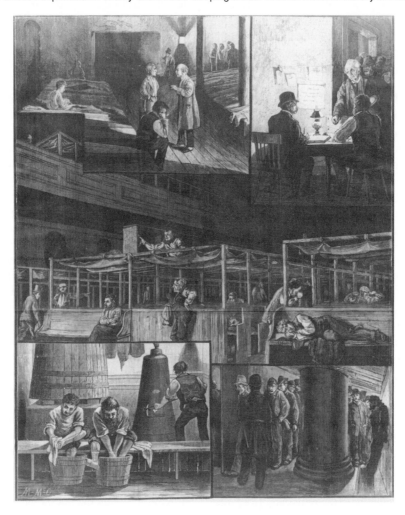

people, the consequence was "shelter poverty"—the inability to meet the need for other necessities after paying the cost of housing. During the 1970s, the number of shelter-poor households increased by 34 percent, or 6.4 million. By 1980, over 25 million households—32 percent of households in the United States—were shelter-poor.

Homelessness   The shock of the 1980s was the realization that many of the people who were shelter-poor in the 1970s were without homes. The most widely quoted estimate was that over the course of a year 3 million Americans were **homeless.** The homeless are defined as those who routinely sleep in bus, train, airport, or subway terminals; in

ISSUES AND CONTROVERSIES
Homelessness and Mental Illness

An especially disturbing dimension of the problem of the homeless is the growing number of the mentally ill in this population. Rescue mission workers estimate that one-third of those who seek help are former mental patients with nowhere else to turn. In the United States, the number of patients in psychiatric wards has been halved since 1970. In some states, two-thirds of the beds have been emptied by court orders allowing mental hospitals to keep only those patients judged a threat to themselves or others. Former Mayor Edward Koch of New York City, which had at least 40,000 homeless people, once complained that many neighborhoods had been turned into "outdoor psychiatric wards."

Los Angeles estimates that, because of the city's warm climate, the number of homeless people in the downtown district doubles in winter to more than 15,000. The county mental health department claims that other communities give one-way bus tickets to Los Angeles to many of their chronically mentally ill homeless as part of a "Greyhound therapy" plan to clear their own communities of the housing burden. Vancouver had a similar experience on Canada's west coast.

Like toxic agents, the homeless are seen by many communities as something to be dumped in other communities. How can communities be supported in taking greater responsibility for the housing of homeless people? How can homelessness be prevented?

abandoned buildings; or outside on steam heating grates and in parks. At any time, from 250,000 to 400,000 people in the United States have no home. About 41 percent of the homeless have chronic physical disorders, 33 percent have psychiatric problems, and 38 percent of the homeless are alcohol or drug abusers. Slightly more than half are minorities, 25 percent women, and 10 percent children aged 15 or less (figure 16-6). Mortality is high. Dozens of the homeless froze to death during the winter of 1984–1985. Twenty died in New York City alone. Many more suffered from pneumonia or tuberculosis. It is likely that Medicaid cuts in the United States, combined with reductions in subsidized low-cost housing, more stringent criteria for Social Security payments, and continuing deinstitutionalization of mental patients will result in continuing homelessness in the future, especially for the mentally ill.

The 1987 Homeless Assistance Act   The growing national embarrassment of homelessness spurred the U.S. Congress to enact the Stuart B. McKinney Homeless Assistance Act, signed into law in July, 1987. The Act provides for a range of services for the homeless, including primary health care services. The hope was that the "seed money" provided by the federal government under this act would get local health care for the homeless programs going and that state and local communities would eventually assume the costs of the programs. However, the total numbers have changed little, and the percentage of homeless who are mentally ill or have alcohol or drug problems remains around 70 percent.

Economic Strategies   Other strategies to ease the housing problem in the United States focus primarily on taxation policies. One such approach would increase the personal income-tax exemption to give low-income taxpayers more discretionary income. Another would eliminate homeowners tax deductions, especially on second homes used for vacation purposes, on the grounds that these deductions primarily subsidize interest rates for high-income taxpayers. A third would put a heavier tax on short-term capital gains from the sale of housing. This would discourage speculative buying and

· · · · · · · · · · · · · · · · · · ·

Figure 16-6

In addition to shelter, other types of services are needed by the homeless. The Covenant House provides a variety of services for homeless teens. *Source:* Ad Council.

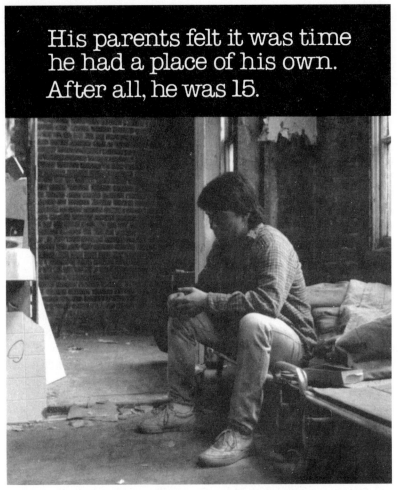

His parents felt it was time he had a place of his own. After all, he was 15.

Every year hundreds of thousands of kids are thrown away. Put out onto the streets. With no job, no money and nowhere to go, these kids turn up in abandoned buildings, alleys and in morgues.

But now there is a number for kids to call. The Covenant House Nineline helps kids with food, clothing, a place to sleep and, most of all, someone to talk to.

To get help in your hometown call our Nineline 1-800-999-9999. It's free, and you can call from anywhere.
Nineline 1-800-999-9999 Anytime. Anywhere.

A Case Study: Housing and Employment Skills

The East Harlem Environmental Extension Service, Inc.* initiated a training, stipend, and field service program for east Harlem residents. The extension service began its training programs with three training cycles of fifteen participants. During training each participant received $80 per week rising to $100. Subjects taught were boiler maintenance, plastering, painting, electrical work, simple plumbing, carpentry, fire prevention, and rodent and pest control. Red Cross first aid training was a key part of the program, and a field manual on health and safety was put to use. The program was linked with family health workers, public health workers, public health nurses, and community health guides.

The program improved the housing in east Harlem and gave the trainees vocational skills that afforded them better opportunities for employment. It showed the way and encouraged other communities to assess their situation and to develop programs that provided improved housing for their citizens. A similar concept demonstrated in Baltimore, Maryland, activated inner city youth enrolled in a community pediatric center to repair broken windows in their neighborhoods. Community leaders have the opportunity to initiate and develop projects for housing betterment.

How might such a program work in your community? What would need to be the same or different to make it work?

_____

*A nonprofit corporation representing housing groups, owners, tenants, and job training organizations working with the Department of Community Medicine of the Mount Sinai School of Medicine and New York City's Board of Education.

selling of real estate for short-term profits, which artificially inflates the cost of housing. A federal housing bank is needed to finance low-income housing at minimal or zero interest rates.

Volunteer Strategies   One strategy that has had wide publicity because of former President Jimmy Carter's active participation is the mobilization of volunteers and local businesses to redevelop neighborhood housing. Through Habitat for Humanity neighbors help neighbors build homes. In NeighborWorks, housing is a community concern of residents and employers (figure 16-7).

OCCUPATIONAL HEALTH ENVIRONMENTS

Workplace environments also are changing and becoming more diverse. By the year 2000 it is anticipated that in North America women will comprise 47 percent of the workforce, minorities 27 percent of the workforce, and that the median age of workers will be 39.2 years. Increasingly the North American economy is moving toward a ser-

vice sector where employment growth is found mostly in small business. Technology allows more workers to conduct business in their homes and cars. Rather than the promise of more leisure time, for many the changes mean more hours, more stress, and a need for new skills. The changing workplace also means needed changes in ways to prevent occupational diseases, injuries, and deaths. Efforts include research and traditional approaches, along with approaches from other disciplines, such as criminal justice and mental health to deal with issues of workplace violence.

Occupational environments must be organized to protect the health of the worker. Work-related injuries and illnesses are as much a social and health burden as they are an economic one. It was estimated in 1993 that work-related injuries in the United States cost $121 billion in medical care, lost productivity, and wages. Modern occupational health has been extended to include nonoccupational and occupational factors that affect the health of workers. Management usually has a legal responsibility for factors affecting the health of workers.

REBUILDING AMERICA'S NEIGHBORHOODS IS EVERYONE'S BUSINESS.

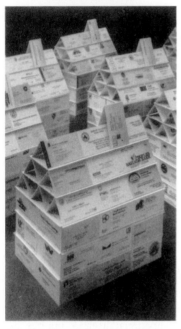

When one neighborhood declines, a whole community can collapse like a house of cards.

That's why a non-profit partnership called NeighborWorks is rebuilding housing and building a stronger community. And that's good for business.

So make it your business to get involved. Write Neighbor-Works, P.O. Box 41406, Baltimore, MD 21203-6406. Or call 1-800-245-6957.

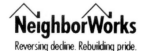

NeighborWorks

Reversing decline. Rebuilding pride.

Ad Council

....
◀ **F i g u r e 1 6 - 7**

The business cards stacked as houses in this photo illustrate the importance of public and private linkages in rebuilding neighborhoods. *Source:* Ad Council.

Attempts to promote the health of workers should be encouraged as a product of collective bargaining, if not as the self-initiating action of management. Although some management voluntarily accepts this responsibility, others are governed entirely by the requirements of the law in dealing with occupational health and safety. Many workers are overlooked in the promotion of industrial health and the community must be concerned. This concern should extend beyond mere legal requirements and codes recognizing minimum responsibility for reducing workplace hazards. It should extend to whatever measures are essential for protection and promotion of the health of every worker.

Epidemiology of Occupational Illness

Progress on the year 2000 Occupational Safety and Health Objectives are mixed (figure 16-8). Two new national objectives were added in 1995. One objective was to reduce the rate of homicides in the workplace and the other to reduce age-adjusted mortality for occupational lung diseases. Adolescents were also added as a special population for reducing work-related injuries.

It is estimated that each year 100,000 Americans die from occupational illnesses and that nearly 400,000 new cases of occupational diseases occur. (These estimates are controversial, but no better ones are available.) When multiple etiological factors are considered, between 10 percent and 20 percent of cancer cases may be related to carcinogens in the workplace.

An occupational health program properly goes beyond the prevention of hazards to physical and mental health and extends into the positive promotion of the health of workers. Health education, rest, recreation, treatment of sudden illness, optical

·····················
Figure 16-8

Status of the Year 2000 Occupational Safety and Health Objectives in the 1995 Middecade Review. *Source: Healthy People 2000: Midcourse Review and 1995 Revisions.* 1996. Boston: Jones and Bartlett Publishers.

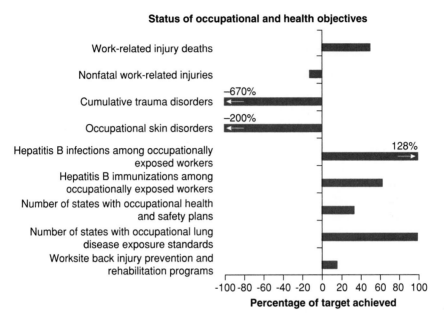

Status of occupational and health objectives

services, and even diagnosis of ailments are aspects of modern occupational health. A competent, trained worker is a valuable asset in industry. The same worker possessing a high level of health is an even more valuable asset. Management is interested in its employees' quality of health for economic reasons, which include concerns with absenteeism, productivity, and morale that relates to satisfaction with working conditions. Some hazards to health are always present in any occupation, operation, plant, or industry. What is important is the degree of danger facing workers. Some hazards are so extreme that they must be eliminated or markedly reduced, while others are of less concern.

Fatalities Work-related injury deaths in the United States had been reduced from 6 to 5 per 100,000 workers by 1993. Workers killed on the job in 1995 were more likely to be wage earners than the self-employed, men (91 percent) than

women (9 percent), and whites (82 percent) rather than all other groups (18 percent). Those in the 35 to 44 age range had the highest rate of fatalities.

Motor vehicle crashes are the leading cause of fatal injury death in the workplace (figure 16-9). One national objective to reduce such deaths encourages employers to mandate the use of occupant protection systems, such as safety belts, during work-related motor vehicle travel. To address the second leading cause of workplace death—homicides and violent acts—a new occupational objective was added to the national agenda in 1995. This objective has particular importance for women in that the leading cause of work-related death among women in the early 1990s was homicide.

Injuries Injuries pose an immediate threat in nearly all occupations, as chapter 13 indicated. Nonfatal injuries at work have fluctuated over the last decade and were at 7.9 per 100 workers in 1993.

Figure 16-9

This figure shows the six main causes of death on the job in 1995, as a percentage of workplace deaths. High death rate from transportation and violence reflect trends in other parts of society. *Source:* Bureau of Labor Statistics.

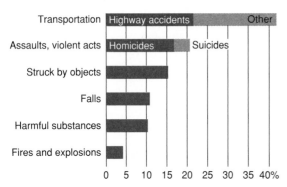

Figure 16-10

This figure shows the groups of workers with the highest rates of on-the-job fatalities in 1995. The overall rate was 5 per 100,000. *Source:* Bureau of Labor Statistics.

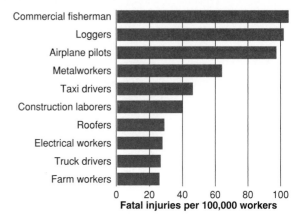

The type and rate of injuries vary by job (figure 16-10). Decreases in fatal injuries were found in mining, construction, transportation, and farm workers, while increases were noted among nursing and personal care workers. There has been a continuing increase at work in cumulative trauma disorders, most notably Carpal Tunnel Syndrome. Although some industries focus only on the safety of their own employees, other industries, such as transportation, also must focus on possible injuries to others, such as passengers or clients.

Dusts, Gases, and Fumes   Dusts, gases, and fumes can be a hazard to the public and to employees (figure 16-11). Fortunately, means are available to reduce these hazards to tolerable levels. Maximum allowable concentration values adopted for various industrial poisons refer to average concentrations that can be tolerated continuously and eight hours per day without impairment to health immediately or in the future.

Dusts are classed as inert, irritating, and toxic. Inert vegetable and animal dusts are present in papermaking, weaving, spinning, and other manufacturing processes that use wool and similar raw materials, but the dangers are not great. Mineral and

Figure 16-11

The potential for industrial fumes to effect the community is vivid in this photograph of children playing in the shadow of industry. *Source:* Photo by Zafar, courtesy World Health Organization.

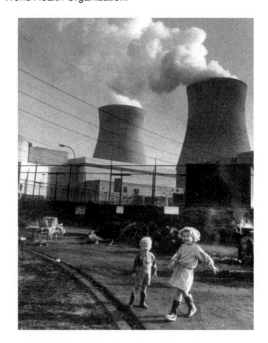

Table 16-2

Major Occuational Hazards and the Estimated Numbers of Workers Exposed in the United States

Potential dangers	Diseases that may result	Workers exposed (U.S.)
Asbestos	White-lung disease (asbestosis); cancer of lungs and lining of lungs; cancer of other organs	Miners; millers; textile, insulation and shipyard workers—estimated 1.6 million exposed
Lead	Kidney disease, anemia; central nervous system damage; sterility; birth defects	Metal grinders; lead-smelter workers; lead storage-battery workers—estimated 835,000 exposed
Arsenic	Lung cancer, skin cancer, liver cancer	Smelter, chemical, oil-refinery workers; pesticide makers and sprayers— estimated 660,000 exposed
Benzene	Leukemia; aplastic anemia	Petrochemical and oil-refinery workers; dye users; distillers; chemists; painters; shoemakers—estimated 600,000 exposed
Cotton dust	Brown-lung disease (byssinosis); chronic bronchitis; emphysema	Textile workers—estimated 600,000 exposed
Coal dust	Blank-lung disease	Coal miners—estimated 208,000 exposed
Coke-oven emissions	Cancer of lungs, kidneys	Coke-oven workers—estimated 30,000 exposed
Radiation (x-rays)	Cancer of thyroid, skin, breast, lungs and bone; leukemia; reproductive effects (spontaneous abortion, genetic damage)	Medical technicians, uranium miners; nuclear power and atomic workers
Vinyl chloride	Cancer of liver, brain, lung	Plastic-industry workers—estimated 10,000 directly exposed.

Source: Occupational Safety and Health Administration; Nuclear Regulatory Commission, U.S. Depts. of Energy, Interior, and Health and Human Services; Health and Welfare Canada.

metallic dusts are more dangerous. Stonecutters, drillers, miners, grinders, and polishers encounter respiratory damage resulting from inert dusts. Granite and quartz dust cause damage to the lungs resulting in *silicosis,* a lung disease that is fatal unless the condition is recognized early and exposure to dust is prevented.

Dusts pose two problems. The first is that of concentration. The second is the important matter of particle size. Concentration and size of dust particles can be measured. Inert and irritating dusts usually can be kept to a minimum. Wet processing reduces the production of dust. Enclosing work that creates dusts, combined with the use of exhaust systems, can reduce dust to a level below the danger point.

Toxic dusts, gases, and fumes such as asbestos, arsenic, lead, benzene, iron oxide, sulfuric acid, carbon monoxide, and manganese pose specific problems of control (table 16-2). Management is usually alert to hazards of this type and is constantly devising procedures to reduce or eliminate these dangers. Research, often with an assist from governmental agencies, is developing measures for the prevention of these industrial hazards. Although the immediate concern is for the worker within the plant, management also has a concern for possible effects on the public. It is usually conceded that no industrial process hazardous to human health is so indispensable to the economy that it could not be eliminated if it cannot be altered sufficiently to protect the health of workers.

Excessive Temperature or Humidity Blast furnaces, smelters, kilns, tanneries, textile mills, laundries, and breweries are examples of industrial processes that make temperature or humidity control difficult. Dermatitis, gastrointestinal disturbances, eye inflammations, and even exhaustion result from atmosphere extremes. Air conditioning can bring atmospheric conditions to tolerable levels. Some workers are physiologically not equipped to tolerate even moderate atmospheric change. Employees who work in buildings with central heating and cooling systems and non-operable windows have little ability to control temperature in their own work space.

Excessive Noise Industry recognizes that noise is more than a health hazard, as it affects production. Noise is an arbitrary descriptor that includes frequency, quality, and loudness of sounds. Loudness is measured in **decibels.** The levels of decibels correspond to the following: whisper, 10 decibels; quiet street, 50 decibels; normal conversation, 50 to 60 decibels; truck or sports car, 90 decibels; pneumatic jackhammer, 95 decibels; loud outdoor motor, 100 decibels; loud power mower, 105 decibels; siren, 125 decibels; riveting, 130 decibels; jet takeoff, 150 decibels. Long doses of 90 decibels or short exposure to a noise of 150 decibels can cause permanent hearing loss.

Infections Infections are a latent hazard in all occupations and are a particularly serious hazard in some industries. Slaughterhouse employees, dairy workers, and others who handle livestock or hides are exposed to such diseases as brucellosis and anthrax. Health care workers may be exposed to the HIV/AIDS virus through unsafe handling and disposal of used needles. Other workers handle substances that serve as media for pathogens of humans. The use of disinfectants and sterilizing methods should prevent most infections in these categories. Medical attention to suspected cases of infection is necessary in industry and elsewhere.

Toxic Chemicals Harmful substances other than gases and fumes can be present in industry (see table 16-2). Chemicals used in plant operations can cause harm to the skin. Chronic poisoning can occur in workers improperly handling materials in routine operations. Knowledge of the presence of these hazards, protective clothing or equipment, and proper regulations governing their handling reduce or nearly eliminate the danger (figure 16-12). Legal regulations and management alertness combine to make poisoning rather rare in modern industry.

Radiation Health hazards of radiation are not a new concern. Luminous paints containing radioactive compounds were recognized as a hazard more than seventy years ago, during World War I; a number of women died after ingesting considerable amounts of radium through the habit of licking the points of their brushes while painting the luminous dials on watches. Today, the use of radioactive products requires special precautions of shielding and the use of personal safety measures such as protective clothing. A necessary safeguard is the use of meters for monitoring the amount of exposure to radiation. Standards for maximum permissible concentration (**MPC**) of radiation have been established for various circumstances.

Disposal of radioactive wastes in the United States is in accordance with standards set by the U.S. Atomic Energy Commission. Sufficient knowledge about radiation hazards is available, and industry is applying this knowledge to prevent any radiation danger to employees or to the public. Opposition to nuclear reactors is partially the usual backlash when new developments are introduced, according to some who work with radioactive materials. For others, however, the concerns about environmental effects and health effects are

••••••••••••••••••••

Figure 16-12

More women, such as these plastic factory workers, are working in industry and coming in contact with hazardous substances. Yet, in most countries, health and safety legislation has a long way to go to guarantee their well-being. *Source:* World Health Organization, photo by P. Almasy.

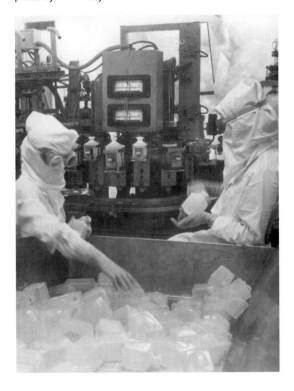

justifiable in the recent memories of nuclear disasters, such as Chernobyl and Bophal and the distant memories of Hiroshima.

Sanitation Proper sanitation measures have long been a concern and accepted responsibility of industry. Industrial sanitation programs are designed to provide conditions that will safeguard the health of employees and provide for maximum production.

A safe and adequate water supply is a first requisite. Industries usually obtain their water from an approved municipal supply. If a private source

is used, the water should be free from cloudiness and contamination and should be tested regularly. A daily test would be called for when threat of contamination is present; once a week can be ample at other times. About twenty gallons per worker per day is necessary for all purposes, although the amount varies with the kind of industry involved. Approved drinking fountains should be placed in convenient locations in the plant, the number depending on the number of workers and the nature of their work.

When an auxiliary water supply is used for fire protection, flushing, and other such purposes, this second supply should be safe for human consumption or so controlled that there will be no possibility that workers will use the unsafe water for drinking or hand washing purposes. Using red or some other color for such faucets or fixtures is a common safeguard.

An approved type of sewage system for liquid wastes is an indispensable sanitation measure. If the plant sewage system cannot be connected to a community system, then provisions must be made for plant sewage disposal. Washrooms must be of good construction with adequate toilets and washbasins. The number of toilet units varies from 1 per 10 workers to 1 per 30 workers. When urinals are installed, only two-thirds as many units are needed.

Washing faucets may be preferred over washbasins because they are less likely to be a means of infection spread. Automatic control of temperatures at 125° F (52° C) is possible with the mixture of hot and cold water running from the same faucet. Liquid soap is preferred because bar soap too easily finds its way to the floor. Shower heads are attached to the wall usually just below average worker chin level.

Illumination Lighting that meets recommended standards reduces accidents and eyestrain and improves efficiency and productive output. Highly detailed work requires more illumination than other kinds of work or open space, such as hallways. It is always important to avoid great contrasts in degree of illumination from one area to another. A ratio of 5 to 1 is preferred, with 10 to 1 the outside limit.

Ventilation Proper ventilation of industrial plants is designed to provide physical comfort by controlling the temperature, humidity, and movement of air. Either natural or artificial means are employed. Removing body heat and moisture in the summer and providing circulation and moderate temperature in the winter are the customary goals. Temperature between 66° and 72° F (19° and 22° C) with a relative humidity of 50 percent, combined with movement of air, provides for physical comfort. Some industries have the problem of removing dusts, gases, vapors, and fumes, for which exhaust systems are employed. If air is recirculated, the ventilation system must be operating efficiently at all times. This requires competent maintenance.

Responsibility for Occupational Health

Management, workers, unions, local government, and the national government have responsibilities in occupational health. Local health departments are rarely equipped to provide the highly technical professional services that occupational health problems demand. Whether the local health department can provide extensive or decidedly limited service, the overall approach must be that of cooperation between all persons and organizations concerned with a particular occupational health problem. Health departments do not enter these situations as a police force but as public servants ready to help remedy existing health problems. Only when industrial management fails to live up to established and accepted standards will the force of legal authority be exercised.

Setting Standards The identification of occupational hazards and illnesses calls for the development of standards for major common health hazards for injury and toxic exposures. Setting and maintaining standards requires increased numbers of health hazard evaluations and routine questioning about occupational health risks by physicians

---

Services and Protection Objectives for Occupational Health and Safety for the Year 2000

Implement occupational safety and health plans in 50 states for the identification, management, and prevention of leading work-related diseases and injuries within the state. (Baseline: 10 states in 1989: 32 states in 1992.*)

Establish in 50 states exposure standards adequate to prevent the major occupational lung diseases to which their worker populations are exposed (byssinosis, asbestosis, coal workers' pneumoconiosis, and silicosis).

Increase to at least 70% the proportion of worksites with 50 or more employees that have implemented programs on worker health and safety.

Establish in 50 states either public health or labor department programs that provide consultation and assistance to small businesses to implement safety and health programs for their employees.

Increase to 75% the proportion of primary care providers who routinely elicit occupational health and safety exposures as a part of patient history and provide relevant counseling.

---

*Public Health Foundation.

---

and other health care providers as part of their patients' medical history. National objectives also relate to increasing workers' knowledge of hazards at their worksite. Educational objectives to increase workers' knowledge of occupational risks include informing workers routinely of their personal exposure measurements, of the results of their health examinations, and about lifestyle behaviors that interact with factors in the work environment to increase risks.

A state or provincial occupational health division may be in the department of health or the department of labor. In either arrangement, the purpose of the occupational health staff is to assist industry with health problems unique to the industry, to conduct surveys, and to enforce regulations relating to occupational health. Teamwork between industry, workers, and official occupational health personnel is the key to effective programs for the promotion of occupational health.

Priorities Allocation of resources for occupational health must be based on considerations of frequency of occurrence, severity of effect, and the likelihood of effective prevention. These three criteria have led to the following list of priorities:

Ten leading work-related diseases and injuries

1. Occupational lung diseases
2. Musculoskeletal injuries
3. Occupational cancers
4. Severe occupational traumatic injuries
5. Occupational cardiovascular diseases
6. Disorders of reproduction
7. Neurotoxic disorders
8. Noise-induced hearing loss
9. Dermatological conditions
10. Psychological disorders

Government Agencies In the United States, two lead government agencies in occupational health are the National Institute for Occupational Safety and Health (NIOSH) and the Occupational Safety and Health Administration (OSHA). **NIOSH** is one of the Centers for Disease Control. It has four basic tasks: (1) respond to requests for investigation of workplace hazards; (2) conduct research to prevent work-related health or safety problems; (3) recommend regulatory actions; (4) train occupational safety and health professionals. **OSHA** is part of the U.S. Department of Labor. Congress declared as its purpose and policy in this act "to assure as far as possible every working man and woman in the Nation safe and healthful working conditions and to preserve our human resources" by encouraging employers and employees in their efforts to reduce the number of occupational safety and health hazards at their places of employment and to institute new and to perfect existing programs for providing safe and healthful working conditions.

Hazard Prevention and Occupational Health Promotion

Components of a comprehensive workplace health program include the implementation of regulatory policies promulgated by federal and state agencies, but also the other channels of influence. Specific interventions follow.

Educational and Informational Measures

Measures that communities and employers or unions can take to support behavior and to increase awareness include the following:

• Reviewing, recommending, initiating, and publicizing occupational health and safety standards and practices necessary for monitoring and surveillance of on-the-job health and safety standards, including environmental health requirements

• Initiating by management, in concert with workers and their representatives, experimental and innovative educational programs relevant to workers' occupational health and safety needs

• Initiating and expanding methods designed to motivate labor and management responsibility for the development and maintenance of a safe and healthful work and community environment

• Developing awareness of the potential interactions between occupational health hazards and lifestyle habits and their effects on health

• Developing worker awareness through electronic and print media, vocational training programs, information from health care providers, campaigns aimed at high-risk worker groups (for example, asbestos workers, newly-employed workers, and elderly workers), and organized labor programs

• Training professional occupational health and safety personnel, including occupational health physicians and nurses, industrial hygienists, toxicologists, and epidemiologists, and including occupational health education in the curricula of medical and nursing schools and in continuing education for health professionals

- Developing awareness in other groups involved with workers or the workplace, including engineers, managers, teachers, social workers, family members, and health care workers
- Developing public awareness of occupational disease and injuries and their high cost to the nation
- Using labeling in simple language to inform workers, employers, health professionals, and the public of occupational hazards, associated risks, and symptoms as appropriate
- Including occupational health as part of the comprehensive health education curricula in high schools

Service Measures Organizational supports for behavior conducive to worker health include the following:

- Implementing well-designed corporate occupational health programs that include preventive and treatment services directed at nonoccupational and occupational health
- Promoting consultation services of governmental agencies to assist small businesses to identify problems and to establish suitable programs for eliminating or controlling these problems
- Encouraging small businesses to form cooperative groups to seek occupational health expertise
- Developing a personal health service delivery system in which the diagnosis and treatment of occupational illnesses and injuries will be coordinated and integrated with other health services that are provided to the worker and his or her family
- Upgrading capabilities of state or provincial and local health departments to participate in occupational health and safety services, including monitoring, surveillance, and consultation to small businesses

Technological Measures Ways to improve the physical environment of the workplace to make it more conducive to health include:

- Improved architectural and engineering design of worksites to prevent injuries
- Control technology to protect workers, including development of safe substitutes for toxic substances, design of process units to eliminate worker exposure, implementation of safe maintenance procedures, and modification of jobs to eliminate harmful physical and mental stress
- Measurement technology to enable quick, accurate, and economical assessment of hazard levels in the workplace by workers, employers, or health professionals (figure 16-13).

Legislative and Regulatory Measures Some of the political and legal strategies possible include:

- Fully implementing laws related to workers' health and provisions for product control
- Recommending, initiating, and evaluating measures designed to improve and expand occupational health and safety legislation, paying particular attention to the possibility of standardizing benefits through a national system of worker's compensation
- Developing criteria and documents recommending standards
- Promulgating new health standards for hazardous substances
- Requiring annual inspections by industrial hygiene compliance officers
- Conducting mandated industrywide studies and health hazard evaluations for carcinogenicity and reproductive effects that could lead to temporary emergency standards
- Changing worker's compensation laws to put stronger economic pressures on employers to reduce hazardous conditions at the worksite

Economic Measures Government agencies can further support improvements through fines and negative publicity for companies with poor health and safety conditions and through tax deduction measures for capital investment in control technology or occupational health programs.

• •
Figure 16-13

Air quality in industry is an international concern. Here officials check that the air quality at a Soviet steel plant conforms to the regulations. *Source:* Photo by Novosti, courtesy World Health Organization.

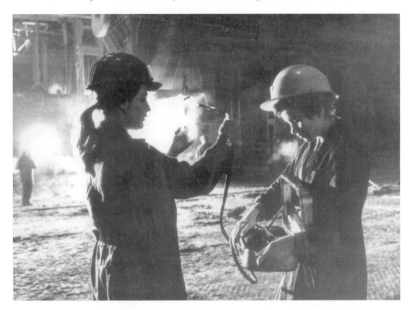

Relative Strength of the Measures Given the broad nature and scope of occupational safety and health problems, the relative strength of the measures varies with the problem at hand, with the nature and adequacy of enforcement efforts and with research capacity. Most occupational health problems require the simultaneous or consecutive application of several types of measures as a comprehensive strategy for hazard eradication. For example, eradication of the asbestos hazard might be achieved by:

• Banning nonessential uses of asbestos
• Substitution of other materials found to be nonhazardous
• Research to determine human exposure during the "life cycle" of the fiber
• Worker education to minimize exposure that may still occur during demolition and repair work

• Rigid enforcement of control standards wherever use of asbestos remains necessary
• Professional education for physicians to assure proper medical help for exposed individuals

This type of eradication program focuses public attention on the problem and goes beyond merely establishing a standard for permissible exposure levels. Finally, better data and better surveillance systems are required if occupational safety and health are to be measurably improved.

OTHER ENVIRONMENTS

Given that 65 percent of the average North American's time is spent inside his or her home, and 22 percent is spent at work, this chapter has already addressed the environments in which adults spend 87 percent of their time. Children, of course, spend a substantial chunk of their time in schools. Future predictions suggests that North Americans will spend increased time at home "cocooning." Of the remaining time, another 6 percent is spent in transit between home and work, leaving a total of only 7 percent at other locations, such as shops, banks, and recreational settings. If exposure time is a criterion of health risk, recreational and other environments pose a limited threat. Schools and public spaces are other important environments of public health concern.

Schools

While adults are exposed to the hazards of occupational environments, children are exposed to the hazards of their school environments. Some of these hazards have been previously addressed in the chapter on children's health, lifestyle concerns, and injury prevention. Here, school structures are highlighted as an environmental issue.

Many of the schools in North America are aging and present the same kinds of environmental concerns as home and occupational environments. By one U.S. estimate, almost one-third of the nation's schools were built before 1950, and 43 percent were built in the 1950s and 1960s. This means that many are due for replacements because of wear and tear or need new configurations to meet safety and technological requirements. The substandard buildings are often in the poorest neighborhoods. Children attending schools with leaking roofs, cracked walls, asbestos exposure, crowded classrooms, and graffiti decorations are not only exposed to health risks, but given a message by the public about the low priority of their education. At the same time there is a record need to renovate old schools and build new ones, voters are increasingly leery of any public expenditures and particularly skeptical about the public schools. Messages about personal health contrast with substandard environments in such schools.

Smoking in Public Places

Some studies indicate that ambient smoke can adversely affect the health of nonsmokers. Thus, reg-

Figure 16-14

A sign of the changing times in smoking policy is this sign at the General Headquarters of the World Health Organization in Geneva, Switzerland. *Source:* World Health Organization.

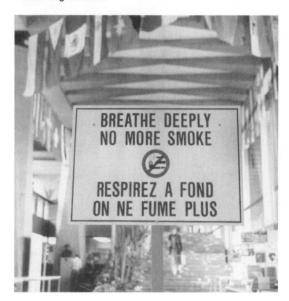

ulating smoking in public places is desirable. Bars and other drinking establishments are notorious for their reputation as smoke-filled places, but restaurants in many parts of the world now offer nonsmoking areas. City and state ordinances require nonsmoking sections in many establishments and ban smoking in some, such as theaters, elevators, public buildings and—increasingly—transport vehicles (figure 16-14).

SUMMARY

People spend over four-fifths of their time in home and work environments. These environments therefore deserve special attention from community health agencies to assure their safety and freedom from serious health risks. Where risks cannot be eliminated, people need to be informed of the risks, of ways to avoid or minimize them, and of tests they can obtain to determine the safety of their environment or to assess their health status in relation to the risks.

Major hazards in residential environments include substandard facilities, crowding, lead paint, and indoor pollution. Building regulations and codes protect the public against some of these hazards, and informed residents can prevent or minimize others through proper ventilation, cleaning, storage, and repainting practices. Population and economic trends have led to increased numbers of people who are homeless, even in Europe and the United States. Deinstitutionalization of the mentally ill has added a particularly vulnerable population to the homeless.

Occupational risks other than injuries, discussed in chapter 13, include dusts, gases, fumes, chemicals, excessive noise, poor ventilation, inadequate lighting, temperature and humidity extremes, infections, and radiation. Employers and workers share the responsibility for reducing occupational hazards, with government setting standards, regulations, and enforcement procedures through laws such as the Occupational Safety and Health Act in the United States. People spend only a small proportion of their time in recreational and other nonresidential, nonoccupational environments, but it can be a high-risk proportion. Public places are increasingly regulated to reduce potential exposure to health risks. Smoking in public places has been banned or restricted in many communities and on some public transportation.

WEB*Links*

http://www.osha.gov
Occupational Safety and Health Administration

http://www.cdc.gov/niosh/homepage.html
National Institute for Occupational Safety and Health

QUESTIONS FOR REVIEW

1. Why is it so difficult to determine scientifically the effect of housing on health?
2. How has improved insulation produced a problem of increased indoor pollution?
3. How do building regulations and zoning codes protect the public's health and safety?
4. What were the major factors leading to the shelter poverty of the 1970s and the homelessness of the 1980s and 1990s?
5. Why should employers want to invest in the health of workers?
6. What factors might account for the improving record of occupational illness and injury in the 1990s?
7. Thinking of the college or university as a workplace, how would you organize efforts to improve the health conditions for workers or students?
8. Why should recreational environments be of any less concern for health purposes than home and work environments?
9. Why has smoking in public places become such an issue?
10. What are the effects of the physical environment in schools on comprehensive school health education programs?

READINGS

American Public Health Association and American Academy of Pediatrics. 1993. *Caring for our children-national health and safety performance standards: guidelines for out-of-home child care programs.* Washington, DC: American Public Health Association. Guidelines for the development and evaluation of the health and safety aspects of family/group daycare homes and childcare centers, beginning with the environmental quality of the care and recreational facilities.

Ross, R. R., and E. M. Altmaier. 1994. *Intervention for Occupational Stress.* Newbury Park, CA: Sage. This book defines the nature of occupational stress and provides information about the emotional, behavioral, psychological, and cognitive symptoms that can occur. Various factors that influence the individual, the work setting, and the larger social context are discussed. Relaxation training, stress management programs, and other coping strategies are explored such as job redesign and career planning.

Shinn, M. 1992. Homelessness: what is a psychologist to do? *Am J Community Psychol* 20:1.

Comparing person-centered and structural explanations for homelessness from data on the distribution of poverty, inadequate and unaffordable housing and 700 families requesting shelter in New York City, this article draws implications for research and action by psychologists.

Weeks, J. L., B. S. Levy, and G. R. Wagner. 1991. *Preventing occupational disease and injury.* Washington, DC: American Public Health Association.

The up-to-date handbook has a public health orientation to occupational disease with strategies for prevention, legal and regulatory resources, worker education and training and an alphabetical listing of disease entities with methods of identification, occurrence, causes, pathophysiology, prevention, and further readings on each.

Williamsen, M. C., and H. De Vries. 1996. Saying "no" to environmental tobacco smoke: Determinants of assertiveness among nonsmoking employees. *Prev Med* 25:575–582.

Nonsmokers' assertiveness can help regulate smoking in worksites by enhancing the salience of nonsmoking norms. This study examined determinants of employees' assertiveness toward smoking colleagues. It is likely that environmental tobacco smoke needs to be perceived as bothersome and harmful for nonsmokers to behave assertively. Worksite education programs could focus more on increasing nonsmokers' awareness of the harmfulness of regular exposure to tobacco smoke at work.

BIBLIOGRAPHY

Baser, M. E. 1992. The development of registries for surveillance of adult lead exposure, 1981 to 1992, *Am J Public Health* 82:1113.

Burrell, R., D. Glaherty, and L. J. Sauers. 1992. *Toxicology of the immune system: a human approach.* New York: Van Nostrand Reinhold.

Consumer Product Safety Commission and American Lung Association. 1990. *Biological pollutants in your home.* Washington, DC: Consumer Product Safety Commission.

Corn, J. K. 1992. *Response to occupational health hazards: An historical perspective.* New York: Van Nostrand Reinhold.

Corner, R. A., G. Kielhofner, F. L. Lin. 1997. Construct validity of a work environment impact scale. *Work* 9:21.

Dolk, H., G. Shaddick, and P. Elliott. 1997. Cancer incidence near radio and television transmitters in Great Britain. *Am J Epidemiol* 145:10.

Eakin, J. M., and N. Weir. 1996. Canadian approaches to the promotion of health in small workplaces. *Can Jour Pub Health* (March-April): 109–13.

Finkelstein, M. M. 1995. Radiographic abnormalities and the risk of lung cancer among workers exposed to silica dust in Ontario. *Can Med Assoc J* 152(1):37.

Fischer, D. B., and A. Boyer. 1993. State activities for prevention of lead poisoning among children—United States, 1992. *MMWR* 42:165.

Guidotti, T. L., and V. M. Clough. 1992. Occupational health concerns of firefighting. *Annu Rev Public Health* 13:151.

Hall, J. R. 1992. *U.S. experience with smoke detectors.* Quincy, MA: National Fire Protection Association.

Lewis, R. J., Sr. 1992. *Sax's dangerous properties of industrial materials.* 8th ed. New York: Van Nostrand Reinhold.

Lovato, C. Y., and L. W. Green. 1990. Maintaining employee participation in workplace health promotion programs. *Health Educ Q* 17:73.

McCauley, L. A. 1998. Chemical mixtures in the workplace. *Am Assoc Occup Health Nurs J* 46:29.

Mood, E. W., ed. 1986. *Housing and health: APHA-CDC recommended minimum housing standards.* Washington, DC: American Public Health Association.

National Institute for Occupational Safety and Health. 1992. *NIOSH health hazard evaluation program.* Pub No 648-004/40829. Atlanta: Centers for Disease Control, Public Health Service, U.S. Government Printing Office.

Ng, C., E. Stone, and P. D. Blanc. 1994. Household chemical exposures: field testing a prevention brochure. *Health Values* 18:24.

Pauls, J. 1991. Safety standards, requirements, and litigation in relation to building use and safety, especially safety from falls involving stairs. *Safety Sci* 14:125.

Rogers, B., and A. R. Cox. 1998. Expanding horizons: integrating environmental health in occupational health nursing. *Am Assoc Occup Health Nurs J* 46:9.

Sciarillo, W. G., G. Alexander, and K. P. Farrell. 1992. Lead exposure and child behavior. *Am J Public Health* 82:1356.

Tarter, S. K., and T. G. Robins. 1990. Chronic noise exposure, high-frequency hearing loss, and hypertension among automotive assembly workers. *J Occup Med* 32:685.

Tenforde, T. S. 1992. Biological interactions and potential health effects of extremely-low-frequency magnetic fields from power lines and other common sources. *Annu Rev Public Health* 13:173.

Toro, P. A., and D. M. McDonnell. 1992. Beliefs, attitudes, and knowledge about homelessness: a survey of the general public. *Am J Community Psychol* 20:53.

Trauma Foundation. 1992. Special issue on housing codes. *Injury Prev Network Newsletter* 9:1.

Upton, A. C., R. E. Shore, and N. H. Harley. 1992. The health effects of low-level ionizing radiation. *Annu Rev Public Health* 13:127.

Wallerstein, N., and H. Rubenstein. 1993. *Teaching about job hazards: a guide for workers and their health providers.* Washington, DC: American Public Health Association.

Webb, G. R., S. Redman, R. W. Sanson-Fisher. 1992. Work injury experience at an industrial worksite. *J Occup Health Safety Austral NZ* 8:143.

Chapter *17*

Control of Atmospheric Pollution

*T*he atmosphere is a blanket for the Earth. Too much blanket or too little, and we're in trouble

—Carl Sagan

Objectives

When you finish this chapter, you should be able to:

- Describe the major sources and the health effects of atmospheric pollution

- Identify the major methods of atmospheric pollution control

- Identify objectives and strategies for environmental protection pertaining to the control of air pollution, radioactivity, and noise in your community

Community actions can affect the health and quality of life of every human population. The burning of coal in China contributes to a parched American sunbelt. The fossil fuels used in North America can contribute decades later to more starvation in sub-Saharan Africa. Carl Sagan's quote reflects an ecological concern: Each individual adds to and takes away from the atmospheric blanket covering you and the entire earth.

Like water, air is a limited and shared resource that knows no national boundaries. It accumulates chemicals, carbon dioxide, and other gases in one geographical region and dumps them as **acid rain** in another or adds to the warming "greenhouse effect" of the atmosphere for the global population.

This chapter offers further evidence of the delicate balance of the environment and how social organization and human behavior, especially since the Industrial Revolution, have upset this balance. The natural history of most life forms, including the human species, evolved over millions of years before human populations had the capacity to affect the environment so vastly. In just the last century or so the human population has imposed a social history so destructive to the environment that people must seek ways to control or compensate for the resultant health effects. In relation to the **atmosphere** this means controlling air pollution, use of radioactive materials, and production of noise.

AIR POLLUTION

We define air pollution as the presence in the **ambient** (surrounding) atmosphere of substances in concentrations sufficient to interfere directly or indirectly with one's comfort, safety, or health, or with the full use of one's property. From the earliest of times pollution from the wastes of human populations has been the main concern, though naturally occurring pollution also can be a threat to health and quality of life.

Epidemiology of Air Pollution

Air pollution arises from industrial exhausts; home heating; incineration; open fires; open dumps; road dust; engine exhaust; crop spraying; construction debris; chemicals, including radon; and other sources. Everyday tools have also come under criticism for their contribution to pollution, including gasoline-powered lawn mowers, leaf blowers, hedge trimmers, snow blowers, and chain saws. These machines produce up to fifty times more air pollution per horsepower than trucks.

Pollutants may be in the form of solids, liquids (vapors), and gases. The atmosphere of a representative industrial area will have about 22 percent of its pollutants from industrial sources; about 10 percent from commercial sources; and the remaining 68 percent from public sources, mostly automobiles. Pollution becomes a problem when a receptor—essentially plant or animal, including a human population—is adversely affected by pollution-related conditions.

Smog **Ozone** pollution produces smog, a persistent problem not only in cities but also in suburbs and rural areas. Ozone in the upper atmosphere protects the earth from harmful solar radiation. In contrast, ozone near the earth's surface is a primary ingredient of smog. Vapors from gasoline, and other organic products mix with atmospheric chemicals in sunlight and are "cooked" to form photochemical smog.

Two basic ingredients in this recipe for pollution are nitrogen oxides and volatile organic compounds (VOCs). Nitrogen oxides come primarily from the incomplete combustion of fossil fuels by motor vehicles and electric power plants. VOCs come from motor vehicles, evaporating solvents, coal burning, chemical and petroleum industries, natural vegetation, and natural events such as volcanic eruptions and forest fires (figure 17-1). Smog accumulates also because of geographic conditions trapping the stagnant air near ground level. The EPA listed Los Angeles, Denver, and Spokane as the three U.S. cities with the worst carbon monoxide pollution in 1996. Meanwhile, more than half of the regions in the United States with unacceptable ozone levels in 1990 had come into the range of federal compliance by 1994 as part of an overall improvement of air quality in most urban areas.

Global Deforestation and the Greenhouse Effect

Since preagricultural times, the world has lost about one-fifth of its forests, from more than 12 billion acres to under 10 billion acres. Each year a tropical forest about the size of Washington State or New Brunswick is cleared from the planet for agricultural or developmental purposes. In the past, much of this loss has been from the developed countries in Europe, Asia, and North America. Now the tropical forests are disappearing most rapidly in Latin America, Asia, and Africa. This loss is considered one of the most serious global problems to some environmental experts because of the role these forests play in regulating the global climate. Through photosynthesis, the forests absorb huge quantities of carbon dioxide. Many scientists believe that if carbon dioxide is not kept in check it will cause significant warming of the earth in a process known as the greenhouse effect.

El Niño, a phenomenon attributed in part to the global climate changes and in turn causing widespread, erratic weather patterns, has spawned several active sites on the Internet:

http://ingrid.ldgo.columbia.edu/SOURCES/
.Indices/ensomonitor.html
This site includes an animated graphic map of the changing conditions and global sea surface temperature anomalies.

http://www.cdc.noaa.gov/~map/maproom/text/
climate pages/sst_olr/old_sst/
sst_9798_anim.shtml
This site is an animated version of how the sea surface temperatures evolved at the equator in 1997. You may need Netscape to view this.

http://www.pmel.noaa.gov/toga-tao/
el-nino/impacts.html
This site outlines some of the impacts of El Niño and La Niña.

Health Effects Human populations suffer an irritating and a direct toxic effect from smog, and some long-term health effects of damage to the outer ozone layer and the warming of the earth's surface. Smog containing ozone causes respiratory

· · · · · · · · · · · · · · · · · · · ·
Figure 17-1

The indirect effects of forest fires on atmospheric pollution are more subtle than the direct effects, but potentially far-reaching. The purposeful destruction of rain forests has even broader effects. The "Smokey the Bear" campaigns have been the most successful over the past several decades of the American public service advertising field in terms of public recognition. *Source:* Advertising Council for Forest Service, U.S. Department of Agriculture, and State Foresters.

Smart Kids Don't Need These Books.

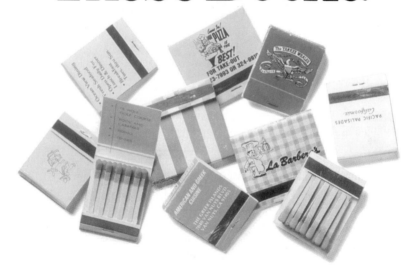

Only you can prevent forest fires.

A Public Service of the Forest Service, USDA, and your State Foresters. **Ad Council**

Photography Henry Bjo

ISSUES AND CONTROVERSIES
Threats to the Earth's Protective Ozone Layer?

Counterclaims to the fears of disaster mount as nations debate their policies for limiting their use of chlorofluorocarbons (CFCs) and carbon fuels and clearing their forests. At issue are the possible restraints these new policies will place on the advances of science, quality of life, and industrial or economic development. Debates between developed and still developing countries center on the relative advantage the developed countries have gained by exploiting these chemicals and resources and the restraint on development the developing countries face if they are to hold back in exploiting their own forests and chemical resources.

One argument is that ozone levels fluctuate from year to year not just with the release of CFCs, methane, and other gases, but also with variable incidence of sunspots. The 11-year cycle in the intensity of sunspots could account for much of the variation observed in the ozone layer over the North Pole region of the earth. These variations have been measured in relation to the 1979 levels, which happen to have been a peak year of ozone thickness. Some debate also surrounds the relative importance of the types of ultraviolet radiation filtered by the ozone layer. Ultraviolet B (UV-B) was thought to be the cause of melanoma—the deadliest form of skin cancer—when the Montreal

Protocol committed the world's industrialized nations to limiting their use of CFCs and other chemicals. UV-A and not UV-B causes melanoma. UV-A is not absorbed by the ozone layer. The rising incidence of melanoma might therefore be related to some other cause such as greater time spent in leisure outdoor activity in more southerly latitudes. UV-B causes a nonfatal squamous cell cancer. One increases one's exposure to UV-B by 10 percent for every sixty miles closer to the equator one dwells. Do these arguments suggest a need to abandon the efforts to control the emissions of gases that reduce the stratospheric ozone cover?

---

problems when air pollution is high. The ingredients of smog also cause environmental damage. Chlorofluorocarbons (CFCs), a type of VOCs, are a family of organic compounds that are nontoxic, long-lived, and nonflammable. While ideal for some uses such as refrigerators and fire extinguishers, their longevity allows them to remain in the atmosphere long enough to rise to the stratosphere. There they break down under intense solar radiation and destroy the ozone. Reduced ozone in the upper atmosphere allows increased ultraviolet radiation to reach the earth, with possible harm to human, animal, and plant populations. In the lower atmospheres the CFCs contribute to global warming. Together with water vapor, carbon dioxide, methane, and nitrous oxide, they absorb infrared radiation, warming the earth's lower atmosphere, soil, and oceans.

The long-term health effects of the CFCs and carbon monoxide in producing health effects re-

mains a point of debate as to their severity (see box). They include skin cancer from ultraviolet rays reaching people more intensely through the thinner ozone layer and a host of secondary effects of global warming. The 1992 international agreement to stop producing ozone-depleting chemicals has begun to reduce the ultraviolet exposures. A Dutch study reported in 1996 that by 2100, controls on the chemicals that attack the Earth's ozone layer would prevent 1.5 million North American cases of skin cancer and another 550,000 in Northern Europe.

The most devastating short-term health effects of air pollution result when a **temperature inversion** occurs. The Denver and Los Angeles areas in the United States are particularly plagued by this problem because of their topography. Surface air normally rises, but during an inversion a layer of warm air resting on top of relatively cool air pins the cool air down much like a lid on a kettle. Smog results when pollution cannot escape.

Based on estimates of harm to human populations from specific levels and types of air pollution, "smog alerts" warn communities on days when air pollution type and level may be hazardous to health. Some effects are acute and can be fatal, while other effects are delayed and may be apparent as chronic diseases only after years of exposure. The acute effects are greater for people who suffer from chronic lung diseases, such as asthma or emphysema, or if they smoke.

Asthma rates in the United States and Canada have surged at least 40 percent since 1982. The trend toward airtight houses and offices creating indoor pollution and allergens accounts for part of this increase in asthma, but atmospheric pollution has contributed to the total impact.

Acute air pollution disasters in the 20th century have included the 1930 Belgium incident where 60 people died as the result of heavy air pollution. In Donora, Pennsylvania, in 1940, a reported 20 people died from pollution. In London in 1952, during a 2-week period of air pollution, about 4,000 more people died than normally would have. And in 1984, a chemical plant in Bhopal, India, accidentally leaked a cloud of methyl isocyanate that killed about 2,000 residents of that city. The 1997 forest fires in Indonesia killed only a few, but thousands of people as far north as Malaysia have suffered acute health effects of the regional air pollution from the smoldering fires. Smog increases death rates by an average of 17 percent in 151 metropolitan areas of the United States. In the most polluted counties of Southern California, research estimates an excess of 275 deaths per year.

Leaks from railroad cars and trucks carrying chemicals have led to local community evacuations in many North American communities. In the air pollution incidents most of those who died had had chronic respiratory or circulatory diseases, and a large proportion were the elderly. The Bhopal chemical tragedy and the transportation accidents illustrate the increasing vulnerability of whole populations to the possibility of industrial or nuclear accidents that could unleash massive doses of air pollutants. Governmental agencies have inherited the onerous responsibility of regulating the construction and safety procedures of such plants.

Three Mile Island in the United States and Chernobyl in the former USSR experienced meltdowns at nuclear power plants. These resulted in the release of nuclear radiation into the atmosphere. In Chernobyl some people died immediately. Sweden continues long-term monitoring of effects of the radioactive cloud from Chernobyl that drifted across northern Europe polluting food chains.

Air pollutants aggravate asthma and other respiratory diseases. Eye, nose, and throat irritations caused by air pollution depend on the individual's sensitivity and the pollutants involved. Irritation of the lungs may make individuals more susceptible to lung infections. Carbon monoxide poisoning may affect heart action adversely and have delayed ill effects on a person. Gastrointestinal disturbances, especially in children, appear to be more prevalent during periods of heavy air pollution. Mexico City has traced some of its diarrheal problems to parasites migrating on particles in the air.

Aesthetic and Economic Aspects Air pollution can damage trees, shrubs, and flowers and ruin crops. Cattle become ill from air pollutants. Air pollution causes damage to residences and other structures. It can interfere with the enjoyment of an otherwise attractive environment. Air pollution can be declared a nuisance on esthetic and health grounds.

Individuals or communities who believe they have been harmed or inconvenienced or have suffered monetary loss from single-source pollution can obtain redress in court. A suit against the firm or persons creating the objectionable air pollution can result in a judgment of monetary compensation for the damage to the plaintiff's person or property. Courts have awarded compensation for harm to cattle resulting from air pollution caused by industrial plants producing aluminum products.

Governments may fine companies for illegally importing chemicals that damage the environment or discharging chemicals into air or water. Governments may also use economic or tax incentives to encourage industries to hasten their conversion of old equipment to newer, cleaner, more environmentally-friendly equipment.

Volcanic Ash   Volcanic ash presents a threat to health in some areas. Not "ash" at all, but pulverized rock, it often contains small pieces of light-weight, expanded lava called **pumice.** A volcano gives advance warning of an eruption, therefore officials usually have time to move populations in the immediate neighborhood to a safer area perhaps twenty or thirty miles away. Long before evacuation is necessary, local and national personnel should have conducted classes and used other means to inform nearby residents of what actions should be taken at the first warning of a volcanic eruption, as in the Mount St. Helen's volcanic activity in the United States. The 1991 eruption of the Mt. Pinatubo volcano in the Philippines forced the evacuation of 16,000 U.S. military personnel, dependents, and civilians from Clark Air Force Base and 20,000 Filipinos living near the volcano. Only two people lost their lives. Proportionate numbers in the Caribbean Island volcanic eruption of 1997 indicate the ability of societies to mobilize for the protection of populations living near active volcanoes, but property damage is almost certain. When residents of a threatened volcanic area refuse to leave, officials may order residents to move. If some families need assistance, officials provide help. All in all, this is a localized problem with relatively low loss of life and few serious injuries. Governmental agencies must assume a major responsibility, but citizen cooperation is essential to saving lives.

Intermittent ash falls may continue over several years after a volcanic eruption. They may cause people to move away from the area, especially those with lung problems.

Air Pollution Control

To control and regulate air pollution by solid particles is least difficult. Various smoke-inspection

Volcanic Winters and Global Air Pollution

New England and New York experienced freezing temperatures and ten inches of snow in the summer of 1816. The summer cold killed much of the green growth in large areas of North America. In Virginia, Thomas Jefferson applied for an emergency bank loan because of his crop failures. England referred to 1816 as "the year without a summer." A typhus epidemic that killed 65,000 people in the British Isles in 1816 was blamed on famine induced by the cold and by crop failures. All of these phenomena were brought about by the eruption in 1815 of Mt. Tambora, a volcano in the Dutch East Indies (now Indonesia). Spewing twenty-five cubic miles of ash into the upper atmosphere, the Tambora eruption was probably the worst in 10,000 years. Mount Vesuvius in Italy is more famous for its sudden burial of an entire city in molten lava during the time of the Roman Empire. The Tambora eruption, however, put a massive cloud of debris into the atmosphere that stayed aloft for months, circled the globe, and blanketed the Northern Hemisphere.

What lessons can you draw from this account of the eruption of Mt. Tambora? Could the great American floods of the Midwest in 1993 be attributed to the Mt. Pinatubo eruption in the Philippines in 1991? Is air pollution confined in its effects to the place of origin? Will the Indonesian forest fires that smoldered for months in 1997 and blanketed much of Southeast Asia with a pale of smoke result in further damage in the years ahead?

devices are available for measuring the density of smoke and other particles in the air (figure 17-2). With established means for measuring smoke pollution, cities have passed ordinances limiting the emission of smoke from industrial plants. Proper firing and design of coal furnaces eliminates 90 percent of their smoke.

Smoke pollution is relatively easy to control. Unfortunately, the most serious air pollutants are carbon dioxide, sulfur oxides, and nitrogen oxides seen increasingly from motor vehicle emissions. These are more difficult to measure and control.

....

Figure 17-2

Measurement of chemical and particulate matter in the air of a square in the heart of Moscow helps inform the necessary control installations on furnaces, incinerators, and dust-producing equipment and procedures. *Source:* Photo by Novosti, courtesy World Health Organization.

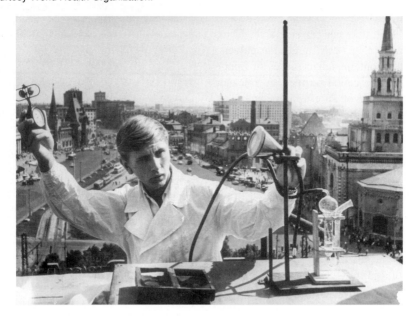

Carbon Dioxide   The most worrisome of the air pollutant gases is carbon dioxide (CO_2), but one hesitates calling this a pollutant because it is essential to the growth of trees and plants. Carbon dioxide molecules trap the heat in the atmosphere much like glass in a greenhouse traps the sun's warmth. The amount of carbon dioxide in the atmosphere has increased 30 percent since human populations began extracting and burning carbon-rich fossil fuels, previously trapped underground for millions of years. Carbon-rich fuels have been driving development since the Industrial Revolution. The concentration of CO_2 in 1750 was 280 parts per million in the 100-kilometers-thick layer of atmosphere blanketing the earth. Today it is 360 parts per million (PPM). The 1995 Intergovernmental Panel on Climate Change predicted that these levels would reach 500 PPM by 2030.

Sulfur Oxides   Pollution from the combustion of sulfur-containing coal and fuel oil is highly injurious to human health, property, and vegetation. Using low-sulfur fuels or removing sulfur from fuels before they are burned reduces pollution. Natural gas, relatively free of sulfur, is preferable to other fuels in terms of reduction of air pollution. Coal is the nemesis, because only a fraction of its sulfur content can be removed before burning. Efforts are directed toward removing the sulfur oxides from the combustion gases before they escape into the air. Sulfur dioxide (SO_2) causes impaired breathing, respiratory illness, alterations in the lungs' defenses, and exacerbation of lung and heart diseases. Those with asthma or chronic lung disease have the worst reactions to sulfur dioxide.

Nitrogen oxides emerge as by-products of combustion processes, including those from automobiles. At present, nitrogen oxide pollution is not as serious a problem as sulfur oxide pollution, but as fuel combustion increases, the nitrogen oxide pollution problem will increase proportionately unless control methods are discovered and implemented. These highly reactive gases play a major role in the formation of ozone and smog. Nitrogen oxides irritate the lungs and lower resistance to respiratory infections such as influenza. Nitrogen dioxide (NO_2) also contributes to acid rain and nitrogen loading of forests and ecosystems.

Lead (Pb) as an atmospheric pollutant has been a serious concern in the past, especially in homes and play areas near roadways or garages where considerable combustion fumes carried lead additives to gasoline. Most of those additives have been removed by law since the introduction of unleaded gasoline in 1975.

Motor vehicle air pollution is partially yielding to newly developed control techniques. Among the methods effective in reducing tailpipe emissions are the modification of fuels and motors to achieve more complete combustion, the injection of air into the exhaust system to oxidize the gases before they reach the tailpipe, and the passage of exhaust gases through afterburners before they are released into the air. Automobile manufacturers apply some of these methods in the form of catalytic converters and exhaust gas recirculation to comply with the standards established by the Clean Air Act.

The International Conferences After noting the poor progress since the Rio Conference of 1992, President Clinton proposed to the meeting of nations in Kyoto, Japan in December, 1997 to cut carbon dioxide emissions by 15 percent to 20 percent by 2010 under the global warming treaty. He proposed a method of "emissions trading," which would allow companies, communities, and nations to get credit for pollution-abatement activities. Canada's Prime Minister Jean Chretian and most European leaders offered more aggressive plans for reduction of greenhouse gases. Canada and the United States are among the

The Double Edge of Public Policy

Automobiles continue to be a major source of air pollution. The highways that carry these vehicles were expanded greatly under the U.S. Highway Act of 1956. Over $50 billion was committed to building more than 40,000 miles of highways. It was the largest public works project in history. This highway construction was in part inspired by fear of nuclear attack during the "red" paranoia of the 1950s. In lobbying Congress for funding, President Eisenhower, a World War II army hero, pointed out that American cities needed broad avenues of escape if threatened by nuclear weapons. By addressing one problem, public escape routes, highways created other problems with congestion, pollution, and the abandonment of inner cities for far-flung suburbs. Today, many lobby for abandoning automobiles in favor of mass public transportation or bicycles. If such transportation solutions are supported, what problems will they solve? What problems are they likely to create?

world's greatest air polluters (figure 17-3). Both countries had increases in their emissions of greenhouse gases in the year before the Kyoto conference. Canada, the United States, and Japan are responsible for 85 percent of the growth in carbon dioxide emissions since 1990.

Legislation In the era when air pollution meant smoke pollution, community ordinances could be enacted to control the problem because the smoke was highly visible and an obvious nuisance that could be smelled or felt in the irritation of eyes. In addition, the degree of smoke pollution could be measured with some precision. Today, air pollution can no longer be regarded as a strictly localized concern. It has become a national and international problem that recognizes no geographical or political boundaries.

U.S. federal air pollution control was first established in 1955 as a consequence of the action of Congress, which passed PL 84-159 "to provide

●●●●●●●●●●●●●●●●●●●●

Figure 17-3

Countries with largest *per capita* contributions to carbon dioxide emissions in the atmosphere in 1994. In *total* metric tons emitted per year, the ten leading countries are, in order, the United States, China, Russia, Japan, Germany, India, Ukraine, the United Kingdom, Canada and Italy. *Source:* Carbon Dioxide International Analysis Center, Oak Ridge National Library, 1995.

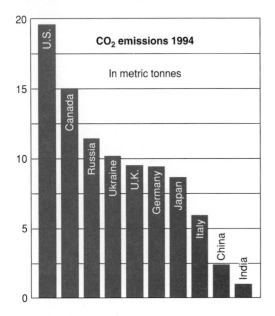

research and technical assistance relating to air pollution control." With the adoption of the **Clean Air Act** in 1963, Congress acknowledged that federal financial assistance is essential for the development of programs to control air pollution. The series of legislative acts and amendments that followed this act of Congress are shown as milestones in the box.

The Clean Air Act was an aggressive piece of legislation that grew out of an era when polls showed that Americans were rating pollution above crime as a serious problem. It was Earth Day, 1970, a time when Girl Scouts wearing gas masks crowded into congressional air quality hearing rooms in support of irate citizens demanding

cleaner air. Declaring air "our most vital resource" and seizing the political initiative to the dismay of Democrats, President Richard Nixon asked Congress in 1970 for sweeping and stringent new clean-air legislation.

Current Issues   Other difficulties plague the Clean Air Act in the political and economic climate of the late 1990s. Some cities—for instance, Los Angeles—will never meet today's air pollution standards unless people there are kept out of their cars by force. Relatively clean areas of the nation must meet even tougher standards designed to prevent them from developing air pollution, causing manufacturers to complain that industrial growth is being hindered in the "sunbelt" (West and South) and communities in the "rust belt" (North) to complain of lost jobs. Different standards for different industries and tougher standards for newer plants tend to encourage the retention of old, inefficient factories. Air pollution has rebounded as a major public issue and a high-priority item on the national agendas of Canada, Mexico, and the United States with the North American Free Trade Agreement (NAFTA).

After two decades of experience, researchers can estimate the number of lives saved by the control of the most dangerous air pollutants—sulfur oxides and particles. Emission restrictions and requirements to burn low-sulfur coal that were imposed on power plants and factories cut the U.S. mortality rate 7 percent, increasing the average life of Americans by a year.

Cost-Benefit Analysis   The problem in determining the effects of pollution on health is that pollutants do their damage over long periods of time. The U.S. Congress dealt with such uncertainties by ordering national standards set low enough to protect the most sensitive people with "an adequate margin of safety" and without regard for what this might cost industry and consumers. That principle was supported by the National Commission on Air Quality, an independent group that studied the act in preparation for the

Milestones in Air Quality and Clean Air Legislation

1775 Sir Percival Potts observed that chimney sweeps develop cancer as a result of their contact with soot, the first recognition of an environment-cancer link.

1864 George Perkins Marsh published *Man and Nature,* first textbook on conservation and human influence on the environment.

1885 Yellowstone, world's first national park, established.

1892 Canada establishes its first national park at Banff, Alberta.

1872 Robert Angus Smith of Scotland provides first description of acid rain.

1905 U.S. Forest Service and National Audubon Society established.

1952 In London 4,000 deaths blamed on smog.

1955 First legislation on air quality, Public Law 84-159, provided research and technical assistance relating to air pollution control.

1962 Rachel Carson published *Silent Spring,* attacking pesticide use and stimulating an environmental movement.

1963 Clean Air Act provided for U.S. federal assistance to states and regions, and encouraged areawide, regional control of air pollution.

1967 Air Quality Act authorized federal intervention to control pollution when a state fails to act. Provided for studies of standards for air pollutants.

1970 This version of the Clean Air Act, the most sweeping in history, led to a vast national cleanup. Pollutants declined sharply enough to increase the life of the average American by a full year. Ordered the automobile industry to cut emissions 90 percent by 1975, a deadline set back repeatedly. National standards set for allowable levels for seven air pollutants (table 17-1). Created EPA.

1972 EPA bans interstate sales of DDT because of its persistence in the environment and its accumulation in the food chain.

1974 Scientists Rowland and Molinas warn that chlorofluorocarbons (CFCs) produced by spray cans and air conditioners are destroying the earth's ozone layer.

1975 Unleaded gasoline introduced, making possible the elimination of the major source of atmospheric lead pollution.

1977 Further amendments, but now the Clean Air initiative began to lose momentum.

1978 President Carter singled out federal clean-air rules as a chief cause of economic inflation.

1979 Nuclear reactor at Three Mile Island in Pennsylvania suffers partial meltdown, but radiation was confined to the reactor dome.

1980s President Reagan eased the standards and control measures as part of wide-ranging **deregulation** of industry. Canada pressured United States on issues of acid rain and other cross-border pollution.

1984 More than 2,000 die and thousands injured by toxic gas from a U.S.-owned industrial plant explosion in Bhopal, India.

1985 Discovery of ozone hole over Antarctica by British scientists.

1986 Chernobyl nuclear reactor explodes, causing thirty-one deaths within days, forcing evacuation of hundreds of square miles in Soviet Ukraine.

1990 New amendments to the Clean Air Act sought to control nearly every important source of air pollution and reduce health and environmental damage caused by acid rain, smog, urban ozone pollution, toxic chemicals, and destruction of the earth's atmospheric

ozone shield. Air Canada became the first smoke-free international airline, followed by Canadian Airlines. Smoking prohibited on all U.S. domestic flights.

1992 First Earth Summit, attended by 178 countries, in Rio de Janeiro. The Global Warming Convention committed these countries to reduction of greenhouse gases. EPA declares second-hand tobacco smoke a human carcinogen and a cause of serious respiratory problems in infants and young children.

1994 Delta Airlines became first U.S. carrier to ban smoking on all international flights.

1995 The United Nations (UN) International Panel on Climate Change acknowledges global warming, reporting that "the balance of evidence suggests that there is a discernible human influence on global climate."

1996 U.S. National Oceanic and Atmospheric Administration study concludes that global campaign to lower production of chemicals that damage the ozone layer had succeeded and that by 2010 the ozone layer will have begun to recover, and by 2050 the ozone "hole" over Antarctica will have closed.

1997 The Environmental Protection Agency (EPA) proposed new air quality standards for particulate matter (e.g., dust and soot) and ozone (smog). These were estimated to provide additional protection to 133 million individuals at elevated risk for lung disease and to save at least $70 billion in health care costs and productivity losses each year. Second Earth Summit held in Kyoto, Japan.

See the EPA web site (http://www.epa.gov/airlinks).

congressional debate. In 1980 the Supreme Court rejected an Environmental Protection Agency (EPA) proposal to use **cost-benefit analysis** in setting new (less restrictive) standards. The commission and the Supreme Court concluded that government must act to control potentially harmful pollutants despite scientific uncertainty about the precise harm they cause, the levels of exposure that cause harm, and the cost. This was the congressional mandate in its "adequate margin of safety" principle.

U.S. industry, the Reagan and Bush administrations, and subsequent Republican Congresses challenged the adequate margin of safety principle. They sought to replace it with a less demanding one that would define a health hazard in terms of "significant risk of adverse effects." The argument is that the air has already been cleaned enough to save most of the lives that could be saved by pollution-control measures, so further expenditures should be limited, with cost to industry and consumers as a consideration. However, asthma deaths have continued to rise.

Scientists believe that for certain dangerous pollutants there is no threshold below which nobody is affected. If this is true, then to meet the congressional mandate could require the closing of many industries. The law will be amended again before that happens. The unions obviously oppose closing of industries, which means that the traditional coalition of Democrats and conservationists has come apart on this issue. Industry, in the meantime, must continue to seek alternative production methods and pollution control devices, because even where there is no direct harm to human life, pollution causes indirect damage to health and the quality of life. **Acid rain,** for example, results from sulfur oxide pollutants carried in rain clouds and can affect marine and plant life, thereby interfering with food chains (see chapter 15).

State and Provincial Programs States and provinces were slow to initiate pollution control programs. Federal legislation and funding helped stimulate provincial and state action. An effective state or provincial air pollution control program requires the following:

- A sanitary authority with status, funds, and research including field studies
- Regional approach to air pollution control
- Calculated program to reduce pollution each year
- Licensing of new industries and new operations based on realistic appraisal of all factors involved
- Industrial zoning based on an intensive study of all factors involved, including the economic benefits to be gained for each proposed industrial installation
- Impartial application of regulations
- A policy permitting changes in regulations, as dictated by experience

Community Programs Few local and regional air pollution control programs in North American cities and counties spend enough on air pollution control. On all levels—federal, state, and local—successful programs are being developed, but some communities have a more serious pollution problem than they had five or ten years ago. National standards of pollution await enforcement of pollution control by communities. Emission standards for pollution control should be applied more rigorously (figure 17-4) and alternative sources of energy should be developed.

Standards The EPA and Environment Canada have set standards for the seven most widespread of the hazardous pollutants (table 17-1). Levels of pollutants measured for the United States and Canada have been reduced. The standard for particles required lowering because only the smallest ones, those that penetrate deep into the lungs, are dangerous. The standard as previously written measures particles of all sizes, including large ones that are trapped in the nose and cause no damage.

Most metropolitan communities that had serious problems in their control of automobile carbon monoxide pollution have made progress. Ozone pollution, however, worsened between 1992 and 1995 averages. Ventura County, California had 22 days exceeding standards, Houston-Galveston,

Figure 17-4

Industrial plants outside cities may have fewer inspections of their equipment and less monitoring of their emissions. *Source:* Photo courtesy World Health Organization and Pan American Health Organization.

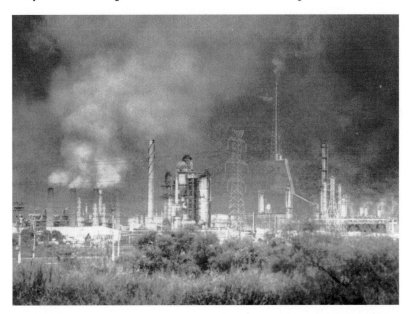

Texas 20 days, Sacramento metro area, California 7 days, New York-New Jersey-Long Island had 5 days, and Baltimore, Philadelphia, and Milwaukee had 4 days exceeding standards.

Besides the seven widespread pollutants for which it has standards, the EPA has identified a group of cancer-causing pollutants that it labels hazardous: asbestos, mercury, beryllium, vinyl chloride, benzene, radionuclides, and arsenic. Of 700 atmospheric contaminants, 47 have been identified as recognized carcinogens (adequate evidence), 42 as suspected carcinogens (limited evidence), 22 as cancer promoters, and 128 as mutagens. These pollutants are emitted in small quantities, but their potential adverse effects on health are more severe than those of the widespread pollutants. The EPA is studying them and has set emission limits for some.

Concern about carcinogenic pollutants is beginning to focus on the growing popularity of diesel automobile engines because, while they emit lower levels of carbon monoxide and hydrocarbons, they emit more nitrogen oxides and 30 to 100 times more particles, which contain some carcinogenic compounds. Nevertheless, the U.S. National Academy of Sciences has found no conclusive evidence that breathing diesel exhaust causes cancer, birth defects, or lung disease in humans, although diesel materials painted on or fed to rats may cause cancer in them. Studies of workers regularly breathing diesel exhaust found no higher rate of cancer among these employees.

Indoor Air Pollution   As buildings are being sealed more tightly to conserve energy, they seal in dangerous pollutants. As is often the case, solving

Table 17-1

The Seven Air Pollutants for Which U.S. Standards Exist, Their Main Sources, and Their Health Effects.

Pollutant	Description	Main sources	Health effects
Ozone	Main component of smog, formed in air when sunlight "cooks" hydrocarbons (like gasoline vapors) and nitrogen oxides from automobiles	Not directly emitted but formed from emissions of automobiles, etc.	Irritation of eyes, nose, throat; impairment of normal lung function
Carbon monoxide	By-product of combustion	Cars and trucks	Weakens heart contractions; reduces oxygen available to body; affects mental function, visual acuity and alertness
Particles	Soot, dust, smoke, fumes, ash, mists, sprays, aerosols, etc.	Power plants, factories, incinerators, open burning construction, road dust	Respiratory and lung damage, in some cases cancer; hastens death
Sulfur dioxide	By-product of burning coal and oil, and of some industrial processes; reacts in air to form sulfuric acid, which can return to earth as "acid rain"	Power plants, factories, space heating boilers	Increases acute and chronic respiratory disease; hastens death
Nitrogen dioxide	By-product of combustion; is "cooked" in the air with hydrocarbons to form ozone (smog); on its own, gives smog its yellow-brown color	Cars, trucks, power plants, factories	Pulmonary swelling; may aggravate chronic bronchitis and emphysema
Hydrocarbons	Incompletely burned and evaporated petroleum products; are "cooked" with nitrogen dioxide to form ozone (smog)	Cars, trucks, power plants, space heating boilers, vapors from gasoline stations	Negligible
Lead	A chemical element	Leaded gasoline	Brain and kidney damage; emotional disorders; death

Source: Adapted from U.S. Environmental Protection Agency.

one problem, energy loss, creates another problem, indoor air pollution (see chapter 16). Tighter insulation prevents the infiltration of outdoor pollutants, but most ventilation systems for smaller and older buildings result in indoor concentrations of inert gases and smaller particles that are as high as or higher than outside levels.

Besides particles from the outside that can become trapped in sealed buildings, including radon, there are many indoor sources of air pollution including gas ranges, smoking cigarettes (figure 17-5), building materials, furnishings, paints, solvents, cleaning agents, and cosmetics. Germs can grow in air conditioning units. Indoor air

Figure 17-5

A mother caresses her infant, but the cigarette threatens the health of both and of others who share the indoor air. After years of growing research evidence, the U.S. Environmental Protection Agency in 1992 declared passive smoking or environmental tobacco smoke a human carcinogen. *Source:* Photo by T. Urban, courtesy World Health Organization.

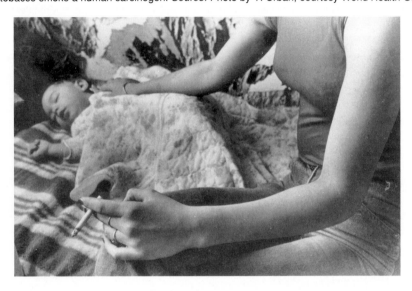

pollution also occurs in airplanes and other sealed spaces.

Common household products emit smog-forming chemicals. Sixteen products account for half of all hydrocarbons (one of two principal ingredients of ozone) from the consumer. These include air fresheners, automotive windshield washer fluids, bathroom and tile cleaners, engine degreasers, floor polishers, furniture maintenance products, general-purpose cleaners, hair sprays, hair mousses, hair-styling gels, glass cleaners, aerosol insect repellents, laundry prewash products, oven cleaners, nail polish removers, and aerosol shaving cream. By far the biggest smog contributor among the sixteen products is hairspray.

One of the ironies of indoor air pollution is that staying indoors is often the recommended solution for outside air pollution (figure 17-6). Furthermore, the average American adult spends about 80 percent of his or her time indoors. Fresh air venti-

lation is a good general solution for most indoor air problems, though this compounds the irony on high pollution days in some cities. Reduction or elimination of pollution sources is the most effective in reducing the health threat.

Asbestos Widely used for its resistance to heat and chemical corrosion, asbestos has over 3,000 uses. Many of these uses are in building products, including insulation, fireproofing, and floor tiles. In the early 1970s the EPA listed asbestos as a hazardous air pollutant and established safety standards for it. Regulations have banned most uses of asbestos (see chapter 16).

When properly maintained, asbestos does not appear to be a health hazard. When it is damaged or deteriorated, however, mineral fibers may become airborne and become a health hazard. Once released into the air, the fibers can remain suspended for days or weeks. If not removed, fibers can pollute

· · · · · · · · · · · · · · · · · · · ·

Figure 17-6

The Pollution Standard Index numbers correspond to the warnings issued to the U.S. and Canadian publics. The United States uses the terms on the left to describe the air quality in media announcements, along with the cautionary statements. The Canadian "Haze Watch" for air quality is published along with the sun intensity indicators to warn people to cover their skin. *Sources:* U.S. Environmental Protection Agency and Ministry of Environment Canada.

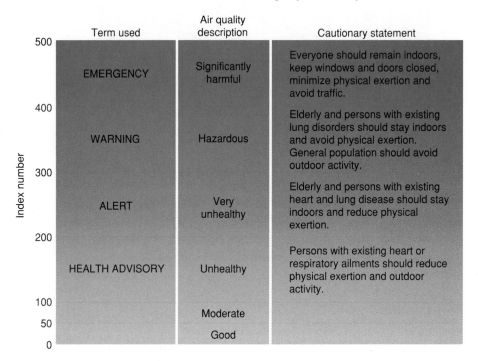

Index number	Term used	Air quality description	Cautionary statement
500			
	EMERGENCY	Significantly harmful	Everyone should remain indoors, keep windows and doors closed, minimize physical exertion and avoid traffic.
400			
	WARNING	Hazardous	Elderly and persons with existing lung disorders should stay indoors and avoid physical exertion. General population should avoid outdoor activity.
300			
	ALERT	Very unhealthy	Elderly and persons with existing heart and lung disease should stay indoors and reduce physical exertion.
200			
	HEALTH ADVISORY	Unhealthy	Persons with existing heart or respiratory ailments should reduce physical exertion and outdoor activity.
100		Moderate	
50		Good	
0			

the building for a lifetime and become airborne whenever dust is stirred up. Asbestos is known to cause asbestosis, a lung disease that is usually fatal, and cancer of the lung, stomach, and chest lining.

Removal of asbestos is not always the answer. Material in good condition and inaccessible may be left until the building is demolished. Some materials may be covered, treated with an encapsulating agent, or repaired. If damaged, deteriorated, or located in areas where it is readily accessible and susceptible to disturbance, it may need to be removed. Only qualified personnel, however, should do removal. The removal process itself can be hazardous to the health of workers and that of building occupants if the asbestos is not handled properly.

Second-Hand Smoke After reviewing the cumulative evidence, the U.S. Environmental Protection Agency declared in 1992 that second-hand tobacco smoke is a human carcinogen and a cause of serious respiratory problems in infants and young children (figure 17-5). The strongly-worded government report concluded that environmental tobacco smoke (ETS) should be added to a select list of the most toxic substances known to cause cancer in humans. The report estimated that 3,000 lung cancer deaths each year and as many as 300,000 lower respiratory tract infections (including bronchitis and pneumonia) among children each year could be attributed to ETS. It also linked ETS to new cases of asthma and to the aggravation of symptoms in some 20 percent of the 2 to 5 million asthmatic children in the United States. The greatest burden, however, as reported in 1995, is heart disease. The majority of deaths caused by secondhand smoke involve heart disease—an estimated 37,000 of the total 53,000 U.S. passive smoking deaths.

Skating Rinks In 1995, an air pollution threat to the public's health was found in the carbon monoxide and nitrogen dioxide left in smaller ice skating rinks and ice hockey arenas by the Zambonis and other internal combustion ice resurfacing machines. Children inhale more of the fumes per body weight. Skaters are at increased risk because the strenuous nature of the activity increases breathing rates. A 1995 survey found air in 40 percent of the 2,500 Canadian community ice rinks exceeded government guidelines for nitrogen dioxide. Large arenas for professional hockey games and ice skating events have enough air space to dissipate the hazardous gases, minimizing the threat to spectators.

RADIATION POLLUTION

Natural sources of radiochemical activity and cosmic radiation have always exposed human populations to "background radiation." All people are exposed to a harmless amount of radioactivity of about 0.1 R (roentgen) per year. Not until the splitting of the atom did radioactive atmospheric pollution become a problem or a threat.

Radioactivity is a natural physical process. Although atoms of most substances are stable, some complex radioactive atoms—known as radioisotopes—are unstable because they have too much energy. They become more stable by releasing extra radiation energy in a process known as radioactive decay. The particles released from this process cannot be seen, smelled, tasted, or heard, but radioactivity is hazardous. Radiation can penetrate human tissue. Depending on the level of exposure the effects on human organs can range from nausea, to localized skin burns, to death.

Epidemiology of Exposure to Radioactivity

Most of the radiation hazard for the public's health still comes from natural sources, as shown in figure 17-7. The housing codes described in chapter 16 seek to control the natural radon seeping into some houses.

Medical and Dental Sources The use of radioactive materials for treatment, research, and other purposes must always be regarded as a potential hazard, but these possible sources of radioactivity are usually well controlled and are not a danger to the public. The immediate danger is to those people working with radioactive materials, and they have the necessary knowledge to use proper shielding and to take other precautions for protecting themselves.

Nuclear Weapons The prevention of nuclear war has been described by some as the ultimate public health problem. The atomic bomb has been used twice as a weapon of war. The United States dropped the bombs on August 6, 1945, in Hiroshima, Japan, and on August 9, 1945, in Nagasaki, Japan. At each site 75,000 people died immediately; many more suffered the effects of radiation-related illnesses and still do.

When nuclear weapons were tested in the atmosphere, explosions sprayed the atmosphere with long-lived radioactive particles. These particles, such as strontium-90 and cesium-137, settled to the earth. Such fallout represents a threat to human life because penetration of body cells by radioactive particles causes ionization of the atoms of cells, particularly cells undergoing division. The extent of damage depends on the dose received and whether it is received externally or internally. For doses received or applied externally, the unit of measurement is the roentgen—the amount of radiation that causes two ionizations per cubic micron. An adult exposed to 1 R would receive about 10 to 17 ionizations over the whole body. A dose of less than 100 R produces no symptoms in a person, but 500 R in one dose

. . . .

Figure 17-7

The distribution of ionizing radiation exposures for the average American shows about 18 percent from sources produced by society. The largest source of natural exposure is radon, partially controllable through building codes and practices. *Source:* National Council on Radiation Protection and Measurements.

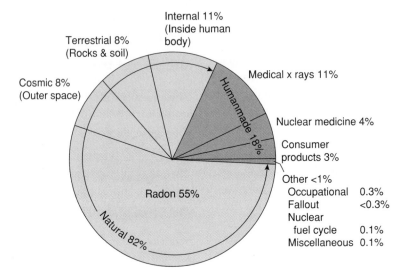

is fatal. The U.S. Atomic Energy Commission reports that the average external dose from nuclear weapons test fallout was from 0.001 to 0.005 R per year, less than 5 percent of the annual dose from background radiation.

Internal dosage is expressed by the strontium unit (SU), equivalent to 0.003 R per year exposure of bone tissue. Internal doses result from ingesting radioactive water, milk, and other foods (figure 17-8). This type of exposure to radioactivity poses a greater health threat than does external exposure. Strontium-90 is chemically similar to calcium and thus is deposited in bone. In young children strontium-90 is distributed throughout the bones, where localized high doses may cause malignancies. In adults the cancellous (spongy) bone is usually affected, causing acute poisoning.

Maximum permissible concentration (**MPC**) has not been established to the satisfaction of scientists in the field of radiation. The U.S. National

Academy of Sciences has proposed 50 SU as the MPC, but the U.S. National Committee on Radiation sets the standard 25 percent higher. The level of radioactive fallout from nuclear tests was greater in the United States than in any other country.

Nuclear arms proliferation among developing countries is a great threat and could become a by-product of nuclear energy technology if the technology is converted to arms by terrorists. The Europeans and New Zealanders have been the most vociferous in objecting to nuclear arms on their territory, but health professionals elsewhere have become increasingly concerned with the health implications of a world faced with the possibility of "the ultimate epidemic." Nuclear disarmament and nonproliferation treaties of Russia, the North Atlantic Treaty Organization, and the United States are hopeful signs. Resistance from some countries such as India, however, has thwarted the ban on nuclear weapons testing.

Figure 17-8

Radiochemical analysis of milk, testing for the presence of strontium 90, has been necessary in regions affected by fallout or leakage from nuclear reactor accidents, nuclear weapon testing, or underground tanks such as those at the Hanford nuclear reservation in Washington State. *Source:* Photo by P. Larsen, courtesy World Health Organization.

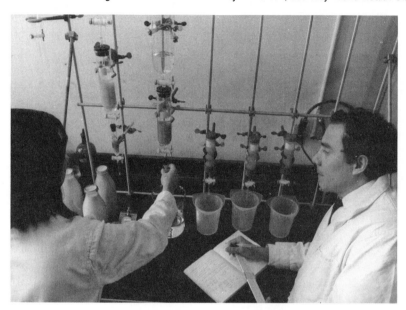

Nuclear Reactors   Energy requirements for development and growing expectations for comfort and convenience are increasing at a rate faster than the rate of population growth. It appears that fossil fuel sources are inadequate and too environmentally unfriendly to meet rising energy needs. The next most readily available source is nuclear energy, which can be converted to electrical energy. To obtain this additional electrical power, governments and public utility companies have developed nuclear reactors. Protesters have raised objections to the proposed plant sites and even to the construction of such plants. They are concerned about the possibility of constant emissions from the reactors, thermopollution from heated water emptied into streams, unsafe disposal of radioactive wastes, and—foremost—accidents that would saturate the atmosphere with lethal radioactive ions. The incident at the Three Mile Island reactor in Pennsylvania and the subsequent Chernobyl incident confirmed the validity of some of these concerns (see Milestones box).

Shielding and the use of other proven methods control emissions of nuclear reactors. Water is cooled before being discharged into streams. Wastes are buried 2,500 feet underground or otherwise rendered distant or relatively harmless to human beings. Accidents that would threaten communities have probabilities close to the order of zero, but Chernobyl demonstrated that "close" is not good enough. Those who work at nuclear plants are the most exposed to any possible danger and the most knowledgeable. These experts who understand the situation tend to minimize any reason for fear. When tapping solar energy becomes more feasible, reducing the need for nuclear reactors, the public will be more reassured.

Nuclear Winter

Based on studies of the Mount Tambora effects of 1816 and on other volcanic and climatological analyses, a group of scientists postulated in 1983 the concept of a disastrous human-made winter caused by nuclear war. The fires and explosions that would follow the detonation of only half of the world's nuclear arsenals would propel at least 180 million tons of smoke and 15 million tons of dust into the atmosphere. These clouds would blanket the earth for at least 6 to 20 weeks, dropping temperatures 18° to 55° F in Europe, North America, and China if the war occurred during spring or summer, or in the Southern Hemisphere if it happened in their spring or summer. The pall of smoke and dust would block out 99 percent of the sunlight, destroying agriculture for at least a year. Famine would be unavoidable for survivors of the war in all parts of the world.

How long a nuclear winter would last is incalculable. The rainfall that might flush the skies could be disrupted by the accumulation of the sun's heat in the upper atmosphere. Even sunlight that did penetrate the blanket of dust would present the additional danger of lethal ultraviolet radiation because much of the protective ozone layer in the upper atmosphere would have been burned away. Given the effects of freezing temperatures; radiation exposure; general air pollution; famine; and the resulting inadequately treated diseases, wounds, and burns (since little medical care would be left available), nuclear winter presents the possibility of human extinction. How might economic globalization affect this scenario?

Electric and Magnetic Fields: A Health Issue?

Over 300,000 miles of power lines stretch across the United States. Electric and magnetic fields exit between the overhead conductors and the ground whenever current flows. Electric and magnetic fields transfer electrical energy to conductive objects, including humans. There is a debate in research about whether these fields independently or in combination cause health problems. A small body of epidemiologic research reports an association between low-level background residential alternating-current magnetic fields and childhood cancer. Regulatory, judicial, and media involvement have raised public awareness and fear on the issue. The challenge is to determine the risk better through solid research and implement ways to avoid it. Until then, we can expect opposition to new transmission facilities, reluctance to buy homes near power lines, labor concerns, and personal damage litigation. Keeping the public informed will be an important public health education responsibility.

cials and special agencies set up to safeguard the public. The public correctly demands constant vigilance to detect and control radiation hazards.

PRESSURED GASES

Gases held under pressure in containers pose direct threats to health and long-term threats to the atmospheric environment.

Fluorocarbon Gases

Fluorocarbon propellants from aerosol spray containers do not decompose chemically in the lower atmosphere because they do not react with any other gases. Rainwater does not remove these propellants from the air so they remain to produce atmospheric effects harmful to human health. Fluorocarbons drift slowly into the upper regions of the stratosphere and release chlorine after being

Surveillance   The federal governments of Canada and the United States, with monitoring stations distributed across North America, keep a close surveillance of nuclear plants and atmospheric radiation and take all possible action to control sources of radiation. Similar agencies in other countries serve this purpose. On the state or provincial and community level, detection and correction of radiation "leaks" from x-ray machines, fluoroscopic equipment, and other sources of radiation is a continuous effort by health offi-

•••••••••••••••••••••

Figure 17-9

Attention on the ozone depletion issue has shifted from fluorocarbon propellant spray cans to refrigerants containing similar ozone-depleting chemicals. Many developing countries have not yet converted their refrigeration systems to the more environmentally safe chemicals. *Source:* Photo by P. Pittet, courtesy World Health Organization, African Regional Office, and Food and Agriculture Organization.

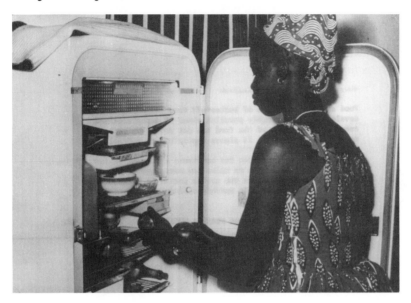

subjected to ultraviolet rays. The released chlorine atoms react with ozone molecules to produce chlorine oxide and oxygen. This reaction in turn decreases the amount of ozone, eventually reducing the ozone concentration by as much as 4 percent. Recovery to normal levels of ozone may take decades. When the ozone level is lowered, more ultraviolet rays reach the earth, which could result in such effects as cancer, particularly of the skin.

The cooling fluid used in most refrigerators and some radiators has a similar effect on the ozone. These are being phased out by treaties signed in 1990 among most Western countries, as the fluorocarbon spray cans have in past years. However, large, Third World countries are just beginning to enjoy the benefits of widespread home refrigeration (figure 17-9). The human respiratory tract can be directly affected by fluorocarbons. In the non-

ciliated part of the nasal junction, fluorocarbon particles move slowly, but particles deposited in the ciliated tissue move more rapidly. Therefore there can be an immediate threat to the lungs of exposed users and possible long-term effects from atmospheric changes created by fluorocarbons.

Few products remain on the market in North America that use fluorocarbon-driven propellants in spray cans. Different types of spray cans such as pump or water-driven sprays have replaced the fluorocarbon containers. The international campaign to ban these products has succeeded in reversing the damage to the ozone layer.

Other Pressurized Gases

Pressurized gases other than fluorocarbons also present dangers. Oxygen in containers can be a fire hazard if released near a flame. Stored in hallways or near vehicles, compressed gas cylinders can be knocked over and explode with devastating results. Rusty cans of ether can be volatile fireballs when kicked. Teenagers sniff aerosol chemicals for a dangerous high. Small children can incur lung damage or poisoning from breathing aerosol fumes. Finally, much of the problem of indoor pollution addressed in chapter 16 is attributable to pressurized gases sprayed or leaked into the contained air spaces of unventilated houses or buildings.

NOISE AND HEAT POLLUTION

Noise and heat are increasingly significant public health concerns. The growing magnitude and complexity of society have brought increases in noise levels to a degree that the public calls for programs to relieve their distress. The global warming trend attributed to the greenhouse gases and the El Niño effect of Pacific Ocean warming have resulted in heat waves and deaths in vulnerable populations.

Epidemiology and Control of Noise

Not all sound is objectionable, nor is all sound classed as noise. Technically, noise is any disturbing sound that interferes with work, comfort, or rest. It is doubtful that deaths have been caused by noise, yet noise can have an adverse effect on health, particularly mental health. Sounds are measured in decibels. Noise over 90 decibels can cause stress, even hearing loss. Prolonged exposure to noise of 85 to 115 decibels have been linked to a variety of mental and social problems.

The urgency of the problem created by noise depends on the frequency of the occurrence, the absolute and the relative loudness, and whether the noise is necessary or unnecessary. The honking of an automobile horn may be objectionable, but the siren of a fire truck may not be. Some sounds that may be objectionable nevertheless must be accepted. For example, as much as the public objects to the roar of jet planes, citizens in certain locations have had to learn to live with this noise. Air-

Figure 17-10

Excessive noise disturbs our environment just as do air, water, or soil pollution. Hearing losses from excessive sound or noise exposure are the most frequently reported occupational injury. *Source:* Winning photograph of the Habitat photo competition, "A Better Way to Live," by Kyoshi Hasaka, Japan, courtesy World Health Organization.

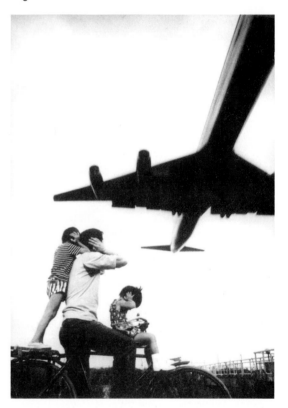

ports change flight schedules and paths to accommodate some citizen complaints (figure 17-10).

Industry Noise Control   Noise represents a problem of some significance in some industries. Exposure to high noise levels can cause deafness. Noises of lower levels can affect workers' efficiency and be otherwise objectionable. Industry usually makes surveys of noise intensities and takes necessary corrective measures, as described in chapter 16. Segregating noisy operations, insulating for sound control, redesigning machinery, and changing operations are among the possible corrective measures. Where noise intensity cannot be avoided, providing workers with ear protectors will safeguard their hearing.

Community Noise Control   Certain noises in the modern community, such as from traffic, street work, construction work, locomotives, and certain industries, may be ever present. The public accepts a certain noise intensity from these sources, but will lodge complaints when the noise rises above a certain level of intensity.

City planning, including restricting industrial or commercial operations to particular zones, is a first measure. Cooperation resulting from communication between the parties concerned is the key to dealing with noise problems that arise and that are not covered by existing ordinances. Community organization efforts should precede court action, but if all other efforts fail, a court injunction will prohibit the offender from continuing the noise nuisance or will order the offender to reduce the noise to a defined, tolerable level.

Noise-control laws have been enacted in various cities. New York enacted the first noise-pollution law in the 1970s. Laws dealing with contemporary noise sources include banning rolling "boom boxes" and cars with megawatt stereos. Limits have been set on car and home alarms in some areas.

Heat Waves as a Health Issue

From July 1 to 13, 1993, the eastern part of the United States suffered a heat wave implicated in 84 deaths in the Philadelphia area alone, especially among elderly and infirm people. Three cases occurring in other parts of the country were described by the centers for Disease Control:

Case 1. A one-year-old infant left sleeping for approximately 75 minutes in the back seat of an automobile with the windows closed was found dead from hyperthermia.

Case 2. On July 7, a 48-year-old woman was found unconscious at her kitchen table in her mobile home. She was pronounced dead on arrival at a local emergency department. Rectal temperature measured at the emergency department after the 20-minute air-conditioned ambulance ride was 108° F (42° C). The windows in the decedent's mobile home were closed and fans turned off when she was discovered. She had been dehydrated the day before when she arrived for her appointment at a local health department clinic.

Case 3. A 68-year-old man, last seen alive on July 5, was found in a slightly decomposed state in his apartment on July 8. Room temperature exceeded 100° F (38° C). Direct cause of death was atherosclerotic heart disease, but hyperthermia was recorded as a contributing factor.

How might these deaths have been prevented at a community level of action?

AIR QUALITY OBJECTIVES

The overall goal of community air quality control programs is to achieve and maintain adequate air quality to avoid adverse effects on human health and welfare and to minimize damage to structures and vegetation, visibility reduction, odor, and other nuisance effects or esthetic insults to the population. Inserting realistic target dates and levels for a given community in place of the levels shown for the year 2000 in table 17-2 should produce appropriate objectives for the community.

The "Midcourse Review" in 1995 of progress on the U.S. air quality objectives gave encouragement, despite the increase in asthma morbidity and mortality over the previous decade. Substantial progress was reported on reducing blood lead levels, particularly among children. The amount of lead in gasoline has declined by 99.9 percent since the introduction in 1975 of unleaded gasoline. A 47 percent reduction in lead used in soldering soft-drink cans and reductions in lead-based paint and plumbing in houses also contributed to this success.

Table 17-2

U.S. National Air Quality Risk Reduction Objectives

A.	B.
Risk reduction objectives Reduce human exposure to criteria air pollutants, as measured by an increase to at least 85% in the proportion of people who live in counties that have not exceeded any Environmental Protection Agency standard for air quality in the previous 12 months. (Baseline: 49.7 in 1988)	Increase to at least 40% the proportion of homes in which homeowners or occupants have tested for radon concentrations and that have either been found to pose minimal risk or have been modified to reduce risk to health. (Baseline: Less than 5% of homes had been tested in 1989; more than 11% in 1993)

Proportion Living in Counties That Have Not Exceeded Criteria Air Pollutant Standards in 1988 for:

Ozone	53.6%
Carbon monoxide	87.8%
Nitrogen dioxide	96.6%
Sulfur dioxide	99.3%
Particulates	89.4%
Lead	99.3%
Total (any of above pollutants)	49.7%

Special population targets

Testing and modification as necessary in:	Baseline	2000 target
11.6a Homes with smokers and former smokers	—	50%
11.6b Homes with children	—	50%

Baseline data sources: Office of Radiation Programs, Environmental Protection Agency; Center for Environmental Health and Injury Control.

Note: An individual living in a county that exceeds an air quality standard may not actually be exposed to unhealthy air. Of all criteria air pollutants, ozone is the most likely to have fairly uniform concentrations throughout an area. Exposure is to criteria air pollutants in ambient air. Due to weather fluctuations, multiyear averages may be the most appropriate way to monitor progress toward this objective.

Baseline data source: Office of Air and Radiation, Environmental Protection Agency.

Implementation of the Clean Air Act has helped increase the proportion of people living in counties that meet EPA standards for air pollution. Figure 17-11 shows the states that have achieved the goal of increasing to 85 percent or more the proportion of their population living in counties meeting EPA standards for the six air pollutants shown in objective A in table 17-2.

Progress is seen also in reduced toxic agents released into the air. Reduced exposure to radon shows slight progress. The proportion of people who report their homes have been tested for radon has more than doubled from less than 5 percent in

1989 to more than 11 percent in 1993. Only three states had adopted construction standards and techniques to minimize radon levels; only two states required disclosure of radon concentrations in conjunction with the sale of property.

Canada has not had national air quality objectives, but has shown progress in reducing exposure to smoking in public places through local bylaws restricting smoking. Figure 17-12 shows the percent of municipalities in Canada with such bylaws in 1995. Restaurant restrictions on smoking are the most common, bus stations least common.

••••••••••••••••••••
Figure 17-11

One of the U.S. air quality objectives was to increase to 85 percent or more the proportion of the population not exposed to six pollutants more than permitted by EPA standards. This map shows the states that have achieved the objective and those at various lower levels of achievement. *Source:* Environmental Protection Agency and U.S. Office of Disease Prevention and Health Promotion.

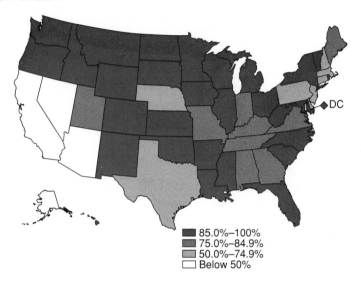

- 85.0%–100%
- 75.0%–84.9%
- 50.0%–74.9%
- Below 50%

••••••••••••••••••••
Figure 17-12

Municipalities with bylaws restricting smoking to designated indoor areas, by location, Canada, 1995. *Source:* Stephens, T. and associates, and Goss Gilroy Inc. *Survey of smoking restrictions in four settings.* 1995. Ottawa: prepared for Health Canada.

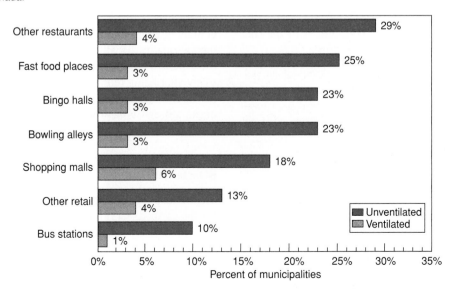

ENVIRONMENTAL PROTECTION AGENCIES

The convergence of concerns about global warming, environmental degradation, sustainability, and environmental health problems led to a strengthening of agencies for the protection and promotion of environmental quality. These agencies are found at all levels of government and are discussed further in chapters 18–20. At the national level in most countries is an agency such as the EPA in the United States. State or provincial agencies are variously named, but a common designation is Department of Environmental Quality. Some metropolitan areas have environmental control departments, but the nature of environmental quality, especially air and water quality, being geographically broad rather than localized, dictates that state or regional bodies serve the needs of populations in matters of environmental control.

State or Provincial Agencies

An unpaid lay commission appointed by the governor or premier usually governs a state or provincial department of environmental quality. The commission appoints a full-time professional director, who in turn appoints the professional staff, subject to approval by the commission. Usually the state or province is divided into districts, and members of the professional staff are assigned to the different districts. Responsibilities of the staff in each district usually are as follows:

- *Air quality:* investigating complaints of air pollution and obtaining necessary corrections; monitoring air quality problems in the district; conducting surveys and collecting samples of air; reviewing and preparing permits for emissions
- *Water quality:* investigating complaints of water pollution and developing necessary controls and enforcement procedures to protect state or provincial water standards; investigating and reviewing proposed waste treatment plant locations; conducting inspections and surveillance

of existing sewage treatment plants and sewage collection systems; conducting inspections and surveillance of existing industrial treatment facilities and waste discharges; preparing waste discharge permits for treatment facilities; conducting water quality basin surveys
- *Solid wastes:* investigating solid waste disposal sites; evaluating proposed sites; preparing permits for solid waste disposal facilities
- *Community and interagency responsibilities:* providing technical assistance and advice to local health departments and officials on such matters as sewage disposal, solid waste disposal, industrial waste disposal, and water quality surveys; consulting with the public, industry representatives, engineers, and city, county, state or provincial, and federal officials regarding plans, programs, and permits related to the design, construction, and operation of sewage treatment facilities, industrial waste treatment facilities, air treatment systems, and solid waste disposal systems; providing public information to local groups on all aspects of environmental quality.

While these state or provincial environmental quality agencies are often separate from the state or provincial health departments, cooperation and a close relationship are important. The magnitude of environmental health problems in contemporary society makes imperative the existence of a self-contained agency to be responsible for environmental quality. Health departments still carry on their traditional functions, perhaps more effectively after being relieved of the many tasks inherent in environmental health programs. Voluntary organizations concerned with the environment also contribute (figure 17-13).

SUMMARY

The atmosphere is a sensitive, protective blanket for the earth, as Carl Sagan warned. Air provides the medium for the transmission of pollutants,

Figure 17-13

Tree planting in urban areas has helped control temperature levels, which reduces the evaporation of water and the production of greenhouse gases. Trees also absorb carbon monoxide. *Source:* The National Arbor Day Foundation.

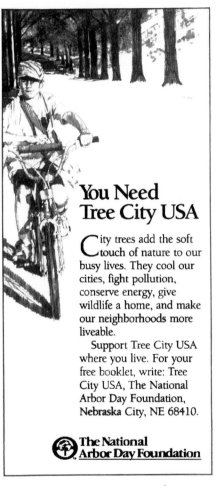

You Need Tree City USA

City trees add the soft touch of nature to our busy lives. They cool our cities, fight pollution, conserve energy, give wildlife a home, and make our neighborhoods more liveable.

Support Tree City USA where you live. For your free booklet, write: Tree City USA, The National Arbor Day Foundation, Nebraska City, NE 68410.

The National Arbor Day Foundation

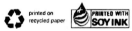

printed on recycled paper — PRINTED WITH SOY INK

radiation, noise and heat, all of which can harm the health of human populations. Cooperation between governmental jurisdictions to control air pollution is essential because it extends across community and national boundaries. The potential for communitywide and worldwide drift of pollutants and clouds of chemicals, dust, or smoke makes the responsibility of each industry, each community, and each nation greater. This has been illustrated most poignantly by the experience of the 1816 "year without a summer," the Bhopal disaster in India in 1984, the Chernobyl nuclear disaster in 1987, and the Indonesian forest fires in 1997.

Problems with radioactivity are attributable to industry, medical care (x-rays), government (nuclear power plants and weapons), and radon gas. Therefore, a small proportion of the exposure of the population at large comes from human sources. Low levels of ionizing radiation can produce delayed effects, such as cancer and genetic anomalies, after a latent period of many years.

As global society becomes increasingly interdependent and populous, and the human capacity to alter the environment greater, the need to control adverse environmental factors becomes more urgent. No one has the right to jeopardize others' welfare by making the environment threatening to health or unpleasant (as in the case of air and noise pollution). The community must impose requirements on its residents for the protection of all. Besides the authority of the community represented in legislative requirements, community officials must provide services that will assist citizens in maintaining the best possible environment from the standpoint of health. Equally important, each citizen should understand his or her responsibility for a healthful environment and be motivated to assume responsibility for the quality of the community's environment. A "blitz" program or cleanup campaign may be justified on occasion but should not be the regular mode of community effort. Constant promotion of environmental health is the effective prescription.

WEB*Links*

http://www.nhes.com
Dr. Patrick Michael's World Climate Report

http://www.ec.gc.ca
Environment Canada

http://www.greenpeace.org
Greenpeace International

http://www.unfccc.de
UN Framework Convention on Climate Change
Secretariat

http://www.worlwatch.org
Worldwatch Institute

QUESTIONS FOR REVIEW

1. Why does air pollution control require cooperation between governmental jurisdictions?
2. How do chemicals, smoke, and ash produce too much "blanket" in the earth's atmosphere?
3. How do chemicals produce too little atmospheric "blanket"?
4. Why does smog accumulate?
5. What role do volcanic eruptions play in the theory of nuclear winter?
6. Why has there been an increased interest in environmental health despite the great advances in the understanding and overall control of environmental pollutants?
7. If an industrial firm that will employ 3,000 people wishes to set up a plant in your community, what measures can protect the health of workers and the community?
8. In the past year, to what radiation dangers have you been exposed?
9. What safeguards and assurances do you get from the burial method of nuclear waste disposal?
10. What questions would you ask if the Department of Energy proposed to put one of the nuclear waste disposal sites in your community?
11. Why is nuclear war referred to as the ultimate epidemic?
12. What are the characteristics of fluorocarbon propellants from aerosol spray cans that enable them to drift to the upper atmosphere and decrease the protective ozone layer?
13. In what ways will the environment of the future be more or less hazardous to human health than the environment of today?
14. How can noise be considered a form of air pollution?
15. Which agencies have jurisdiction over environmental controls in your community?

READINGS

Keating, M. 1996. *Canada and the State of the Planet.* Oxford: Oxford University Press.
North Americans face increasing threats of environmental changes such as the thinning of the ozone layer, deforestation, extinction of animal and plant species. This book explains the main elements of those changes in a clear, non-partisan way.

O'Riordan, M. C., and A. P. Brown. 1997. Ionizing radiation. In *Oxford textbook of public health,* edited by R. Detels, W. W. Holland, J. McEwen, and G. S. Omenn. 3d ed. Vol. 2. Oxford: Oxford Medical.
This review of the public health aspects of radiation covers quantities and units of measurement, sources of ionizing radiation, exposure to radon, biological action of ionizing radiation, carcinogenic and genetic effects of radiation, principles of radiological protection, and radiation accidents.

Steenland, K., and D. A. Savitz. eds. 1997. *Topics in environmental epidemiology.* New York: Oxford University Press.
Defines environmental epidemiology as the study of the health consequences of exposures that are involuntary and that occur in the air, water, diet, or soil. Topics include particulates and mortality, respiratory diseases and lung function; nitrogen dioxide and ozone as these affect lung function; passive smoking and middle ear diseases, childhood asthma, sudden infant death syndrome, lung cancer, and heart disease.

Upton, A. C. 1997. Radiological sciences. In *Oxford textbook of public health,* edited by R. Detels, W. W. Holland, J. McEwen, and G. S. Omenn. 3d ed. Vol. 2. Oxford: Oxford Medical.
This review of radiological issues and methods covers the characteristics of electromagnetic waves, including ionizing and nonionizing radiations, and electromagnetic fields, and studies of acute effects.

BIBLIOGRAPHY

Baxter, L. A., F. J. Finch, and Q. Yu. 1997. Comparing estimates of the effects of air pollution on human mortality obtained using different regression methodologies. *Risk Anal* 17:273.

Chen, J-D, J-D Wang, and W-I Chao. 1997. Effects of occupational and nonoccupational factors on liver function tests in workers exposed to solvent mixtures. *Arch Environ Health.* 52:270.

Deadman, J-E, B. G. Armstrong, and G. Theriault. 1996. Exposure to 60-Hz magnetic and electric fields at a Canadian electric utility. *Scan J Work, Environ & Health* 22:415.

Feychting, M., U. Forssen, and B. Floderus. 1997. Occupational and Residential Magnetic Field Exposure and Leukemia and Central Nervous System Tumors. *Epidem* 8:384.

Flodin, U., J. Ziegler, and O. Axelson. 1996. Bronchial asthma and air pollution at workplaces. *Scan J Work, Environ & Health* 22:451.

Fresh Approaches to Fresh Air. 1997. *Am Demographics* 19:64.

Friis, R. H., and T. A. Sellers. 1997. *Epidemiology for public health practice.* Frederick, MD: Aspen Publishers, Inc.

Goldstein, B. D., and M. R. Greenberg. 1997. Toxicology and environmental health. In *Oxford textbook of public health,* edited by R. Detels, W. W. Holland, J. McEwen, and G. S. Omenn. 3d ed. Vol. 2. Oxford: Oxford Medical.

Goren, A., and E. Yehudit. 1996. Introduction: Proceedings of the Workshop on Air Pollution and Health in the New Middle East, Jerusalem, Israel. *Public Health Reviews* 25(July 2):3.

Griffiths, R., and P. Saunders. 1997. Reducing environmental risk. In *Oxford textbook of public health,* edited by R. Detels, W. W. Holland, J. McEwen, and G. S. Omenn. 3d ed. Vol. 3. Oxford: Oxford Medical.

Hine, D. W., C. Summers, and A. McKenzie-Richer. 1997. Public opposition to a proposed nuclear waste repository in Canada: an investigation of cultural and economic effects. *Risk Anal* 17:293.

Hoffman, W., H. Dieckmann, and I. Schmitz-Feuerhake. 1997. A cluster of childhood leukemia near a nuclear reactor in Northern Germany. *Arch Environ Health* 52:275.

Katsouyanni, K. 1997. Short-term effects of air pollution on health: A European approach using epidemiologic time series data. The APHEA project. *Public Health Reviews* 25:7.

Kromhout, H., D. P. Loomis, D. A. Savitz. 1997. Sensitivity of the Relation between Cumulative Magnetic Field Exposure and Brain Cancer Mortality to Choice of Monitoring Data Grouping Scheme. *Epidem* 8:442.

Lipfert, F. W. 1997. Perspective: Air pollution and human health: perspectives for the '90s and Beyond. *Risk Anal* 17:137.

Melamed, S., P. Froom, and J. Ribak. 1997. Industrial noise exposure, noise annoyance, and serum lipid levels in blue-collar workers—the CORDIS Study. *Arch Environ Health* 52:292.

Moolgavkar, S. H., E. G. Luebeck, and E. L. Anderson. 1997. Air pollution and hospital admissions for respiratory causes in Minneapolis-St. Paul and Birmingham. *Epidem* 8:364.

Omenn, G. S., and E. M. Faustman. 1997. Risk assessment, risk communication, and risk management. In *Oxford textbook of public health,* edited by R. Detels, W. W. Holland, J. McEwen, and G. S. Omenn. 3d ed. Vol. 2. Oxford: Oxford Medical.

Orlebeke, J. F., D. L. Knol, and F. C. Verhulst. 1997. Increase in child behavior problems resulting from maternal smoking during pregnancy. *Arch Environ Health* 52:317.

Owens, J. W. 1997. Life-cycle assessment in relation to risk assessment: an evolving perspective. *Risk Anal* 17:359.

Schell, L. M., A. D. Stark, and W. A. Grattan. 1997. Blood lead level, by year and season, among pregnant women. *Arch Environ Health* 52:286.

Schwartz, J. 1997. Air pollution and hospital admissions for cardiovascular disease in Tucson. *Epidem* 8:371.

Singleton, C. R., and M. S. Legator. 1997. Symposium survey: initial, critical step in a comprehensive community health study plan. Editorial. *Arch Environ Health* 52:255.

Sjoberg, L., and B-M Drottz-Sjoberg. 1997. Physical and managed risk of nuclear waste. *Risk: Health, Safety & Environ* 8:115.

Toomingas, A. 1996. Provocation of the electromagnetic distress syndrome. *Scan J Work, Environ & Health* 22:457.

Part Five

HEALTH ORGANIZATION, RESOURCES, AND SERVICES

We direct community and population health action at the three modifiable components of the health field concept introduced in part 1 of this book: lifestyle, environment, and organized health services. Part 2 showed how these applied at various stages of the life span, from infancy to old age. Part 3 presented health promotion strategies directed primarily at the lifestyle or behavioral determinants of health, and part 4 discussed environmental strategies to protect health. This concluding part 5 describes the organization and deployment of resources and services necessary to plan, implement, and evaluate community and population health strategies. Resources and services are described first in the broader global and national context, then in the state, provincial, or regional context. The final chapter describes the local community and personal health services that emerge from these broader systems, but also that provide the grassroots source of innovation and populist influence on the broader systems.

Chapter *18*

World and National Context of Community Health Services

*T*hink globally; act locally.

—Anonymous

*T*he pursuit of health is inseparable from the struggle for a fairer, more caring society.

—David Werner, health activist and author of *Where There is No Doctor*

Objectives

When you finish this chapter, you should be able to:

- Identify the sources of authority in national and international health agencies and actions

- Describe the placement of typical governmental functions at the national level and how they support community health and national health objectives

- Identify and be able to contact major agencies, foundations, and associations supporting community health at national and international levels

---

Community and population health services have historical, philosophical, scientific, political, and economic roots. The historical conditions affecting a community's health services reflect not only the history of that community and its immigrant populations, but national and global philosophies, such as those that define health services as a right and community self-determination and self-sufficiency as ideals. Health science is universal by definition, although its application needs contextual sensitivity. National and international politics and economics determine the resources available to com-

munities. They set the foundation for the authority and capability of communities to provide services to meet their own health needs and to build on their strengths.

This chapter begins with a review of international organizations influencing health. It then moves to the U.S. federal government to examine the wide range of national influences on health, and closes with a look at the roles of professional organizations and foundations. These agencies change structure and focus over time to accomplish their mission within available resources. To

· · · · · · · · · · · · · · · · · · · ·
Figure 18-1

Primary health care is the first level of contact for individuals, the family, and the community with the national health system. It brings health care as close as possible to where people live and work, whether it is in the developed countries of North America or this rural village in Papua New Guinea. *Source:* Photo by D. Anand, courtesy World Health Organization.

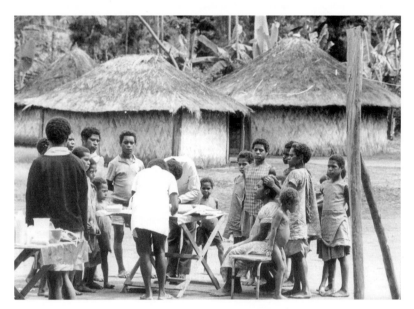

keep abreast of these changes and to retrieve health information tailored to your community, some key web sites for organizations reviewed here are included at the end of this chapter.

GLOBAL STRATEGY OF HEALTH FOR ALL

The Declaration of Alma-Ata contains the clearest and most widely accepted articulation of a basic set of values for health, as these relate to world development. The principles were articulated in a 1978 conference sponsored by the World Health Organization and the United Nations Children's Fund (WHO/UNICEF). Most countries, including the United States and Canada, endorsed the Declaration. It acknowledges health as a human right, not a privilege, and ties health status to economic and social status (see box titled "Declaration of

Alma-Ata, Summary"). It establishes health as a common concern of all countries and shaped WHO policy for the 1980s and 1990s. Included in these principles is primary health care for all people by the year 2000 (figure 18-1). The principle of participation in the declaration is what makes national and international health resources more relevant to and supportive of community health. It continues to guide the policies and programs of the World Health Organization and many of its member countries into the twenty-first century.

OFFICIAL INTERNATIONAL HEALTH ORGANIZATIONS

For more than a century, health scientists of the world have worked cooperatively and harmoniously in promoting the health of all people. National interests have given way to world interests.

Declaration of Alma-Ata, Summary

Article I: "Health . . . is a fundamental human right and . . . the attainment of the highest possible level of health is a most important worldwide social goal whose realization requires the action of many other social and economic sectors in addition to the health sector."

Article II: "The existing gross inequality in the health status of the people, particularly between developed and developing countries as well as within countries, is politically, socially, and economically unacceptable and is, therefore, of common concern to all countries."

Article III: "Economic and social development, based on a New International Economic Order, is of basic importance to the fullest attainment of health for all and to the reduction of the gap between the health status of the developing and the developed countries. The promotion and protection of the health of the people is essential to sustained economic and social development and contributes to a better quality of life and to world peace."

Article IV: "The people have the right and the duty to participate individually and collectively in the planning and implementation of their health care."

Article V: "Governments have a responsibility for the health of their people which can be fulfilled only by the provision of adequate health and social measures. A main social target of governments, international organizations, and the whole world community in the coming decades should be the attainment by all peoples of the world by the year 2000 of a level of health that will permit them to lead a socially and economically productive life. Primary health care is the key to attaining this target as part of the development in the spirit of social justice."

The basic philosophy of Primary Health Care (PHC) is described under the Declaration of Alma-Ata as follows:

Article VI: "Primary health care is essential health care based on practical, scientifically sound, and socially acceptable methods and technology made universally accessible to individuals and families through their full participation and at a cost that the community and country can afford to maintain at every stage of their development in the spirit of self-reliance and self-determination . . . ."

The development of PHC is clearly identified not only as a national priority for developing countries, but as an international mission in Article IX of the Declaration:

"All countries should cooperate in a spirit of partnership and service to ensure primary health care for all people since the attainment of health by people in any one country directly concerns and benefits every other country."

Exchange of health knowledge, loan of the services of experts, and united efforts in preventing the spread of disease have characterized the international activities of public health personnel everywhere (see box on p. 555). In the early years of international health activities, health personnel directed nearly all attention to the control of communicable diseases. Programs have expanded, however, to encompass the entire spectrum of health promotion. International organizations have placed the rights of children and women, and progress toward social development, at the center of the international health agenda.

World Health Organization

Progress toward human rights, sustainable development, and health for all requires a sustained political will and the marshalling of adequate resources. The World Health Organization (WHO) has been a focal point for international cooperation on health for nearly fifty years.

Origins The International Health Conference that convened in New York City on June 19, 1946, ushered in a new era in health cooperation. Representatives from the member states of the United Nations and observers from thirteen countries that were not members attended the conference. At the closing session on June 22, delegates approved and signed the final instruments for the creation of the World Health Organization. They included a protocol providing for the absorption by WHO of the International Office of Public Health and the League of Nations Health Section. The constitution of

Milestones in World Health Cooperation

1830 Cholera pandemic spread across Europe.

1851 First International Sanitary Conference was initiated to discuss measures against the importation of plague into Europe.

1892 Limiting focus on cholera, International Sanitary Convention passed.

1897 International conventions for prevention of plague were adopted.

1902 Pan American Health Organization (PAHO) created as International Sanitary Bureau

1907 L'Office International d'Hygiene Publique created in Paris.

1919 League of Nations created in Geneva with the Health Organization of the League of Nations.

1926 International Sanitary Convention revised to encompass measures for prevention and control of smallpox and typhus.

1935 International Sanitary Convention for aerial navigation.

1938 Conseil Sanitaire, Maritime et Quarantinaire at Alexandria handed over to Egypt, later became WHO Regional Office for the Eastern Mediterranean.

1945 United Nations Conference on International Organization in San Francisco approved resolution to establish new, autonomous, international health organization.

1946 Constitution for World Health Organization (WHO) approved at International Health Conference in New York.

1947 WHO Interim Commission organized first international health cooperation to assist Egypt in cholera epidemic.

1948 WHO Constitution ratified on April 7, now celebrated each year as World Health Day. First World Health Assembly held with fifty-five member governments.

1950 The International Office of Public Health absorbed by the WHO under the United Nations.

1973 Twenty-sixth World Health Assembly, noting widespread dissatisfaction with health services and the need for radical changes, decided that WHO should collaborate with, not "assist," its member states in developing national health care systems.

1974 Expanded Program on Immunization launched by WHO.

1977 Health for All by the Year 2000 set as a target "to permit all people to lead a socially and economically productive life."

1978 Alma-Ata Declaration on Primary Health Care adopted as the key to attaining Health for All.

1979 United Nations General Assembly affirms that health is a powerful lever for socioeconomic development and peace.

1980 Worldwide eradication of smallpox certified by Global Commission.

1981 United Nations General Assembly endorsed Global Strategy for Health for All by the Year 2000 and urged other international organizations to collaborate with WHO.

1986 WHO designated dracunculiasis (guinea worm disease) as the next disease scheduled to be eradicated (by 1995) after smallpox.

1987 Global Program on AIDS launched with WHO.

1988 On fortieth anniversary of WHO, resolution adopted to eradicate poliomyelitis by 2000.

1991 Pandemic of cholera spread across South and Central America, requires renewal of cooperation that led to first International Sanitary Conference in 1851.

1993 World Conference on Human Rights, Vienna.

1995 United Nations Fourth World conference on Women, Beijing.

1996 Second United Nations Conference on Human Settlements (Habitat II), Istanbul.

1997 Second Environmental Summit Conference in Kyoto, Japan.

WHO came into force on April 7, 1948, to enable cooperation among the sixty-one member governments and with others to promote the health of all people. That date, commemorated each year as World Health Day, made WHO an intergovernmental organization within the United Nations system. It has grown to 190 Member States.

Purpose The founding principles of WHO, which include a widely quoted definition of health, are set forth in the preamble of its constitution:

> Health is a state of complete physical, mental, and social well-being and not merely the absence of disease or infirmity.
>
> The enjoyment of the highest attainable standard of health is one of the fundamental rights of every human being without distinction of race, religion, political belief, or economic or social conditions.
>
> The health of all peoples is fundamental to the attainment of peace and security and is dependent upon the fullest cooperation of individuals and states.
>
> The achievement of any state in the promotion and protection of health is of value to all.
>
> Unequal development in different countries in the promotion of health and control of disease, especially communicable disease, is a common danger.
>
> Healthy development of the child is of basic importance: the ability to live harmoniously in a changing total environment is essential to such development.
>
> The extension to all peoples of the benefits of medical, psychological, and all related knowledge is essential to the fullest attainment of health.
>
> Informed opinion and active cooperation on the part of the public are of the utmost importance in the improvement of the health of the people.
>
> Governments have a responsibility for the health of their peoples that can be fulfilled only by the provision of adequate health and social measures.

Financing WHO raises its budget by assessing Member States according to a formula, with a limitation that no nation shall pay more than 25 percent of the total assessment. In addition, the organization receives funds from various other sources, such as the Pan American Health Organization, and voluntary contributions from governments, institutions, and individuals.

Organization The organization of WHO reflects its democratic quality, where legislation, administration, and services are under the direction of the 190 Member States. Many services by Member States are contributed without any cost to the organization.

The World Health Assembly is the legislative branch of WHO. Delegates of the Member States and nongovernmental associate members meet annually in Geneva, Switzerland (figure 18-2), where WHO is headquartered. The World Health Assembly establishes policy and decides on the program and budget for the next year.

The executive board, composed of thirty-one persons qualified in health matters, meets at least twice a year to advise and act for the assembly. Each year the assembly elects eight governments to designate members to serve for three years on this board of directors.

The secretariat designates the professional management of WHO. The director-general is the chief executive. The secretariat is organized into three departments: advisory services, central technical services, and administration and finance.

Regions provide for decentralized organization and operation. For WHO purposes, the world is divided into six regions, each with its own organization consisting of a regional committee composed of delegates from governments in the region, and a regional office that administers WHO-aided projects and supervises the staff in the various projects. Regional offices of WHO are logically distributed as shown in figure 18-3. Each regional office has its own staff and method of operation. In addition, there are more than 1,000 health-related institutions around the world designated officially as WHO collaborating centers.

Advisory panels consist of more than 12,000 scientists, health administrators, and educators from many nations. These panels provide expert advice in their respective fields. Committees of

· · · · · · · · · · · · · · · · · · · ·
Figure 18-2
Annual meeting of the World Health Assembly in the Palais des Nations in Geneva, Switzerland. *Source:* World Health Organization.

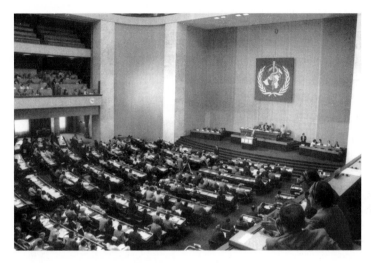

· · · · · · · · · · · · · · · · · · · ·
Figure 18-3
Six World Health Organization regional offices and the areas they serve. *Source:* World Health Organization.

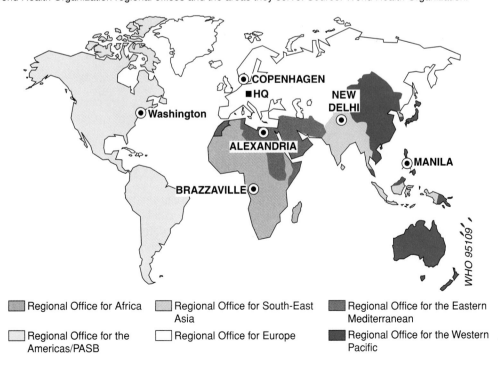

experts are chosen from these panels to provide the necessary expertise to deal with particular health problems.

Functions of WHO   The main functions of WHO are to give worldwide guidance in the field of health; to cooperate with governments to strengthen the planning, management, and evaluation of national health programs; and to develop and transfer appropriate health technology, information, and standards for human health. To meet the objectives of its charter, WHO recognizes specific functions as its responsibilities.

1. International health—to act as the directing and coordinating authority on world health (figure 18-4)
2. International conventions—to propose conventions, agreements, and regulations and make recommendations concerning international health matters
3. International standards—to develop, establish, and promote international standards for food, biological, pharmaceutical, and similar products
4. Nongovernmental organizations—to promote cooperation among scientific and professional groups that contribute to the advancement of science
5. Research—to promote and conduct research in health
6. Public health—to study and report on public health and medical care from preventive and curative points of view, including hospital services and social security
7. Primary health services—to assist governments, upon request, in strengthening primary health care services
8. Maternal and child health—to promote maternal and child health and welfare and to foster the ability to live harmoniously in a changing environment
9. Diseases—to stimulate and advance work to eradicate epidemic, endemic, and other disease
10. Diagnosis—to standardize diagnostic procedures as necessary

Figure 18-4

An outstanding success of the coordinating authority of World Health Organization was the eradication of small pox by 1980. This two-year-old girl is one of the last cases of smallpox discovered in Bangladesh, and therefore one of the last known cases of the more virulent form of small pox variola major. WHO keeps a global reserve of smallpox vaccine, sufficient for 300 million persons. *Source:* Photo by Dr. Tarantola, courtesy World Health Organization.

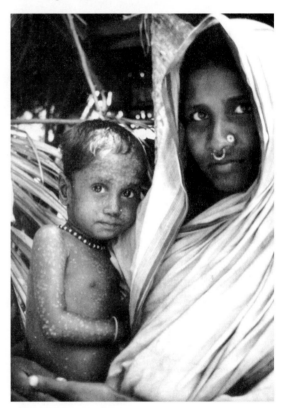

11. Living conditions—to promote the improvement of nutrition, housing, sanitation, recreation, economic, or working conditions, and other aspects of environmental hygiene
12. Accidents—to promote the prevention of accidental injuries
13. Mental health—to foster activities in mental health, especially those affecting human relations

14. Education—to promote improved standards of teaching and training in health, medical, and related professions

WHO is helping many nations to solve their health problems. In collaborating with a nation, it is always the objective of WHO to build the nation's capacity by training its personnel so that eventually outside help will not be needed. In some cases the services of WHO are merely advisory, but in many instances the organization's personnel are on the scene to do the job that is necessary. WHO also operates closely with the United Nations Children's Fund (UNICEF); the United Nations Specialized Agencies, especially the Food and Agriculture Organization (FAO); the United Nations Educational, Scientific and Cultural Organization (UNESCO); the United Nations Development Program (UNDP); and the International Labor Organization (ILO).

Pan American Health Organization

The mission of the Pan American Health Organization (**PAHO**) is to cooperate technically with its Member Countries and to stimulate cooperation among them in order that, while maintaining a healthy environment and charting a course to sustainable human development, the peoples of the Americas may achieve health for all and by all.

Origins The Second International Conference of the American Republics in Mexico City in 1902 formally organized the International Sanitary Office. The fifth such conference, which met in Santiago, Chile, in 1911, changed the name to Pan American Sanitary Bureau.

Accomplishments From its inception the Pan American Sanitary Bureau devoted its attention primarily to the control of communicable diseases. The participating nations cooperated with each other by exchanging vital statistics reports, exchanging health information on travelers, reporting new advances in disease control, exchanging knowledge on advances in sanitation procedures, training health personnel, and making technical experts available to other nations on a consulting basis. The Pan American Sanitary Bureau, now known as the Pan American Health Organization, is integrated with WHO as its regional office for the Americas.

Since PAHO was founded at the turn of the century, one of the most spectacular accomplishments was the eradication of smallpox from the Western Hemisphere in 1973. The Americas were the first region to succeed in the global campaign against the disease. Other significant accomplishments include reducing the incidence of other communicable diseases, cutting the infant mortality rate in half between 1960 and 1980, reducing the incidence of major childhood diseases as a prime cause of death through a hemispherewide immunization campaign, increasing life expectancy, providing safe water and basic sanitation, and improving nutrition.

For a majority of the people living in the Americas, however, disease and health risks still cast dark shadows over the future. More than one-third of the people in Latin America and the Caribbean have no access to clean water. More than two-thirds have no access to basic sanitation and 40 percent of this population has no access to health care.

Much work remains to be done to extend health services to those millions lacking them; to provide clean water, basic sanitation, adequate immunization (figure 18-5), and good nutrition; and to achieve prevention, early detection, and cure of disease. PAHO and its member governments are committed to meeting that challenge and making the universal right to health a reality in the Americas.

Priorities and Objectives To provide all citizens access to primary health care, PAHO's member countries have identified priority health areas and specific strategies for developing their infrastructures. Priorities include increased life expectancy, reduction of infant mortality, immunization of all infants, provision of safe drinking water, development of sewage services in all

· · · · · · · · · · · · · · · · · · · ·
Figure 18-5

In communities where technology is limited, such as this village in Mexico, health personnel using microphones and loud-hailers ask parents of small children whether they had been immunized. *Source:* Photo by L. Taylor, courtesy World Health Organization

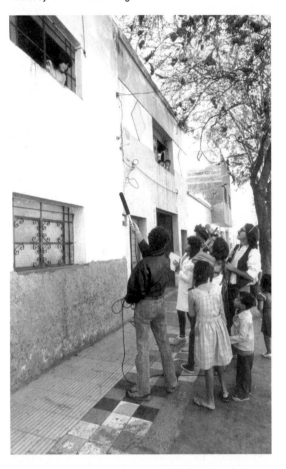

areas, and extension of health services to all. Elements of national strategies from Member Countries have been incorporated into hemispherewide strategies and a basic plan of action. The plan for meeting these goals emphasizes health promotion and disease prevention, combined with health restoration, rehabilitation, and improvements in the environment.

SOURCES OF AUTHORITY IN HEALTH

These international organizations have little **authority** in matters of health and, instead, depend on cooperation among nations for their influence. The authority of national governments in matters of health varies from country to country, depending on whether the country is under constitutional, imperial, or martial law. At one extreme, constitutions that create a republic, federation, or commonwealth of disparate states tend to reserve most powers for the states and grant only essential powers for the *common* good to the central government. This is the case, for example, in Australia, Canada, the United Kingdom, and the United States. At the other extreme, small countries, some monarchies, many socialist countries, and countries under martial law tend to centralize power at the national level and depend on state or local governmental bodies merely to carry out central plans and directives. Most countries swing between these extremes during their history.

Centralized Functions and Powers

The U.S. federal government provides many indispensable health services, as will be outlined in this chapter. Although the U.S. Constitution grants the federal government no *direct* authority to engage in public health activities, authority to promote health is conferred by general clauses concerning federal responsibilities. The British North America Act of 1867 similarly established Canada with a clear division of responsibility between federal and provincial governments, leaving jurisdiction over most health matters to the provinces. The many health functions carried on by the U.S. and Canadian federal governments derive their authority from the few specific centralized powers of the federal government. These powers are typical of those reserved by nations at the federal or central level.

Regulation of Interstate Commerce   Most national charters reserve the right to regulate interstate commerce. In the United States, Australia, and Canada, this provision gives Congress or

Parliament the right to pass legislation controlling shipment and quality of foods and drugs and governing movement of people and livestock on interstate carriers. Control of insects, air pollution, stream pollution, and other health threats becomes a federal function under the authority to regulate interstate commerce.

Taxing Power   Health-compromising products are taxed in most countries. In the case of the United States, Congress controls narcotics, alcohol, and tobacco by requiring a tax for a permit to possess and sell narcotics and a tax on each transaction for the sale of cigarettes and alcohol. Oddly, the courts have held that these particular measures are primarily for revenue rather than for regulatory purposes.

Postal Power   The United States and some other national governments prohibit the use of the mail in any frauds, including health frauds. Misbranded or fraudulent drugs, patent medicines, and foods cannot legally be shipped through the mail, nor can any promotional material relating to fraudulent drugs or foods.

Patent Authority   Many national governments require that any newly developed drug or medicine to be distributed to the public must be registered or patented. International copyright and patent codes have ensured some uniformity among nations on patents, but the procedures for approval of drugs for marketing vary widely among countries.

Treaty-Making Power   National governments enter into agreements with other nations for control of communicable diseases, regulation of sanitary conditions, exchange of health information, and other health matters that are international in nature.

National War Power   National governments have the authority to protect and maintain the health of personnel in their armed forces.

Local Authority   National governments have the responsibility to govern and to provide health services for local populations in federal trust territories, such as Canberra in Australia and the District of Columbia in the United States. The authority to govern the District of Columbia carries an implied responsibility for the health of residents of the District.

Power to Appropriate Money   Responsibility for the general welfare, together with the right to create agencies, forms the great umbrella under which most federal health activities operate. Appropriating money for health agencies of the national, state or provincial, and local governments; for the construction of hospitals; for research; for health personnel training; for stream pollution control; and for other health projects has been the major contribution of national governments to health.

Power to Create Agencies   Responsibility for the general welfare has enabled national governments to set up agencies to deal with each health problem that arises (figure 18-6). For example, within each of the U.S. federal executive departments there exist bureaus, divisions, or branches directly or indirectly concerned with some aspect of health.

OFFICIAL FEDERAL HEALTH AGENCIES

Countries as large as Australia, Canada, and the United States have various federal ministries, departments, bureaus, and other agencies engaged in some sphere of health work. In most cases health is a partial or subordinate function of the agency. For example, the U.S. Department of Health and Human Services is concerned not only with health, but also with welfare, housing, and a host of other human services. Arguments can be made about the relationship of health to such services, but no particular overall organizational relationship exists between these agencies. When cooperation does occur, it arises from the administrators involved or

· · · · · · · · · · · · · · · · · · · ·
Figure 18-6

One of the levers by which a nation shapes the health of its residents is the development of research and service agencies. This scientist works at the Norwegian Cancer Registry, an agency established in that country to contribute to the nationwide effort against cancer.
Source: Photo by P. Boucas, courtesy World Health Organization.

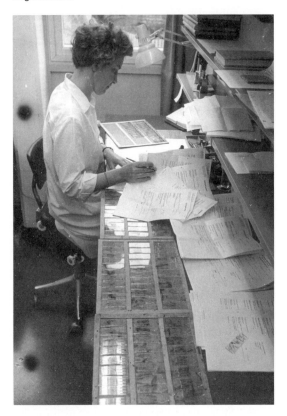

occasionally by legislative requirement for joint action and pooling of resources.

The assignment of health functions to government agencies sometimes appears unrelated to agency purposes. For example, health departments in many states were assigned responsibilities for administering Medicaid services. This responsibility pulled them away from traditional community health and prevention services toward health care

services. In other cases, government agencies appear to be a composite of special interests. This can occur when groups succeed in having a certain health program assigned to a particular agency. Once the program has been lodged with a certain agency, the special interest group will guard the agency's prerogative.

Most of the federal agencies with health functions are concerned with special problems or serve special groups. In the United States the Public Health Service is one of the few federal agencies that truly deals with general health protection and health promotion. All others contribute one or more of the health services of the jigsaw puzzle referred to as the federal health program (figure 18-7).

U.S. Executive Departments with Health Services

In most national governments, every executive department or ministry has one or more branches directly or indirectly involved in health work. In almost every instance, health is not a sole or principal concern of the department or ministry. For the purpose of the present discussion, only a limited number of agencies in each executive department of the U.S. federal government will be identified and their health activity indicated. These U.S. agencies provide direct health services, regulatory services, advisory services, and grants-in-aid; and they loan personnel, conduct special studies, disseminate information, conduct research, and provide other services related to their primary mission. Similar departments exist in most other countries as "ministries." The larger size of the United States means it has more specialized agencies that would be combined in most other countries under broader headings.

Department of Health and Human Services (DHHS) The DHHS is the government's principal agency for protecting the health and providing essential human services, especially for those who are least able to help themselves. The department is continually restructuring its operating divisions.

· · · · · · · · · · · · · · · · · · · ·

Figure 18-7

Spread across many different departments and agencies, federal programs contribute variously to the nation's health as evidenced by the effects of regulatory changes in the last decades.

Government works

Ruling	Source*	Result
Safety belts: required in all cars since 1968	NHTSA	5,300 lives of front-seat occupants saved in 1993 alone. If all front-seat occupants had worn their belts, more than 14,000 lives would have been saved in 1993.
Air bags: starting in 1997 all new cars must have dual air bags	NHTSA, 1989, 1991	470 lives saved in 1993, even though the devices were in few cars. Eventually, when all cars are equipped with dual air bags, the devices are expected to save thousands of lives each year.
Car windshields: since 1960 glass must be laminated and securely mounted	NHTSA	100 lives saved each year, plus an estimated 39,000 serious facial lacerations and 8,000 fractures prevented.
Antilock brakes for big trucks: required as of 1995	NHTSA	500 lives saved each year, plus 27,000 injuries prevented.
Food labeling: complete, standardized nutritional information on all packaged foods	FDA, 1992–3	Better dietary decisions, especially concerning processed foods; benefits include decreased rates of cancer, heart disease, and other chronic diseases and will far exceed the costs of labeling.
Asprin labels: must warn against Reye's disease in children with flu symptoms	FDA, 1986	Reye's disease (which can cause brain damage or death) is now rare; formerly affected 2,200 to 4,200 children each year.
Air-quality standards: industry required to reduce auto, power plant, factory emissions	EPA, 1970	Air pollution reduced overall by 24%.
Lead in gasoline: progressively eliminated	EPA, 1970	Levels of lead in the air phased down by 98% since 1970, though vehicle miles traveled have more than doubled. (Lead is a pervasive and deadly pollutant that particularly threatens children.)

Source: *NHTSA is the U.S. National Highway Traffic Safety Administration. FDA is the Food and Drug Administration. EPA is the Environmental Protection Agency. This chart is based on data from Public Citizen.

DHHS Regional Offices

Region	Area	Office Location
1	Connecticut, Maine, Massachusetts, New Hampshire, Rhode Island, Vermont	Boston, MA
2	New Jersey, New York, Puerto Rico, Virgin Islands	New York, NY
3	Delaware, Maryland, Pennsylvania, Virginia, West Virginia, District of Columbia	Philadelphia, PA
4	Alabama, Florida, Georgia, Kentucky, Mississippi, North Carolina, South Carolina, Tennessee	Atlanta, GA
5	Illinois, Indiana, Michigan, Minnesota, Ohio, Wisconsin	Chicago, IL
6	Arkansas, Louisiana, New Mexico, Oklahoma, Texas	Dallas, TX
7	Iowa, Kansas, Missouri, Nebraska	Kansas City, MO
8	Colorado, Montana, North Dakota, South Dakota, Utah, Wyoming	Denver, CO
9	Arizona, California, Hawaii, Nevada, American Samoa, Guam, Trust Territory of the Pacific	San Francisco, CA
10	Alaska, Idaho, Oregon, Washington	Seattle, WA

As of 1998, there were twelve agencies within DHHS that reported directly to the Secretary. Some of these agencies are primarily concerned with health, such as the Centers for Disease Control and Prevention, while others have a health component, but are devoted primarily to other human services, such as the Administration on Aging. For administration closer to the grass roots, DHHS has ten regional offices (see box above). Most divisions of the DHHS have offices and personnel in these regional headquarters. The organization and functions of this Department and its constituent units will be presented in more detail following a brief account of the health-related activities of the remaining departments of the executive branch of the federal government.

Department of Agriculture (USDA) This department administers a variety of programs with prevention components, including food and nutrition programs. An example of interdepartmental cooperation is the USDA and DHHS joint publication every five years of *The Dietary Guidelines for Americans.* The guidelines set standards for nutrition programs offered by the department. Other

prevention activities include food safety, family health, and nutrition education.

Food and Consumer Service (FCS)—ensures access to nutritious and healthful diets for citizens through food assistance programs and nutrition education. This service administers fifteen food assistance programs that serve one in six Americans. The goals of the service are to provide needy persons with access to a more nutritious diet, to improve the eating habits of children, and to help farmers by providing an outlet for the distribution of food purchased under farmer assistance authorities.

Food Safety and Inspection Service (FSIS)—ensures the safety of meat and poultry products through such activities as inspection of animal carcasses at slaughter sites; laboratory testing for pathogens and foreign matter in meat and poultry; analysis of critical control points in food production; and consultation with consumers, educators, researchers, and the media.

Cooperative State Research, Education, and Extension Service—is USDA's direct educational network for food and nutrition information. It's mission emphasizes partnerships with the public and private sectors to increase and provide access to scientific knowledge; strengthen the capabilities of land-grant and other institutions in research, higher education, and extension; increase access to and use of improved communication and network systems; and promote informed decision making by producers, families, communities, and other customers.

Department of Commerce Research is conducted by this department on fishery resources and the safety, quality, and identity of fishery products through the National Oceanic and Atmospheric Administration (NOAA). This agency and the Food and Drug Administration jointly developed a Voluntary Seafood Inspection Program to ensure the safety, wholesomeness, and proper labeling of seafood products.

Department of Defense The initial health promotion program launched by this department in 1986 focuses on the improvement and maintenance of military readiness and enhancement of the quality of life for the department's personnel and other beneficiaries. Programs are focused on key risk reduction areas, including smoking prevention, exercise, nutrition, stress management, alcohol and drug abuse, and early identification of hypertension. Each of the armed services has implemented physical fitness programs. A strong policy against drug abuse has been established. A long history of efforts to control sexually transmitted diseases has met with varied success. New programs deal with the Gulf War syndrome and include establishment of a defense women's health resource clearinghouse.

Department of Education Among the seven current priorities of this department is that every school will be strong, safe, drug-free, and disciplined. This program is the federal government's primary vehicle for reducing drug, alcohol, and tobacco use, and violence, through education and prevention activities in schools. Grants from this department allow states and communities to tailor drug and violence prevention activities to

local needs. National programs are directed to communities with severe drug and violence problems and include program evaluation and information dissemination.

Department of Energy Within this department the Office of Environment, Safety, and Health InfoCenter facilitates access to quality environment, safety, and health information providing multimedia access to federal, industry, and international information sources.

Department of Housing and Urban Development This department contributes to community health through the provision of decent, safe, and sanitary housing to program participants. A program to prevent lead-based poisoning involves research, testing, and abatement of lead-based paint in public and private housing. Community and economic development programs set minimum property standards for housing design and construction to reduce the potential risk to public health from human-made and natural hazards and irritations, such as toxic dumps, power lines, and drainage canals. The McKinney Homeless Housing Assistance Program provides funds to enable homeless persons to find housing and supportive services.

Department of the Interior This department is committed to restoring and maintaining the health of federally managed lands, waters, and renewable resources; preserving natural and cultural heritage; providing recreational opportunities; protecting diverse plant and animal species; conserving resources of American Indian and Alaska Native tribes; and providing scientific information for resource decision making.

Department of Justice Funding, technical assistance, and training are provided in areas such as crime prevention and control, consumer protection, drug abuse prevention, family violence, gang activities, child physical and sexual abuse, and HIV/AIDS as it relates to the criminal justice system. Drug prevention programs include those

• •

Figure 18-8

The National Crime Prevention program, sponsored by the Department of Justice, features McGruff the Crime Dog, who urges youth to prevent violence. This message also supports the safe school priorities of the Department of Education. *Source:* The Ad Council and the Department of Justice

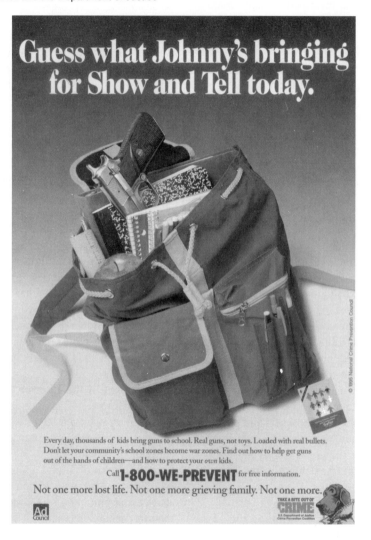

for high-risk youth; multiservice, neighborhood-based programs for youth and their families; and the National Citizens' Crime Prevention Program (see figure 18-8). These programs are designed to complement the supply-side strategies of interdiction and law enforcement to reduce drug smuggling and drug selling. Other Justice Department health-related programs include those for missing and exploited children and assistance to victims of crime.

Department of Labor Several preventive and rehabilitative health programs of this department involve the development of health and safety standards to protect workers exposed to work-related hazards, provision of information to employers and employees to gain compliance with these standards, enforcement of standards, and compensation programs for those injured or made ill at work.

Occupational Safety and Health Administration (OSHA)—develops, enforces, and educates about safety and health standards intended to provide workers with job environments as free as feasible from health and safety hazards. Workplace inspections are accompanied by citations and penalties for violations. Health standards are set to protect workers against a wide variety of chemicals. Since it was created in 1970, the overall workplace death rate has been cut in half, a statistic for which OSHA takes some credit.

Mine Safety and Health Administration (MSHA)—develops and enforces safety and health rules for mining and mineral processing operations from two-person sand and gravel pits to large underground coal mines. MSHA makes at least four complete inspections of all underground operations yearly and at least two surface mine inspections a year.

Department of State This department uses diplomacy as a principal means to defend national interests, respond to crises, and achieve international goals. Included among its responsibilities are international concern for human and worker rights, biodiversity, inspections for animal and plant health, conservation, and refugee status.

Department of Transportation (DOT) The mission of this department is to ensure a fast, safe, efficient, accessible and convenient transportation system that meets vital national interests and enhances the quality of life for today and into the future (figure 18-9).

National Highway Traffic Safety Administration sets safety standards for motor vehicles; conducts public information programs (figure 18-10);

....

Figure 18-9

This poignant public information ad sponsored by the Department of Transportation reminds the public about the consequence of drinking and driving. *Source:* The Ad Council and the Department of Transportation.

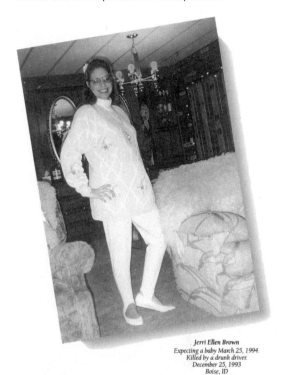

Jerri Ellen Brown
Expecting a baby March 25, 1994.
Killed by a drunk driver.
December 25, 1993
Boise, ID

If you don't stop someone from driving drunk, who will? Do whatever it takes.

FRIENDS DON'T LET FRIENDS DRIVE DRUNK.

and implements other programs to reduce deaths, injuries, and economic losses resulting from traffic accidents. Programs in this administration include the use of seat belts and child safety seats, reduction of alcohol-related fatalities, pedestrian safety, motorcycle safety, and prevention of trauma and injury.

Federal Highway Administration—has a mission to reduce deaths, injuries, and economic losses resulting from motor vehicle crashes. This

•••••••••••••••••••

Figure 18-10

In this public information ad, the Environmental Protection Agency worked with private and international agencies to create a strong statement about the state of the national and international waters. *Source:* The Ad Council and the EPA

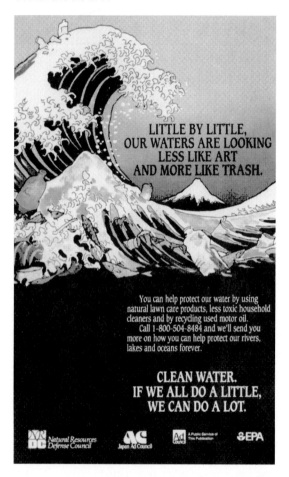

is accomplished by setting and enforcing safe performance standards for motor vehicles and items of motor vehicle equipment, and through grants to state and local governments. It has broadened its regulation of commercial motor vehicle safety through such actions as removing unsafe and un-

qualified drivers from the highways. Commercial motor vehicles operating in interstate commerce must pass, at least annually, a thorough inspection to comply with federal standards.

Federal Aviation Administration (FAA)—contributes to reduction of aviation injuries through a comprehensive regulatory program that includes the design, manufacture, operation, and maintenance of aircraft, their component systems, and spare parts. This administration also operates the nation's air traffic control system.

Other prevention-related programs of DOT include protection of the marine environment and boating safety by the Coast Guard; railroad standards and safety; and urban mass transportation services, which enable the elderly and handicapped to use public transportation through specially equipped vehicles.

Department of the Treasury   Certain regulatory and law enforcement agencies of the Treasury Department, such as the Bureau of Alcohol, Tobacco, and Firearms (ATF), provide health-related prevention activities. DHHS and the ATF work together on the labeling of ingredients and substances that may pose a public health problem. Other programs include the health-warning labeling of alcoholic beverages and testing for the contamination or alteration of alcoholic beverages. Through testing, the ATF has found problems such as the presence of pesticides and methanol in alcoholic beverages, leading to product recall.

Department of Veteran Affairs (VA)   The former Veterans Administration was elevated to department status in 1989. It established a National Center for Health Promotion and Disease Prevention in 1995 to monitor and encourage VA activities that provide, evaluate, and improve preventive medicine services. The center serves as a resource for inquiry about health promotion strategies, VA policy and model programs, and educational programs. Each VA medical center and independent outpatient clinic engages in prevention programs.

Independent U.S. Federal Agencies and Health Services

Environmental Protection Agency (EPA)   The EPA protects human health and safeguards the air, water, and land through a variety of standard setting, monitoring, enforcement, education (see figure 18-10), and research activities. Major programs address air quality, water quality (including safe drinking water), pesticides, solid waste, toxic substances, the protection of groundwater and wetlands, climate change, and environmental hazards in homes. Among the activities of this agency are collection of a broad range of environmental statistics, an initiative to label consumers products promoting more environmentally friendly choices, establishment of measurable environmental goals similar to those established for health, and a home page on global warming. The EPA works with industry, the military, and other governmental organizations to ensure the lowest achievable levels of emission of chlorofluorocarbons (CFCs) and halons to prevent further destruction of the ozone layer.

Consumer Product Safety Commission   The Commission was created in 1972 to protect consumers from unreasonable risks of injuries and deaths associated with consumer products. Over 15,000 types of consumer products fall within the Commission's jurisdiction including cigarette lighters, swimming pools and hot tubs, toys with choking hazards, playground equipment, riding lawn mowers, gas detection, poison prevention, chemical hazards, and heat tapes. The Commission identifies products that present the more serious safety problems and deals with them on a priority basis. Identification of such products is aided by the National Electronic Injury Surveillance System, a cooperative effort with selected hospitals that provide data about product-related injuries treated in emergency rooms across the country.

Other Agencies   A considerable number of other somewhat independent federal agencies provide health services to a significant degree. From a long list, a few of these agencies are identified as examples.

Federal Trade Commission (FTC)—control of deceptive advertising of foods, drugs, cosmetics, and devices shipped in interstate commerce

National Academy of Sciences—is a private, nonprofit society of scholars that advises the federal government on scientific and technical matters. It includes the Institute of Medicine and the National Research Council. Both publish reports of their committees, which carry out studies on issues of national and international health importance.

National Science Foundation—development of fundamental research in biological, physical, medical, and health sciences

Scores of federal agencies are engaged in health work. In each case the service is significant—in some, essential. The principal health organizations in the U.S. federal government, however, are located in the Department of Health and Human Services, covered in more detail in the following section.

U.S. DEPARTMENT OF HEALTH AND HUMAN SERVICES

Having reviewed a wide range of health-related services across the U.S. government, this section provides more detail on the federal government's principal agency to protect health—the U.S. Department of Health and Human Services (DHHS). In 1997, the department operated on a budget of $354 billion, employed 59,000 people, and supported over 300 programs. Two major divisions within DHHS are the Public Health Service Operation Divisions and the Human Services Operating Divisions (figure 18-11). The following is a discussion on the health-related services, primarily located within the Office of the Assistant Secretary for Health and the Public Health Service Operating Division.

• •

Figure 18-11

Frequent reorganization of the Department of Health and Human Services (DHHS) makes it difficult for the organizational chart to keep up. This latest version of the chart (March 1996) shows the main agencies of the DHHS, but not the operating divisions of the Public Health Services and Human Services. *Source:* DHHS.

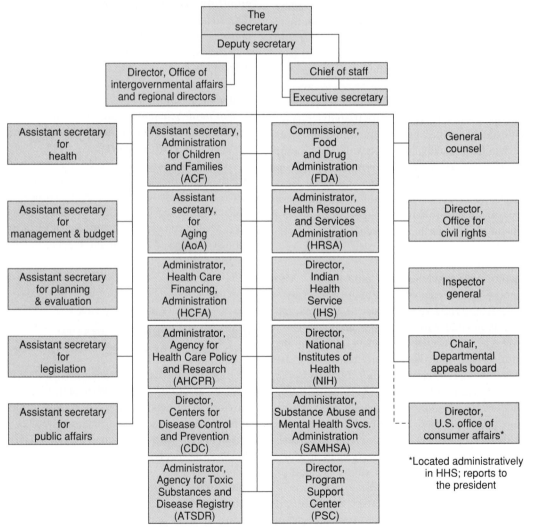

**Organization chart
U.S. Department of Health and Human Services**

Office of the Assistant Secretary for Health

The Office of Public Health and Science is under the direction of the Assistant Secretary for Health. This office serves as the focal point for leadership and coordination across the Department for public health and science. The Assistant Secretary's Office consists of a number of offices including those directed toward health promotion, physical fitness, and HIV/AIDS.

Office of Disease Prevention and Health Promotion (ODPHP)

Created as the Office of Health Information and Health Promotion by legislation in 1974, the renamed ODPHP has provided leadership in stimulating, coordinating, and unifying national disease prevention and health promotion strategies among federal, state, and local agencies, and major private and voluntary organizations. Included among the activities of this office are the National Health Objectives (the year 2000 objectives are used throughout this text); various net links between sources of health information and professionals and consumers, dietary guidelines, drug policy; and healthy community, workplace, and school initiatives. A few of these are selectively reviewed in the following sections.

Healthy People Initiative—launched in 1979 with publication of the first *Surgeon General's Report on Health Promotion and Disease Prevention.* The ODPHP coordinates a massive effort to develop, track, and report on quantifiable, ten-year objectives for disease prevention and health promotion, such as those first released for 1990 and a decade later for the year 2000. This last set of objectives involved links among all DHHS agencies and more than six-hundred national organizations, business groups, and state agencies. The year 2000 objectives have three broad goals: (1) increase the span of healthy life for Americans; (2) reduce health disparities among Americans; (3) achieve access to preventive services for all Americans. To help meet these goals, 300 specific objectives are set in twenty-two separate priority areas. These include health promotion, health protection, and preventive services, with specific objectives for age groups and special populations.

Clearinghouse and Web Links—The ODPHP operates the National Health Information Center (NHIC) to provide a central health information referral service for consumers and professionals. The NHIC is a key component of the interagency support for Healthfinder, a gateway web site linking consumers and professionals to health and human services information from the federal government and its many partners.

Public Health Functions—To strengthen the nation's public health infrastructure, efforts are undertaken to marshal consensus on essential services of public health, document public health expenditure, assess public health data capacity, and identify workforce capacities and needs (figure 18-12).

Office of HIV/AIDS Policy

In advising the Secretary on appropriate and timely policies for HIV/AIDS, activities of this office have included integration of the array of HIV/AIDS prevention services, review of needle exchange programs, and evaluation of the impact of HIV/AIDS provider education and training programs.

President's Council on Physical Fitness

The Council coordinates and promotes opportunities in physical activity, fitness, and sports with activities such as the President's Challenge Physical Fitness Test, summer fun programs, and 4-H projects.

Other staff offices that advise the assistant secretary on prevention issues, policies, and programs in targeted areas include the Office of Women's Health, Office of Emergency Preparedness, Office of International and Refugee Health, Office of Minority Health, and Office of Population Affairs (OPA). Also reporting directly to the Assistant Secretary for Health is the Surgeon General and the Public Health Service.

• •

Figure 18-12

Working together, the government, professional associations, and foundations produced these shared understandings about the mission and work of public health. *Source:* American Public Health Association.

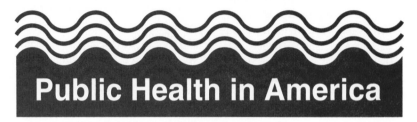

Public Health in America

Vision:

Healthy people in healthy communities

Mission:

Promote physical and mental health and prevent disease, injury, and disability

Public health
- Prevents epidemics and the spread of disease
- Protects against environmental hazards
- Prevents injuries
- Promotes and encourages healthy behaviors
- Responds to disasters and assists communities in recovery
- Assures the quality and accessibility of health services

Essential public health services
- Monitor health status to identify community health problems
- Diagnose and investigate health problems and health hazards in the community
- Inform, educate, and empower people about health issues
- Mobilize community partnerships to identify and solve health problems
- Develop policies and plans that support individual and community health efforts
- Enforce laws and regulations that protect health and ensure safety
- Link people to needed personal health services and assure the provision of health care when otherwise unavailable
- Assure a competent public health and personal health care workforce
- Evaluate effectiveness, accessibility, and quality of personal and population-based health services
- Research for new insights and innovative solutions to health problems

Adopted: Fall 1994, Source: Public Health Functions Steering Committee, Members (July 1995):
American Public Health Association • Association of Schools of Public Health • Association of State and Territorial Health Officials • Environment Council of the States • National Association of County and City Health Officials • National Association of State Alcohol and Drug Abuse Directors • National Association of State Mental Health Program Directors • Public Health Foundation • U.S. Public Health Service—*Agency for Health Care Policy and Research* • *Centers for Disease Control and Prevention* • *Food and Drug Administration* • *Health Resources and Services Administration* • *Indian Health Services* • *National Institutes of Health* • *Office of the Assistant Secretary for Health* • *Substance Abuse and Mental Health Services Administration*

ISSUES AND CONTROVERSIES
Immigrant and Refugee Health

Not since the early years of the twentieth century have Canada and the United States received such high numbers of immigrants as in the last decades. The differences between the immigration waves then and now is that the early immigrants to the American "melting pot" and the Canadian "mosaic" were primarily from Europe, especially the British Isles. Today the immigrants come predominantly from Latin America and Asia. The language and cultural differences are greater and, for many of today's refugees such as the "boat people" from Vietnam, Cambodia, Haiti, and Cuba, the burden of prior disease, malnutrition, and physical and mental suffering is greater. While some immigrants arrive in great poverty, some have brought great wealth to their new countries, such as those emigrating from Hong Kong before its reannexation by China.

What lessons might be learned from North America's previous immigration waves in caring for the new immigrants and protecting the health of the resident population? What do students preparing today for careers in the health professions need to learn about multicultural health services? What is the role of the federal government, as distinct from the role of communities, in immigrant and refugee health?

Public Health Service Operating Divisions

History   What began in 1798 as the Marine Hospital Service in the Treasury Department evolved into the Public Health and Marine Hospital Service in 1902. In 1912 the name was changed to the U.S. Public Health Service (PHS). The responsibilities of the agency have increased dramatically over the years. In 1917 it was charged with responsibility for the physical and mental examinations of all immigrants to the United States. By 1929 the medical care of federal prisoners and narcotic addicts became a responsibility of the Public Health Service. In the same year a program in mental hygiene was launched. The Social Security Act of 1935 further extended the responsibilities of the Public Health Service. Grants-in-aid to states to strengthen local and state health departments were administered by the Public Health Service.

A series of congressional acts continued to increase the functions of the Public Health Service, such as the National Cancer Act in 1937, followed by the Venereal Disease Control Act a year later. In 1939 the U.S. Public Health Service was moved from the Treasury Department to the Federal Security Agencies. The landmark Public Health Law enacted in 1944 provided for an expansion, reorganization, and consolidation of the agency and a revision of laws relating to public health. When the Department of Health, Education, and Welfare was established in 1953, the Public Health Service became a part of the new department.

In 1980, the Department of Education was created, and the Department of Health, Education, and Welfare was renamed the Department of Health and Human Services (DHHS). The Assistant Secretary for Health is the administrative head of the eight divisions of the Public Health Service. The head of the Commissioned Corps of Uniformed Public Health Service Offices is the Surgeon General.

Mission   The mission of the PHS, broadly stated, is to protect and advance the health of the American people by:

- conducting and supporting biomedical, behavioral, and health services research and communicating research results to health professionals and the public;
- preventing and controlling disease, identifying health hazards, and promoting healthful behaviors for the nation's citizens;

- monitoring the adequacy of health personnel and facilities available to serve the nation's needs;
- improving the organization and delivery of health services and bringing good health care within the reach of all Americans;
- ensuring that drugs and medical devices are safe and effective and protecting the public from unsafe foods and unnecessary exposure to radiation;
- administering block grants to the states for preventive health and health services; alcohol, drug abuse, and mental health services; maternal and child health services; and
- Working with other nations and international agencies on global health problems and their solutions.

Organization Over time the Public Health Service has contained numerous offices, bureaus, centers, institutes, and divisions that change their names, locations, or functions to some degree with every major health bill passed by Congress. They grow, shrink, split, or disappear with each year's appropriations. Of the sixty-two units of DHHS that were listed in the 1973 edition of this book, only a few still existed under the same administrative division and with the same name twenty-five years later. The mission and activities of the current eight PHS units are highlighted in the following sections.

Centers for Disease Control and Prevention (CDC) Based in Atlanta, this agency emerged in 1946 dedicated to control of disease. Over the years, the Centers for Disease Control has met other threats to health, here and abroad. Its most recent change in 1993 officially added *prevention* to its name. The mission of the CDC is to promote health and quality of life by preventing and controlling disease, injury, and disability. The eleven centers, institutes, and offices of CDC employ approximately 6,900 employees in 170 occupations including epidemiologists, microbiologists, entomologists, physicists, toxicologists, chemists,

physicians, nurses, dentists, public health advisors, pharmacologists, veterinarians, health education specialists, writers, statisticians, social scientists, environmental engineers, industrial hygienists, skilled technicians, and administrative and support personnel.

Celebrating its fiftieth anniversary in 1996, the CDC identified five priorities in public health for the next century: strengthen essential public health services, expand capacity to respond to urgent health threats, develop nationwide prevention strategies, promote women's health, and invest in the health of youth. These priorities reflect changing national health concerns. For example, when CDC was founded in 1946 it was concerned with controlling new and exotic diseases from the South Pacific potentially brought back by service personnel following the war. Fifty years later the agency is dealing with new and reemerging diseases such as hantaviruses or strains of tuberculosis resistant to drugs. Another example of change is that from infectious diseases and immunization programs to a broader health focus on noninfectious threats to health, such as domestic violence. The health of women and youth have come into sharper focus with family planning and infertility programs and an epidemiologic analysis of risk-taking behavior of school-aged youth.

CDC works closely with state and local health departments in developing and operating disease control programs, such as those for sexually transmitted diseases, childhood immunization, diabetes control, and community water fluoridation. Also provided are laboratory diagnostic services for unusual problems. CDC supplies rare vaccines, immunoglobulins, and therapeutic drugs that are not otherwise available for preventing and treating uncommon diseases. Annually, CDC personnel assist state health departments in investigating disease outbreaks. The investigation of contaminated food from a church supper in Maryland in 1997 that lead to two deaths and over 600 affected people is a good example of these cooperative efforts; other examples are the investigations of toxic shock syndrome, Reye's syndrome, Lyme disease, and acquired immunodeficiency syndrome (AIDS). CDC trains state and local health officials in epidemic control and in operating local disease prevention and health promotion programs. It is the lead agency for working with the states and communities to track and implement *Healthy People 2000* objectives.

On the international front, CDC works with governments of other nations and with the World Health Organization to help track and control diseases before they can spread from one country to another. Through the exchange of epidemiological information, health authorities throughout the United States and the world are able to take quick action in response to outbreaks, epidemics, and natural disasters. Programs focus on decreasing morbidity and mortality among infants and children, preventing the spread of HIV/AIDS infection, improving conditions for refugees, and strengthening public health capacities overseas. For example, CDC administers a national quarantine program carried out not only at U.S. ports of entry but also at strategic locations overseas, to protect the United States against the introduction of diseases from other countries. It also provides assistance and consultation when needed in the case of epidemics, as requested by health administrations of other nations.

CDC has been active in assessing special health-related problems, such as the impact on health of the volcanic eruption of Mount St. Helens, the health consequences of the nuclear accident at Three Mile Island, the potential risks associated with toxic waste disposal, and the effects of heat waves on communities. CDC cooperates with federal, state, and local officials in carrying out designated activities related to health effects of exposure to toxic substances. Scientists at CDC's National Institute for Occupational Safety and Health (NIOSH) conduct laboratory research and epidemiological studies to determine hazards in the working environment and steps that should be taken to eliminate them. NIOSH recommends acceptable exposure limits for toxic substances and harmful physical agents that workers may en-

counter; it also evaluates health conditions at specific work sites in response to requests from employers or employees.

An inaccurate laboratory diagnosis can be as great a threat to health as an untreated disease or an industrial hazard, which is why CDC monitors the licensing and certification of clinical laboratories and administers a comprehensive program to improve the nation's laboratory service.

CDC's health education activities seek to develop better ways of educating people about their health through school systems, health care providers, community organizations, and other channels. CDC has educational programs in HIV/AIDS, family planning, smoking cessation, exercise, and violence prevention. CDC is also undertaking a series of activities to ensure that prevention is a key component of health care delivery systems through managed care organizations.

National Institutes of Health In 1887 the Marine Hospital Service founded a research laboratory at the Marine Hospital, Staten Island, New York. In 1891 the name was changed to Hygienic Laboratory, and the unit was moved to Washington, D.C. In 1930 the Hygienic Laboratory became the National Institutes of Health (NIH) and moved to Bethesda, Maryland.

The mission of the NIH is the development of new knowledge for the prevention and control of disease (figure 18-13). A broad, complex program is designed to meet the needs in biomedical science. The NIH includes eighteen Institutes of Health, each with its own medical or health focus (see box). The focus of these institutes reflects not only physiological logic, but political pressure. The emphasis on the production of new knowledge through research has been balanced with the dissemination of knowledge through public education campaigns. Although scientists in the laboratories and clinical centers of the NIH carry on part of the program of research, most of the research is done by others through grants administered by the NIH. About 90 percent of the institute's **appropriation** of nearly $13 billion yearly goes

....
Figure 18-13

Basic research of the National Institutes of Health (NIH) is applied in public awareness campaigns such as this one about cholesterol levels and implications for heart disease. *Source:* National Heart, Lung, and Blood Institute.

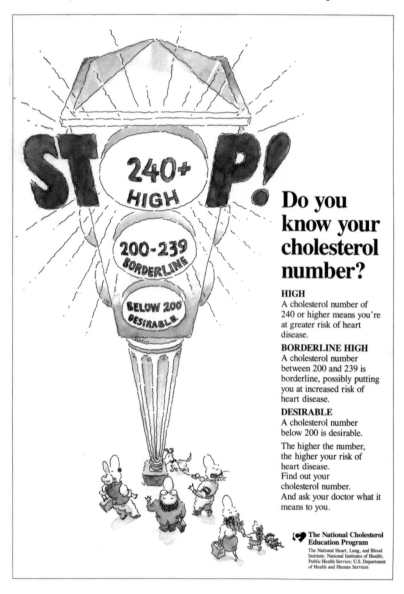

National Institutes of Health

The National Institutes of Health is a federation of organizations that includes eighteen institutes of health, each with its own medical or health focus:

National Cancer Institute (NCI)
National Eye Institute (NEI)
National Heart, Lung, and Blood Institute (NHLBI)
National Human Genome Research Institute (NHGRI)
National Institute of Aging (NIA)
National Institute on Alcohol Abuse and Alcoholism (NIAAA)
National Institute of Allergy and Infectious Diseases (NIAID)
National Institute of Arthritis and Musculoskeletal and Skin Diseases (NIAMS)
National Institute of Child Health and Human Development (NICHD)
National Institute on Deafness and Other Communication Disorders (NIDCD)
National Institute of Dental Research (NIDR)
National Institute of Diabetes and Digestive and Kidney Diseases (NDDK)
National Institute on Drug Abuse (NIDA)
National Institute of Environmental Health Sciences (NIEHS)
National Institute of General Medical Sciences (NIGMS)
National Institute of Mental Health (NIMH)
National Institute of Neurological Disorders and Stroke (NINDS)
National Institute of Nursing Research (NINR)

to the **extramural** program of grants to scientists and research institutions throughout the nation and the world.

The grants program is planned to provide a continuous supply of competent scientists in biomedical disciplines. In addition to the training grants, fellowships, and traineeships, the program also provides facilities; equipment; and other resources, including computers and primate centers. Basic research cuts across several of the traditional biomedical areas. Special attention is given to national trends and to neglected areas of research.

The NIH has an international research program that seeks to make use of the abilities of qualified scientists the world over. Grants have been made to scientists in various health disciplines in many countries. The NIH has also provided opportunities for promising young American scientists to work abroad as members of established research groups. No foreign grants are made unless they are of a high value and are related to health objectives of value to the United States. Nobel Prize awards in medicine and physiology have been made to foreign investigators who were working under grants from the NIH.

The NIH makes contracts with foreign institutions to conduct research and provides fellowships to American scientists to study at foreign research centers of excellence. NIH also promotes a visiting program that brings distinguished scientists to the United States to work in the NIH laboratories or the John E. Fogarty International Center.

NIH finances research in hospitals, medical schools, and nonprofit research centers. All together, it underwrites about 40 percent of the biomedical research done in the United States.

Food and Drug Administration (FDA) The FDA is one of our nation's oldest consumer protection agencies. It regulates products that run the gamut of modern life, including food, drugs, the nation's blood supply, vaccines, food and drugs for animals, cosmetics, heart pacemakers, x-ray machines, and microwave ovens. It is estimated that the FDA regulates products that account for twenty-five cents of every dollar spent by consumers. The work of the FDA's scientists—physicians, chemists, nutritionists, microbiologists, pharmacologists—forms the basis of its regulatory activities. The FDA monitors the manufacture, import, transport, storage, and sale of nearly $1 trillion worth of products each year at the cost of about $3 per person.

Three areas of FDA services include inspections and legal sanctions, scientific expertise, and product safety. FDA investigators and inspectors visit more than 15,000 facilities each year to assure product quality and truth in labeling. If products do not meet requirements, the FDA can encourage the firm to voluntarily correct the problem or bring legal sanctions if necessary. The fastest way to remove unsafe products is a recall, such as those that make headlines for automobiles or children's toys. About 3,000 products a year are removed from the market. The scientific expertise of the agency backs up legal cases and assesses risks for new drugs and medical devices. In deciding whether to approve new drugs, the FDA examines results of studies done by the manufacturer, rather than conducting its own research. Among the many activities the FDA undertakes to protect the safety and wholesomeness of food are to set labeling standards to help consumers know what is in the foods they buy.

Substance Abuse and Mental Health Services Administration (SAMHSA)   The administration was created in 1992 through reorganization of the former Alcohol, Drug Abuse, and Mental Health Administration (ADAMHA). The administration has lead responsibility for the federal government's support and conduct of research on mental illness, substance abuse, and addictive disorders. SAMHSA's mission is to improve the quality and availability of prevention, treatment, and rehabilitation services to reduce illness, death, disability, and cost to society resulting from substance abuse and mental illnesses.

Centers operating within the administration focus on different targets. The Center for Mental Health Services leads national efforts to demonstrate, evaluate, and disseminate service delivery models to treat mental illness, promote mental health, and prevent the development or worsening of mental illness when possible. The Center for Substance Abuse Prevention provides national leadership in the federal effort to prevent alcohol, tobacco, and illicit drug problems fostering the development of comprehensive, culturally appropriate prevention policies and systems. The Center for Substance Abuse Treatment seeks to expand the availability of effective treatment and recovery

services for alcohol and drug problems. In addition to these centers the administration operates the National Clearinghouse for Alcohol and Drug Information (NCADI), and the Knowledge Exchange Network (KEN).

Agency for Toxic Substances and Disease Registry (ATSDR)   The ATSDR was created in 1980 by the Comprehensive Environmental Response, Compensation, and Liability Act, commonly known as the Superfund. Its mission is to prevent the exposure to hazardous substances from waste sites. The work of the agency is carried out through research at potentially hazardous Superfund sites, development of databases to profile and link exposure to substances and subsequent health and environmental effects, and dissemination of scientific information about the health effects of exposure to hazardous substances.

Indian Health Service (IHS)   The IHS assists in developing the capacity to staff and manage health programs for American Indians and Alaska Natives. Capacity development includes training, technical assistance, and human resource development. The Service also helps tribes coordinate health planning, obtain and use health resources available through the government, design and operate comprehensive health care services, and develop community sanitation facilities.

The IHS provides health care for approximately 1.4 million American Indians and Alaska Natives through a network of thirty-seven hospitals and more than one-hundred other health facilities. Among the prevention focuses of the IHS are maternal and child health, child abuse and neglect, community injury control, fluoridation, and substance abuse prevention.

Health Resources and Services Administration (HRSA)   Leadership is provided by this Administration to promote access to health care services, primarily through programs that increase the availability and accessibility of community health resources. Priority programs are those that improve

··················

Figure 18-14

This public awareness campaign is specifically targeted to encourage organ donation among diverse population groups. *Source:* Ad Council

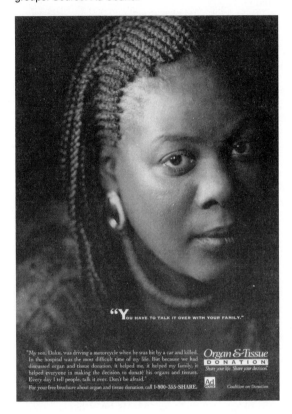

"**Y**OU HAVE TO TALK IT OVER WITH YOUR FAMILY."

"My son, Daku, was driving a motorcycle when he was hit by a car and killed. In the hospital was the most difficult time of my life. But because we had discussed organ and tissue donation, it helped me, it helped my family, it helped everyone in making the decision to donate his organs and tissues. Every day I tell people, talk it over. Don't be afraid." For your free brochure about organ and tissue donation, call 1-800-355-SHARE.

Organ & Tissue
DONATION
Share your life. Share your decision.

Coalition on Donation

the availability of primary care for the medically underserved and for specific at-risk populations.

Among the health-related services provided is the Healthy Start Initiative, which involves collaboration of the administration with states and communities to reduce infant mortality. Other responsibilities include administration of the National Organ Transplant Program (figure 18-14); support of states to plan and deliver health care to the underserved urban and rural area residents, migrant workers, and the homeless; assistance in ensuring health and workplace standards for federal employees; and provision of services for HIV/AIDS

patients, including education and construction of nonacute care facilities.

The administration provides leadership in health resources through the education, distribution, and use of health professionals, including increasing the number of minorities in all health professions. The National Health Service Core provides primary care physicians, psychiatrists, dentists, and other health professionals to underserved areas in return for scholarship or loan repayment. AmeriCorps is a new national initiative that involves people of all ages and backgrounds in strengthening America's communities through service. Over 20,000 AmeriCorps members serve full- or part-time in more than three-hundred-fifty programs nationwide. In exchange for service, members receive education awards.

Agency for Health Care Policy and Research (AHCPR) Established in 1989, the agency serves as the federal focal point for health services research to enhance the quality of patient care services. The broad goals of the agency are to promote improvements in clinical practice and patient outcomes through more appropriate and effective health care services; to promote improvements in the financing, organization, and delivery of health care services; and to increase access to quality care. Among the Agency's activities are support for conferences on primary care research, support and dissemination of health policy research, and the provision of pre- and postdoctoral support for academic training and for research concerning health services research methods and problems.

Human Services Operating Divisions

Although the human services divisions of the Department of Health and Human Services is not strictly focused on health, as are the preceding agencies within the Public Health Service, it does provide health-related services. These agencies are highlighted in the following sections.

Health Care Financing Administration (HCFA) Medicare and Medicaid, legislated in

ISSUES AND CONTROVERSIES
Politics and the Poor

The theme of economic independence that runs throughout programs in this administration reflects the economic realities and political debates of our times. Changes in the executive and legislative branches of the government lead to renewed debate as to whether these types of social service programs, in the long run, promote independence or dependence in their recipients. For example, in 1996 when the Administration for Children and Families replaced a program for *Aid to Families with Dependent Children (AFDC)* with *Temporary Assistance for Needy Families (TANF)*, more than a name change was involved. The existence of multiple generations of a family on social services is used by some as an argument for the dependence fostered by such programs. The desperate plight of homeless children and the disabled who are unable to care for themselves are evidence to others of the need for such services.

How these debates are resolved will shape the structure and programs offered by the government. In what ways do national programs help or hurt those they intend to assist? How do national decisions to care for the poor impact your community?

1966, culminated a quarter century of legislative efforts to ensure that no elderly, disabled, or poor American need forego basic health care because of cost. These programs, described in greater detail in chapter 21, are managed by the Health Care Financing Administration. **Medicare** provides low-cost health insurance for 37 million elderly and disabled persons. **Medicaid,** jointly funded by federal and state governments, provides almost free health coverage for 36 million low-income persons, including 17.6 million children. Medicaid also pays for nursing home coverage for low-income elderly, covering almost half of the total national spending for nursing home care. The Health Care Financing Administration also develops and enforces standards to ensure high-quality health care for health services financed by federal funds.

Administration for Children and Families (ACF) Established in 1991, this Administration provides leadership in the implementation of assistance and services programs designed to promote family stability, self-sufficiency, responsibility, and economic security. The sixty programs operated by this administration, including Head Start and Temporary Assistance for Needy Families, focus on improving the health and well-being of low-income families, neglected and abused children and youth, Native Americans, and individuals with lifelong disabilities. These targeted populations are those at special risk in the *Year 2000 Objectives for the Nation's Health.*

Administration of Aging (AoA) The AoA was established to provide a focal point in government for the concerns and needs of older people and to coordinate federal policies that affect them. It supports community-based nutrition and companionship programs, such as "Meals on Wheels," transportation services, legal aid, homemaker and home health services, residential repair, and recreational activities for older people. A primary goal of programs for the elderly is to provide supportive services in the community that will enable them to lead fully independent lives, avoid unnecessary institutionalization, and be a part of the community.

NATIONAL PROFESSIONAL HEALTH ORGANIZATIONS

In addition to national government agencies, there are numerous national professional societies or associations concerned with health. Professional health organizations have a common purpose to uphold professional standards and to serve society better through their united efforts. The basic preparation of future practitioners and the continuing professional education of current practitioners is of concern to these organizations. While the primary purpose of a professional society is to promote the interests of the profession and its members, its image and prestige depend on its service to the public. What best serves the public should be in the best interests of the professional organization. Examples of the more prominent community health professional societies follow, but many more allied and specialty health professional groups are active in each country and many states.

American Medical Association

The American Medical Association (AMA) was founded in 1847. Its constitution states that "the object of the Association is to promote the art of medicine and the betterment of public health." The association aims to serve physicians and their patients by establishing and promoting ethical, educational, and clinical standards for the medical profession. It advocates what it claims to be "the highest principle of all—the integrity of the physician/patient relationship."

The AMA is a federation of state societies, and these in turn are made up of county societies, which means that the national organization is an association of state societies rather than of individual practitioners. The AMA strives to improve the quality of medical service by informing members of advancements in medicine and related fields. It has had programs and committees investigating possible fraud in drugs, foods, cosmetics, and related products that might jeopardize the health of the public. The AMA also participates in the accreditation of hospitals.

The *Journal of the American Medical Association* is a weekly publication and is regarded as a leading journal in its field. The AMA also publishes health-related pamphlet material for distribution.

The AMA has lent its considerable political weight to numerous community health issues. It helped pass the legislation that eventually eliminated smoking on domestic commercial airline flights. It supported legislation that would outlaw plastic handguns that could not be detected in airport metal detectors and another bill that would require a seven-day waiting period and background check on handgun purchasers. The association worked to protect it's "highest principle" in attempts at national health care reform. For some this principle clashed with principles necessary to provide universal health care. These and other lobbying efforts are directed toward protection of the public and of the interests of physicians.

American Dental Association

The American Dental Association was formed in 1860 to advance the dental profession by raising the quality of dental education and dental practice. The association is the profession's agency for keeping practitioners informed of new developments in equipment, procedures, and techniques.

In its early years the American Dental Association was an organization of individual dental practitioners; later it became an association of state societies, which in turn are composed of representatives from county societies. The American Dental Association publishes the *Journal of the American Dental Association* and a yearly index of periodical dental literature. The association also publishes pamphlets for distribution to patients.

American Public Health Association

The American Public Health Association (APHA) is the oldest and largest organization of public health professionals in the world, representing more than 50,000 members from over fifty occupations of public health. The Association and its members have been influencing policies and setting priorities in public health since it was established in 1872. It celebrated its one-hundred-twenty-fifth anniversary in Indianapolis at its annual convention in 1997.

The American Public Health Association carries on a wide variety of activities through over twenty sections: laboratory, alcohol, tobacco and other drugs, health administration, community health planning and policy development, statistics, environment, radiological health, food and nutrition, international health, maternal and child health, public health education and health promotion, gerontological health, social work, population and family planning, public health nursing, epidemiology, school health education and services, oral health, mental health, occupational safety and health, pediatric health, vision care, and medical care.

The association has developed standards and procedures that have been widely accepted and adopted, including methods for the inspection of water and sewage, guidelines for the operation of swimming pools, diagnostic reagents and procedures, the appraisal of local health work, a model health code for cities, and standards for the accreditation of public health training. The association conducts surveys and other studies for government agencies. Its publication, the *American Journal of Public Health,* is issued each month. In addition, the association publishes *The Nation's Health,* a monthly newsletter, pamphlets, and special reports.

American Nurses Association

Since 1896, when nurses first banded together to form their national professional organization, the American Nurses Association has represented registered nurses in setting standards of practice, standards of education, and standards for nursing services (figure 18-15). An ethical conduct guide was adopted by the association in 1950 as the Code for Nurses. Standards of practice in specialized areas of nursing and advocacy for the baccalaureate degree as the appropriate entry level preparation for nurses have been reflected in the credentialing and licensure procedures for nurses and accreditation procedures for nursing schools and nursing services. ANA publications number over two-hundred. The *American Journal of Nursing* is published monthly. *The American Nurse,* a monthly newspaper, keeps the fifty constituent state nurses' associations in communication with each other.

Figure 18-15

The American Nurses Association, like other professional associations, serves as a focal point for interests and standards of its members. This public service ad was developed to raise interest in nursing as a career choice. *Source:* Ad Council.

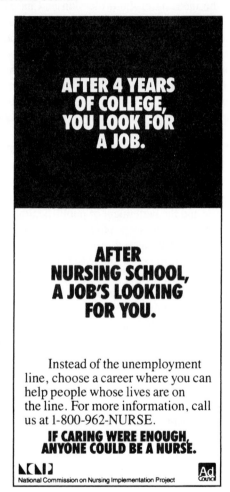

Canadian Public Health Association

The Canadian Public Health Association (CPHA), incorporated in 1912 as a national nonprofit association, serves approximately twenty-five community health disciplines in conducting and supporting national and international health programs.

CPHA works in partnership with federal and provincial government departments, international agencies, and nongovernmental organizations in conducting research and programs. Representing public health in Canada, the membership believes in universal and equitable access to the basic conditions necessary to achieve health for Canadians. The mission of the association is "to constitute a special national resource in Canada that advocates for the improvement and maintenance of personal and community health according to the public health principles of disease prevention, health promotion and protection, and healthy public policy."

CPHA publishes the *Canadian Journal of Public Health,* and various newsletters and materials. The CPHA Health Resources Centre is the Canadian distributor of WHO publications and various books of interest to community health professionals. Affiliated with CPHA are the Canadian Society for International Health and the Canadian Association for Teachers of Community Health.

Society for Public Health Education

The Society for Public Health Education was formed in 1958 as the Society of Public Health Educators. Its change in name reflects its commitment to promotion of health education of the public, which transcends the interests of its professional members. With a membership of less than two thousand, the society has been remarkably effective in influencing national policy related to health education, including the Health Information and Promotion Act of 1976 (PL 94-317). The society publishes *Health Education and Behavior* (formerly *Health Education Quarterly*), *SoPHE News and Views,* and meets annually in conjunction with the American Public Health Association.

American Alliance for Health, Physical Education, Recreation and Dance

The American Alliance for Health, Physical Education, Recreation and Dance began in 1885 as the American Association for the Advancement of Physical Education. It became a department of the National Education Association in 1937.

"Alliance" refers to its several constituent organizations, including the Association for the Advancement of Health Education. Several areas of alliance activity are related to health; these include school nursing, school medical service, health teaching, nutrition education, dental health, mental health, and recreation. The alliance recommends program standards for communities. It publishes the monthly *Journal of Physical Education, Recreation and Dance, Journal of Health Education* and *Research Quarterly for Exercise and Sport.*

HEALTH FOUNDATIONS

Many philanthropic foundations engage in community and population health programs. Some foundations are international in scope; others are national or even limited to a state, region, or city. Some have broad programs and operate in a variety of fields; others are specific in their activities and tend to concentrate on relatively few projects. A proliferation of new community health foundations has been spawned by the sale of community nonprofit hospitals. Five foundations will be described as examples of the different types that engage in health projects.

Rockefeller Foundation

The Rockefeller Foundation was chartered in 1913 under the laws of the state of New York for the purpose of "promoting the well-being of mankind throughout the world." In its organization the foundation carries out work in five areas: (1) international health, (2) medical sciences, (3) natural sciences, (4) social sciences, and (5) humanities.

The international health effort is an operating agency with its own laboratories and staff of scientists. Three phases of work have been pursued: (1) control of specific diseases such as yellow fever, tuberculosis, and influenza; (2) aid to health departments; and (3) health demonstrations, aid to selected schools, public health education, and grants of postgraduate fellowships in public health. Out of the research laboratories of the foundation have come many significant contributions in the treatment of yellow fever, typhus, influenza, and malaria. The other divisions of the Rockefeller Foundation support university, laboratory, and other research groups.

Commonwealth Fund

The Commonwealth Fund was founded in 1918 with a simple but meaningful objective: "To do something for the welfare of mankind." Activities have included health, medical education and research, education, and mental hygiene. The fund has been instrumental in advancing public health practices and procedures through research, improved teaching in medical schools, extension of public health services to rural communities, provision and improvement of hospital facilities, and strengthening of mental health services in the United States and Great Britain.

W. K. Kellogg Foundation

The W. K. Kellogg Foundation was established in 1930 to "help people to help themselves" and for "the promotion of health, education, and the welfare of mankind, but principally of children and youth, directly or indirectly, without regard to sex, race, creed, or nationality." A functional problem solving approach has been used rather than one of research or relief. As one of the largest philanthropic organizations, the foundation has remained true to its philosophical foundations by addressing significant human issues with direct, pragmatic answers. From modest beginnings, with programs relating to the health and educational needs of children in south-central Michigan, the foundation has grown to a position of national and international prominence for its contributions in meeting social goals. For many years the Foundation funded projects in many countries, but now limit grants outside the United States and Latin America to the Kellogg International Fellowship Program. Current program interests include coordinated cost effective health services, a wholesome food supply, and adult continuing education.

Ford Foundation

Founded in 1936 by automobile manufacturer Henry Ford and his son Edsel, the Ford Foundation devoted most of its resources prior to 1950 to charitable and educational institutions in Michigan. Since becoming a national and international foundation with headquarters in New York, it has distributed billions to organizations and individuals in 100 countries. The Foundation provides grants and loans to projects that strengthen democratic values, reduce poverty and injustice, promote international cooperation, and advance human achievement. In national affairs, it has supported educational institutions and helped establish the Public Broadcasting Service. It has also provided assistance for minorities through educational support and community action, housing, and job training. In international affairs, the foundation makes grants to developing countries to help build institutions needed for long-range growth. Some of its most notable contributions have been in family planning programs through the Population Council.

Robert Wood Johnson Foundation

The Robert Wood Johnson Foundation began its work on the national scene in 1972, with offices just outside Princeton, New Jersey. Foundation grants put primary emphasis on improving access to general medical and dental care. The statistics on access have improved considerably, so two additional priorities have been added: (1) support for research programs to make health care more effective and more affordable; and (2) support for research, development, and demonstration projects that show promise of helping large numbers of people avoid disabilities and maintain or regain maximum possible functioning in their everyday lives.

VOLUNTARY HEALTH ORGANIZATIONS

Voluntary health organizations perform a unique and important role in the promotion of health in every U.S. state and in most nations. No health program is complete in the sense that it serves every individual who could benefit from the program. Thus there is a need for these organizations to expand and intensify their services. Furthermore, there are areas of health needs that receive little attention and less service. Perhaps the National Foundation for Infantile Paralysis (now the March of Dimes Birth Defects Foundation) charted the course that all existing voluntary and official agencies might consider. When the agency's original goal of preventing poliomyelitis was nearly achieved, the agency directed its attention and energies to other health problems in need of solution, such as the prevention of birth defects. Voluntary health organizations will be described in the remaining chapters.

SUMMARY

This chapter casts the subject of community and population health services in the broader context of the global and national structures. At the global level, the structures supporting community health services include various philanthropic foundations and international agencies representing multigovernmental concerns. Several of the United Nations' agencies carry health responsibilities, but chief among these is the World Health Organization. Of its six regional offices, the Pan American Health Organization represents the governments of North, Central, and South America and the Caribbean. These international agencies depend on collaboration and cooperation to achieve health goals. The most significant recent development in international health-related agencies has been renewed commitment to community health services, epitomized by the Alma-Ata Declaration on Primary Health Care and the WHO global policy goal of "Health for All by the Year 2000."

National or federal structures exist to support community health through the allocation of responsibilities to various agencies and levels of government. In most republics, this authority comes from a constitution reserving certain generic powers for the central or federal government. Many federal governments, such as those of Australia, Canada, and the United States, leave the majority of specific health responsibilities to the states or provinces. Numerous federal agencies in the United States carry health authority and health-related responsibilities. Chief among these is the Department of Health and Human Services (DHHS), comparable to Health Canada in that country and to the ministries of health in most countries. Within DHHS, the chief responsibility for health lies with the eight agencies formerly constituting the Public Health Service. Programs throughout multiple organizations of the PHS are directed toward achievement of the *Year 2000 Health Objectives* discussed in the early chapters of this book. Within the Public Health Service, the major agency having direct relationships with states and communities is the Centers for Disease Control and Prevention.

Foundations and voluntary health agencies have made a significant contribution to health in Western nations and the world. Each agency is free to choose its own course of action and is sufficiently flexible to adjust to changing conditions and needs. These agencies tend to specialize and demonstrate what can be done in a specific field of health. In theory, when this has been accomplished, the task or field is taken over by an official health agency and the need for the voluntary agency no longer exists. In practice, few voluntary agencies are ever dissolved, and overlapping of programs exists to some degree.

WEB *Links*

http://www.hc-sc.gc.ca
Health Canada

http://www.uncle-sam.com/guide_index.html
Internet Guide to the U.S. Government

http://www.hhs.gov
United States Department of Health and Human Services home page

http://www.cdc.gov
Centers for Disease Control and Prevention home page

http://nhic-nt.health.org
National Health Information Center home page

http://www.cihi.ca
Canadian Institute for Health Information

http://www.epa.gov
United States Environmental Protection Agency

QUESTIONS FOR REVIEW

1. How does the government use its taxing power in matters of health?
2. Why is it difficult to recall any time that you or any member of your family received a direct health service from a federal agency?
3. What are your reasons for or against establishing the U.S. Public Health Service as an independent agency?
4. What is the significance of the fact that 95 percent of the professional public health people in the United States are nonmedical people?
5. Why should appropriations for health represent investments rather than expenditures?
6. What justification is there for the NIH subsidizing the research of scientists in other countries?
7. In your judgment, what specific health problem is most in need of more extensive and intensive research?
8. What examples of health issue programs can you find running through multiple federal agencies, for example heart disease or health promotion?
9. Considering the current DHHS organization chart, if you were to reorganize the jigsaw puzzle of the federal health programs what would you suggest?
10. What voice does a local medical practitioner have in the policies of the AMA?
11. Which of the professional health organizations do you regard as most public-spirited and least self-interested? Why?
12. Why do most Western nations give far more to WHO than they receive? What is your comment?
13. Why does WHO place so much emphasis on communicable disease control in view of the recent technological advances in this field?

14. Why is it so important that WHO place primary emphasis on helping nations to help themselves?

READINGS

Chapman, S., and D. Lupton. 1994. *The fight for public health: principles and practice of media advocacy.* London: BMJ Publishing Group.

This book examines public health news and case studies of the strategic use of news and the mass media to advocate for public health policies.

Evans, R. G., M. L. Barer, and T. R. Marmor. 1994. *Why are some people healthy and others not? The determinants of health of populations.* New York: Aldine de Gruyter.

This book has had a major influence on the organization and developing policies in public health and health care for Canada, and its influence on the U.S. thinking about "producing health" versus "consuming health care" is growing.

Lee, P., and D. Paxman. 1997. Reinventing public health. *Ann Rev Public Health* 18:1.

From the Office of the Assistant Secretary of Health and the Office of Public Health and Science, this review of the current state of public health in light of the social, political, economic, scientific, and technological changes buffeting the United States gives perspective to the contents of the chapter you have just completed.

Vladeck, B. C., and K. M. King. 1995. Medicare at 30: preparing for the future. *J Am Med Assoc* 274:259.

The first of a series of articles in this issue of *JAMA* recounts the events since 1965, when only 50 percent of the U.S. elderly population had health insurance, to now when over 97 percent are insured. Ways in which Medicare provides vital support to the American health care infrastructure, expenditures, trends and the future of Medicare are discussed.

World Health Organization. 1997. *Tobacco or health: a global status report.* Geneva: World Health Organization.

This WHO report documents the current situation of the tobacco epidemic in most countries of the world, trends over the past two decades, industry practices, national control policies, ranking of countries according to key indicators of the tobacco situation, production and use.

BIBLIOGRAPHY

Airhihenbuwa, C. O. 1995. *Health and Culture: Beyond the Western Paradigm.* Newbury Park, CA: Sage.

Bennett, A., and O. Adams, eds. 1993. *Looking north for health: what we can learn from Canada's health care system.* San Francisco: Jossey-Bass.

Brown, L. D., ed. 1991. *Health policy and the disadvantaged.* Durham, NC: Duke University Press.

Coyte, P. C. 1990. Comparative health systems, Canada. *Adv Health Econ Health Serv Res* 1(suppl):103.

Crichton, A., D. Hsu, and S. Tsang. 1990. *Canada's health care system: its funding and organization.* Ottawa: Canadian Hospital Association Press.

Dignan, M., R. Michielutte, K. Blinson, H. B. Wells, L. D. Case, P. Sharp, S. Davis, J. Konen, and R. P. McQuellon. 1996. Effectiveness of health education to increase screening for cervical cancer among eastern-band Cherokee Indian women in North Carolina. *J National Can Inst* 88:1670.

El Bindari-Hamad, A., and D. L. Smith. 1992. *Primary health care reviews: guidelines and methods.* Ottawa: Canadian Public Health Association Health Resources Centre.

Farley, C. 1997. Evaluation of a four-year bicycle helmet promotion campaign in Quebec aimed at children ages 8 to 12: Impact on attitudes, norms and behaviours. *Can J Public Health* 88(1): 62.

Hancock, T. 1993. The evolution, impact and significance of the Healthy Cities/Healthy Communities movement. *J Public Health Policy* 14:5.

Healthy people 2000: national health promotion and disease prevention objectives. 1990. Washington, DC: U.S. Department of Health and Human Services, Government Printing Office.

Kimball, A. M., S. Berkley, and H. Gayle. 1995. International Aspects of the AIDS/HIV Epidemic. *Ann Rev Public Health* 16:253.

Laitakari, J., S. Miilunpalo, and I. Vuori. 1997. The process and methods of health counseling by primary health care personnel in Finland: A national survey. *Patient Educ Couns* 30:61.

Lauren, P. G. 1996. Between pandemonium and order: assessing international organizations and multiethnic societies. *Am Behavioral Scientist* 40:66.

Mantell, J. E., A. T. DiVittis, and M. I. Auerbach. 1997. *Evaluating HIV prevention interventions.* New York: Plenum Press.

McCain, T. A., and A. Hollifield. 1995. A national network in the global village: U.S. policy goals for an international network. *Social Sci Computer Rev* 13:183.

Monekosso, G. L. 1993. African universities as partners in community health development. *J Community Health* 18:127.

National Highway Traffic Safety Administration. 1990. *Protecting our own: community child passenger safety programs.* 2d ed. Washington, DC: U.S. Department of Transportation.

Nutbeam D., and M. Wise. 1996. Planning for Health for All: international experience in setting health goals and targets. *Health Promotion Internat* 11:219.

Nyamwaya, D. 1996. Impediments to health promotion in developing countries: the way forward. *Health Promotion Internat* 11:175.

Oxman, A. D., M. A. Thomson, D. A. Davis, and R. B. Haynes. 1995. No magic bullets: A systematic review of 102 trials of interventions to improve professional practice. *Can Med Assoc J* 153:1423.

Pan American Health Organization. 1992. *The crisis of public health: reflections for the debate.* Ottawa: Canadian Public Health Association Resources Centre.

Pollitt, P. A. 1996. From National Negro Health Week to National Public Health Week. *J Community Health* 21:401.

Ragan, E. 1996. Global immunization: Is a child's life worth $15? *Can Med Assoc J* 155:1492.

Rimer, B. K. 1995. Audiences and messages for breast and cervical cancer screenings. *Wellness Perspectives: Research, Theory Prac* 11:13.

Sanders-Phillips, K. 1996. Correlates of health promotion behaviors in low-income black women and Latinas. *Am J Prev Med* 12:450.

Schaalma, H. P., G. Kok, R. J. Bosker, G. S. Parcel, L. Peters, J. Poelman, J. Reinders. 1996. Planned development and evaluation of AIDS/STD education for secondary school students in the Netherlands: Short-term effects. *Health Educ Quar* 23:469.

Selby-Harrington, M., J. R. Sorenson, D. Quade, S. C. Stearns, A. S. Tesh, and P. L. N. Donat. 1995. Increasing Medicaid child health screenings: The effectiveness of mailed pamphlets, phone calls, and home visits. *Am J Public Health* 85:1412.

Simons Morton, B. G., W. H. Greene, N. H. Gottlieb. 1995. *Introduction to health education and health promotion.* 2d ed. Prospect Heights, IL: Waveland Press, Inc.

Stevenson, M., S. Jones, D. Cross, P. Howat, and M. Hall. 1996. The child pedestrian injury prevention project. *Health Prom J Austral* 6:32.

The world almanac and book of facts 1997. 1996. Mahwah, NJ: World Almanac Books.

Timmreck, T. C. 1995. *Planning, Program Development, and Evaluation: A handbook for health promotion, aging, and health services.* Boston: Jones & Bartlett Publishers.

U.S. Bureau of the Census. 1996. *Statistical abstract of the United States.* 116th ed. Washington, DC: U.S. Department of Commerce.

U.S. Department of Health and Human Services. 1996. *Planned Approach to Community Health: guide for the local coordinator.* Atlanta, GA: U.S. Department of Health and Human Services, Centers for Disease Control and Prevention, National Center for Chronic Disease Prevention and Health Promotion.

Willemsen, M. C. 1997. *Kicking the habit: The effectiveness of smoking cessation programs in Dutch worksites.* The Netherlands: University of Maastricht.

Wong, M. L., R. Chan, J. Lee, D. Koh, and C. Wong C. 1996. Controlled evaluation of a behavioural intervention programme on condom use and gonorrhoea incidence among sex workers in Singapore. *Health Educ Res* 11:423.

World Health Organization. 1993. *Implementation of the global strategy for Health for All by the Year 2000: second evaluation.* Geneva: World Health Organization.

Wyatt, D. 1995. Comments. On providing a truly international perspective. *Soc Sci Med* 41:1623.

Chapter *19*

State or Provincial Health Organizations, Resources, and Services

A *state without some means of change is without the means of its conservation.*

—Edmund Burke, Reflections on the Revolution in France, 1790.

I *f public health is to maintain the reputation it now enjoys, it will be because in everything we do, behind everything we say as the basis for every program decision—we are willing to see faces.*

—William H. Foege, M.D., former director, Centers for Disease Control

Objectives

When you finish this chapter, you should be able to:

- Identify the source and extent of state or provincial authority for health-related functions

- Describe the organization, resources, and services typical of state or provincial health agencies

- Describe ways in which states or provinces plan and promote health legislation

---

In this chapter you go a step closer to home, from the global and national context of community and population health to the state or provincial context. You should become increasingly aware of the constitutional and legal frameworks within which community and population health operate. You should recognize the resources available to your community from higher levels of organization at the state or provincial and national level. The most effective community health programs are those that take full advantage of such resources while developing their own local resources and self-sufficiency.

The term **federalism** means the opposite of what it might appear to mean. It does not mean more power to the central government of federated states. It pertains to the recognition of the common values but vast differences between the states or provinces in their needs and their traditions (figure 19-1). Likewise, communities must understand

589

....

Figure 19-1

The variations across jurisdictions like states, provinces, and school districts can be illustrated most clearly in the statistics on a highly volatile subject such as tobacco control. Here the percentage of schools with total bans on smoking varied across the provinces and territories of Canada from 10 percent to 72 percent in 1990 and from 15 percent to 93 percent in 1995. Federalism and federal policy in health must take these variations into account, as states and provinces must take variations among school districts into account. *Source:* Thomas Stephens and Associates and Goss Gilroy Inc. Survey of Smoking Restrictions in Four Settings. Prepared from Health Canada, August 1995.

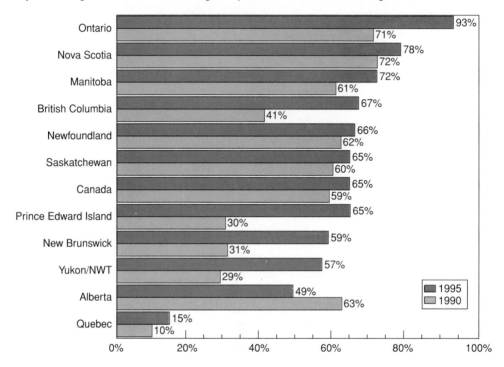

their own local needs and demand their share of state and national resources.

The "New Federalism" of the last two decades of the twentieth century in North America sought to return many of the rights to states or provinces that federal agencies seemed to have usurped. Unfortunately, the transfer of responsibility back to states did not carry with it the transfer of resources. The U.S. and Canadian federal contributions to the states and provinces declined during this period. With this decrease in federal contribution, tax revolts at home, rising health costs, and increasing demands from entitlement programs, state and provincial governments across North America face challenges to provide health care and prevention programs.

States have been at the forefront of pushing the United States toward health care reform, just as the provinces have been the source of innovation in the Canadian health experience. In the 1992 presidential election health care reform was a key issue, but the Clinton administration was unable to pass the reform package it proposed to Congress. Reform was beaten back by health insurance industry advertising and a public frightened by the prospect of losing their choice of personal physicians.

Health reform barely surfaced in the 1996 election. In Canada, the electorate sent Members of Parliament back to Ottawa and the provincial capitals with a clear message that preserving the health care system was their highest priority. Prevention and federal responsibility to states or provinces were key issues in the reform debates of both countries.

CLOSER TO HOME

One argument for decentralization from federal to state or provincial and local levels is to make services and the allocation of resources more sensitive to the needs of the people intended to be served—the "faces" referred to by Dr. Foege in the quotation at the beginning of this chapter. Program requirements for public health agencies differ depending on the characteristics of the population served. For example, state populations range from a low of a half million in Alaska to nearly 30 million in California. Rural populations vary from 7 percent in California to 68 percent in Vermont. Public health agencies often care for the most needy of the population, who range from a low of 6 percent below the poverty line in New Hampshire to a high of 25 percent in Mississippi. These different population characteristics place different demands on the nature, location, and administration of public health programs.

Health planning and resources are coordinated in most countries at some level between the local community and the national agencies responsible for public health. This intermediate level is the provincial or state health agency (SHA), usually named the provincial Ministry of Health or the state Department of Health.* The state constitution provides the SHA with broad functions. The state constitution also permits or directs the state legislature to pass supplemental statutory provisions. In Australia and Canada state ministers of health also sit as elected legislators of parliament. In small

countries, such as Ireland, the county or a district functions as the equivalent of a state or province.

In Canada and other countries following more closely the British tradition, the Ministry of Health has broader responsibilities for direct financing and management of large parts of the medical care system. The part of the provincial Ministry of Health that matches the SHA in the United States is usually under a medical officer of health (MOH). Our reference to SHAs in the remainder of this chapter generally encompasses the MOH part of provincial ministries of health.

State and provincial health agencies seek to develop a long-range, equitable, comprehensive, and balanced approach to the diverse needs of many communities. Political changes with periodic elections, however, make long-range planning difficult. Changes in government leadership often break the continuity of long-range plans and allocation schemes designed to reduce inequities among local communities and population groups.

If states or provinces allow each community to have complete autonomy in addressing short-range health concerns of local interest groups, the programs will tend to serve only their most affluent or the most politically influential.

Provincial and state agencies support the local health department. They provide the services of experts when requested or needed for an important local health problem. The SHAs also provide local health departments with laboratory services and with equipment and facilities for special surveys and other purposes. Devices for measuring air pollution and other types of equipment are made available by the state to local authorities for the protection or promotion of community health.

The SHA acts as the link between national health agencies and local health departments. Federal health funds are allocated by the SHA to the local health agencies. Through the SHA, community health departments are able to obtain the services of national or federal health experts to solve unique or difficult health problems or to deal with an emergency when summary action is required.

*We will use the abbreviation SHA to refer broadly to health agencies at the state (United States or Australia) and provincial (most other countries) level.

HEALTH AUTHORITY, LAW, AND RESPONSIBILITY

Woodrow Wilson defined law as "that portion of the established thought and habit which has gained distinct and formal recognition in the shape of uniform rules backed by the authority and power of government." More concisely, laws are crystallized public opinion. They express health policy and establish implementation procedures.

Public health applies **statutory law** and **common law** to protect and prevent against injury and disease and to promote health. All sources of public health law have some impact on health. Laws can play positive and negative roles in relation to public health. Positive roles are those that protect health, provide access to health services, or assure the quantity and quality of health care. Negative roles include restricting or ignoring such services. Laws must be balanced with ethical concerns and informed by scientific and epidemiological evidence.

Sovereignty, or ultimate authority, in matters of health rests with the people. Most democracies vest this authority in local and state or provincial governments to pass such legislation and take such action as may be necessary to promote the health and general welfare of the people. As stated by James Madison, who more than anyone set the tone of the U.S. Constitution, the state in the United States has virtually unlimited authority to do what is necessary to promote the greatest good for the greatest number of people. Similarly in Canada, provinces have the primary authority in matters of health and each province administers its own health system.

There is but one limitation on the state's power to pass legislation regarding health matters—a statute may not violate or be inconsistent with the provisions of the U.S. Constitution. In the exercise of the state's police power in matters of health, the action taken must be *reasonable* and *constitutional.* In the case of Canadian provinces, they may not violate the Charter of Rights.

Delegation of Authority

The people of a state approve a constitution, which in some cases mentions health only in providing that the legislature set up health agencies and pass laws to protect and promote the public's health. In some states in the United States the constitution delineates in detail what the state health organization and services shall be. Most public health authorities agree that the state constitution should contain broad, general provisions granting to the state legislature authority to establish the necessary health agencies, their responsibilities, and their powers. This type of general constitutional provision would provide for changes through legislation as needs arise.

In some states, notably California, the people's impatience with the legislative process has led to numerous health initiatives by referendum on the state ballot. These have included an increase in cigarette taxes to pay for more health education and smoking prevention programs and health care to help pay for the medical costs incurred by tobacco use (see figure 19-1).

Legislators in most states and provinces choose to delegate much of their health authority to state or regional boards of health to pass health regulations, standards, and requirements, with the provision that the health boards must restrict themselves to health matters. In effect the state or provincial board of health acts as a quasilegislative body. The legislature also charges the health board with the responsibility for the enforcement of these regulations, which have the force of law.

Statutory Authority

The U.S. Constitution   Historically, the states came first as colonies that united and created the federal government to serve specific purposes. The Constitution is a grant of authority by the states to the federal government, but with reservations. The reservations are expressed in the Tenth Amendment: "The powers not delegated to the United States by the Constitution, nor prohibited by it to the States, are reserved to the States respectively, or to the people." The word **health** does not appear in the Constitution. Nor is there any reference to public health. Thus the control of public health is primarily a state function as discussed in the previous chapter.

State Constitutions and Legislation Fundamentally promotion of public health is the function of the state. Governments have long recognized health as a basic human condition that government has an inherent obligation, right, and power to protect and promote. From colonial times states and provinces have taken measures to safeguard and promote the health of their citizens. This authority is vested in the states' **police power,** which the courts and the federal government recognize.

Common Law A heritage from Great Britain, the common law derives from custom or court decision rather than from formally enacted statutes. Based on practice and experience, common law interprets a present situation in terms of past court decisions. Some health problems or controversies may be adjudicated on the basis of custom or past practice. To this extent the common law represents a source of public health law.

Police Power

Police power is the authority of the people, vested in government, to enact laws, within constitutional limits, to promote and protect the peace, health, comfort, safety, order, morality, and general welfare of the people. This means the authority to promote the welfare of the public, which may sometimes necessitate restraining freedom and regulating the use of property. The police power is based on the concept of the greatest good for the greatest number of people and may operate to the inconvenience and even distress of certain individuals. All persons, business firms, and corporations must regulate their conduct subject to the police power.

Historically, the focus of public health was the protection of the public from the threats of diseases affecting large numbers of people, either communicated from infected animals or individuals or threats from identifiable environmental factors. With the increased emphasis on disease prevention and health promotion, threats to health have been identified from a wide variety of sources. The use of legal powers to protect a group of people, such as a ban on smoking in public places, can be interpreted as infringement on the individual rights of others. These kinds of debates related to public health law occur also around the use of motorcycle helmets, seat belts, emission controls on cars, and other laws intended to protect the greater good.

Limits Any *reasonable* action taken under the shield of police power will tend to be upheld unless contrary to U.S. constitutional or Canadian Charter of Rights provisions. The First, Fourth, Sixth, and Fourteenth Amendments to the U.S. Constitution safeguard the personal rights of the citizen. Although the Constitution guarantees freedom of religious belief, such a guarantee does not invalidate a school board regulation requiring students to have a health examination or to be immunized before admission to school. Likewise it is a valid exercise of the police power for a state or provincial law to require marriage license applicants to have a physician's statement certifying that they are free from certain sexually transmitted diseases.

ORGANIZATION OF STATE AND PROVINCIAL HEALTH

In four states in the United States the state constitution names the department responsible for the activities necessary to protect and promote health and specifies its functions. In the remaining states the state constitution delegates this authority to the state legislature. Massachusetts established the first state health board in the United States in 1869. (Local official health agencies had operated for more than a century prior to the creation of the Massachusetts State Board of Health.) No two states have precisely the same structure for their health programs. In most states the governor appoints the head of the SHA to a cabinet-level position.

Health Agencies in the State or Province

Each state or province has official health agencies and voluntary health agencies. An **official health agency** or service is one supported by tax funds and recognized as a governmental agency or service. Examples of such agencies are the Minnesota Department of Public Health, the Maryland Department of Health and Mental Hygiene, and the British Columbia Ministry of Health. Official health agencies have staffs appointed by some official governmental body. The staff members are government employees and may be classified as officials, also referred to less kindly as bureaucrats or technocrats.

A **voluntary health agency** is one supported entirely or primarily by financial contributions from citizens and private organizations. These agencies may bid on and accept government contracts to perform health services. Examples of such agencies are the American Lung Association, the American Cancer Society, the Canadian Cancer Society, and the Canadian Heart and Stroke Foundation. Full-time, salaried, professional personnel perform the services of voluntary health agencies at the state level. Most of the recognized voluntary health agencies in the United States and Canada have a national organization with state or provincial divisions and local chapters or affiliates. The effective, principal sphere of operation of most voluntary agencies is at the state or provincial level where funds are raised, programs are planned, and services are developed. Some of the funds raised in the state or province are contributed to the national office, and some may be channeled to the local chapters or affiliates.

Official Agencies Serving Health

Each of the fifty states, the District of Columbia, eight U.S. territories, and the ten provinces and two territories of Canada has a government agency responsible for the administration of public health services. Depending on how activities in a state are organized, public health responsibilities and authority may not be located in the SHA. For example, some SHAs are the state mental health authority and most SHAs in the United States have a separate lead agency for environmental health and protection.

Various other official agencies also engage in health promotion and environmental health protection. Most of these agencies provide health as a secondary service or an incidental activity. Educational and agricultural agencies, for example, produce health benefits as a by-product of the primary activities of the agency. Nevertheless the composite activities of these agencies amount to a significant contribution to health and quality of life.

Two or more agencies may carry on the same health function. This duplication usually results from long-established custom or priority and political patronage or protectionism. On the state or provincial level and the local and national levels, agencies multiply and often outgrow their original purpose, so they create new activities to justify their continuing existence rather than put themselves out of business.

SHAs are usually organized in one of two ways: as a freestanding independent agency responsible directly to the governor, premier or the board of health, or as a component of a superagency. Figure 19-2 shows an example of a state, Massachusetts, with a freestanding independent state health agency. The Massachusetts Commissioner of Health reports directly to the Governor of Massachusetts.

Figure 19-3 shows a superagency structure in Delaware where the Commissioner of Public Health heads one of many subagencies reporting through two bureaucratic layers to the governor. For a comparison of SHA organization charts, see web sites at end of this chapter. In a state larger

Figure 19-2

Massachusetts Department of Health's organization chart illustrates the typical structure of a state health agency with a freestanding, independent relationship to the governor of the state. Issues with high priority such as Narcotics and Dangerous Drugs often have a staff office to give them freer access to several of the line agencies below the director or commissioner. *Source:* Centers for Disease Control. 1991. *Profile of state and territorial public health systems: United States, 1990.* Atlanta: U.S. Department of Health and Human Services. For updates and detailed descriptions of the divisions, the Department's website URL is http://www.magnet.state.ma.us\dph\dphorg2htm.

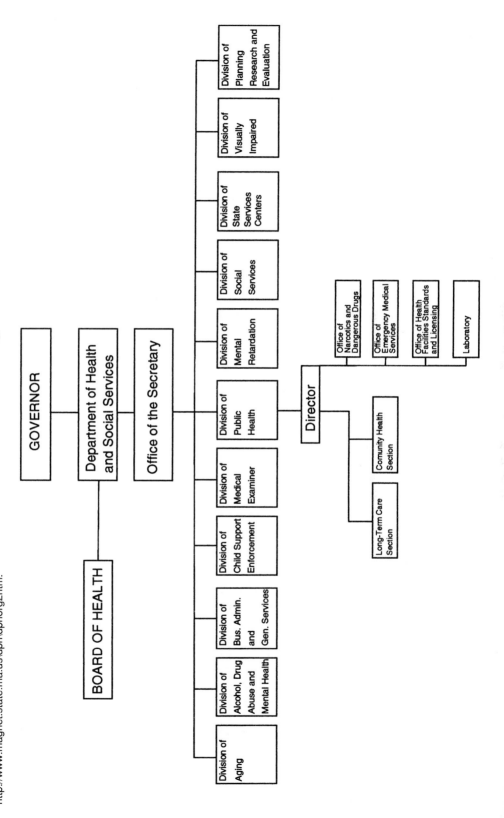

The Delaware Division of Public Health is located two layers deep in the superagency Department of Health and Social Services. Many of the usual functions of a state health agency, such as aging, alcohol, and drug abuse, reside in other agencies at the same level. *Source:* Centers for Disease Control. 1991. *Profile of state and territorial public health systems: United States, 1990.* Atlanta: U.S. Department of Health and Human Services. For updates and descriptions of the divisions, go to htttp://www.state.de.u/sovern/agencies/dhss

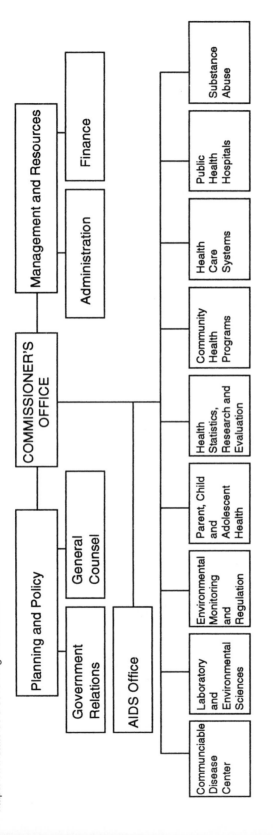

than Delaware this would put the public health program at some disadvantage in competing for state resources.

To note all the other state or provincial agencies that perform health services to some degree would produce an almost interminable list. The agencies and organizations found in most states and provinces will indicate the spectrum. In many cases the title of the agency gives some indication of the nature of its health function. These may include agencies named Department or Ministry of:

- Agriculture
- Education
- Labor and Industry
- Welfare or Social Services
- Conservation or Environment
- Mental Health or Mental Hygiene
- Motor Vehicles
- Public Safety
- Civil Service and Registration
- State Institutions
- Parks and Recreation
- Drug and Alcohol Agencies or Substance Abuse Prevention
- Higher Education, Postsecondary Education, or Universities and Colleges

They also include boards and councils such as the Board of Health; the Governor's Council on Physical Fitness; Industrial Inquiry; Water Resources; and examining and licensing boards for medicine, dentistry, nursing, medical laboratory, podiatry, pharmacy, and other allied health professions.

Cooperation with Other Sectors

Combining agencies and coordinating services can result in a reduction in costs and in an improvement in services. In large states, however, consolidation sometimes creates overly complex and confusing bureaucracies. The preferred strategy in recent years has been to build coalitions or partnerships of public, voluntary, and private sector organizations (see box).

The U.S. objectives for the nation for 1990 and 2000 in disease prevention and health promotion captured the imagination of many health professionals and the collaborative commitment of some organizations outside the health sector. Canada did not develop national objectives except in relation to tobacco, injury control, and child health. As of 1997, most of the U.S. states and Canadian provinces had completed their own turn-of-the-century health objectives. In the United States, these were based usually on the national objectives, matching the twenty-two priority areas of the Healthy People 2000 initiative (figure 19-4). The eight states without their own year 2000 objectives had committed to statewide assessments of their disease prevention and health promotion progress in relation to the national objectives.

Health professionals and official health agencies alone could not accomplish most of these objectives. Attaining them requires the active participation of other sectors, other professionals, and other institutions than those primarily identified with health. It is remarkable that health objectives draw any attention at all, considering their remote and sober character. They hardly have the siren call raised by the devastating epidemics of the past. They scarcely compete even with economic concerns, much less with threats of global environmental degradation. It is little wonder, then, that other sectors and the public at large often respond with indifference when called on to help achieve the national, state, or provincial objectives in disease prevention and health promotion.

Building on Shared Needs and Values Several advantages and benefits of the health goals and the partnerships that formed around them seem to explain the developing interest in health promotion that has been shown within the health sector. They helped build a common language for disease prevention and health promotion. They gave increased visibility and public awareness to the importance of disease prevention and health promotion needs and efforts. They focused media

ISSUES AND CONTROVERSIES
Caveats for Coalitions Revisited

Many grants from federal government agencies to states and provinces, and from them or from foundations to communities require the grantee to have a coalition. As a condition of even applying for the grant the state, provincial or regional agency must have a coalition of organizations committed to cooperate in the planning, execution, and evaluation of the grant program. Let us revisit the caveats presented in Chapter 2 on undertaking the development and maintenance of a coalition:

- The willingness of each member or organization to join a coalition does not include a willingness to be coordinated with each of the others.
- Conflicts of interest inevitably arise between some of the individuals representing their organizations and the needs or goals of the coalition.
- The larger organizations may resist having an equal vote with smaller organizations in the coalition.
- Representatives from other sectors (e.g., education, recreation)

often believe that investments in the field of health, which usually has more resources than their own sector, siphons their resources for little gain to their sector.
- Opposition from health agencies to letting another sector assume the leadership in matters concerning health.
- Some organizations at the state or provincial level do not have the authority to make deals with other organizations without the approval of their national parent organization.
- So much effort and resources sometimes go into the tasks of building and maintaining the coalition that little energy and funds are left for actually carrying out a program together.
- Coalitions serve best in achieving a shared vision and broad goals on what needs to be accomplished, and in allocating responsibility to specific organizations or paired partnerships of organizations to develop more specific plans and to carry out specific actions. They usu-

ally function with greater difficulty as instruments of implementation.
- The people who come to coalition meetings as representatives of their organizations often have too little authority to make decisions for their organizations without consulting with their supervisors, so decision making at coalition meetings often ends in stalemates. Decisions often must be deferred to the next meeting.

How would you overcome some of these difficulties in organizing and maintaining a coalition? Should foundations and federal granting agencies require state or provincial organizations to have interorganizational or intersectoral coalitions as a condition of receiving grants in aid?

For web sites concerning coalitions see:

http://futurehealth.ucsf.edu
Community Campus-Partnerships for Health

http://www.healthycities.org
Coalition for Healthier Cities & Communities

attention and health education activities around specific priorities. They provided a framework for policy and legislation with greater specificity and concreteness than legislators had seen in health promotion. Finally, they provided a mechanism to increase communication and program coordination within the state health department and with other agencies and sectors.

The specific appeals for other sectors to become involved in the disease prevention and health promotion initiatives were two. One is the

perceived demand of the public; the second is the possibility that support could contribute to other goals that they seek.

Sensing a public demand for health promotion, many organizations outside the health field have taken up health-related programs. Business and industry, in particular, have risen to the challenge of consumer demand, providing health, nutrition, and fitness products and services. Many companies have begun to offer health promotion programs or facilities for their employees. Some have justified

· · · · · · · · · · · · · · · · · · · ·
Figure 19-4

By 1995, forty-two states and territories (including the District of Columbia and Guam) had completed their year 2000 objectives and plans for disease prevention and health promotion programs in line with the *Healthy People 2000* document of the U.S. Department of Health and Human Services. The distribution of state objectives by the twenty-two priority areas of the national document is shown here. *Source:* U.S. Department of Health and Human Services. 1996. *Healthy People 2000 Midcourse Review and 1995 Revisions.* Boston: Jones and Bartlett Publishers.

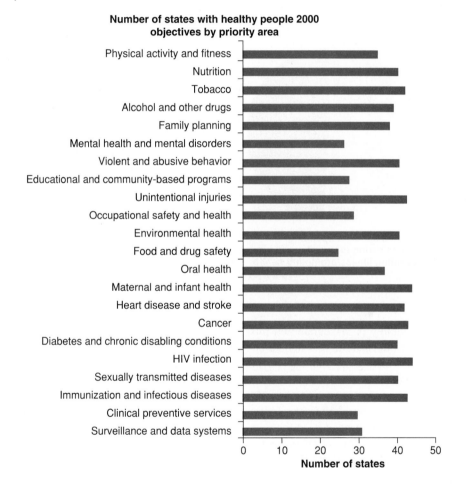

Number of states with healthy people 2000 objectives by priority area

these expenditures on the grounds that such programs provide the organization a competitive edge in attracting and holding the best employees.

How did this consumer demand come about? Can it be sustained or even nurtured to gain further support from other sectors? At least part of the answer to these questions lies in an enlightened public (figure 19-5). Continuing health information and education programs produce increased consumer discretion in matters of health. Increased interest and discretion in turn stimulate commercial and news media to provide yet more information,

· · · · · · · · · · · · · · · · · · · ·

Figure 19-5

A 1996 survey of Californians showed dissatisfaction with the way health dollars are spent. More than one in three supports spending a greater share on preventing illness and promoting health. *Source:* The California Wellness Foundation's Health Improvement Initiative. 1997. *Spending for health: Californians speak out about priorities for health spending. "Living Well" statewide survey series.* Sacramento: Conducted by the Field Institute in cooperation with the California Center for Health Improvement.

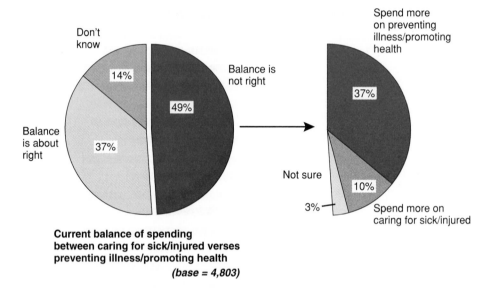

Current balance of spending between caring for sick/injured verses preventing illness/promoting health
(base = 4,803)

some of which inevitably is inaccurate and misleading. Conflicting information stirs debate and controversy, further whetting the public's appetite for more health information and education.

One disadvantage of this growing market for health ideas is the consequent glutting of information. Some of the innocent bystanders in the withering crossfire of health information despair at ever avoiding all the risks to health that are reported by the media. The public pleads for relief from this tumult. Nowhere does the cooperation of health organizations in various sectors promise greater relief for the public than in the development of consensus on selected health messages and the dissemination of joint communications. *The Dietary Guidelines for Americans,* for example, were such a joint formulation by the U.S. Department of Agriculture and the U.S. Department of Health and Human Services. The health goals for

individual states and provinces offer even greater potential for consensus than do national health goals.

Linking Health to Other Goals The second motive accounting for interest shown by other sectors in health promotion is the possibility that it might contribute to their own mission, which is something other than health. In the business sector the hope of many executives—and the conviction of some—is that their employee health promotion programs will contribute to improved morale, greater productivity, and reduced health insurance claims (see figure 19-6). Some even support these programs with no conviction that they will influence health, so strong is their belief that the programs will improve morale and productivity. These alternative "bottom lines" should remind health professionals that the cooperation of other

····················

Figure 19-6

Organizations at the state or provincial level, besides health agencies, sometimes see ways in which they can support or promote health objectives relevant to their own objectives. The Insurance Corporation of British Columbia, which insures automobiles and crash liability, sponsored this ad. Any company or vendor such as a sports stadium owner can put their own logo at the bottom of the ad. *Source:* Courtesy Insurance Corporation of British Columbia.

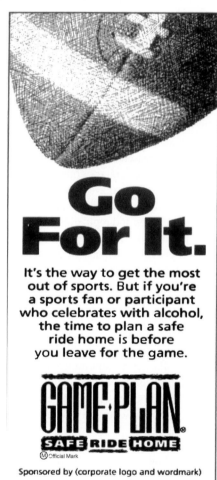

Sponsored by (corporate logo and wordmark)

The Coordination Paradox of Health Promotion Today

Not since the nineteenth century has medical care been more irrelevant to the task of improving the public's health. Medicine, more and more miraculously, restores the health of ailing individuals. Its organization and resources bend mostly to this task, with very little time or financing left for the task of promoting health. The health professions know what must be done to improve health—hence they have the ability to state achievable objectives for the year 2000. They are, however, helpless by themselves to achieve most of these objectives. Success depends on reaching people where their daily decisions about environment and lifestyle are influenced and made. This means reaching them in schools, at worksites, and in other nonmedical settings in the community.

Some health professionals assume that a wave of the coordinating wand will bring disparate interests into line if only the wand is waved at a high bureaucratic level. Such wishful thinking has given the health care sector the mistaken impression that other sectors of human services are all too willing to set their own priorities aside if presented with a health problem requiring attention. Perhaps there was once a time when coordination was easier, when epidemics were threatening enough to galvanize concerted community action, but this is very seldom the case now. Most disease is chronic and privately degenerative rather than acute and publicly communicable.

What must be done to gain the cooperation of other sectors and to build statewide coalitions for health promotion? Why do agencies need to coordinate and collaborate in population health matters? What prevents them from, or makes them resistant to, cooperation?

Health professionals sometimes lose sight of the fact that for most people health is not a terminal value. Rather, people seek health as an instrumental means to gain other ends. Similarly for organizations whose mission is not health, health promotion can nevertheless serve as a means to achieve their ends. The education sector provides

sectors depends on an ability to translate the objectives into terms that relate to these sectors' economic goals or other nonhealth outcomes.

an example of the need to shift the "health-for-its-own-sake" orientation of the objectives for disease prevention and health promotion. Schools are leaping to the task of raising the cognitive learning scores of children in basic subjects. This has resulted in abandoning certain courses, often including health education. Health promotion in the schools and in other community settings that reach children can contribute to children's greater alertness and improved cognitive performance in basic subjects. Presenting this thesis to the education sector should make it possible to regain the schools' cooperation in health promotion for productivity motives. The productivity of schools depends on average daily attendance, not unlike the productivity needs of industry in supporting health programs for their employees to reduce absenteeism.

State Board of Health

State boards or councils of health are used for citizen input into the operation of the SHA in 40 states. State health boards or councils function in a policymaking capacity in 21 states, in an advisory capacity in 17, and in both capacities in 2 states. The usual practice is to appoint a board of about 9 members. Board members are appointed by the governor—subject to approval by the legislature—and serve without pay but are reimbursed for personal expenses in connection with their duties, such as attending meetings and participating in special functions. Board members usually are appointed for terms of 6 years, with terms staggered to provide for changes in board membership yet still ensure desirable continuity.

The board is not generally composed of health specialists but ideally is made up of a cross-section of the population of the state and is representative of various interests, geographical areas, and backgrounds. The board's role is to reflect the viewpoints, interpretations, desires, and needs of the public. There could be no objection to having a physician on the board, but to have the membership dominated by health professionals would defeat the purpose for which the board is created.

Just as education policies are left to non-experts in education rather than to professional academicians, lay citizens with the viewpoint and judgment of the general public decide general health policies. Services of experts are provided to the board by the professional staff of the health department and other consultants as needed.

Powers of the Board of Health   The state board of health has such powers and functions as have been granted to it by the state or provincial constitution and the legislature. Seven acknowledged powers of any board of health include code making, quasi-judicial powers, administration, investigation, supervision and consultation, education, and coordination with other health agencies.

Making health codes is a quasi-legislative function. The professional health staff usually recommends rules and regulations for consideration by the Board. Once passed these rules and regulations are assembled into a sanitary code. This code has the effect of law. Courts have upheld the power of the board to enact binding rules and regulations, providing these rules and regulations do not go beyond the bounds of health matters or the U.S. Constitution or Bill of Rights. In Canada, provincial parliaments can pass emergency laws that go beyond the Charter of Rights as long as they are time limited.

The state board has authority to summon before it anyone alleged to have violated state or provincial health regulations. The board has the further recognized authority to summon witnesses. The board may hold hearings before granting or revoking a license. In all cases the citizen concerned has the right to appeal in court any adverse action of the board.

State or Provincial Director of Health   Administrative functions of the state or provincial board of health are delegated to the full-time staff of health specialists. In Australia, Canada, and many Asian, African, South American, and European countries, the chief provincial health officer is called the minister of health. In most states of the United States the chief administrator is called the health commissioner, although "health officer," "health director," "secretary of health," and other titles are used. In some states of the United States the board elects the commissioner; in others the governor appoints the commissioner. Nearly half the states require that the head of the SHA have an M.D. degree. In Canada, the Minister of Health is an elected member of the provincial parliament. As a politician, the Minister seldom is expected to have a health science degree or even to have a background in health. The Minister, therefore, usually appoints a Medical Officer of Health to oversee the public health functions of the Ministry.

Top leadership positions other than the Director or Medical Officer of Health tend to be filled by nonphysicians, although SHAs usually have physicians on staff or access to input from physicians with preparation and experience in public health. The Commissioner or Minister has certain recognized responsibilities:

- general administration;
- recommendation of health legislation, rules, and regulations for consideration by the board;
- appointment of personnel;
- preparation of the budget;
- supervision of divisions or bureaus;
- enforcement of health rules and regulations; and
- coordination of relationships with official agencies, organizations, and the public.

Organization

The structures of state or provincial health department or ministries vary (see figures 19-2 and 19-3). Just below the top administrative officer (health commissioner, officer, or minister of health) are the primary administrative units, usually called *divisions*. Divisions, in turn, are divided into *bureaus* or *sections*. There may be further subdivisions, but this would be necessary only in departments in heavily populated states or provinces. A populous state or provincial

health agency may have ten divisions, whereas a small one may have only half as many. Each division, bureau, or section has a director or chief. In most instances, the title of the division or bureau, as shown in figure 19-2, indicates the function or areas of health service. A state or province with highly dispersed populations over a vast geography might have regional branches or field offices.

The distribution of program effort can be illustrated by reviewing the functions of the units of a typical state or provincial health agency.

FUNCTIONS OF A STATE OR PROVINCIAL HEALTH AGENCY

To accomplish their usual mission of promoting and protecting health and preventing illness and injury, SHAs have three core functions outlined by the National Academy of Science's Committee on the Future of Public Health: assessment, policy, and assurance.

- First, public health agencies *assess* community health status and whether the community has adequate resources to address the problems identified. Surveillance of disease and injury rates, risk factors in the population, and risk conditions in the environment employ epidemiological methods to determine where action is needed to prevent, promote, or protect health.
- Second, they use the data gathered to develop health *policy,* and to recommend and organize programs to carry out those policies.
- Third, they must *assure* that the necessary, high quality, effective services are available. This function includes a responsibility for quality assurance through licensing and other certification and monitoring mechanisms.

The typical grouping of activities to carry out these functions tend to fall under the rubrics following. The first series of functions relate to the life cycle outlined in chapters 5-8 in Part 2 of this book.

Maternal and Child Health

After environmental control of communicable diseases, one of the first public health services in every country, state, and province is maternal and child health services. State and federal governments established these services jointly in the United States under Title V of the Social Security Act early in the twentieth century (see chapter 5). The Maternal and Child Health Services program identifies the health needs of women of childbearing age and children and addresses those needs through a broad range of programs with a diversity of services. Family health services include maternity clinics for prenatal and postpartum care, child health clinics, and diagnostic and evaluation centers for handicapped children. Speech and hearing programs train individuals in screening techniques; check audiometers for correct calibration; and maintain a statewide registry of all audiometers, all firms that calibrate audiometers, and all persons who use audiometers for screening or diagnostic purposes.

Other programs include family planning; nutrition education and consultation; the Supplemental Food Program for Women, Infants, and Children (WIC); projects for children and youth; intensive-care nursery projects for high-risk infants; and vision care programs. WIC funds from the U.S. Department of Agriculture make up the largest contribution to state health agency funds from federal agencies other than health, amounting to as much as 20 percent for some state health agencies.

Handicapped children's programs

If a handicapped child's parents are unable to afford adequate medical care, the Crippled Children's Services program (also under Title V in the U.S. Social Security Act) provides the necessary hospital care and specialized medical services to treat the malady. Handicapping conditions included are bone, joint, muscle, or nerve defects or deformities, congenital heart defects, and cystic fibrosis (figure 19-7).

······················
Figure 19-7

Cystic fibrosis is the most common serious genetic disorder in people of European descent. Patient and parents are counseled on the management of cystic fibrosis under programs supported by state and provincial governments. *Source:* Photo from Queen's University, Belfast, courtesy World Health Organization.

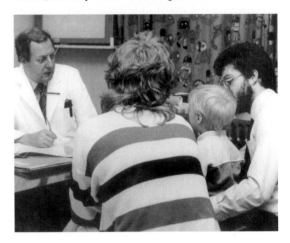

Emergency medical services

For the adolescent and young adult populations, provincial and state health functions offer as their main line of services the provisions for policy and assurance of emergency care for injury. These emergency medical services apply to heart attack victims in older ages and to childhood injuries. Legislation usually assigns responsibility to the SHA for many aspects of an emergency medical services system. Functions of the SHA include ambulance vehicle licensing and inspection, ambulance consultation, emergency medical communications, standards for 911 medical response (figure 19-8), ambulance attendant testing and certification, and ambulance personnel and vehicle-registry. These functions apply to routine and disaster situations. State **disaster plans** are sometimes coordinated under this functional unit (figure 19-9).

....
Figure 19-8

State and provincial health agencies set standards for and oversee the effective implementation of emergency response capabilities, including the medical aspects of 911 telephone services and ambulance response to such emergencies. *Source:* U.S. Fire Administration and National Highway Traffic Safety Administration.

LEARN TO USE THIS LIFE-SAVING DEVICE.
KNOW YOUR LOCAL EMERGENCY NUMBERS.

There's been a crash. Someone is hurt. Do you know how to call for help?

Keep emergency numbers by your phone for medical help, police and fire services. The right number gets help on the way *faster*.

For medical emergencies, contact

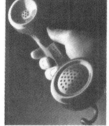

EMS, Emergency Medical Services. One call connects you to a whole emergency medical team—ambulance, paramedics, physicians and nurses—who are specially trained to help people who are hurt or sick.

Your phone can help save time, and lives, in an emergency. Know how to use it.

 United States Fire Administration

 the *right* EMS call EMERGENCY MEDICAL SERVICES ...*when seconds count.*

 National Highway Traffic Safety Administration

....
Figure 19-9

In states and provinces with remote populations, rescue by air may be the only way to safety or emergency treatment in disasters or medical crises. "Medivac" by helicopter for crash victims on clogged freeways also has become a standard emergency medical service in some states, provinces, and municipalities. *Source:* Pan American Health Organization, courtesy World Health Organization.

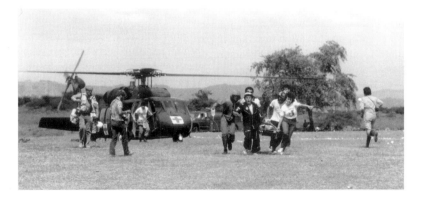

. . . .

Figure 19-10

Screening programs for chronic diseases and risk factors such as hypertension have been given increasing attention and support by state and provincial health departments. Some remain controversial as to their cost-effectiveness for younger adults. *Source:* Photo by J. Vizcarra, courtesy Pan American Health Organization, World Health Organization.

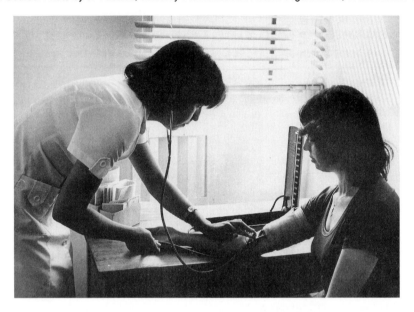

Chronic Diseases

State or provincial cancer and heart disease programs provide community screening services, consultation, and educational resources. For example, cancer information services and tumor registry programs augment community activities with centralized computer capabilities. Ongoing care of the cancer patient is encouraged through a systematic follow-up system. Morbidity and survival data are supplied for use in continuing education programs. Workshops are held to promote the development of community cancer programs and to coordinate follow-up for cancer patients.

Educational services are provided to teach individuals about the warning signs of cancer and the hazards of smoking. The SHA usually coordinates an interagency council on smoking and health.

The state or provincial chronic diseases division assists residents who have end-stage renal disease and require life-sustaining dialysis treatments or a kidney transplant. This is usually a state rather than local program because many communities cannot afford the high cost of kidney dialysis.

Chronic disease screening programs include services for cholesterol, hypertension, diabetes, and breast cancer screening and detection. The object of screening activities is early recognition and treatment. Individuals identified as possibly having an abnormal condition or suspicious sign, such as elevated blood pressure or cholesterol, are referred to the physician of their choice for medical evaluation and treatment (figure 19-10).

The Federal-Provincial Heart Health Program in Canada, the National High Blood Pressure and Cholesterol programs in the United States, and various tobacco control programs in both countries emphasize primary prevention and health promotion through public health education, taxation on tobacco products, and consultation to local health agencies.

Policies and laws such as controlled access of alcohol and tobacco to minors and smoke-free environments are passed ideally at the state or provincial level to minimize the unequal competition for customers between local jurisdictions. Unfortunately, the tobacco lobby is much stronger at the state or provincial level to block such legislation, so most laws and ordinances controlling tobacco product sales and smoking restrictions are passed at the local level. When enacted in state or provincial legislatures, they sometimes carry provisions that preclude more aggressive legislation at local levels.

Public Health Nursing

The state or province provides leadership to public health nurses through consultation, teaching, and demonstration. Emphasis is placed on providing a high quality of health care that accommodates a variety of cultural patterns and individual health needs. Public health nursing services are offered in community settings such as homes, schools, industrial plants, clinics, and public health centers. These services may include bedside care in the home, teaching health maintenance and prevention of illness, providing for early detection of illness, and obtaining appropriate medical care for citizens.

Provincial or state professional nursing staff help local public health nurses to keep their knowledge and practical skills current with scientific developments and progress in the medical and nursing fields. This assistance is partially accomplished through the development of continuing education courses and in-service education for nurses. Planning and helping to implement new and improved methods of delivering nursing care in collaboration with other members of the health care team is another function of the state. Nursing consultation is provided to public health regional offices, local health departments, public schools, schools of nursing, and other professional workers and interested individuals as requested.

Local Health Services

In-service training to local personnel maintains and updates such skills as budget preparation, general record keeping and maintenance of tuberculosis registers, birth and death records, and morbidity statistics. Financial aid also is given to help local departments provide the vital services required by their communities. Some small or sparsely populated counties even contract with the state for direct state provision of local health services, especially those that require more specialized skills or equipment.

Communicable Disease Services

The state or provincial agency coordinates disease control activities that cross local boundaries. It conducts the routine morbidity surveillance of specified reportable diseases occurring in the state. This function includes collecting and tabulating reported data and preparing graphic representation and written interpretation of communicable disease morbidity occurrence and trends. Educational support for the control of infectious diseases is given by developing and distributing booklets, pamphlets, technical literature, video and audio training materials and manuals, presenting on-the-job training programs to selected audiences, and providing consultation upon request. These surveillance and information services are especially helpful in facilitating interaction with and support of immunization programs and sexually transmitted disease (STD) control programs.

HIV/AIDS, hepatitis, and STD control programs typically include comprehensive medical, nursing, educational, epidemiological (interview contact and case follow-up), and laboratory services for public and private agencies offering medical services to HIV/AIDS and STD patients. The state or province supports these through morbidity reporting and epidemiological control systems to ensure location of contacts. The state or province also tries to assure access to and quality of HIV/AIDS and STD clinics or other treatment facilities. It conducts educational programs to communicate relevant health information to people at risk, with the dual objectives of preventing exposure to infection and motivating infected individuals to seek early medical care and to cooperate in locating contacts. The state or province also seeks to involve the private medical community in all aspects of HIV/AIDS, hepatitis, and STD control. With the HIV/AIDS epidemic and widespread problems of infected needle use by addicts, these programs dominate the state expenditures in communicable diseases, surpassing immunization in public health expenditures of states and provinces.

The provincial or state immunization service develops and implements programs designed to raise immunization levels in the entire population. The SHA maintains continuous surveillance over the proper application of daycare center and school immunization laws and provides vaccinations where no local mechanisms exist. Vaccines distributed free of charge by some SHAs to local health departments and district agencies help to maintain high immunization levels across the state. Many states and provinces operate an extensive direct-mail program in which parents of newborn children are reminded and encouraged to start immunizations soon after the child's birth and to complete them shortly after the first birthday.

Some provinces in Canada routinely provide for home visits to new mothers and infants. Parents return business reply cards when immunizations are started and completed. Those parents who do not respond may be contacted by a field staff member who discusses the importance of the preventive aspects of immunizations with parents by telephone or in their homes. The aides also receive referrals each month of nonimmunized preschool children identified through the U.S. Early Periodic Screening, Detection and Treatment program (EPSDT).

Tuberculosis Services

Early civilizations recorded tuberculosis as one of the oldest communicable diseases. Modern science has developed effective methods to prevent and treat tuberculosis. The decrease of past decades in tuberculosis cases has leveled off, indicating the emergence of antibiotic-resistant strains, immigration of refugee populations, and failure to complete short-course therapy. This highlights the need for state agencies to continue to monitor communicable diseases such as tuberculosis, at a time when many communities cannot justify maintaining a local staff dedicated to tuberculosis control. The U.S. Department of Health and Human Services has targeted tuberculosis for eradication; it falls to the SHA, then to:

- Find and successfully treat all infectious cases of tuberculosis;
- Prevent disease spread by early detection and treatment of tuberculosis infections; and
- Insure the completion of prescribed treatment, because failure to follow the regimen to completion results in many of the relapses and the development of antibiotic strains.

To reduce the prevalence of tuberculosis, SHAs seek to ensure that more patients who are detected complete the prescribed treatment. They cooperate with local authorities in assuring coordinated care and careful monitoring of ambulatory patients. Persons suspected of having tuberculosis and contacts of known cases are examined, and infected persons at high risk of developing tuberculosis are given preventive treatment. The state or province provides direct services in some communities; in other areas, they support local health agencies.

Epidemiology

We defined epidemiology in chapter 3 as the study of the distribution of disease and the determinants of disease frequency in human populations. It is no longer restricted to the study of epidemics or infectious diseases. It applies today as much to the chronic diseases. Public health is grounded in epidemiology, and in turn epidemiology is grounded in four disciplines: clinical medicine, pathology, demography, and biostatistics. It uses sociological and ecological perspectives to study populations. The SHA's professional staff

●●●●●●●●●●●●●●●●●●●●●
Figure 19-11

State and provincial laboratories provide for the more specialized testing that local agencies might not be able to afford, such as this extractor for chromosomal disorders, and for enforcement of standards applied in private laboratories. *Source:* Photo by P. Almasy, courtesy World Health Organization.

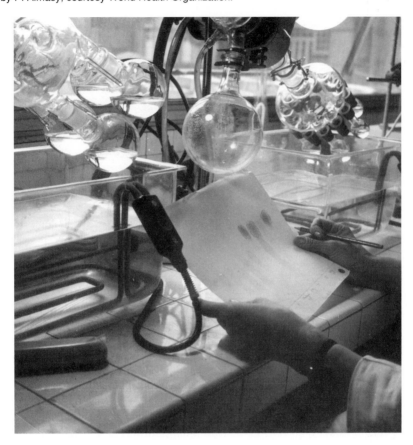

therefore must have competence in these several areas and in the art of applied epidemiological investigation.

Epidemiological methods are employed daily by the staffs of the SHA for planning and evaluation of particular programs. The SHA's epidemiology division is charged with carrying out epidemiological investigations of disease problems and stands available to assist in investigations conducted in the state or province by other public health units.

Laboratories

The division or bureau of laboratories provides an essential service of the SHA. It remains one of the least-known agencies to people outside the health professions. **Laboratory services** are provided for communicable disease control, chronic disease detection and control, environmental protection, dental health, genetic testing (figure 19-11), and many other public health activities. In addition, the laboratories serve as general diagnostic centers for private physicians, particularly for procedures that

••••••••••••••••••••
Figure 19-12

State and provincial health agencies have responsibility for hospital licensure and certification to ensure that high standards are maintained in medical facilities. *Source:* Photo by J. Vizcarra, Pan American Health Organization, courtesy World Health Organization.

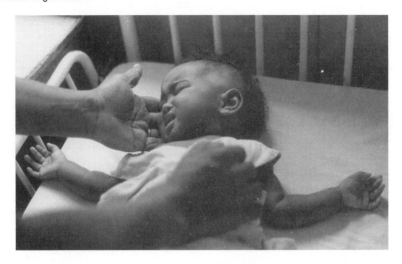

are beyond the scope or capabilities of private and local medical laboratories. Millions of samples and specimens are processed and tested in the state laboratories. As a result of these tests, hundreds of thousands of citizens are assured of prompt, accurate diagnosis and treatment by their private physician or local public health clinic.

Veterinary Public Health

The veterinary public health service conducts vector and zoonosis control programs responsible for the detection, investigation, and eradication of animal diseases that can be transmitted to human populations. Rabies, several types of encephalitis (sleeping sickness), ornithosis (a poultry disease), and psittacosis (parrot fever) are just a few examples of such diseases, many of which can be fatal to humans and to animals. The veterinary public health service also conducts the state meat and poultry inspection program to ensure the health of food animals and the safety and wholesomeness of fresh meats and poultry processed or sold in the

state or province, as described in chapter 15. Meat-processing establishments, rendering plants, animal-food manufacturing plants, kennels, and zoos are inspected periodically and sometimes without warning to the proprietors.

Hospital Licensure and Certification

To achieve and to maintain high standards in the quality of medical facilities (figure 19-12), states and provincial agencies survey and certify hospitals, home health agencies, independent laboratories, rehabilitation facilities, end-stage renal disease facilities, and physical therapists in independent practice. They also inspect and certify suppliers of x-ray and other equipment or services to participants in the provincial health care program or the federal Medicare or Medicaid programs. The hospital licensure and certification division usually has an intra-agency agreement with the long-term care division to survey skilled nursing facilities that participate in the Medicare program.

States and provinces also set and enforce standards for safety and sanitation in licensed general hospitals; state medical hospitals; state and private mental hospitals; and state schools for the retarded, deaf, and blind.

The state is also responsible for conducting appropriate United States Public Health Service proficiency examinations for selected health care personnel. The proficiency examinations provide an additional way for health care personnel to be considered qualified for Medicare purposes. States conduct proficiency examinations for clinical laboratory technicians, cytotechnologists, vocational nurses who have received licenses by waiver, and physical therapists in independent practice. These exams measure skills of selected health personnel against required standards.

Managed Care Organizations

Managed care is represented in the United States by a variety of new health insurance and prepaid health care arrangements and the older health maintenance organizations (HMOs). They are designed to offer the public an alternative to the traditional fee-for-service system. They differ from health insurance companies in that services are provided through contracts with specific providers of medical service, such as a group of doctors, a hospital, and an affiliated pharmacy. HMOs and other managed care organizations offer a broad range of health services, from routine physical exams to the most sophisticated surgical procedures. (See chapter 21 for a more complete description of managed care.) Variations on traditional medical practice such as preferred provider organizations (PPOs) and designated provider organizations (DPOs) have emerged. States regulate and certify managed care organizations. They evaluate the quality of care being provided by these groups and make recommendations for or against certification to a state board of insurance and to the federal government.

Ethics and Medical Disclosure Panels

The health ethics or medical disclosure panel in most states is composed of physicians, lawyers, social scientists, and ethicists. The panel, often selected and staffed by the state department of health, determines what risks and hazards are involved in medical care, surgical procedures, and research projects. They judge the adequacy of procedures proposed by health care providers to disclose these risks to their patients. Informed consent procedures required by various federal laws have placed greater medical decision-making power in the hands of patients and families and consumers of health insurance and other health products.

Vital Statistics

States and provinces record some of the most significant events in the lives of citizens. These include marriage, birth of a child, and death. Maintaining such records was one of the earliest duties assigned to state and provincial health departments. Processing records of births, marriages, divorces, and deaths requires the services of skilled statisticians. Laws require physicians to notify their local health officials of any cases of selected communicable diseases diagnosed in their practice. Local health officials, in turn, forward records that the province or state compiles in statistical tables to analyze patterns of occurrence and to detect outbreaks that can be contained before they become epidemics. Statistical analyses are essential in many kinds of governmental planning. For example, knowing where people are choosing to live will help determine where health facilities need to be located; knowing what diseases and injuries are occurring most often, and where, helps to plan control programs. Dozens of similar analyses enable the state government to serve its communities more effectively.

Long-Term Care

The state provides for facility licensing, Medicare and Medicaid certification actions, quality-of-care assurance and consultation, classifications of patient care, periodic medical reviews, and utilization reviews. The quality of care provided to the sick elderly and the physical plant safety of long-term

· ·
Figure 19-13

State and provincial agencies oversee the regulation of long-term care and the quality of services of home health care providers. With growing proportions of populations in the age groups requiring these services, this function of state health agencies (SHAs) may be expected to grow and to be increasingly watched by the mature children of the aging parents. *Source:* Copyrighted photo by Kim Griffiths, Edmonton, courtesy Alberta Heritage Foundation for Medical Research.

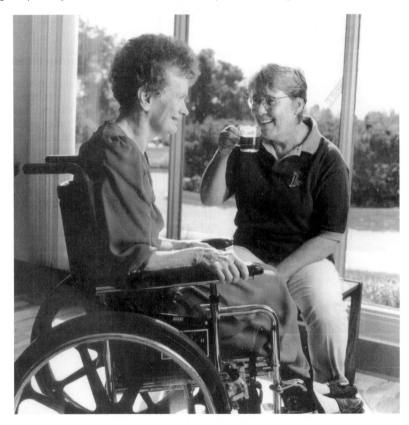

care facilities are regulated by the state. Reviews of records and on-site visits compare a facility against established standards (figure 19-13).

State and Provincial Health Planning

The SHA is usually the state agency designated by the governor as the state health planning and resource development agency in compliance with the U.S. National Health Planning and Resources Development Act of 1974. This makes the department responsible for performing all health planning and resource development functions on the state level and for developing an annual state health plan and state medical facilities plan. This function will be further described later in this chapter.

In Canada, the Medical Officer of Health for most provinces has the health planning responsibility, setting long-range health goals and targets, assessing progress toward these, and reducing inequities between population groups.

• •
Figure 19-14

State or provincial health agencies carry out food processing inspections because most manufacturers ship their products beyond the community. Milk is given particular attention because of the several points at which it could be contaminated from the dairy to processing, to bottle or packaging, to storage, to market or restaurant, to consumer. *Source:* Photo by J. Vizcarra, Pan American Health Organization, courtesy World Health Organization.

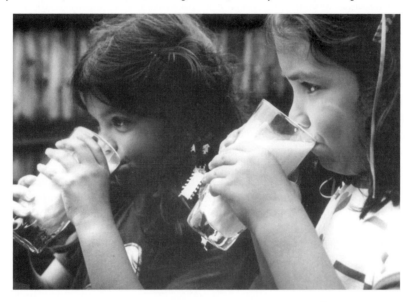

Consumer Health Protection

Most SHA product safety programs protect the public through inspection of manufacturing and distribution facilities where hazardous substances are made or handled. They also establish appropriate regulations, identify potentially hazardous products, and enforce proper labeling, and, in some cases, the banning of products that are unnecessarily or extremely hazardous to the public. The product safety programs have directed their attention particularly toward the flammability of fabrics (especially children's clothing), aerosol sprays, cleaners, polishers, lead-based paint, and other common household products.

The province or state enforces laws that deal with the regulation of milk and milk products (figure 19-14). State personnel, in cooperation with local health department regulatory officials, rou-

tinely inspect all dairies, milk and dairy product processors, milk storage and transportation facilities, single-service container manufacturers, and retail outlets where milk or milk products are sold. The National Conference on Interstate Milk Shipments, by reciprocal agreements between states, provides assurance that all Grade "A" milk and milk products transferred between states are produced and processed in conformance with regulatory standards set forth in the U.S. Public Health Service Grade "A" Pasteurized Milk ordinance.

It is the statutory responsibility of states to administer and enforce those laws designed to assure the consumer of safe foods, drugs, and cosmetics. Surveillance and compliance inspections are made of the operations and premises of all food, drug, and cosmetic manufacturers, wholesalers, repackers, distributors, and retailers. Raw materials and finished products are sampled for laboratory analysis to ensure compliance with acceptable standards.

Natural disasters impose a special responsibility on states or provinces for the consumer health protection program. State personnel stand ready to move into disaster areas to determine whether disaster-exposed food and drugs should be used or discarded.

Provincial and state health agencies also have shellfish sanitation control programs. These enforce state laws to ensure the wholesomeness and safety of shellfish harvested and processed in coastal jurisdictions or sold in other areas. Program staff perform sanitary surveys, collect samples, and evaluate the water quality in shellfish harvesting areas along the coast; inspect harvesting boats and docking areas; inspect, certify, and license processing plants; and prepare maps indicating safe harvesting areas for shellfish. Most inland provinces and states do not have such a specialized program, but those in coastal areas have a responsibility for the control of salmonellosis outbreaks in their own populations and in their export markets.

Environmental Health

Water quality and the safety of toxic waste dumps are among the environmental health concerns of SHAs. For water, this includes the surveillance of the construction, operation, and maintenance of public drinking water supply systems because they usually serve more than one local jurisdiction. SHAs also monitor toxic waste dumps. The state operates a certification program that assists in developing and coordinating training courses for water supply and wastewater system operators. The SHA reviews plans for new public water systems and for major improvements to existing systems to certify that they meet current standards. Likewise, the SHA reviews chemical and bacteriological records of water systems to ensure compliance with standards.

The state or province maintains chemical and bacteriological records of water samples collected periodically from its public water systems. They make recommendations for improvements to the water system officials responsible. The state or province initiates enforcement action when necessary and provides technical information and assistance to municipal officials and water system owners and operators. States and provinces also maintain air quality standards through inspection and control of emissions from factories and automobiles.

Administrative Services

The management functions of the SHA programs include the official fiscal and budgetary functions and controls and data processing, general plant supervision, and sometimes public health education. Funds received and expended by the department are recorded and accounting reports prepared. Budget reports are also prepared on warehousing, shipping and receiving, property management, maintenance of buildings and grounds, utilities, equipment maintenance, the central library facilities, the department's payroll, and on-premises food services for department employees.

The SHA's data processing services usually operate twenty-four hours a day (figure 19-15). Thousands of computer runs made each month draw on and feed into a library of hundreds of computer tapes. If it were not for the data-processing capabilities of the state health department, many of the programs would be impossible to administer, and countless other programs would be far less effective than they are. To cite an earlier example, the immunization program uses birth certificates, recorded by the vital statistics bureau, as the source of names and addresses of families with newborn children. The SHA computer then automatically prints form letters to the infants' parents to remind them at each of the stages of development (2 months, 4 months, 6 months, etc., as shown in figure 5-10) to have their babies immunized. Copies of the names and addresses go to local health departments for follow-up (figure 19-16). Most of this would not be feasible without computers.

Besides accounting for funds received and spent, the SHA must plan for future needs and translate those needs into specific budget figures.

••••••••••••••••••••

Figure 19-15

Computers have made possible the storage; rapid retrieval; transfer between state and local officials; and analysis of millions of records, including birth, marriage, and death certificates, communicable disease reports, chronic disease registries, behavioral risk survey questionnaires, and financial reports. *Source:* Photo by T. Farcus, courtesy World Health Organization.

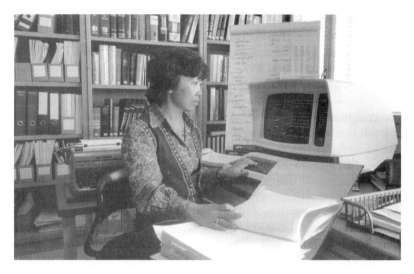

••••••••••••••••••••

Figure 19-16

State and provincial health agencies help keep child immunizations by local health agencies on schedule by sending computer-generated letters at each of the points after birth when the selected immunization should occur (see figure 5-10). This example of state-local collaboration is made possible by computer facilities in state and provincial agencies. *Source:* Photo by James Martin, courtesy Missouri Department of Health.

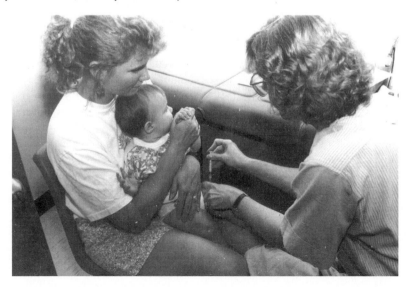

Each departmental or ministry budget is submitted to the state legislature or to the provincial Parliament annually or biennially.

Public Health Education

SHA programs rely heavily on education to help accomplish their purpose in preventing disease and injury. The public health education division employs professional writers, editors, artists, health educators, social scientists, and other personnel to assist the other divisions in carrying out their responsibilities. With the growing emphasis on lifestyle causes of chronic diseases and injury and on other determinants of health that require an informed electorate to support changes in policies, some of these units have been renamed health promotion divisions.

Most SHAs also publish dozens of new pamphlets, brochures, booklets, posters, and other pieces of literature each year. They distribute weekly press releases, newspaper columns, and five-minute radio programs or thirty-second radio or TV spots as public service announcements for radio and television. They also maintain a web site and some operate telephone information or hotlines.

Most SHAs maintain a video and film library to supply tapes and prints to schools, clubs, and individuals, usually on a free-loan basis. Some agencies have their own printing plant to produce the millions of pieces of literature, including essential records and reporting forms, used by local health departments and private physicians.

The public health education unit also provides staff training for public health personnel at the state and local levels. Major courses or conferences are conducted each year and are supplemented by occasional one-day training sessions and on-site consultations.

FINANCES OF STATE AND PROVINCIAL HEALTH AGENCIES

Provinces and states spend an average of 20 percent of their budgets on health-related programs (figure 19-17). The overall state costs for health continued to increase in 1997, the largest component of which was the medically-oriented Medicaid costs. The cost-controls on medical spending and the introduction of managed care for Medicaid populations resulted in the first year of leveling off of expenditures in 1997. The Medicaid expenditures, primarily for the poor and disabled, now account for some 11 percent of state spending; twenty-five years ago it was only 3 percent.

With decreased contributions from the federal government, states and provinces are often faced with doing less rather than picking up a larger share of health costs. States pay an average of 45 percent of health costs; the federal government 30 percent; and the remaining costs are supported by local government, fees, reimbursements, and other sources. At 30 percent the federal government picks up a larger percentage of state health costs than the average of 17 percent the federal government contributes to state and local budgets. This is largely because of Medicaid entitlement programs for which the federal government passed the laws that oblige shared financing.

In Canada, federal cost sharing with provinces for medical care is justified partly on the grounds that the federal government has much greater taxation powers than the provinces, and partly on the basis of a national commitment to achieve greater equity among provinces.

Most federal funds reside in **block grants** in the United States, or tax revenue transfers in Canada, giving the state or province considerable discretion in allocating the fund to programs according to its priorities.

Block grants from U.S. Department of Health and Human Services sources for state-administered public health programs cover specific areas mandated by laws passed before the grouped categorical grants were converted to block grants. These include, in order of magnitude:

- the maternal and child health portion of Title V of the Social Security Act;
- the crippled children's portion of Title V;
- comprehensive public health services block grants;

····················
Figure 19-17

California state expenditures in a recent year shows nearly 30 percent of the total going to health and welfare and nearly the same amount to primary and secondary education. *Source: State and local government finance in California: a primer. 1996. Sacramento: The California Budget Project.*

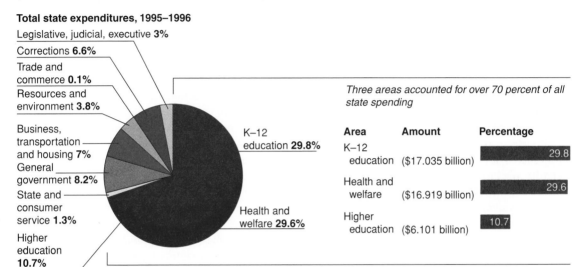

Total state expenditures, 1995–1996

Legislative, judicial, executive **3%**

Corrections **6.6%**

Trade and commerce **0.1%**

Resources and environment **3.8%**

Business, transportation and housing **7%**

General government **8.2%**

State and consumer service **1.3%**

Higher education **10.7%**

K–12 education **29.8%**

Health and welfare **29.6%**

Three areas accounted for over 70 percent of all state spending

Area	Amount	Percentage	
K–12 education	($17.035 billion)		29.8
Health and welfare	($16.919 billion)		29.6
Higher education	($6.101 billion)		10.7

- family-planning grants under Title X of the Public Health Service Act; and
- AIDS education funds from the Centers for Disease Control.

The largest single federal funding source is the Supplemental Food Program for Women, Infants and Children (WIC), administered by the U.S. Department of Agriculture.

APPRAISAL OF OFFICIAL STATE AND PROVINCIAL HEALTH SERVICES

Activities of the typical North American SHA have been presented here to provide a sense of the different state or provincial health services and programs. The functions should provide a more complete picture of the areas of responsibility and emphasis in U.S. state health departments than do the organizational charts in figures 19-2 and 19-3. Organizational charts can be deceptive because the boxes are approximately the same size, giving the

illusion that the programs and services are of similar scope. The examination of budgets or expenditure figures for each program or service can help to provide additional insight into their relative magnitude and scope.

As a support service to many programs, health education funds should be set aside within the program budgets. This often is not the case, however, even though the programs require health education services. Hence certain basic functions such as health education sometimes end up with no budget, and their expenditures, if any, are from left-over funds.

As provincial and state health services have expanded and technology has advanced, the health of the public has improved, diseases have been prevented, and deaths have been postponed. A full appraisal of the value and significance of the official state and provincial health services would have to consider that many of the health services and programs do not deal with life-and-death matters but contribute to the quality of life.

For provincial and state health services, four cardinal needs exist. The first is the need for sufficient funds to do adequately what should be done in health promotion. A second need is to obtain better data relevant to the chronic diseases, many of which are related to lifestyle. A third need is to integrate or at least coordinate the health functions of state agencies that provide health services in some form. The state or provincial health, agriculture, education, labor, automobile and drivers' licensing agencies, traffic safety and mass transit or transportation agencies, and other agencies that have health functions must work closely together to allocate responsibility for overlapping health programs. They in turn must provide the fourth need by working closely with nongovernmental and nonhealth organizations, recognizing that many of these also receive federal health grants to complement official state and local health agency programs.

The British North American Act of 1867 and the Constitution of Canada place the mandate for health with the provinces. The federal government collects from provincial citizens' personal income taxes and General Service Taxes (GST) on purchases. Then, through equalization payments favoring the poorer provinces and through transfer payments, the federal government redistributes that income to the provinces. Transfer payments provide for specific health services and hospital insurance. The provinces fund a comprehensive range of health services from their federal share and from their other sources of revenue such as sales taxes and corporate taxes. In disease prevention and health promotion the provinces build on federal policy and leadership, but each follows its own strategy, methods, and funding priorities. Examples from a few of the provinces will illustrate.

Health Education and Health Promotion

The Canadian initiatives in health promotion tend to subscribe more than the U.S. Healthy People initiatives to the definitions of health and health promotion promulgated by the World Health Organization. Indeed, much of the WHO approach to

health promotion owes its origins to Canadian initiatives and to the Ottawa Charter for Health Promotion from the First International Conference on Health Promotion held in Canada with WHO cosponsorship. The three functions most health promotion programs in the Canadian provinces seek to serve are to increase public awareness; to improve the capacity of individuals, families, and communities to address health issues through self-care and mutual aid; and to create social and physical environments that support health.

California and Massachusetts have had the most aggressive antitobacco campaigns in North America, dedicating earmarked taxes on tobacco products to the programs. New Brunswick has an animated cartoon program broadcast on television to raise awareness of risk factors and their role in cardiovascular diseases. This is one of several Canadian federal-provincial initiatives in heart health, but the only one among the provinces that emphasizes a broad mass media approach to heart health. Neighboring Prince Edward Island has developed school health curriculum modules to help children understand the hazards of smoking. British Columbia has a school-based program for alcohol and drug abuse prevention, based on the PRECEDE model (see chapter 4), that places a prevention worker in each school to assist teachers and the community to coordinate their efforts. Many of the U.S. states and some Canadian provinces, notably Ontario, have supported local health agencies in applying the Planned Approach To Community Health (PATCH) strategy for planning health promotion and disease prevention programs. These specific examples show how states and provinces have played a role between federal and local efforts in health education and health promotion.

Strengthening Capacity Newfoundland's HIV/AIDS prevention program combines mass media advertisements for public awareness with a specific media advocacy strategy to promote public support for preventive efforts and to mobilize key government decision makers. It also supports educational programs to provide training for youth in decision making and other social skills that would enable them to resist peer pressures. Needle-exchange programs in some twenty-five cities across Canada are sponsored by provincial or municipal governments, compared with only a dozen or so cities with needle-exchange programs in the United States. The development of seniors' wellness councils in Nova Scotia is another example of strengthening community capacity, in this case to address the neglected needs of the growing population of elderly people. In the Northwest Territories more than fifty health representatives have been trained to work with the far north communities with their aboriginal populations spread over several thousand square miles and with their ten official languages. The Healthy Schools programs of some states and provinces seek to actively engage school children in identifying their own health issues, to reach consensus, and to take collective action to deal with those issues. Similar programs for Healthy Workplaces and Healthy Communities work with employees and community residents.

Supportive Environments

Beyond the actions individuals and organizations can be supported to take, policies must be developed at the state or provincial level and through municipal and district levels to create healthful living conditions and to make healthful personal choices the easier choices for individuals. In Manitoba, for example, a coalition of churches, food banks, and antipoverty groups work with the provincial and local governments to address problems of food security and accessibility. Alberta's injury prevention initiative uses a similar coalition approach to affect policies and to support programs for safer environments. New tobacco legislation in British Columbia, Manitoba, and Ontario has sought to tighten the accessibility of tobacco to minors and to add to the tobacco tax on cigarettes. The Healthy Community movement ("Villes et Villages" in Quebec), based on the WHO Healthy Cities model, seeks to engage community residents, policymakers, and leaders from various sectors in collaborative efforts to change health-related policies. They also seek to improve living conditions and to advocate for and with the most vulnerable populations in their communities.

Canada has not developed national and provincial objectives for disease prevention and health promotion as thoroughly as the United States. However, a few Canadian provinces have been more aggressive than most American states in going beyond risk-factor objectives to set broader goals relating to the social determinants of health and mandatory standards. The Ontario Provincial Health Act (see box) and the British Columbia *New Directions* policy the *New Challenges* goals are exemplary. The British Columbia initiative includes a major emphasis on decentralizing the provincial roles to give greater decision-making authority to community health councils and regional health boards. The theme of British Columbia's provincial initiative is "bringing health closer to home."

The Comprehensive Health Planning Act of 1966 and the Partnership for Health Amendments of 1967 were enacted in the United States to establish comprehensive planning for health services, the health workforce, and health facilities essential at every level of government. It sought also to strengthen the leadership and capabilities of the SHAs and to broaden and make more feasible and relevant federal support of state and community health services. This legislation was superseded by the National Health Planning and Resources Development Act of 1974.

The U.S. federal budgets during the 1980s eliminated the support for state health planning. The state and area health planning agencies already had been weakened, and most have now been closed, by federal repeal of the Act. It is unlikely that Congress will restore funds to rebuild the planning agencies. Thus the state and local health departments once again must turn to their own devices to bring some order into the chaos of the burgeoning American medical and hospital "nonsystem" of care, which emphasizes high technology treatment for the insured rather than primary health care, prevention, and health promotion for all.

The Ontario Provincial Health Act

After several years of preparation and following wide consultation, the Health Protection and Promotion Act was proclaimed in 1984 to the Ontario Legislature. The Honourable Keith Norton, Minister of Health, spoke of how the new act represented a great stride forward for public health, calling it "the most progressive public health legislation in North America."

The focus of the act is "on the promotion of healthy lifestyles and the prevention of illness." Replacing the Public Health Act, enacted more than one-hundred years ago, the new act was designed to prepare boards of health to exercise leadership in the era of disease prevention and health promotion. At the heart of the act is the establishment of minimum program re-

quirements, or **mandatory programs,** which all local or district boards of health must ensure are available in health units.

Programs currently offered by boards of health did not change radically as a result of the new act, but they were subject to the mandatory programs requirements. For example, the preventive dentistry mandatory program must provide preventive dental services to the community and provide dental health education, oral hygiene instruction, and fluoride rinse programs to school children.

Mandatory programs are provided in the following areas: community sanitation, communicable disease control, preventive dentistry, family health, home care ser-

vices, nutrition, and public health education. Finally, public health education will be a component of all of the preceding programs. Boards of health may add other services and programs to supplement those that are mandatory.

In addition to mandatory programs, the Health Protection and Promotion Act broke new ground in several other areas of public health. For example, it formally recognizes the role boards of health play in occupational and environmental health matters. To this end, the act created the legislative ground for the close working relationship that must exist between the Ministries of Health, Environment, and Labour. The Act was renewed with minor revisions in 1997.

An Example of State and Provincial Planning Processes

The Epidemiological Assessment Recognizing that each state's problems, needs, and circumstances differ from those of other states, the state health planning process allows for the systematic assessment of those needs and circumstances within the state. This leads to an identification of the leading causes of death, illness, injury, and disability. Most states set their priorities for health action on the basis of mortality rankings rather than morbidity, injury, or disability rates. This leads to a typical set of priorities that places heart disease and cancer high on the ratings of importance. Comparing their statistics with other states, some states also conclude that they can do much better in controlling infant mortality or congenital anomalies, even though these do not show up among the leading causes of death. Through this process of statistical analysis and comparison, different states arrive at different priorities (figure 19-18).

Behavioral Risk-Factor Surveys For those health priorities for which behavioral or lifestyle risk factors determine most of the premature deaths, a second level of state planning draws upon the available data on the distribution of these risk factors in the population. Most states conduct behavioral risk-factor surveys periodically to track trends in the most important behavioral risk factors. Tabulations of those risk-factor surveys by CDC allow a state like West Virginia, for example, to note that its rate of smokeless tobacco use at 8.2 percent is number one among the states. Such data enable a state to shift its priorities for purposes of primary prevention or health promotion. Depending only on mortality data would mean that the actions a state can take on chronic disease control comes twenty years too late to take preventive action. Using trends and comparisons in risk-factor data allows West Virginia to take some action on smokeless tobacco even though its mortality rates for cancer are not exceptionally high.

····················

Figure 19-18

The assessment of vital statistics for a state or province will result in different priorities in the health plans of different states and provinces. *Source:* Office of Disease Prevention and Health Promotion, U.S. Department of Health and Human Services.

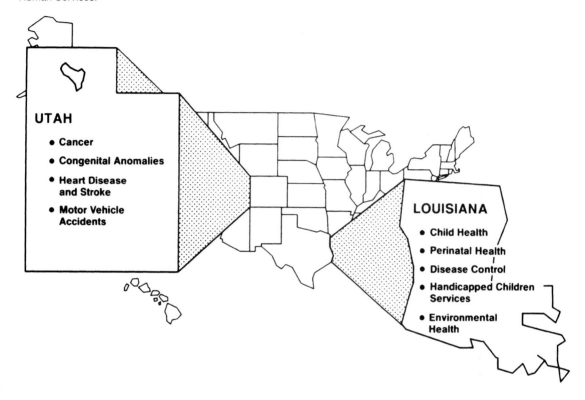

Setting Goals and Targets   A third phase of state or provincial planning for health is the establishment of quantitative objectives that reflect the potential for change in the mortality rates and the risk-factor prevalence rates. Such objectives can be stated for the province or state as a whole and for specific subpopulations such as males and females, urban and rural, teenagers and adults, whites and others. The form of the objectives, as outlined in chapter 4, is "how much (usually a percent reduction) of what (usually a mortality rate or a risk factor) will be achieved by when (year) in which population." West Virginia, for example, might set its objective for smokeless

tobacco control as follows: "To reduce the use of smokeless tobacco to 2 percent by 2005 among 15- to 19-year-old males." Setting such objectives presents an opportunity to engage a wide range of professionals, experts, interest groups, and sectors other than health. Here is where the process of consensus building can be most valuable. Obtaining agreement on objectives gives concerned parties a shared direction and commitment. Coordination of subsequent implementation plans then becomes much easier. Once objectives have been stated in quantified terms and with definite target dates, the allocation of resources can be made strategically.

SUMMARY

The provinces and states provide a wide variety of health-related programs and services that touch all aspects of daily life from the sanitation of the milk poured on cereals in the morning to the quality of air inhaled during the day. State and provincial agencies record the births and deaths scanned by citizens in their daily newspaper. That information lays the basis for health services. Protection against rabid animals (figure 19-19), surveillance of quality health care, and inspection of food are distant and "silent" services that get little public attention until problems arise. When the flood of 1993 disabled the water supply to whole cities in Iowa or the contaminated bottled fruit juices caused the deaths of children in California, Washington, and British Columbia in 1997, the quiet daily services of state and provincial agencies moved to the headlines. Public health services are vital to protect and promote health and to prevent disease and injury.

The provinces and states play a pivotal role in achievement of the national and provincial health objectives and implementing national health policies. Strategies for achieving such objectives can be implemented more readily at the state or provincial level than at the national level for several reasons. First, the breadth of authority in health matters is greater at the state or provincial level than at the national level. The opportunity through personal acquaintance or contact for cooperation between various sectors, such as education and health, is also greater at the state or provincial level. Furthermore, states have wider latitude in their use of federal funds under the block grants, as provinces have with federal transfers in health services. For all these reasons, state or provincial action is required for the integration of services and the cooperation of sectors necessary for effective implementation of disease prevention and health promotion programs that address the new complexities of lifestyle and the environment.

At the turn of the century state and provincial governments across North America are cutting back on basic services, due in part to reduced

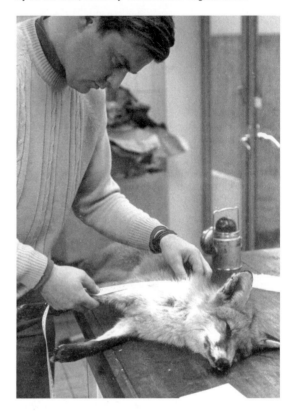

Figure 19-19

State and provincial health department veterinarians conduct examinations of foxes and other wildlife suspected of rabies, thereby protecting the domestic animals and human populations of the state or province. *Source:* Photo by E. Schwab, courtesy World Health Organization.

federal support and deficit economies. They find themselves in a position of cutting services that affect health—such as education and public safety—at the same time that costs are rising for health insurance and publicly supported medical services. The typical functions of most state and provincial health departments, the progressive initiatives of some, and the demise of the comprehensive health planning experiment, point ultimately to the community as the final arbiter of health needs and objectives appropriate to a population—the subject of the next chapter.

WEB*Links*

State Health Departments in the United States
Alabama—**http://www.alapubhealth.org**
Alaska—**http://health.hss.state.ak.us/dph/dph_home.htm**
Arizona—**http://www.hs.state.az.us/**
California—**http://www.dhs.cahwnet.gov/**
Colorado—**http://www.state.co.us/gov_dir/cdphe_dir/cdphehom.html**
Connecticut—**http://www.ctstateu.cdu/~dph/**
Florida—**http://www.state.fl.us/hrs_hsi/**
Georgia—**http://www.ph.dhr.state.ga.us/**
Hawaii—**http://www.hawaii.gov/health/index.html**
Idaho—**http://www.state.id.us/dhw**
Illinois—**http://www.idph.state.il.us**
Iowa—**http://www.idph.state.ia.us**
Kansas—**http://www.ink.org/public/kdhe/**
Louisiana—**http://www.state.la.us/index.htm**
Maine—**http://www.me.us/dhs/boh/boh001.htm**
Maryland—**http://www.charm,net/~epi9/**
Massachusetts—**http://www.magnet.state.ma.us\dph\dphorg2.htm**
Michigan—**http://www.mdmh.state.mi.us/**
Minnesota—**http://www.health.state.mn.us/**
Mississippi—**http://www.msdh.state.ms.us/**
Missouri—**http://www.health.state.mo.us/**
Montana—**http://www.mt.gov/**
North Carolina—**http://www.ehnr.state.nc.us/EHNR/**
New Jersey—**http://www.state.nj.us/**
New York—**http://www.health.state.ny.us/**
North Dakota—**http://www.chs.health.state.nd.us/ndhd/**
Ohio—**http://www.odn.ohio.gov/ohio/health/index.htmlx**
Oklahoma—**http://www.health.state.ok.us/**
Oregon—**gopher://gopher.state.or.us:70/11/.d148.dir**
Pennsylvania—**http://www.state.pa.us/PA_Exec/Health**
Rhode Island—**http://www.sec.state.ri.us/STDEPT/sd29.htm**
South Carolina—**http://www.state.sc.us/dhec/**
South Dakota—**http://www.state.sd.us/state/executive/doh/doh.html**
Tennessee—**http://www.state.tn.us/health/**
Texas—**http://www.tdh.state.tx.us/**
Utah—**http://hlunix.hl.state.ut.us/**
Virginia—**http://www.vdh.state.va.us/**
Washington—**http://www.doh.wa.gov/**
Wisconsin—**http://www.dhfs.state.wi.us/**
Wyoming—**http://wdhfs.state.w.us/health/home.htm**

Canadian Provincial and Territorial Ministries of Health and related sites
Prince Edward Island—**http://www.gov.pe.ca/hss/index.html**
Newfoundland—**http://www.gov.nf.ca/**
New Brunswick—**http://www.gov.nb.ca/hcs/**
Quebec—**http://www.msss.gouv.qc.ca/**
Ontario—**http://www.gov.on.ca/health/index.html**
Manitoba—**http://www.gov.mb.ca/health/index.html**
Alberta—**http://www.health.gov.ab.ca/**
University of Alberta directory of Canadian sites—**http://bugs.uah.ualberta.ca/welcome.htm**
British Columbia—**http://www.gov.bc.ca/**
University of British Columbia links—**http://www.ihpr.ubc.ca**

QUESTIONS FOR REVIEW

1. To what extent is the SHA or provincial ministry of health the "intermediary" health organization?
2. Is the state or provincial authority over the health of the people in your country too great or not great enough? Why?
3. What check does the public have to prevent health authorities from being too powerful and arrogant?
4. Why should residents always have the right to appeal to a court when they believe that they have been unjustly dealt with by health officials?
5. What health functions does your state or provincial department of agriculture engage in?
6. How do you explain that local health departments were formed long before state health departments were established?
7. How does your state or provincial decision-making body relate to local decision-makers on health matters?
8. Should the state or provincial board of health be composed entirely of physicians?
9. Who is your health commissioner or minister of health, what has been his or her professional preparation and experience, and for how many years has he or she been in the position?
10. When was the last time you or any member of your family received direct service from personnel of your state or provincial health department?
11. What are some health problems in your area on which the state or provincial health department should be conducting research?
12. What service now required of or otherwise carried on by your state or provincial health department should not be a part of the department's activities?

13. What consolidations of official health services have taken place in your state or province in the last ten years?
14. How has health planning affected the health of the people in your community?
15. Why did the U.S. Congress enact laws to regulate health planning in states and regions?

READINGS

Bodenhorn, K. A., and L. D. Kemper. 1997. *Spending for health: Californians speak out about priorities for health spending.* Sacramento: California Center for Health Improvement.

As part of the California Wellness Foundation's series on surveys of opinions of Californians on key policy issues and programs or services affecting their health, this report examines the fiscal issues of perceived costs and benefits of public and private spending for health. Web site is http://www.webcom.com/ cchi/

Funnell, R., K. Oldenfield, and V. Speller. 1995. *Toward healthier alliances: a tool for planning, evaluating and developing healthy alliances.* London: Health Education Authority.

This manual outlines practical steps and indicators for the building and maintenance of coalitions for health planning at the regional level.

Healthy Iowans 2000 Midcourse Revisions. 1996. Des Moines: Iowa Department of Public Health.

The state of Iowa organized its objectives in disease prevention and health promotion around the same 22 priority areas as Healthy People 2000 and included 132 goals and 338 action steps. This report found at mid-decade that most of the action steps scheduled to be implemented by 1995 had been partially or fully completed. It also reports on revisions in the original goals to accelerate and document the state's progress.

Healthy Rhode Islanders 2000 Mid-Course Review. 1996. Providence: Rhode Island Department of Health.

With its state motto of "Hope" this state of nearly 1 million people had 25 objectives for the year 2000 in health promotion and disease prevention, seven of which had seen substantial improvement by 1995, eight had seen some improvement, three had no improvement, whereas objectives in substance abuse prevention and nutrition moved in a negative direction.

Stoto, M. A., L. W. Green, and L. A. Bailey, eds. 1997. *Linking research and public health practice: a review of CDC's program of Centers for Research and*

Demonstration of Health Promotion and Disease Prevention. Washington, DC: National Academy Press.

This report of a committee of the Institute of Medicine, National Academy of Sciences, emphasizes the relationships needed between schools of public health and state health agencies if the benefits of research centers are to be fully realized in the regions in which these centers are located.

BIBLIOGRAPHY

Ackman, D. M., D. M. Ackman, and M. Flynn. 1996. Assessment of surveillance for meningoccal disease in New York State. *Am J Epid* 144:78.

Adlaf, E. M., F. J. Ivis, and G. W. Walsh. 1996. Enduring resurgence or statistical blip? recent trends from the Ontario Student Drug Use Survey. *Can J Public Health* 87:189.

Alabama Department of Public Health. 1991. *Healthy Alabama 2000: health promotion and disease prevention objectives for the year 2000.* Montgomery, AL: The Department.

American Public Health Association. 1992. *America's public health report card: a state-by-state report on the health of the public.* Washington, DC: The Association.

Boscarino, J. A., and R. J. Diclemente. 1996. AIDS knowledge, teaching comfort, and support for AIDS education among school teachers: a statewide survey. *AIDS Educ & Prev* 8:267.

Butler, J. T. 1995. The Delaware School Health Advisory Committee. *J School Health* 65:60.

Cahill, K. M. 1996. The role of health in New York State under the governorship of Hugh Carey. *J Community Health* 21:1.

Federal, Provincial and Territorial Advisory Committee on Population Health. 1996. *Report on the health of Canadians: Technical appendix.* Ottawa: Health Canada Communications and Consultation Directorate.

Glanz, K., B. Lankenau, and T. Schmid. 1995. Environmental and policy approaches to cardiovascular disease prevention through nutrition: opportunities for state and local action. *Health Educ Q* 22:512.

Goldstein, A. O., and N. S. Bearman. 1996. State tobacco lobbyists and organizations in the United States: crossed lines. *Am J Public Health* 86:1137.

Habbick, B. F., J. L. Nanson, and A. L. Schulman. 1996. Fetal Alcohol Syndrome in Saskatchewan: Unchanged Incidence in a 20-year Period. *Can J Public Health* 87:204.

Hawthorne, G. 1996. The social impact of Life Education: estimating drug use prevalence among Victorian primary school students and the statewide effect of the Life Education programme. *Addiction* 91:1151.

Jackson, D. M., M. L. Rivo, and T. M. Henderson. 1995. State legislative strategies to improve the supply and distribution of generalist physicians, 1985 to 1992. *Am J Public Health* 85:405.

Johnson, J. L., P. A. Ratner, and J. L. Bottorff. 1995. Urban-rural differences in the health promoting behaviours of Albertans. *Can J Public Health* 86:103.

Johnson, M. M., T. G. Hislop, and A. Lai. 1996. Compliance with the screening mammography program of British Columbia: will she return? *Can J Public Health* 87:176.

Kann, L., C. W. Warren, and L. J. Kolbe. 1993. Youth Risk Behavior Surveillance—United States, 1993. *J School Health* 163:119.

Kaye, G., and T. Wolff, eds. 1997. *From the ground up: a workbook on coalition building and community development.* 2nd edition. Amherst, MA: AHEC/Community Partners.

Leo, A. 1996. Interview: a circle of healing, a circle of hope—healthcare reform the Northwest Territories way. *Leadership in Health Serv* 5(3):4.

Li, J., G. S. Birkhead, and F. B. Coles. 1996. Impact of institution size, staffing patterns, and infection control practices on communicable disease outbreaks in New York State nursing. *Am J Epid* 143:1042.

Lillquist, P. P., M. Haenlein, and C. Mettlin. 1994. Cancer control planning and establishment of priorities for intervention by a state health department. *Pub Health Rep* 109:791.

Macdonald, A. J., S. A. Roberecki, and N. L. Cosway. 1996. Influenza immunization surveillance in rural Manitoba. *Can J Public Health* 87:163.

Margolis, L. H., M. Kotelchuck, A. L. Ware. 1995. Validity of the Maternal and Child Health Services Block Grant as an indicator of state infant mortality reduction initiatives. *Am J Prev Med* 11:40.

Matthews, M. K., K. Webber, and M. Laryea. 1995. Infant feeding practices in Newfoundland and Labrador. *Can J Pub Health* 86:296.

McCombs, S. B., I. M. Onorato, and K. G. Castro. 1996. Tuberculosis surveillance in the United States: case definitions used by state health departments. *Am J Public Health* 86:728.

Nelson-Simley, K., and L. Erickson. 1995. The Nebraska "Network of Drug-Free Youth" Program. *J School Health* 65:49.

Nolan, L., and V. Goel. 1995. Sociodemographic factors related to breastfeeding in Ontario: results from the Ontario Health Survey. *Can J Pub Health* 86:309.

Paine-Andrews, A., K. J. Harris, S. B. Fawcett, K. P. Richter, R. K. Lewis, V. T. Francisco, J. Johnston, and S. Coen. 1997. Evaluating a statewide partnership for reducing risks for chronic diseases. *J Community Health* 22:343.

Rush, B., S. Tyas, and G. Martin. 1996. Substance abuse treatment for Ontario residents in the United States. *Addiction* 91:671.

Sullivan, M. J. L., and Y. Scattolon. 1995. Health policy planning: a look at consumer involvement in Nova Scotia. *Can J Pub Health* 86:317.

Wright, J. W., ed. 1997. *The New York Times 1998 Almanac.* New York: Penguin Books Ltd.

Zieve, A. M. 1996. Public Health & The Law: FDA's proposed regulation of the sale and promotion of tobacco products to minors. *Public Health Rep* 111:280.

Chapter *20*

Local Health Organizations, Services, and Resources

⋮ *R* *ain does not fall on one roof alone.*

—Cameroonian Proverb

Objectives

When you finish this chapter, you should be able to:

- Identify the sources and scope of local authority related to community health

- Describe the organization and components of local health services

- Participate in the planning and evaluation of local health services

---

Closer to home than states or provinces, local communities pursue some health goals that states or provinces are too distant to appreciate. Communities also perform functions that individuals and families cannot attain by themselves. These goals must be pursued through collective action. Some individual needs can be met better or more equitably on a community or cooperative basis. In today's complex society, no one is totally self-sufficient in dealing with all threats to health. To facilitate and supplement what the individual does in health promotion, and to bring local, state or provincial, and national resources to bear on health problems, official and voluntary health organizations have been established on the local level to function independently and cooperatively.

LOCAL RESPONSIBILITY

Need, demand, custom, and gradual development have led society to accept responsibility, as a community, for certain health services on behalf of all residents and visitors. As the population grows and tends to concentrate in urban and suburban areas, new health problems develop, and most of the long-standing community health problems become more complex and more difficult to manage. With each increase in the complexity of community health problems, society has advanced its technology to cope.

Accepted responsibilities of local organizations and services include the following environmental protections: a safe, ample water supply; a safe milk supply; regulation of food establishments; waste disposal; control of air pollution, insects, and rats; and nuisance elimination. Preventive

626

Figure 20-1

Among the wide range of health-related services provided at the local level are immunizations for humans, and rabies and other vaccines for animals. With health certificates in hand, this family assures health protection not only for the puppy, but themselves and the community. *Source:* Photo by J. Blancou, courtesy World Health Organization.

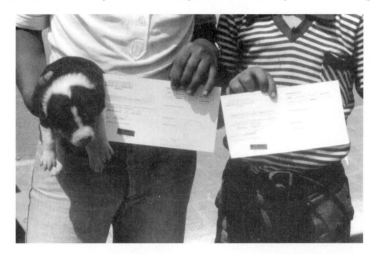

health services include screening and referral for detection of genetic and chronic diseases; immunizations for communicable disease control; maternal, infant, child, adult, and senior citizen health promotion; mental health services; nutrition education; and laboratory services and other services that are specific for certain communities or subpopulations (figure 20-1). Supporting services for all these are collection and recording of vital statistics, health education, and laboratory services.

LOCAL PUBLIC HEALTH AUTHORITY

Public health law in the United States and Canada derives from several sources. It is implemented at multiple levels. The closer to a community the source of a public health law, the greater is its enforcement by and presumed value to the community. Locally passed laws are more likely to be sensitive to local needs and customs, and more likely to have the support of local populations.

Delegated Authority   As noted in the previous chapter, the control of public health is primarily a state or provincial function. State legislatures have the authority to delegate enforcement power to counties and cities to exercise within their own territorial boundaries. They may do this by granting **"home rule"** to counties and municipalities. A city may present a proposed city charter to the state legislature for consideration; if the legislature approves, it grants this charter and home rule to the city. This enables counties and cities to pass health ordinances and regulations to be effective within their own geographical boundaries. Community standards may be higher than state standards, but not lower. Generally counties and cities adopt the same health standards and regulations found in the state sanitary code.

Jurisdiction   Any official health department has **jurisdiction** over all persons and things within its boundaries. A state law may extend the jurisdiction of a county or city health department beyond the county or city boundaries. Even in the absence

· ·
Figure 20-2

Relationships between state health agencies and local health departments reflect the diversity of patterns based on history and political traditions of the various states and their degrees of home rule or local control. *Source:* Centers for Disease Control. 1991. *Profile of state and territorial public health systems: United States, 1991.* Atlanta: U.S. Department of Health and Human Services.

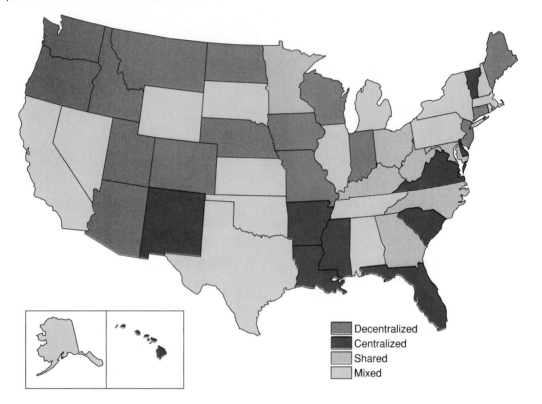

Decentralized
Centralized
Shared
Mixed

of such law, a local health department may take action to correct a problem outside its territory if its own citizens are affected. The state health department can assume jurisdiction in a health dispute or health problem involving two or more cities or two or more counties.

Organization of Authority The most effective governmental unit to exercise public health powers differs among the states and provinces. Those in which there is strong local control resist centralized public health authority (figure 20-2). The state and local authorities are under constant review in many jurisdictions.

LOCAL PUBLIC HEALTH ORGANIZATIONS

Multiple layers of government exist at the local level, which affect public health. Those discussed here include county government, the local board of health, and the **local public health agency** (LPHA). Depending on the size of the area served, these layers may be collapsed or highly stratified to develop public health policies and provide services. Some local areas depend on the state health agency for services (figure 20-3).

· · · · · · · · · · · · · · · · · · · ·
Figure 20-3

Percentages of U.S. population residing in areas served by local health departments (LHDs) or state health agencies in lieu of LHDs, or neither. *Source:* Public Health Foundation and Centers for Disease Control and Prevention.

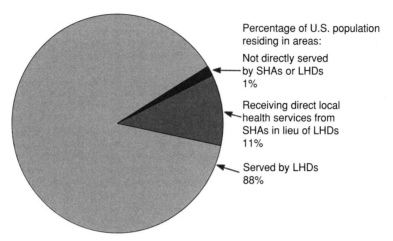

Percentage of U.S. population residing in areas:

Not directly served by SHAs or LHDs
1%

Receiving direct local health services from SHAs in lieu of LHDs
11%

Served by LHDs
88%

County Government

Authority to establish a LPHA in the United States is delegated by the state legislature to the legislative body of the county or parish. About 70 percent of counties have a county commission form of government structure. The commission consists of an elected board, ranging from two to over one-hundred members. A hallmark of the commission form of government is that commissioners share administrative responsibility with other independently elected officers such as the county clerk, auditor, assessor, treasurer, sheriff, and coroner. The commission is concerned with all matters of county government, including health.

The county commission usually appoints the county board of health. State statutes may specify how to choose the board of health and the type and number of people to serve. In some instances a county supervisor or commissioner may be appointed to the county board of health. This arrangement can promote coordination between the board of supervisors and the board of health. In other states the members of the county board of health must be from outside the membership of the county commissioners.

The county commission has legislative powers that may include passing ordinances and adopting budgets, and administrative powers that many include supervising county departments, including health. The "home rule" option in thirty-two states provides counties with an opportunity to enact a "local constitution," which gives the county authority and power to levy taxes to pay for all county services and activities, including those of the local public health agency.

Local Board of Health

Local boards of health are used in most states to provide local input into or control of the operation of the LPHA. In nearly three-quarters of the local public health agencies, the local board of health operates at the county level. In other areas the board may be at the city or town level or in some combined city and county combination. These local boards are concerned with the health needs of the citizens in the counties or cities they serve.

Although not controlled by the state boards of health, the local boards may work with the state and other local boards on matters of health policy and services.

Appointed by the county commission, the local board of health may be composed of five, seven, nine, or any other number of members. Too small a membership may not provide adequate representation of the diverse public interests, and too large a number of members may create a debating assembly. Term of office varies from three to six years, and terms are staggered to provide for continuity and replacement. Many segments of the population have members on the board to assure that a cross-section of the population is represented. Usually at least one physician serves on the board, but no one profession should dominate the membership. A chairperson is elected by the board from among its own members. The county health officer usually serves as an **ex officio** member or as executive secretary of the board.

The local board of health has administrative, legislative, and quasijudicial functions. Among its administrative responsibilities, in forty-eight states the board appoints a health officer or director who provides leadership for the LPHA. Minnesota and Rhode Island have no local health officers. In twenty-two states local health officers are required to have a medical degree; many health officers also have preparation in public health. The board may also approve professional staff appointed by the director. The local board of health votes on the budget, as recommended by the director, and then sends the budget to the county commission for approval. The commission has responsibility for the entire county budget, including that portion relating to health.

Legislative functions of the local board of health begin with the adoption of a sanitary code. This code, prepared by the professional staff, is usually the state sanitary code modified to fit the county situation. The county standards can be more rigid than those of the state, but not less rigid. This county code has the effect of law. The board amends it from time to time as conditions require.

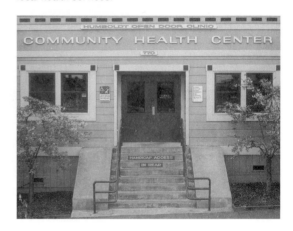

Figure 20-4

The Community Health Center in Humboldt County California is one of thousands of such centers providing local health services.

Quasijudicial powers of the local board of health are inherent in the authority of the board to hold hearings preliminary to granting or revoking a license. The board has the authority to summon people to appear before it in cases where health regulations have been violated. Any decision by the board may be appealed to the courts by any citizen who believes that the decision was unjust.

Local Public Health Agency

LPHA Organization   County governments are the most common type of local government structure within which the local public health agency operates. There are nearly 3,000 LPHAs across the United States (figure 20-4). Approximately 65 percent of LPHAs serve populations with fewer than 50,000 citizens. LPHAs provide 72 percent of services at the county level, 11 percent at the town level, and the remainder have combined city and county, multicounty, or multicity arrangements. Contrasting forms of organization are found between Massachusetts and California. The former state has only one county health department

· · · · · · · · · · · · · · · · · · · ·
Figure 20-5

Types of local health departments (LPHAs) by jurisdiction in Massachusetts reflect the mixed forms of local government carried over from Colonial times. *Source:* Centers for Disease Control. 1991. *Profile of state and territorial public health systems: United States, 1991.* Atlanta: U.S. Department of Health and Human Services.

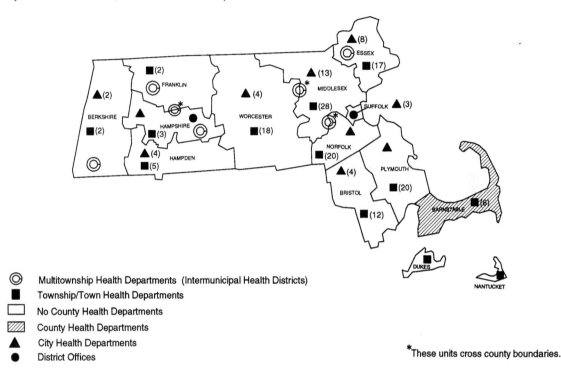

◎   Multitownship Health Departments (Intermunicipal Health Districts)
■   Township/Town Health Departments
▭   No County Health Departments
▨   County Health Departments
▲   City Health Departments
●   District Offices

*These units cross county boundaries.

(figure 20-5). California has nearly all LPHAs organized at the county level, except two at the city level (figure 20-6).

Some of the larger cities such as New York, Los Angeles, and Houston have a city health department that functions as the LPHA. In the early development of official health agencies in Europe and North America, it was the city health department that was in most evidence. Baltimore established the first city health department in the United States in 1798. Nearly all U.S. cities had a health department of some description by the midtwentieth century. With the spread of the population, the county became an increasingly functional level for providing public health services. In many situations smaller city health departments consolidate

with county health departments. A city of 30,000 in a county of 70,000 will usually depend on a county health department rather than support a separate city department.

LPHA Personnel   The health officer appointed by the local health board is usually the administrator for the LPHA. The health program of the LPHA is carried on by salaried professional personnel. The number of the staff depends on size of the local public health area, the population, special health problems involved, resources, and the public's view of the importance of the work of the health department. In consideration of these varied criteria, the number of staff in LPHAs varies from one person to 26,000.

· ·

Figure 20-6

California has uniformly distributed county health departments. The three field offices enable the state health department to maintain field staff in three regions of the state, in addition to Sacramento. City health departments in San Jose and Los Angeles (San Francisco is a city-county combination) serve their special urban needs in large, dispersed counties. *Source:* Centers for Disease Control. 1991. *Profile of state and territorial public health systems: United States, 1991.* Atlanta: U.S. Department of Health and Human Services.

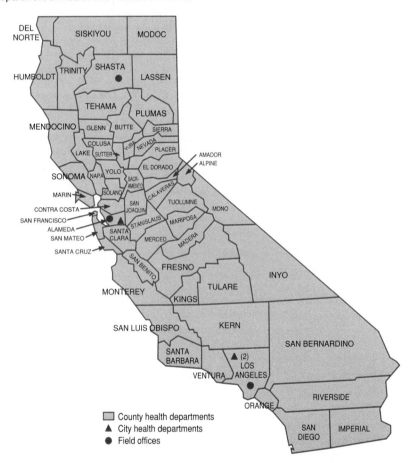

In the past the local health agency in smaller areas consisted of a part-time health officer, a quarantine officer, a sanitarian, and a clerk. Activities largely involved enforcing isolation and quarantine for the purpose of communicable disease control and inspection of unsanitary conditions.

Some small communities still have part-time health officers who are not trained in public health, who are political appointees, and who regard their public health duties as a side line to their medical practice. Fortunately, this situation now gives way to professionally staffed local public health agencies.

Forty-six percent of the LPHAs report a staff of nine or fewer full-time employees. Typically the majority of LPHAs serving fewer than 25,000 people

Figure 20-7

Health educators extend the work of the local health agency through linking health policy and research with local concerns, priorities, and culture. Here a health educator meets with a group of students in the school setting to discuss AIDS. *Source:* Photo by E. Mandelmann, courtesy World Health Organization.

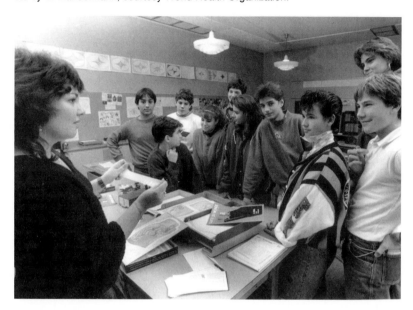

employ a clerical worker (89 percent), a registered nurse (83 percent), and an engineer (65 percent). The employment of a clerk or administrative assistant is economically sound because it relieves the director of many routine, time-consuming tasks and increases the number of people that can be served. LPHAs serving up to 50,000 persons also report employing a physician (65 percent). LPHAs serving up to 100,000 persons may employ a health educator (54 percent) (figure 20-7), and a nutritionist or dietician (67 percent).

LPHA Finances Total expenditures for LPHAs are difficult to compare and interpret because of variations in their organization, responsibilities, and programs. Acceptable and adequate funding will depend on the problems of the community, the public's perception of the importance of these problems and their causes, the efficiency of the

organizations addressing them in raising local funds or obtaining state or federal grants, and the policies of the state (SHA) in passing federal funds through to the LPHA (figure 20-8).

For economic reasons a population of 50,000 has long been regarded as the minimum unit for which a local health department should be established. Smaller populations can either contract for services from the state or unite two or more sparsely populated areas into an LPHA with at least 50,000 people. There have been debates about the minimum LPHA population, especially as two-thirds of LPHAs serve fewer than 50,000.

LOCAL PUBLIC HEALTH SERVICES

Direct health services to the people of the community are provided by the full-time professional staff. General and specific services vary greatly

· · · · · · · · · · · · · · · · · ·

Figure 20-8

Block grants from federal to state and from state to local agencies have maximum flexibility for allocation to various programs. Other grants, and especially contracts, have highly specific purposes that leave the recipient agency little discretion in their allocation. *Source:* Office of Disease Prevention and Health Promotion, U.S. Department of Health and Human Services.

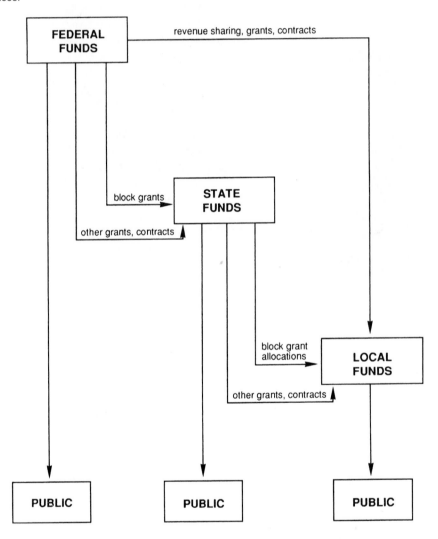

among LPHAs within a state and from one state to another. A state legislature may require LPHAs to perform special services. For example, one state requires the LPHA to make medical investigations of death and child abuse, while another state may require neither service. In many instances LPHAs may be providing the same service, but under different titles. For example, a service may be called family health in one LPHA and maternal and child health in another. To cite all types of service given

Ten Organizational Practices or Processes that Must Be Carried Out by a Component of the Public Health System in Each Locality

ASSESSMENT
1. *Assess* the health needs of the community.
2. *Investigate* the occurrence of health effects and health hazards in the community.
3. *Analyze* the determinants of identified health needs.

POLICY DEVELOPMENT
4. *Advocate* for public health, build constituencies, and identify resources in the community.
5. *Set priorities* among health needs.
6. *Develop plans* and policies to address priority health needs.

ASSURANCE
7. *Manage* resources and develop organizational structure.
8. *Implement* programs.
9. *Evaluate* programs and provide quality assurance.
10. *Inform and educate* the public.

by LPHAs would be to list unusual, rare, and minor services, along with those considered essential. The core functions and services discussed in the following pages are provided by nearly all full-time LPHAs (see box).

Vital Statistics

Biostatistics, public health statistics, human biometrics, and other terms designate public health recordkeeping. Vital statistics concern the vital facts of human existence, such as births, marriages, disease incidence, and deaths. For the health staff, vital statistics point out the health needs of the city or county and the strengths and weaknesses of the health program. Health data accrue from registration and enumeration.

Registration of certain health information is required by law and health regulations. Physicians must report to the LPHA cases of certain communicable diseases. To make reporting easy, physicians are provided with a simple form on which the physician can quickly record pertinent data and can mail postage-free. Birth, death, and marriage records usually come from the county clerk.

Enumeration of health data usually requires that the health staff actively collect information. Health examinations, dental examinations, and water samples provide important information. Special surveys and studies also yield data regarded as important by the health staff, especially in relation to lifestyles that influence chronic disease and injury rates.

Health statistics, not an end in themselves but a means to an end, can reveal health conditions, health levels, health needs, and health problems. Certain rates per year are of particular health significance. (See chapter 3.)

Communicable Disease Control

Constant vigilance is necessary for communicable disease control. Programs can be planned and effectively administered so that epidemics do not occur and so that the number of outbreaks of communicable disease is held to a minimum. Such a control program requires certain preventive measures: (1) immunization; (2) public health education; (3) protection of water, milk, and other food supplies; (4) promotion of sanitation; and (5) control of carriers of disease. Control measures must concentrate on infected persons and their environment and entail (1) recognition of the disease (figure 20-9), (2) prompt reporting of all cases, (3) isolation procedures, (4) quarantine when warranted, and (5) decontamination.

In a national survey, more LPHAs reported the provision of immunizations than any other public health service (figure 20-10). Other communicable disease control measures rank among the most frequently provided services of LPHAs.

• • • • • • • • • • • • • • • • • • •

Figure 20-9

Control of communicable diseases includes
the smear test for gonorrhoea. The
temporary embarrassment of undergoing
such a test is a small trade-off against
individual health and community protection.
Source: Photo by T. Farkas, courtesy World
Health Organization.

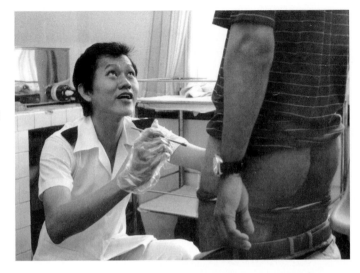

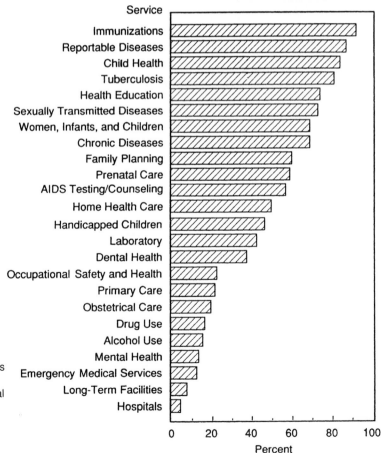

• • • • • • • • • • • • • • • • • • •

Figure 20-10

Percent distribution of selected services
reported by 2,263 local health
departments (LPHAs). *Source:* National
Association of County Health Officials.
1990. *Selected characteristics of local
health departments—United States,
1989. MMWR 39:609.*

Maternal and Child Health

In maternal health promotion certain direct measures are taken to safeguard the health of the expectant mother, fetus, and later the newborn infant. These include promotion of prenatal care, postnatal care, and adequate delivery facilities. Indirect means of promoting maternal health include education for family members, maternity benefits, daycare, and family planning. The LPHA provides education and some direct services for women and children. Direct services may include family planning, immunization, and well-baby clinics. In some communities the current organization of health service in the United States places tension between public health agencies providing these services free to women and children and medical practitioners who charge for these services. The preventive nature of the services and the low income of most recipients enables such services to be provided.

Public health nurses are key personnel in maternal and infant health. Prenatal visits may be made to high-risk mothers to provide education and counseling. Liaisons with hospitals identify new mothers in need of follow-up services. The public health nurse may do follow-up visits in homes to teach families about infant care and well-being. Families are assisted to understand the particular health needs and health problems of the infant; encouraged to have the infant examined at regular intervals by a physician; helped to secure medical diagnosis and treatment for the infant when such needs are indicated; and taught about good nutrition, feeding, and parenting practices. The LPHA receives its funding for maternal and child health services from the Women, Infants, and Children (WIC) program of the U.S. Department of Agriculture and the community block grants. The LPHA has an obligation to cooperate with all recognized agencies, including schools, that contribute to child health.

Chronic Disease Control

Many if not most of the organic diseases of the late years have their genesis in middle age or even early adulthood. Accordingly, adult health promotion gives emphasis to the middle years of life and to the elderly (figure 20-11). Indeed, preventive efforts directed toward the younger age groups can yield the most productive dividends. A constructive adult health promotional program ideally concentrates on the following three health factors:

1. Periodic screening and examination
2. Correction of all remediable disorders
3. Health education that emphasizes moderation in use of alcohol, avoiding infection, diagnosis and treatment of infection and other symptoms immediately when they occur, nonsmoking, exercise, proper diet, coping with stress, and checking with a physician when any abnormal condition persists

Community organization on the part of the health department calls for getting adults examined and assuring proper follow-up of those screened. Cooperation with the medical society, industry, labor unions, and service organizations backed by a good promotional program through various media is required (see chapters 4, 6, 7, and 12).

Mental Health Promotion

Major emphasis in mental health promotion is placed on the mental health of the normal individual. The modern mental health program offers individual and group counseling, seminars, institutes, hot lines, demonstrations, lectures, web sites, and other services. Psychiatric, psychological, and social work services are available to normal individuals, families, people with minor disturbances, delinquents, people with serious emotional problems, the disordered, people with alcohol- or drug-related problems, and those in the process of rehabilitation (see chapter 9). That a city, county, or district health department provides a mental health center where a person may go for consultation is extremely significant for citizens in the community. Some LPHAs integrate their drug and alcohol abuse education and substance abuse treatment programs into their mental

••••••••••••••••••••

Figure 20-11

A visiting nurse provides screening and chronic disease counseling. Homes visits also offer the opportunity to work with seniors to identify potential safety hazards, for example, falls. *Source:* Photo by Marsha Burkes, courtesy University of Texas Health Science Center at Houston.

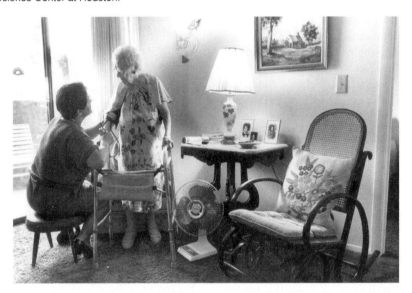

health programs and services. They are supported by mass media and hot line services directly from the federal government and voluntary agencies (figure 20-12).

Environmental Health Protection

Sanitarians are primarily occupied with public sanitation but provide consulting services when requested by householders. Home sanitation is encouraged through continuous educational measures. Most of the sanitarian's time and attention is directed to the inspection and appraisal of public water supplies, food services, milk and milk products, sewage disposal, public buildings, swimming pools, insect infestation, and industrial operations. Preventing disease is the primary goal of the sanitation program, but promotion of an esthetic environment is usually a secondary benefit. (See chapters 13 to 16.)

Laboratory Service

Most LPHAs in sparsely populated counties do not have their own laboratories but depend on the centralized laboratory of the state health department (see chapter 19) or a local laboratory in a hospital or a clinic. Water plant operators are usually competent to run bacteriological and chlorine examinations of water. Even without its own laboratory a county health department can improvise sufficiently to provide limited laboratory service.

Having a local health department laboratory has many advantages in convenience and reduced time for running laboratory tests. Communicable disease control by means of laboratory tests requires promptness. Diagnostic tests, water and milk examinations, and food contamination tests can be done promptly in the local health department laboratory.

. . . .
Figure 20-12

The American Mental Health Fund and other community agencies have formed coalitions to not only promote mental health, but address stereotypes of mental illness. *Source:* American Mental Health Fund and Advertising Council.

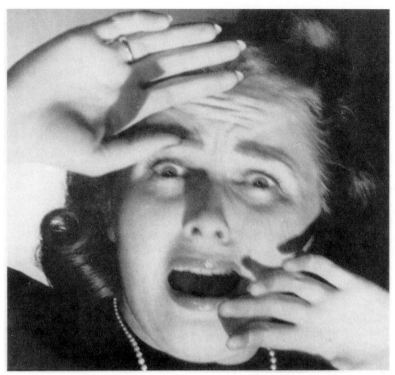

Dental Public Health

The most effective strategy for reducing dental caries and lost teeth is fluoridation of community water supplies. At an estimated cost of $1 per child per year, fluoridation remains the least expensive caries prevention measure. Every dollar spent for fluoridation will save $50 in dental bills. The benefits accrue to adults as well as children. Fluoride occurs naturally in most water, but usually at less than optimum levels. Since the introduction in 1945 of the practice of fluoridating community water supplies, there has been a steady increase in the number of people using water with levels of fluoride high enough to be significant for dental health. The national objective for 2000 is to assure that "at least 75% of the population on community water systems should be receiving the benefits of optimally fluoridated water." This is an example of a year 2000 objective that is lower than the previous objective set for 1990. The target for community water supplies was lowered because of increasing amounts of fluoride consumed by the public in soft drinks and other processed foods.

In addition to working on the fluoridation issue, some local health departments provide direct dental care to indigent populations, many conduct fluoride rinse programs for schoolchildren, and most support dental health education in the schools.

Health Education

The base of the pyramid called community health is public health education, and the breadth and stability of the base largely determines the height to which the pyramid can rise. Health education is effective to the extent that it constructively affects people's health knowledge, health attitudes, and health practices. To be effective, public health education must win public *acceptance* of a program or practice, arouse a *desire* in people to benefit from it, obtain the *involvement* of the people in the program or practice, and support *maintenance* of changes in public health practice.

Public health education targets different segments of the population for different purposes.

Direct communications with people whose health behavior places them at risk seek to inform them about and gain their acceptance of a program or practice and to increase their motivation to benefit from it. Indirect communications through parents, teachers, officials, employers, membership organizations, and peers are designed to provide a supportive social environment and reinforcement for behavior conducive to health. Additional communications directed to organizations such as service clubs, church groups, parent-teacher organizations, labor unions, health agencies, insurance companies, child study organizations, parent groups, and neighborhood organizations are designed to enable and facilitate good health habits by organizing community resources required for the health behavior to occur (figure 20-13)

Public health education is beset by many obstacles, particularly false advertising, quackery, cultism, superstition, professional and public indifference, and the human tendency to seek the easiest solution to every health problem. However a well-organized and effectively administered community health education program can have a substantial influence on the health of the community's population.

The head of the community health education or health promotion program has professional preparation as a community health education specialist. This person may supervise a number of organized units and individuals who have contributions to make. All members of the local health department staff engage in health education as part of their professional activities. The health educator coordinates the educational efforts of the staff, provides consultation, and initiates action that will involve other staff members of the department and other agencies in the community and lay self-help groups.

Voluntary health agencies; child health councils; schools; the medical society; the dental society; and a number of other organizations in the city, county, or district each contribute to health education. Imaginative, sensitive, and persistent leadership from the health department is required

····················

Figure 20-13

A coalition of legal, commercial, academic, and public health agencies supports alcohol-free drinks as an option for college-age youth. *Source:* Gwynedd Health Authority, North Wales.

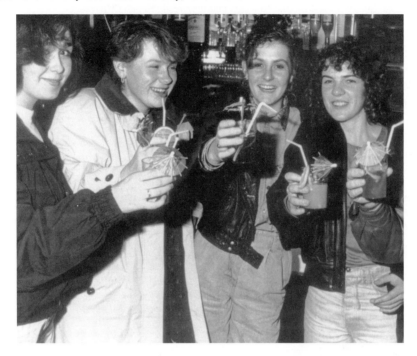

to get all of these organizations and individuals contributing in a coordinated way.

Numerous services and materials constitute the methods used in community health education. Each medium makes its own contribution, but it is the composite effect of a coordinated program that achieves the goal of a health-educated public (see chapters 4 and 11).

Nuisance Abatement

Health departments take all possible action to prevent nuisances by passing regulations declaring certain conditions to constitute nuisances. Such action is taken by state boards of health and local boards of health. A public health or environmental **nuisance** is one detrimental to the physical or mental health of one person or a large number of people. Although most nuisances are not health threats, some nuisances are potential health threats, such as water pollution, improper sewage disposal, air pollution, contaminated milk, food other than milk, lead paint in housing, rat infestation, stagnant water allowing for insect breeding, and excessive noise (figure 20-14).

If a nuisance cannot be corrected by negotiation, action to abate it may be taken by a private citizen or a public health official. Courts recognize three classes of nuisances: private, public, and mixed. A nuisance that affects, injures, or damages only one individual or relatively few people, such as sewage from a septic tank flowing onto neighboring property, may be declared to be a private nuisance if the offended citizen takes court action. **Abatement** of a private nuisance may

••••••••••••••••••••

Figure 20-14

Excessive noise can be a public or private nuisance. This chart shows the different noise levels of various settings and sources, as measured in decibels and sound pressure. Local standards for noise levels may exceed, but not be lower than, state regulations. *Source:* Poster by Bruel & Kjaer, courtesy World Health Organization.

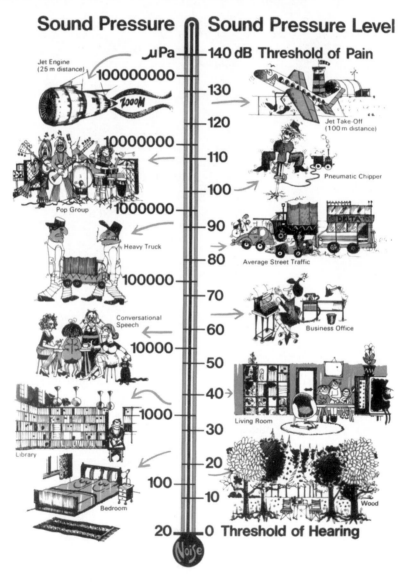

occur following a formal complaint or may require a suit for damages.

A nuisance that affects, injures, or damages a considerable number of people, for example a plant emitting objectionable fumes affecting a neighborhood, could be considered a public nuisance. A group of citizens may file court action or may request local health officials to take action in a court of equity. The court may issue an **injunction** forbidding the continuance of the condition, or may order the defendant to reduce the degree of offensiveness of the condition. Immediate action is sometimes necessary, and there is not always sufficient time to resort to court action. In this event quick abatement is the remedy.

Other Local Public Health Services

Through legislative requirement, local pressure, custom, or even coincidence, a local health agency may be engaged in one or more unique services not included in the usual list of responsibilities. Some local health agencies are responsible for the medical investigation of deaths of unknown cause. Child abuse cases and inspection of foster care homes may be referred to the health agency. Other kinds of unique activities of different LPHAs include speech, occupational and physical therapies, and fielding questions about community resources. Someone must perform these services, but if these activities interfere with the effective performance of the basic public health functions, the public may lose more in health protection than it gains in social services.

Coalitions for Community Health

On the city, metropolitan, county, or district level, health coalitions have been valuable in coordinating the health activities of various agencies and individuals. Coalitions usually have no official status but are voluntary and composed of representatives from various organizations and groups having common health interests or goals. Coalitions usually have from ten to thirty members, with representatives from such groups as voluntary health agencies, the medical profession, the

dental profession, parent-teacher organizations, labor unions, chambers of commerce, women's organizations, church groups, social agencies, universities, law enforcement, and various other groups. The coalition usually represents a cross section of the organizations serving various population groups and can make known the health needs of the people. It can make recommendations to the LPHA and can be called on to support certain of its activities. Housing the coalition has sometimes been a function of the United Way, but more often the coalition has an office in one of the participating organizations.

A community coalition can provide a valuable community service so long as it considers the overall health needs of the people and strives to support and supplement the health department. It serves as a health promoting force in the community and provides for broad involvement in public health, but it may have problems (see p. 598).

COMMUNITY HEALTH PROFESSIONALS

Health programs, offered by local public health agencies, are often provided by professionals specially trained in the field of public health. The core functions of public health are assessment, assurance, and policy development focused on health promotion and disease prevention at the community level, which may include environmental, physical and mental health, and primary care. Appendix A identifies and describes areas of community health specialization. Appendix B lists common job titles in public and community health.

Community health professionals differ from those trained in personal health services by their emphasis on prevention over cure, populations over individuals, and community rather than clinical settings. A nurse, for example, working in the neonatal intensive care unit of a hospital is highly trained to work with the special equipment needed to save the life of a premature infant and to support the family in time of crisis. A community health nurse works to assure that mothers receive adequate prenatal care and education to reduce the

Table 20-1

Projected Supply of Economically Active Public Health Graduates for Selected Categories of the Professional Health Workforce for Community Health, United States, 1990–2000

Area of specialization*	Estimated number of graduates economically active in the specialty[†]	
	1990	2000
Biomedical and laboratory sciences	1,673	2,164
Biostatistics	2,787	3,606
Environmental sciences	7,247	9,377
Epidemiology	5,575	7,213
Health education	3,902	5,049
Health services administration	15,609	20,196
Nutrition	2,787	3,606
Occupational safety and health	1,115	1,443
Public health practice and program management	6,690	8,655
Other	8,362	10,819
TOTAL	55,747	72,128

Based on estimates and assumptions in Hall, T. L., R. S. Jackson, and W. B. Parsons. 1980. *Schools of public health, trends in graduate education.* DHHS Pub. No. (HRA) 80–45. Washington, DC: Division of Associated Health Professions, Public Health Service.
*See Appendix A of this text for description of the areas of specialization with illustrative jobs and job settings.
[†]Based on adjustments that eliminate most Canadian and other foreign graduates and the double counting that might result from persons with two or more degrees from schools of public health.

chances of premature birth and low-birthweight babies. Both nurses are concerned about maternal and child health; the emphasis is different.

As the nation turns toward health care reform, greater emphasis on disease prevention, health promotion, and population health is universally acknowledged. The application of community health values, principles, knowledge, and technologies is essential to realize the benefits of effective health care reform. Many of the national goals adopted as part of *Healthy People 2000* will depend on an adequate supply of those trained in community health. A 1993 report by the Bureau of Health Professions in the U.S. Department of Health and Human Services determined that there is a need for well-trained community health professionals, especially in the disciplines of epidemi-

ology, biostatistics, environmental health, nutrition, and nursing (table 20-1).

Much of the preparation of today's community health professionals focuses on schools of public health, preventive medicine programs in medical schools, public health nursing programs, and specialty public health or community health programs in a variety of disciplines. The community health emphasis is already seen in the preparation of an increasing number of health professionals.

THE EVOLUTION OF COMMUNITY HEALTH PLANNING AND SERVICES

Most countries subsidize local health services from state or national revenues. In the United States, this subsidy may be given directly or indirectly to

ISSUES AND CONTROVERSIES
Politics and Planning

Politics shape how federal monies are used to support communities. At some points in history, federal money has been ear-marked directly for the community to deal with particular social issues, such as health issues or voting rights. At other times, federal money has been distributed to states to decide how best to spend it. Where do you stand on direct and indirect federal support for community health? Does your position vary by population, economic status, or type of health issue?

communities as diagrammed in figure 20-8. In these various subsidy routes, politics, planning, and programs mix, as decisions are made about *who* has a say, *which* health objectives have priority, *what* services will be directed toward their achievement, and *how many* resources should be expended.

Politics and the Distribution of Health Resources

Building the Infrastructure In the United States, the first major federal subsidies to states were grants-in-aid for maternal and child health programs and to state and local governments for the establishment and development of health departments (Titles V and VI of the 1935 Social Security Act). Then came the Hill-Burton Hospital Survey and Construction Act of 1946, which assisted more than 3,800 communities to build hospitals, extended care and rehabilitation facilities, and public health centers. The National Institutes of Health was also developed during this postwar period of federal investment, contributing over $14 billion toward the development and support of biomedical and health related research. Support for health personnel development also began during this period, providing traineeships for public health specialists, most of whom were already employed in community health agencies but without formal training in public health.

By the early 1960s there was considerable disillusionment with the results of these massive investments in the three major areas of national health resources—facilities, knowledge, and personnel. The United States had reached the highest level of per capita expenditures for health in the world, but American health services and health statistics rated poorly among those of developed nations—in infant death rates, in the percentage of mothers who died in childbirth, in life expectancy, and in the death rate of males in their middle years.

The previous investment period had succeeded in building a massive health and medical care complex, but this complex had failed to adjust its structure appropriately to trends in the distribution of illness, demands for services, specialization of practitioners, development of more sophisticated medical equipment, and demands of office and hospital personnel for competitive wages. Physicians and hospitals clung tenaciously to traditions of individualism, endeavoring to be all things to their patients despite the obvious need to pool specialized facilities and services. Rural areas most notably were still without community health services.

Comprehensive Community Health By the mid-1960s the United States had entered a period of ferment in the evolution of national health policy. New emphasis was placed on community health services and consumer participation in health planning. This shift toward comprehensive health services was exemplified in mental health and maternal and child health services. In 1963

President Kennedy signed the Community Mental Health Centers Act. This act differed from earlier construction assistance acts in that it required centers to provide comprehensive services including outpatient care, consultation, and education. Approximately four-hundred community mental health centers had been established by 1970. The innovations resulting from this comprehensive approach marked a new direction in organizational arrangements, such as citizen participation and a community education orientation. These centers contributed to enormous shifts in the care of the mentally ill and public attitudes toward mental health. Those suffering from mental illness were no longer removed to distant state institutions. They were returned closer to home for care.

Also in 1963 the Maternal and Child Health and Mental Retardation Acts provided for similarly comprehensive, community-based approaches for high-risk, low-income groups. Prenatal care received as high priority attention as did delivery services and postnatal care. These services were combined into Maternal and Child Health (MCH) block grants in the 1980s.

Neighborhood Health Centers   The Economic Opportunity Act of 1964 supported research, demonstration, and training for Neighborhood Health Centers. These grants resulted in widespread use of health care teams, indigenous community workers, and community health aides. Most significantly, from an educational perspective, serious attention was given to participation of the poor in the planning and evaluation of services. By mid-1969 about fifty projects had been funded, a drop in the bucket in relation to the needs and legitimate demands of the poor, but again significant in terms of the concepts demonstrated. Federal support for Neighborhood Health Centers declined in the 1970s.

Community Action Programs   The Economic Opportunity Act of 1964 also created Community Action Programs, which moved consumer participation from a matter of voluntary action to a mat-

ter of public policy. Community action was suddenly defined in legal terms, which carried new opportunities and new obligations for the poor. "Maximum feasible participation" was further mandated by PL 89-749 in 1965 (authorizing the establishment of Comprehensive Health Planning Agencies) and in the Model Cities Demonstration Act of 1966.

For all the good intentions behind the consumer participation movement, its legislated implementation was misunderstood or misused by many professionals. The "maximum feasible misunderstanding," as characterized by Senator Daniel Patrick Moynihan a few years later, was the co-optation of consumer participants into managerial functions. This undermined the intent of the legislation and left many volunteer participants feeling exploited and suspicious of governmental purposes.

Regional Medical Programs   The Regional Medical Program Act of 1965 needs to be read critically for its messages of professional protection in a time of increased community demands for participation. For example, the purposes of this Act were (1) to establish regional cooperative arrangements among medical schools, research institutions, and hospitals for research, training, and demonstrations projects in heart disease, cancer, and stroke; (2) to afford the medical profession the opportunity of making the latest advances in diagnosis and treatment more widely available; and (3) to improve the availability of health personnel and facilities, "without interfering with the patterns, or the methods of financing, of patient care or professional practice, or with the administration of hospitals, and in cooperation with practicing physicians, medical center officials, hospital administrators, and representatives from appropriate voluntary health agencies."

Note particularly the hesitation in this legislation to offend or challenge the medical establishment. This crippling clause made no mention of official (state or local) health agencies and no mention of health professionals or paraprofessionals other than

••••••••••••••••••••••
Figure 20-15

During the 1980s, there was a consistent reduction in the amount of direct aid to cities. A portion of this reduction was to be picked up as block grants to states. *Source:* National League of Cities.

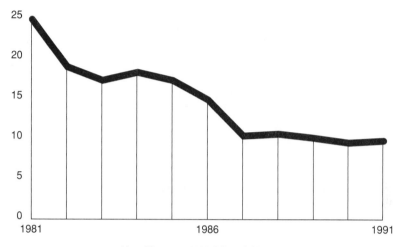

Note: These are 1982 dollars, in billions.

those of the hospital "establishment." The Regional Medical Programs were phased out in 1976 with the advent of regional Health Systems Agencies (HSAs).

National Health Planning and Resources Development Act of 1974   Under a later federal health planning program, consumers participated in local and state efforts to correct many deficiencies and inequities in the delivery of health care. The National Health Planning and Resources Development Act of 1974 provided for a majority of consumers (51 percent to 60 percent) to serve on two major planning bodies—the more than two-hundred HSAs, and the Statewide Health Coordinating Councils. These bodies, together with the State Health Planning and Resources Development Agencies, had broad authority over the allocation and development of health resources, including personnel, facilities, and services. Congress repealed this Act ten years later, after the Reagan administration systematically eliminated its budget support for the state and area health planning agencies (figure 20-15).

Healthy Communities 2000: Model Standards
Contemporary federal support for community health planning includes Model Standards for healthy communities. Developed cooperatively between the federal government (CDC) and the American Public Health Association, these standards intend to help local and state agencies determine their own public health priorities and to establish objectives compatible with the national objectives for the year 2000.

While many local communities share the vision of national objectives for disease prevention and health promotion, they lack blueprints to translate and implement these ideas in their own situations. The Model Standards help with this translation by the use of planning tools such as APEXPH (Assessment Protocol for Excellence in Public Health) and PATCH (Planned Approach To Community Health). APEXPH is a process for use by local health departments to assist them in better meeting the public health needs of their communities. PATCH is a community health promotion methodology that involves and enables communities to plan, implement, and evaluate programs. The

Eleven Steps for Model Standards

Assess and determine the role of the public health agency within the community

Assess the lead health agency's organizational capacity

Develop an agency plan to build the necessary organizational capacity

Assess the community's organizational and power structures

Organize the community to build a stronger constituency for public health and establish a partnership for public health

Assess the health needs and available resources

Determine local priorities and available resources

Select outcome and process objectives that are compatible with local priorities and the Healthy People 2000 objectives

Develop communitywide intervention strategies

Develop and implement a plan of action

planning process for Model Standards differs from some community planning efforts in the past by linking communities nationally in a structured process to achieve identifiable local and national health goals.

The Future of Participatory Planning

A look back allows an understanding of the various ways in which planning and politics shape health objectives and the distribution of health services and the resources. Remnants of various approaches to health-planning have survived and influence current approaches. Through the Model Standards and other planning processes, consumers continue to contribute to decisions that will help produce a more rational, responsive, effective, and equitable health care system. Participatory planning involves consumers in dealing with the unintended effects of past planning decisions, such as deinstitutionalization of the men-

tally ill, and involve them in future decision making. Good planning can, for example, help strike a better balance between the emphasis in health care on crisis intervention for the treatment and the need for prevention and health maintenance. Consumers can help restrain hospitals in acquiring expensive equipment. Instead of having the latest technology, the community may focus on equity in health care. Other problems also can be alleviated through more effective planning for the production and use of community health resources and services. Consider, for example, the following facts concerning the present U.S. system of health care.

- In general, inner-city areas and remote rural sections are served by too few physicians.
- Primary care is often available only after the patient endures a long wait in a crowded waiting room or drives long distances to see a physician.
- The affluent areas of cities have built more hospitals than needed.
- The costs of medical care have been rising rapidly. Part of this increase is attributable to the poor location of health care facilities and the costs of staffing and equipping these facilities.

Active consumer leadership in health planning can help produce a more immediate and tangible impact on patients through improved service and staffing patterns; more equitable fees; a mechanism to respond to patient grievances; improved physical facilities; and, above all, care that protects the dignity and well-being of the individual patient. These and other issues of personal health care will be addressed in chapter 21.

For the individual consumer, participation—not co-optation—in health planning can yield benefits beyond promoting improvements in the health care system. Many consumers who have served on planning boards in the past report a deep sense of community involvement that has enriched their lives. Others found they had increased their effectiveness in other community activities.

In one respect, health planning is an educational process for the community. It is a way of making citizens, public officials, and health care providers aware of community needs, perceptions, and better ways of allocating health resources. By including a nonprovider perspective, consumers can help create a climate in which community interests take precedence over special interests of dominant professions and institutions.

VOLUNTARY HEALTH AGENCIES

Voluntary health agencies are the focus in this chapter on local health services, in contrast with professional health organizations and health foundations discussed in chapter 18. The latter tend to function at the national rather than local level and have relatively fewer local affiliates to provide direct support to community health programs. Foundations tend to identify neither with the voluntary, private sector, nor with the official, public sector, but refer to their niche as the "independent sector." Voluntary health agencies have a clear community commitment, in organizational structure with local affiliates and program focus.

Nontax-supported, voluntary health agencies provide opportunities for communities to fulfill needs beyond the scope or resources of official agencies. These voluntary health organizations have pioneered in promoting health programs and in demonstrating the contributions to health improvement that can be made. Frequently, when a voluntary health organization or a foundation demonstrates what can be done, the official agencies then enter the field and supplement the functions or services of the voluntary organization.

In the late nineteenth and early twentieth centuries, governmental agencies took action reluctantly on existing health problems. They were slow to use available means for dealing with these problems and to develop new measures for disease prevention and control. Voluntary groups organized in response to the clear need to take progressive action to solve problems of disease prevention and control. Many such organizations have been formed, several of which will be discussed as representative of the types of voluntary health agencies that have served the public over the past half century or more at national and community levels.

Lung Associations

Founded in 1904 as the National Association for the Study and Prevention of Tuberculosis, the American Lung Association was the first voluntary agency of the educational, promotional type. From the outset, education was the foundation of this association's program, based on the premise that, while it is essential to extend knowledge through scientific research, such knowledge serves few unless it is available to the public, medical practitioners, health personnel, and patients on the widest possible basis.

With the tuberculosis problem largely under control, in 1973 the American Lung Association turned much of its attention and efforts to the problem of asthma, tobacco control (figure 20-16), and environmental health. The American Thoracic Society is a subsidiary of the American Lung Association composed of physicians and researchers who are specialists in **thoracic** diseases.

The association's program operates primarily on the community level. This emphasis has been responsible for much of the success of the program. Every state and local American Lung Association provides programs on asthma and smoking, and offers professional and consumer information on lung cancer, emphysema, influenza, pneumonia, tuberculosis, allergies, and air pollution. In addition, the association sponsors summer camps for youth with asthma, workplace programs, radon testing, and programs for diverse communities, such as the African-American Tobacco Use Prevention Project in Faith Communities. The Association has an intensive and extensive research program. Financing of the association's program is primarily through Christmas Seal campaigns.

Cancer Associations

The American Cancer Society, Inc. was founded in 1913 "to disseminate knowledge concerning the

· ·

Figure 20-16

Lung cancer is gradually replacing breast cancer as the number one cause of cancer deaths among women in the industrialized world. Many voluntary health agencies direct programs at youth to reduce lung cancer trends such as the Smoke-Free Class of 2000 sponsored by the American Lung Association and the Starting Free: Good Air for Me programs sponsored by the American Cancer Society. *Source:* Photo by Zafar, courtesy World Health Organization.

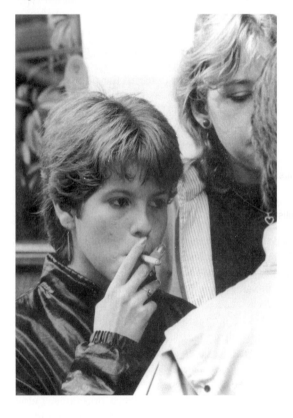

symptoms, diagnosis, treatment, and prevention of cancer; to investigate the conditions under which cancer is found; and to compile statistics in regard thereto." The society was established largely through the efforts of medical professionals, although the work of the organization has been carried on largely by lay people. Australia, Canada and other countries have counterpart associations called Cancer Foundations.

Educational programs designed by cancer agencies inform the public that cancer in its early stage can be cured; that early diagnosis is of primary importance, and that prompt, scientific treatment is the acknowledged method of cure. The educational campaigns often use an impersonal approach in an effort to avoid arousing fear of cancer. The agencies offer a wide array of patient services, prevention and detection programs, school health programs and special events.

In addition to public health education, cancer agencies encouraged health departments to expand their cancer programs; stimulated medical schools to extend their work in cancer research; and helped organize a National Advisory Cancer Council, which influenced the passage of the National Cancer Act and the creation of the National Cancer Institute as a part of the U.S. Public Health Service. Together with the American Lung Association and the American Heart Association, the American Cancer Society joined forces to create the National Interagency Council on Smoking.

The state affiliate of the society is called a "division" and, to use Michigan as an example, is titled American Cancer Society, Inc., Michigan Division. Operation of the program is basically on the county level and enlists the active participation of lay people in a program of health education.

Income of the American Cancer Society is derived from donations, dues, endowments, and legacies. In many instances citizens losing a family member because of cancer assign life insurance benefits to the society. The official publications of the society are *Cancer—A Journal of the American Cancer Society, CA—A Cancer Journal for Clinicians,* and *Cancer News.*

The March of Dimes Birth Defects Foundation

Founded in 1938 as the National Foundation for Infantile Paralysis, the March of Dimes Birth Defects Foundation has made substantial contributions to the health field. President Franklin D. Roosevelt, stricken by poliomyelitis, helped establish the foundation and, thereby, gave great impetus to

March of Dimes (MOD) Milestones

These selected milestones show how this foundation expanded its focus to birth defects following successful support for a polio vaccine. The full list of milestones is available on the Foundations website at http://www.midimes.org/about/mstones.htm.

1938   President Franklin Delano Roosevelt established the National Foundation for Infantile Paralysis; Comedian Eddie Cantor coins the phrase "March of Dimes," which becomes synonymous with the foundation.

1939   First MOD chapter established in Ohio.

1949   Project began to determine the number of polio virus types needed for a vaccine. Dr. Jonas Salk headed a participating laboratory.

1951   Scientists supported by MOD identified the three crucial polio virus types.

1953   Salk published the first report confirming the feasibility of a killed-virus vaccine for polio.

1954   MOD grantees received Nobel Prize for developing a method to grow polio virus; MOD began field trials of Salk vaccine with 1,830,000 school children.

1955   Results of field trials proved the Salk vaccine was "safe, potent and effective."

1958   MOD expanded concern for health of America's children by initiating the first concerted efforts to prevent birth defects.

1960   First MOD Birth Defects Center opened at Children's Hospital; MOD established The Salk Institute for Biological Studies; first global conference on birth defects brought together 480 scientists from twenty-six countries.

1961   Test developed to screen newborns for phenylketonuria, an inherited cause of mental retardation.

1962   Sabin oral polio vaccine, developed with support from the MOD, was licensed.

1969   MOD grantee shared the Nobel Prize for showing how genes direct normal development.

1973   Fetal alcohol syndrome, a specific pattern of birth defects, linked directly to alcohol consumption by pregnant women.

1979   Foundation officially changed name to March of Dimes Birth Defects Foundation.

1982   MOD launched "Babies and You," a workplace, prenatal education program.

1989   MOD launched its nationwide Campaign for Healthier Babies.

1996   FDA approved fortification of enriched grain products with folic acid, following three years of advocacy efforts by the MOD.

the organization. From its start, the foundation was financed through the March of Dimes program. Children saved allowances and contributed their own dimes during community drives.

Financial assistance from the March of Dimes was instrumental in demonstrating the effectiveness of the Salk vaccine in the 1954 poliomyelitis vaccine field trial. This assistance resulted in the shortest elapsed time between the discovery of a preventive measure and its widespread use. With success in supporting an effective vaccine for poliomyelitis, the March of Dimes expanded its efforts to the prevention of birth defects in 1958 (see box).

With several state chapters and more than nine-hundred local chapters, the March of Dimes sponsors programs concentrated on the prevention of birth defects, including prenatal care; teenage pregnancy prevention; and reduction of smoking, drug use, and alcohol use by pregnant women. The present program also includes investigation into birth defects (congenital defects) and genetic and nutritional disorders of the newborn.

Local chapters that are branches of the national organization give direct medical assistance and raise funds to maintain national and local activities. A considerable part of the funds raised locally remains in the community to promote the local program. Contemporary fund raising includes "Walkathons" and other community events.

Heart Associations

Originally formed as a scientific and professional organization of physicians interested in heart disease, the American Heart Association was reorganized in 1948 as a voluntary health agency with thousands of nonprofessional members affiliated with their state associations. The objective of the association is to prevent and control heart disease through research, professional education, public education, and community service. Canada and other countries have counterpart organizations called Heart and Stroke Foundations.

State or provincial and local heart associations have a large corps of volunteers who work together to plan and execute the associations' programs. The state heart association has a professional staff, which provides consultation services and works with the professional and lay volunteers in planning and implementing the education and fund-raising aspects of the program. Funds are raised by state or provincial drives and come from voluntary contributions, endowments, and legacies. Most of the Canadian and American Heart Association funds go into heart research or an allied activity.

The associations provide a wide range of programs and services including smoking cessation, nutrition, and weight control programs; speakers' bureaus; school health programs; community service programs to train volunteers in blood pressure measurement; and work simplification programs that demonstrate methods to help people who have had heart attacks organize their work in a manner that will limit stress and fatigue. The associations maintain information and referral services that include directories of cardiac services. The website provides extensive consumer information.

The Red Cross

The international Red Cross and Red Crescent societies have been most notable for their disaster relief and wartime care of casualties. The Red Cross was founded in 1881 in accordance with the Geneva Treaty of 1864, ratified by the United States in 1882, thanks to the efforts of Clara Barton. The purpose of the international organization is to protect life and health and to ensure respect for the human being. It seeks to prevent and alleviate human suffering impartially by not discriminating as to nationality, race, religious beliefs, class, or political opinions in its efforts.

The American Red Cross has a quasigovernmental status because it is incorporated under a charter granted by Congress in 1900. The president of the United States is president of the American Red Cross, an affiliate of the international organization, which has 127 national Red Cross societies. The organization provides a wide array of services including those directed at armed forces emergency, blood and tissue banking, disaster, health and safety, international, and youth. In times of peace, the American affiliate has established health centers, helped to conduct public health surveys, sponsored health demonstration projects and first aid and water safety programs and provided public health nursing service for rural areas that were not otherwise served. In 1981 the American Red Cross adopted a new set of priorities emphasizing health promotion and disease prevention. Its blood banking program has been most salient in recent years because of the HIV/AIDS epidemic. During natural disasters such as the San Francisco earthquake in 1989, Hurricane Andrew in 1992, and the great Midwest floods of 1993, the Red Cross provided relief efforts and organized volunteers to help the local victims.

The Red Cross works closely with private and governmental agencies at all levels—international (figure 20-17), national, state, and community, as a matter of policy. County chapters are formed but operate under the supervision of the national office, which establishes policies and must approve all local projects.

Figure 20-17

International Red Cross Societies work cooperatively with other international agencies on a range of activities from large scale international relief efforts to sponsoring a poster contest on the inclusive theme of "Friendship between disabled and other children." *Source:* World Health Organization.

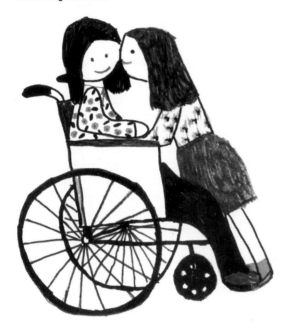

The National Urban League

Health has been a core program activity of the National Urban League since 1910. During its early years the National Urban League published a monthly health education bulletin, and for more than twenty years it stimulated local efforts such as dental clinics, immunization programs, tuberculosis screening, well-baby clinics, and a variety of convalescent care programs through its Annual Health Education Week.

Frustrated in its attempt to eliminate discrimination in employment in the health professions and in health facilities, the National Urban League, led by Dr. Montague Cobb, joined forces with the National Medical Association, the National Association for the Advancement of Colored People (NAACP), and the Medico-Chirurgical Society. This coalition spearheaded a vigorous attack on hospital discrimination between the late 1950s and the mid-1960s.

In 1962 the National Urban League adopted a policy statement supportive of family planning in the interest of strengthening family life and reducing individual and family dependency on welfare. This was a courageous move at a time when family planning was viewed by some black activists as **genocide.**

The National Urban League has identified health promotion and disease prevention as the area in which nonmedical community-based organizations can play a significant and strategic role in improving the health status of black Americans. Projects sponsored by the League have included evaluations of consumer health education and training programs, a study of health personnel resources and facilities, a poison control project, the development of allied health careers curricula in traditionally black colleges, dental services for preschool children, and a sickle-cell education/ screening program. Current programs also focus on healthy cities, families, retired persons, child health, and HIV/AIDS. The National Urban League firmly supports legislation for comprehensive and universal national health insurance and improvement of health services in local communities. The league continues to address these crucial issues through public testimony and participation in organized, broad-based coalitions.

Other Nonprofit Organizations

The national offices of these and other voluntary health agencies have attempted to ensure that new health legislation and special federal initiatives addressing community health provide for the participation of nonmedical community-based organizations. Therefore future health programs in such areas as high blood pressure education, HIV/AIDS, cancer education and screening, physical fitness, and nutrition will be more likely to provide for local outreach information and education activity.

Community-based organizations such as heart associations and National Urban League affiliates can qualify to operate funded programs in these health care areas. Funding, for the most part, must be obtained at the state level. This makes it particularly important for local affiliates of voluntary health agencies to stay abreast of statewide planning and the allocation of health funds to the local level from block grants at the state level.

SCHOOL HEALTH PROGRAM

The school health program, although dedicated to and supported by the education sector, should be considered as part of the community health program and therefore be integrated with it. The health of children and adults should be the concern of schools because they can contribute to and benefit from the health of both. Nearly 70 percent of all deaths—those caused by heart disease, cancer, and stroke—are linked to bad health habits established early in life.

School health programs include health services, health instruction, and a healthful environment. Health services provide appraisal and remediation of existing health-related conditions and prevention of future health problems. Health instruction addresses the future health of children through planned and incidental instruction. Healthful school environments include a sanitary and safe physical environment. It also incorporates consideration of the mental health of students and teachers. Administrators, teachers, parents, cafeteria workers, and the custodial staff are potential contributors to a healthful school environment.

Schools play a role in communicable and chronic disease control. Schools have the legal authority and the responsibility to take reasonable measures for promoting immunization. Courts have upheld the right of local boards of education to require immunization as a condition for school admission. Early recognition of infectious disease in schools depends on recognition by the teacher and confirmation by the school nurse. During an epidemic schools work cooperatively with the local public health agency and are governed by the regulation and recommendations of the LPHA. Although schools would seem to have a lesser role in chronic disease control, the most important risk factors for such diseases develop at young ages and track into adult life. Comprehensive school health education plays an important role in preventing these risk factors (see box on p. 656 and figure 20-18).

WORKSITE HEALTH PROMOTION PROGRAMS

Employers have specific responsibilities by law for the protection of workers from illness or injury that could result from the work environment. These were outlined in chapter 16. As a member of the community, the employer also has an opportunity to promote the health of workers, their families, and the community through policies and provisions that enable employees to have greater access to health services and health enhancing facilities. Specifically, screening programs and employee wellness programs have become increasingly common in large worksites around the United States. As an adjunct to community health programs, these sites provide the equivalent opportunity for adult health that schools provide for child health.

Scope of Worksite Health Promotion Programs

A national survey of worksites with fifty or more employees found that two-thirds had one or more health promotion programs, facilities, or services. More than half of these had been started within the five years preceding the survey. The types of programs ranged from health risk assessment (30 percent) to smoking cessation (36 percent), blood pressure control and treatment (16 percent), exercise and fitness (22 percent), weight control (15 percent), nutrition education (17 percent), stress management (27 percent), back problem prevention and care (28 percent), and off-the-job injury prevention education (20 percent).

Figure 20-18

The PRECEDE planning model outlined in chapters 4 and 12 was applied in a school-based community project to reduce heart disease risk factors in children. It produced significant improvements in several behavioral and physical measures of risk. *Source:* From Bush, P. J. 1989. *Am J Epidemiol* 129:466. Reproduced with permission.

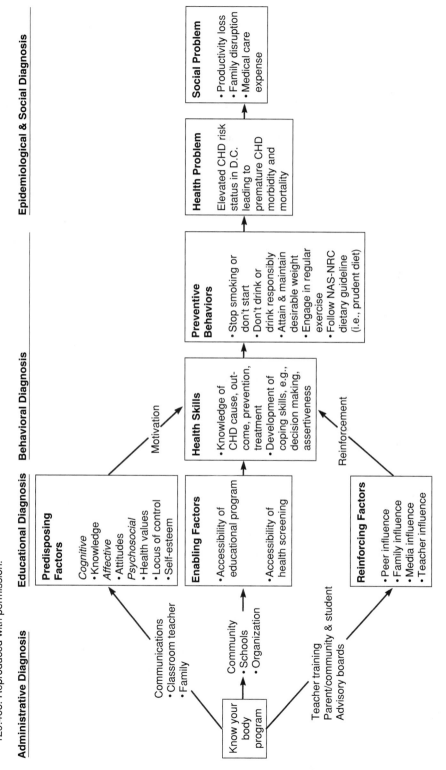

Case Study of a "Know Your Body" Program

A systematic application of the planning principles outlined in chapter 4 were applied in Washington, DC with black children in grades 4 to 6 who were attending nine District of Columbia elementary schools. The social problems of black children in these schools were those associated with poverty, as shown in figure 20-18. This schematic diagram also shows how the diagnostic planning model outlined in chapter 4 was applied to identify the epidemiological relationships; the behavioral risk factors; and preventive behaviors determining the health problems, the health skills that could influence the preventive behaviors, and the educational factors that a coordinated school program could influence to improve health skills (reading from right to left in figure 20-18). At the end of two years of intervention, results indicated that the program significantly reduced blood pressures, postexercise pulse recovery rates, cholesterol levels, and smoking. Significant improvements were found also for health knowledge and attitudes toward smoking. Schools need not develop their own health curriculum and teaching materials from scratch. Numerous model curricula and media are produced by organizations such as the American Health Foundation ("Know Your Body"), the voluntary health associations, and various state and federal health agencies.

Issues in Worksite Health Promotion

Despite their popularity with employees and their growing acceptance as a responsibility by employers, many health professionals have expressed concerns about the worksite wellness programs. The rapid development and diffusion of these programs have taken on the features of a social movement. Professionals who have devoted their careers to worker protection through the regulatory and collective bargaining routes express concern that the worksite health promotion programs could divert resources and attention from the prevention of occupational hazards in the work environment or the working conditions. Other health professionals worry that the scientific bases for promoting some of the lifestyle modifications in these programs have not been sufficiently validated.

Another issue that must be addressed in the further development of the worksite health promotion movement is the extent to which the programs reach the people who need them most. The programs have usually served "white collar" (executive, professional, and managerial) personnel and to a lesser extent "pink collar"(clerical) workers. They have barely penetrated the "blue collar" stratum of workers. Furthermore, the intensity of the programs has been limited by the problem of release time from work, hours of availability during the workday, and the cost of maintaining the programs. These limitations have resulted in variable participation rates and low maintenance rates. These problems plague all community health promotion programs, but the presumed advantage of the worksite in overcoming some of these problems has been less than complete.

EVALUATION

It is difficult to measure the effectiveness or value of community, school, and worksite health programs in terms of lives saved, illnesses prevented, and health improved. Inferential means of appraising a health program are based on the assumption that if a health or teaching staff provides certain activities or services, certain health benefits accrue to the public. This inference is based on independent studies, which have shown that certain services and activities produce certain public health results. This approach to evaluation is simply an accounting of services rendered, however. Many public health and education professionals evaluate by specifying the services a health department or a school should provide and then measuring the amount or proficiency of these services, rather than their effects. This approach to evaluation is called **quality assurance** or quality control.

Full-time city, county, or district health agencies provide direct health services that can be measured. These services provide various means for reducing the incidence of disease, lowering the death rate, reducing invalidism and dependency, preventing disabilities, correcting remediable defects, decreasing wage losses, reducing hospital and medical costs, and reducing hazards to health and life. Some agencies attempt to get periodic measures of these outcomes to appraise their programs.

In the final analysis the evaluation of community health services is greatly complicated by the relationship of health outcomes with aspects of poverty, culture, and the environment over which community health agencies, schools, and worksites have limited control. These relationships must be acknowledged and addressed by the community.

SUMMARY

Populations derive most of their local authority in health matters from the state and from common law. The state or province delegates much of its authority to the community, then exercises its rights of regulation over the quality of services delivered by the community health agency. The community establishes a health board at the municipal, county, or (in some states and Canada) district level to look after its interests. In 1974 the U.S. federal government introduced additional levels of planning authority with the establishment of Health Systems Agencies (HSAs), but most of these have not survived the cuts in federal subsidies for their funding in the 1980s. Model Standards for communities provide opportunities for local public health agencies to link local areas with national objectives in disease prevention and health promotion.

Community health agencies include the official local public health agency, other official agencies having health responsibilities, private organizations with proprietary interests in health, and a variety of voluntary agencies that address health concerns. Coordination of these entities is accomplished through United Way agencies or other health councils, sometimes staffed by official health department personnel.

The minimum services provided by the official community health agency include vital statistics record-keeping, maternal and child health care, communicable and chronic disease control, mental health services, laboratory services, and health education.

Consumers have an obviously deep and primary interest in community health services. The health professions alone cannot be the sufficient guardians of that interest. Consumers must have effective representation—wherever possible, a majority—in the policymaking processes of major health facilities and organizations. This representation must reflect all aspects of the community, including cultural, racial, and linguistic diversity. Special emphasis should be placed on meaningful representation of the poor and minority groups.

WEB*Links*

County and City Associations
http://www.astho.org Association of State and Territorial Health Officials
http://www.nachc.com National Association of Community Health Centers
http://www.naccho.org National Association of County and City Health Officials
http://www.apha.org/science/model/msmain.html
Healthy People 2000: Model Standards
http://www.phf.org Public Health Foundation
http://indyunix.iupui.edu/citynet/cnet.html
Healthy Cities

Voluntary Associations

http://www.arthritis.org/ Arthritis Foundation
http://www.cancer.org American Cancer Society
http://www.amhrt.org/ American Heart Association
http://www.lungusa.org/ American Lung Association
http://www.nf.lung.ca/ Canadian Lung Association
http://www.modimes.org March of Dimes
http://www.nul.org/ National Urban League
http://www.redcross.org/ American Red Cross
http://www.glen-net.ca/ccs/ Canadian Cancer Society

School Health

http://www.ed.gov/DrugFree U.S. Department
of Education
http://www.hc-sc.gc.ca/main/hc/web/datahpsb/
children/english/sec1-2.htm Bibliography on
comprehensive school health education
http://activeliving.ca/activeliving/cahperd/index.html
Canadian Association for Health Promotion, Education,
Recreation and Dance
http://www.hc-sc.gc.ca/main/hc/web/datahpsb/
children/english/sec1-3.htm/ Canadian Association
for School Health
http://www.aahperd.org/aahe/ American
Association for Health Education
http://www.lung.ca/resource.html Canadian Lung
Association school health resources
http://www.nchec.org/ National Commission for
Health Education Credentialing, Inc.

QUESTIONS FOR REVIEW

1. About one-tenth of the counties (and parishes) in the United States are without a full-time health department. What is the explanation for this situation?
2. If you lived in a county or parish without a full-time health department, what measures would you take to obtain full-time public health service?
3. What is "home rule"? Does it apply only to health matters?
4. Is it just or unjust that some people get more service than others from the county health department?
5. Which level of health department in the United States—federal, state, or local—is most likely to give service to the individual citizen?
6. Why aren't laws and regulations passed identifying as nuisances all conditions and practices that might cause hurt, injury, or inconvenience to people?

7. If a local health department refuses to take action to stop a condition that citizens regard as a nuisance, what action can the citizens take?
8. Why should there not be only medical doctors on the county board of health?
9. Why should decisions by the county board of health be subject to appeal to a court?
10. Why is it illogical to say that one position on the county health staff is more important to the public than is another?
11. Why does public health education employ a variety of media and methods of communication?
12. In matters of health, why are schools concerned with more than just health education in the classroom?
13. One of the purposes of the "Regional Medical Programs" in the mid-1960's was "to afford the medical profession the opportunity of making available to patients the latest advances" in health care. What does this statement say about power relationships between health professionals and citizens in health care? Did this Act support health as a right or a privilege?
14. What evidence can you present that people in the United States and Canada have better health today than those who lived there at the turn of the century, and what has been the contribution of official and voluntary health agencies?
15. How can development of worksite health promotion involve blue collar workers in the planning?
16. School and community health workers are often separated in not only their training programs, but in practice by the type of organization in which they work. What bridges can be built among health professionals—not just their organizations—to contribute to community health?

READINGS

Airhihenbuwa, C. O. 1995. *Health and culture: beyond the Western paradigm.* Newbury Park, CA: Sage.
In this book, a health educator explores the additional features required to make models such as Precede-Proceed more adaptable to local ethnic variations; developing countries; and Third-World or traditional cultures, communities and populations.
Goodman, R. M., and A. Wandersman. 1994. FORECAST: a formative approach to evaluating community coalitions and community-based initiatives.

J Community Psychol Mongraph Series CSAP Spec Issue: 6.

Formative evaluation enables local practitioners to influence project planning, development, and implementation. The method proposed in this article uses a combination of conceptual modeling of the logic or causal assumptions underlying a program and evaluation methods to assess the ways in which the coalition organized for the program addresses the presumed causes of the problem and the actions required to correct those causes.

MacDougall, H. 1990. *Activists and advocates. Toronto's health department, 1883–1983.* Toronto and Oxford: Dundurn Press.

This chronicle of the history of the City of Toronto Department of Public Health during its first hundred years captures the spirit of the public health movement during the latter nineteenth and early twentieth centuries, and how local citizens and health professionals advocated and worked for better community living conditions and life-styles.

Mantell, J. E., A. T. DiVittis, and M. I. Auerbach. 1997. *Evaluating HIV prevention interventions.* New York: Plenum Press.

This book outlines experience and recommendations for the monitoring and evaluation of HIV/AIDS prevention programs in community and clinical settings. Specifically suggests ways to apply the Precede-Proceed model in developing these local programs.

BIBLIOGRAPHY

Bailey, P. H., E. E. Rukholm, R. Vanderlee, and J. Hyland. 1994. A heart health survey at the worksite: The first step to effective programming. *AAOHN Journal* 42:9.

Bellingham, R. 1994. *Critical Issues in Worksite Health Promotion.* New York: Macmillan Publishing Co.

Berger, D., M. Inkelas, S. Myhre, and A. Mishler. 1994. Developing health education materials for inner-city low literacy parents. *Publ Health Rep* 109:168.

Boothroyd, P., L. W. Green, C. Hertzman, J. Lynam, J. McIntosh, W. Rees, S. M. Singer, M. Wackernagel, and R. Woollard. 1994. Tools for sustainability: Iteration and implementation. Chap. 10 in *Ecological Public Health: From Vision to Practice,* edited by Cordia Chu and Rod Simpson. Toronto: Centre for Health Promotion, University of Toronto.

Breckon, D. J., J. R. Harvey, and R. B. Lancaster. 1994. *Community health education: settings, roles, and skills for the 21st Century.* 3d ed. Gaithersberg, MD: Aspen Publishers, Inc.

British Columbia Ministry of Health, Community Health Division. 1994. *School-Based Prevention Model Handbook.* Victoria: BC Ministry of Health.

Cottrell, R. R., E. Capwell, and J. Brannan. 1995. Comprehensive school health conferences: the Ohio evaluation model. *Wellness Perspec* 11(4):55.

Cottrell, R. R., E. Capwell, and J. Brannan. 1995. A follow-up evaluation of non-returning teams to the Ohio Comprehensive School Health Conference. *J Wellness Perspec* 12(1):1.

Farthing, M. 1994. Health education needs of a Hutterite Colony. *Canadian Nurse/L'Infirmiere Canadienne* 90(7):20.

Frankish, C. J., and L. W. Green. 1994. Organizational and community change as the scientific basis for disease prevention and health promotion policy. In *Advances in Medical Sociology, Volume IV: A Reconsideration of Health Behavior Change Models,* edited by Gary L. Albrecht. Greenwich, CT: JAI Press Inc.

Garvin, T. 1995. "We're Strong Women" - Building a community-university research partnership. *Geoforum* 26:273.

Gilbert, G. G., and R. G. Sawyer. 1994. *Health Education: Creating Strategies for School and Community Health.* Boston & London: Jones & Bartlett Publishers.

Green, L. W., and C. J. Frankish. 1994. Theories and principles of health education applied to asthma. *Chest* 106(4, Suppl.); 219S.

Johnson, C. C., C. R. Powers, W. Bao, D. W. Harsha, and G. S. Berenson. 1994. Cardiovascular risk factors of elementary school teachers in a low socio-economic area of a metropolitan city: the Heart Smart Program. *Health Educ Res* 9:183.

Keintz, M. K., L. Fleisher, and B. K. Rimer. 1994. Reaching mothers of preschool-aged children with a targeted quit smoking intervention. *J Community Health* 19(1):25.

Kloos, H. 1995. Human behavior, health education and schistosomiasis control—a review. *Soc Sci Med* 40:1497.

Kreuter, M. W. 1992. PATCH: its origin, basic concepts, and links to contemporary public health policy. *J Health Educ* 23:135.

Kristal, A. R., R. E. Patterson, K. Glanz, J. Heimendinger, J. R. Hebert, Z. Feng, and C. Probart.

1995. Psychosocial correlates of healthful diets: baseline results from the Working Well study. *Prev Med* 24:221.

Kroger, F. 1994. Toward a healthy public. *Am Behavioral Sci* 38:215.

Lefebvre, R. C., L. Doner, C. Johnston, K. Loughrey, G. I. Balch, and S. M. Sutton. 1995. Use of database marketing and consumer-based health communication in message design: An example from the Office of Cancer Communications' 5 a Day for Better Health program. Chap. 12 in *Designing health messages: approaches from communication theory and public health practice,* edited by E. Maibach and R. L. Parrott. Thousand Oaks: Sage Publications Inc.

Mansour, A. A., and S. A. Hassan. 1994. Factors that influence women's nutrition knowledge in Saudi Arabia. *Health Care for Women Internat* 15:213.

Mathews, K., K. Everett, J. Binedell, and M. Steinberg. 1995. Learning to listen: formative research in the development of AIDS education for secondary school students. *Soc Sci Med* 41:1715.

McGowan, P., and L. W. Green. 1995. Arthritis self-management in Native populations of British Columbia: An application of health promotion and participatory research principles in chronic disease control. *Can J Aging* 14(suppl. 1):201.

McKenzie, J. F., and R. R. Pinger. 1997. *An introduction to community health.* Boston: Jones & Bartlett Publishing Co.

McKenzie, T. L., J. E. Alcaraz, and J. F. Sallis. 1994. Assessing children's liking for activity units in an elementary school physical education curriculum. *J Teaching Phys Educ* 13:206.

Morrison, S. D., and S. Dorfman. 1994. PRECEDE model as a framework for using health education in the prevention of diarrhea infant mortality in rural Mexico. *Eta Sigma Gamma Monogr Series* 12:41.

Nguyen, M. N., R. Grignon, M. Tremblay, and L. Delisle. 1995. Behavioral diagnosis of 30 to 60 year-old men in the Fabreville Heart Health Program. *J Community Health* 20:257.

O'Loughlin, J., G. Paradis, N. Kishchuk, K. Gray-Donald, L. Renaud, P. Fines, and T. Barnett. 1995. Coeur en santé St. Henri - a heart health promotion programme in Montreal, Canada: design and methods for evaluation. *J Epidem & Community Health* 49:495.

Paradis, G., J. O'Loughlin, M. Elliott, P. Masson, L. Renaud, G. Sacks-Silver, and G. Lampron. 1995. Coeur en sant± St. Henri - a heart health promotion programme in a low income, low education neighbourhood in Montreal, Canada: theoretical model and early field experience. *J Epidem & Community Health* 49:503.

Parks, C. P. 1995. Gang behavior in the schools: reality or myth? *Educational Psychol Rev* 7:41.

Pucci, L. G. 1994. "Naturally Smoke Free": a support program for facilitating worksite smoking control policy implementation in Sweden. *Health Prom Internat* 9:177.

Reichelt, P. A. 1995. Musculoskeletal injury: ergonomics and physical fitness in firefighters. *Occupational Med* 10:735.

Rimer, B. K. 1995. Audience and messages for breast and cervical cancer screenings. *Wellness Perspec* 11(2):13.

Rimer, B. K., C. T. Orleans, L. Fleisher, S. Cristinzio, N. Resch, J. Telepchak, M. K. Keintz. 1994. Does tailoring matter? The impact of a tailored guide on ratings and short-term smoking-related outcomes for older smokers. *Health Educ Res, Theory & Prac* 9(1):69.

Schumann, D. A., and W. H. Mosley. 1994. The household production of health: Introduction. *Soc Sci Med* 38:201.

Spruijt-Metz, D. 1995. Personal incentives as determinants of adolescent health behavior: the meaning of behavior. *Health Educ Res* 10:355.

Stivers, C. 1994. Drug prevention in Zuni, New Mexico: Creation of a teen center as an alternative to alcohol and drug use. *J Community Health* 19:343.

Turner, L. W., M. Sutherland, G. J. Harris, and M. Barber. 1995. Cardiovascular health promotion in North Florida African-American churches. *Health Values* 19(2):3.

Wortel, E., G. H. deGeus, G. Kok, and C. van Woerkum. 1994. Injury control in pre-school children: a review of parental safety measures and the behavioural determinants. *Health Educ Res* 9:201.

Chapter *21*

Personal Health Care Services and Resources

*O*ne of the first duties of the physician is to educate the masses not to take medicine.

—Sir William Osler, M.D.

*T*he greatest medications are those that are swallowed by the mind.

—Mohan Singh

Objectives

When you finish this chapter, you should be able to:

- Identify issues and the sources of protection for consumers of health services and health products

- Analyze major trends in personal health care resources, including types of

personnel and facilities available in a community

- Describe the major features of the personal health care systems of at least two other countries

Nations spending the most for training of physicians and other health care personnel, and for hospitals and other medical facilities, do not necessarily have the greatest life expectancy or the highest level of health. This paradox can be attributed to two factors. The first is the tendency of people and communities to expose themselves to risks in lifestyle and in the environment, as outlined in parts 2, 3, and 4 of this book. The second has been the difficulty in bringing the citizen who needs medical, dental, and other health care services together with the necessary service. The people who need health care the most often fail to receive the care they need.

The foregoing chapters analyzed health promotion, protection, and services at the community level. This chapter focuses on health and medical care at the individual level. A common bond between the health of the community and the individual is **primary health care.** As the World Health Organization and UNICEF declared in the Alma-Ata (see chapter 18), health of the individual and community are interwoven. Primary health care acknowledges health as a fundamental human right requiring support from all sectors of society. It concerns the health of the whole person, including the environment, and not just the illness of isolated body parts. Primary health care includes self-care education, health promotion, health resources and services for the whole person in the community context, and protection from fraudulent practices that rob the most vulnerable.

CONSUMER HEALTH PROTECTION

Millions of people are victims of ignorance in matters relating to self-care and the use of health products and services. Confidence in scientific fact and personal responsibility must replace health superstitions, fads, hopelessness, recklessness, and the gullible acceptance of extravagant claims and outright quackery. A primary requirement is recognition that health does not come in a package or in a clinic. It comes with a style of life, with protective measures in the environment, and with the appropriate and timely use of self-care products and health services.

Health Fraud

Quackery connotes selling a worthless treatment (whether the seller believes in its worth or not). **Health fraud** implies intent to deceive. Some promoters of quackery are sincere, but mistaken about the value of their products. Others are cynical manipulators intent on fame and a fast buck through fraud. Quacks may use worthless, unorthodox, or unproved treatments to cure or prevent disease by ineffective procedures, nostrums, and diagnostic and therapeutic devices. "Quack" comes from "*kwaksalver,*" Dutch for a boastful, and not necessarily reliable, peddler of salves. Rembrandt titled his drawing of a street vendor of nostrums with this word in 1635. **Nostrums** are unauthorized, secret, or patented substances or devices for which quacks or advertisers make false therapeutic claims.

Populations inadequately educated in matters of health protection, especially where scientific medicine has lost touch with people's needs, allow quacks to operate. Many people have emotional needs not adequately met by physicians and other licensed practitioners. Health fraud flourishes in such settings.

The appeals have changed little since pitchmen in the frontier sold "golden elixir" from the back of a horse-drawn wagon. The U.S. Food and Drug Administration (FDA) has identified nine categories in which medical fraud is most frequent: figure enhancers, arthritis and pain relievers, sleeping aids, hair and scalp treatments, youth prolongers, sex aids, pure air and water devices, disease diagnosers, and cure-alls. The fitness movement and HIV/AIDS have brought out a whole new generation of health fraud and quackery. Today's promotional methods differ in their range, using telephone banks and computer-generated lists to help find opportune targets, particularly the victims of arthritis and cancer.

One argument justifies quackery on grounds that it makes people feel good or gives them options in hopeless situations. Users of useless treatments, however, lose valuable time in seeking valid treatment. Others may experience dangerous treatments. Still others lose hope when they feel duped or experience guilt that their illness was caused by a lack of "natural harmony" with their body. All lose money.

Varieties of health fraud include drug and cosmetic, food and nutrition, and electrical and mechanical. Some quacks use all three, but others operate only one form as long as it is profitable and they can avoid legal prosecution.

Drug and Cosmetic Quackery Some proprietary drugs mask pain and distress and therefore delay the point at which the person finally seeks medical diagnosis (figure 21-1). Such delay can be critical with signs or symptoms related to conditions such as heart disease or cancer. Drug quackery exists in many forms—rejuvenation nostrums, blood purifiers, hay fever remedies, breast developers, sex vitalizers, nerve tonics, and concoctions that claim to "cure" the range of chronic ailments including cancer and arthritis. Cosmetic quackery appears as skin "foods," hormone creams, "complex vitamin creams for a complex world," skin restorers, geriatric cosmetics, salves, tablets, and every conceivable potion. These nostrums usually

••••••••••••••••••

Figure 21-1

Quackery preys on those aspects of health and medical needs for which people seek pain relief or simpler solutions than those offered by conventional medicine and "official" health advice. Particular targets include arthritis, fitness, weight loss, cancer, HIV/AIDS, and beauty or sexual attractiveness. *Source:* Photo courtesy Alberta Heritage Foundation for Medical Research.

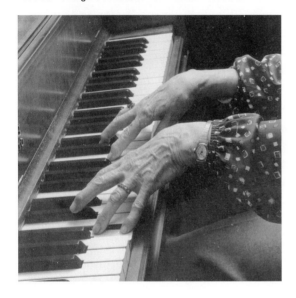

do nothing. They sometimes do harm directly or indirectly if they mask signs or symptoms that need medical attention such as skin rashes, lesions, lumps, or discoloration.

Nutrition and Weight-Loss Quackery   Stores and catalogues have offered "health foods" for centuries as natural foods, organic foods, exotic foods, miracle foods, bee products, and other dietary cure-alls. "Nutrition experts" and "health lecturers" write best-selling books on food fads. Nutrition education has failed when food and nutrition quacks find a clientele eager to pay exorbitant prices for the same foods available at regular food markets at less than half their cost. Those in the multibillion-dollar weight loss industry who promise quick and painless weight loss while

eating all one wants without exercise, have a ready audience in the increasingly overweight population. Too many people want their weight loss as fast and convenient as their foods. Some nutritionists and consumer advocates have devoted their careers to developing a marketplace more conducive to consumer awareness of the contents and relative price and value of the foods they buy (see box on p. 665).

Anti-Aging Quackery   Baby-boomers, poised to swell the ranks of older Americans and Canadians, have become a rapidly growing market for those who sell magical or miracle potions or advice for staving off the aging process. Many of the advice books are well-intended self-help and self-care manuals, but they usually oversimplify the task of staying fit and healthy in old age. They also overpromise the hope of reversing the inevitability of the aging process. Titles seen in recent years include "Stop Aging Now!," "Earl Mindell's Anti-Aging Bible," "Ageless Body, Timeless Mind," "Dr. Mollen's Anti-Aging Diet," "Reversing Human Aging," and "Stay Young the Melatonin Way." The search for the fountain of youth has changed only in the new forms of the mythical fountain (from blood of young men transfused to old men in the Middle Ages, to plastic surgery, to hormone and vitamin supplements) and in the absolute and relative numbers of older people. Though many of the antiaging books are written by physicians and are based on research, the research (such as that on Melatonin and antioxidants) is often weak or not yet sufficiently replicated to be taken as evidence worthy of the claims made for the methods they promote. The best advice remains the selection of lifestyle habits that provide the best chance of being healthy while one grows old. However the work of exercise and other self-care practices seems too tedious to the many who seek shortcuts.

Electronic and Mechanical Nostrums   Quacks often lease rather than sell fraudulent devices. This can be a clever bit of strategy from the

The Hippocratic Oath

I swear by Apollo the physician, by Aesculapius, Hygeia and Panacea, and all the gods and goddesses, to keep to the best of my ability and judgment the following Oath: To reckon him who taught me this Art (of medicine) as dear to me as my own parents; to share my goods with him; to look upon his children as my own brothers; to teach them this Art if they so desire without fee or written promise; to impart a knowledge of the Art to my sons and the sons of the master who taught me, and to such disciples as have bound themselves to the rules of the profession—but to no others. I will prescribe regimen for the good of my patients to the best of my ability and judgment, and do harm to nobody. I will give no deadly medicine to anyone, even if it is requested, nor give advice that might result in death. Nor will I give a woman a pessary to produce abortion.

With purity and holiness will I practice my Art. I will not cut persons suffering from kidney stone but will leave this to be done by specialists in that Art. Whatever houses I visit, I shall enter only for the good of my patients, abstaining from any willful evil-doing and corruption, and especially from the se-

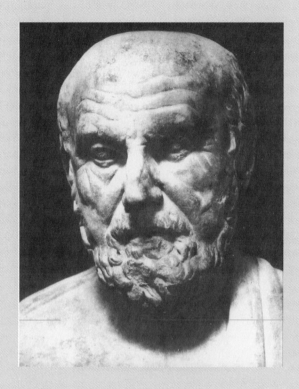

duction of women or men, whether they be free or slaves. All that may come to my knowledge in the exercise of my profession or in daily commerce with men, which ought not to be spread abroad, I will keep

secret and never reveal. If I keep this Oath faithfully, may I long enjoy life and the practice of my Art, respected by all men in all times. But should I swerve from it or violate it, may the reverse be my lot!

legal standpoint and from the sales angle. Charms, crystals, "galvanic" belts, amulets, "radionized" water, water purifiers, radioactive ore, and other devices with equally mysterious designations are offered to the public and readily bought or rented by people who are desperate. The term "electronic" is to devices as the term "organic" is to foods and "secret formula" is to cosmetics. These features make the product appear advantageous.

Advertising Quacks use advertising and testimonials, but not in reputable scientific journals. The basis of most quack treatment is "secret," which makes the source unknowable and untestable. They use the name of a high-sounding organization, often a "foundation," and the endorsements of actors, writers, athletes, politicians, or look-alikes for any of these. Quacks usually refuse inspection, contend that "the medical establishment" is persecuting them, and, when challenged, promise to

Esther Peterson (1906–1997): Consumer Advocate and Protector

In her years in the Old Executive Office Building, across from the White House, Esther Peterson served the American consumer and pioneered innovations in consumer protection that have influenced laws and regulations in countries around the world. She served the U.S. federal administrations of John F. Kennedy, Lyndon B. Johnson, and Jimmy Carter. She continued after her posts as Special White House Advisor on Consumer Affairs working for businesses as Vice President for Consumer Affairs for Giant Food, Inc., the largest supermarket chain in the Baltimore-Washington area. She later served as consumer advisor to the National Association of Professional Insurance Agents where she concerned herself with the problems of older people while also serving on the Board of the Consumers Union.

Ms. Peterson received a bachelor's degree from Brigham Young University in 1927 and a master's from Columbia Teachers' College in 1930. She began her career in a series of teaching positions in the 1930s, then a series of jobs with unions in the 1940s and 1950s. President Kennedy appointed her Assistant Secretary of Labor and Director of the Women's Bureau in 1961. This agency administered the labor laws concerning women. President Johnson brought her into the White House as a special advisor on consumer affairs. Between government appointments in the 1970s and after serving the Carter Administration in a similar capacity in the early 1980s, she developed a new career as consumer advocate within industry, working for Giant Food. She persuaded the supermarket to disclose what seafood had been previously frozen and to try nutritional labeling on its private products, comparing calories and proteins. She convinced them also to use open dating to indicate clearly to the consumer, not just in code for the clerks stocking the shelves, when perishable products should be sold. These practices, now commonplace and required by law in many places, were new to the retail food industry.

make their methods or drugs available to health authorities—but they seldom follow through on such a promise. Cultists, hypnotists, arthritis "specialists," and purveyors of devices use dramatic "health lectures," "clinics," late night "infomercials," and demonstrations. Communication media rules permit the advertising of products under freedom of speech protections. The Food and Drug Administration may intervene when the advertisement makes a direct claim of health benefits that have not been established by the FDA.

Insurance Fraud   With the aging of populations, insurance fraud has become more frequent and more noticeable as families seek to cash or redeem policies held for many years. After a two-year investigation, for example, Florida officials in 1997 concluded that the Prudential Insurance Company of America, the largest insurer in the United States, had deliberately cheated its customers for more than thirteen years. The investigative report said the company had "trained its agents to mislead, misrepresent and defraud policyholders." They presented some life insurance policies to customers as pensions and long-term health care programs. Agents targeted the elderly. Health insurance fraud has been widespread in selling supplemental plans for those covered by Medicare, in misrepresenting the benefits of such plans, and in charging the federal government inappropriately for services provided to Medicare beneficiaries.

Protection of Consumers

People reasonably expect protection by their governmental agencies so that they are not victims of the fraudulent claims of health charlatans. Legal agencies afford this protection after the fact. Professional organizations offer more proactive help by setting standards and developing or managing mechanisms of "quality control."

Consumers need two kinds of information. One is information for **informed consent** (whether or not to use a product, submit to a medical or surgical procedure, or take a medication). The other is information for safe and effective use of a product or service after the initial decision to use it has been made. At the very minimum, a consumer has the right to information about risks and benefits associated with any product or procedure. It is appropriate for governments and institutions to establish some core, or "floor," of information that should be available to their citizens or members. The prescribing physician and pharmacist can best decide what information and how to relay it in the case of prescribed medications (figure 21-2). Government agencies must regulate the information required in the advertising and packaging of nonprescription drugs. Prescribed and nonprescribed drugs may require a **patient package insert** to be enclosed with the medication package to inform the user of the possible side effects of the drug.

Nutritional Labeling of Food   Progressive legislation in the 1970s gave consumer protection a new lease on life. Food labeling laws passed by the U.S. Congress in the 1970s and again in the early 1990s represented a fundamental shift in regulatory philosophy that put more information and power in the hands of consumers (see box, p. 665). Deregulation in the 1980s left the 1970's laws only partially implemented, but the new food labels mandated in the 1990s made each packaged food product a source of essential nutrient information. Efforts were made to make the labels less confusing to the average consumer. When a product describes itself as "lite" or "light," does it have fewer calories, lower fat, less sodium, a fluffy texture, scant seasoning, or less breading than similar products? Laws now define what producers may call "light," but many consumers remain confused on this and other terms. While trying to understand current products, consumers face an average of 12,000 new food products annually. Most of these change their labels regularly to emphasize newness or innovation in the product. Information

about food contents also needs extension to the daily scramble of 46 million people who eat in fast food restaurants.

The Nutrition and Labeling and Education Act of 1990 enabled consumers to find complete nutrition information on most packaged foods, raw produce, and fish. The rules make it possible to compare serving sizes for similar items. They clearly define descriptor claims such as "lite" and "low calorie." They regulate health messages to ensure that they are supported by scientific evidence. They also make ingredient statements more informative (see chapter 12).

It is impossible to list in the space of a label everything that consumers might need to know. Health educators usually agree that the effect of a labeling program depends on information made available to consumers in other ways. Consumers need a foundation of knowledge from schooling and general consumer education to use labels effectively and to comprehend other messages at point of purchase or point of use.

Generic Drugs   The FDA's compilation in 1980 of the Approved Drug Products List gave American consumers another protection. Generic drug products are those sold under their established chemical name. They often sell for less than brand-name products. Consumers pay higher prices when they buy prescription drugs under their brand names when therapeutically equivalent drugs are available for less.

The Approved Drug Products List includes the thousands of prescription drug products that the FDA believes to be therapeutically equivalent to others within a therapeutic category based on criteria proposed for evaluation of therapeutic equivalency. Consumers can save when the pharmacist dispenses an available lower-cost drug product. For example, a patient prescribed ampicillin, a common antibiotic, can save money if the pharmacist dispenses a generic ampicillin product, knowing that the FDA has approved it as therapeutically equivalent to higher-priced brand-name versions. Prescription drugs also cost more in the United

· · · · · · · · · · · · · · · · · · · ·
Figure 21-2

The best protection against the misuse of prescription drugs is patient education. This campaign appeals to physicians to talk to their patients about medications and to parents to talk to their physician, their pharmacist, and their children. *Source:* National Council on Patient Information and Education.

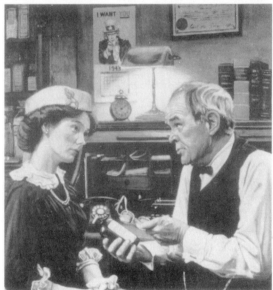

What Is a Food Additive?

A food additive is any substance added to food. Legally, the term refers to "any substance the intended use of which results or may reasonably be expected to result—directly or indirectly—in its becoming a component or otherwise affecting the characteristics of any food." This definition includes any substance used in the production, processing, treatment, packaging, transportation, or storage of food.

If a substance is added to a food for a specific purpose in that food, it is referred to as a *direct additive*. For example, the low-calorie sweetener aspartame, used in beverages, puddings, yogurt, chewing gum, and other foods, is considered a direct additive. Many direct additives are identified on the ingredient label of foods.

Indirect food additives are those that become part of the food in trace amounts due to its packaging, storage, or other handling. For instance, minute amounts of packaging substances may find their way into foods during storage. Food packaging manufacturers must prove to the U.S. Food and Drug Administration (FDA) that materials coming in contact with food are safe before they are permitted for use in such a manner.

Source: U.S. Food and Drug Administration, Washington, DC. For further information call 301-827-4420.

States than in Canada. Only one in five drugs cost more in Canada than in the United States.

Patient Protection Act of 1997   The U.S. Congress passed legislation in 1997 that provides several protections for consumers of health care and making health plan and insurance companies more accountable to patients and their families.

- **Access to emergency services.** Establishes a toll-free number, available twenty-four hours a day, for preauthorization of emergency visits, and requires health plan companies to consider clear criteria before denying services or coverage.
- **Disclosure of financial incentives to providers to limit or deny care.** Health plan companies (managed care, HMOs, health insurers) must provide enrollees with information in English, Spanish, Vietnamese, and Hmong about methods of reimbursement. This provision is aimed particularly at the practices of some managed care providers of giving financial rewards or incentives to the physicians and hospitals to limit the number of days of hospitalization, the number of tests, and other costly aspects of care.

- **Access to specialists.** Consumers will have access to procedures used by HMOs to determine access to specialist care and visits to their doctor if the enrollee changes plans or if the doctor leaves the plan.
- **Ban on gag clauses for whistle-blowers.** Protects health care workers when speaking out against health plan company policies and advocating for their patients.
- **Exclusive contracts are prohibited.** Keeps health plan companies from demanding exclusive contracts for their medical providers.
- **Simple billing.** When a patient is required to pay any portion of a bill, excluding flat copayments, the health plan must provide an explicit and easy-to-understand invoice. This means that any deductible portions of any medical bill must show the details of what the patient is required to pay and why.
- **Consumer oversight.** A consumer advisory board composed of "true consumers" (people who are not profiting in some way from the provision of medical or nursing services) will be responsible for making recommendations to the state legislature on patient protections and educating the public on health care issues.

- **Disclosure of executive salaries.** Health plans must make public the company's five highest paid salaries.
- **Provider identification.** Any licensed health care provider must wear a nametag.

Consumer Protection Agencies

The U.S. Food and Drug Administration and the Health Protection Branch of Health Canada
As described in chapters 15 and 18, the FDA conducts thousands of inspections and court actions per year in the United States. Health Canada's Health Protection Branch performs the same functions for Canada. Some of the actions involve seizure of harmful products and requests for injunctions restraining persons from continuing a practice or selling products hazardous to public health. These agencies also test products; set standards; pass on claims; investigate imports; and cooperate with state or provincial and local officials in matters of food and drug production, marketing, adulteration, and contamination.

The Federal Trade Commission The Federal Trade Commission (FTC) has authority over false advertising and deceptive practices in the United States. Following complaints, the commission investigates and may issue orders to the offending person or firm to cease and desist from continuing the practice. Many people accept the validity of advertisements for health products on the belief that they must be factually correct or such health protection agencies as the FDA and FTC would not permit them to appear. Without complaints from health professionals or consumers, however, much false advertising never comes to the attention of these agencies.

The Postal Service Most countries prevent the use of the mail service for the shipment and sale of deceptive, adulterated, contaminated, or fraudulent foods, drugs, cosmetics, or devices. A professional or consumer complaint is sufficient to initiate an investigation, followed by legal action when appropriate. In 1997, the U.S. Postal Inspection Ser-

vice joined with the FTC and others in a campaign to collect and review fraudulent mail to shut down the scams before they become widespread. Telemarketing fraud usually originates with a phony offer or sweepstakes notice that comes in the mail. Respondents to the mailed offers become the victims then of telemarketing phone calls, followed by the use of the mails again to collect their money. The antifraud campaign will mobilize volunteers to collect, sort, and analyze suspicious mail and pass it on to law enforcement officials.

The Consumer Product Safety Commission
The Consumer Product Safety Commission (CPSC) evaluates the safety of consumer goods in the United States. The box titled "Consumer Products Safety Alert" illustrates the frequency and types of *Safety Alerts* issued by the CPSC in two recent years. Some systems that assist the CPSC in assessing injury rates include a computerized compilation of emergency room records, coroners' reports, and consumer hot lines. Depending on the degree of hazard assessed, actions taken by the CPSC include (1) working through voluntary standards organizations, (2) information and education campaigns, (3) mandatory labeling, (4) banning, and (5) recall. The first two approaches involve some costs and may meet with industry resistance. The last three are the most expensive, generally meet with the greatest resistance, and are reserved for products that pose the greatest hazards.

Nongovernmental Professional and Voluntary Agencies Professional associations of physicians, nurses, and health educators, among others, have advocated and educated on behalf of the public and personal health care or health product consumers. The American Medical Association (AMA), for example, has variously supported a Bureau of Investigation, a Council on Foods and Nutrition, and a Committee on Cosmetics. Such units work with state medical associations to carry out examinations of clinical or experimental evidence, biopsy or autopsy data, drug samples, and publication of results of studies.

Consumer Product Safety Alert

These Consumer Product Safety Alerts about some hazards to children were published in recent years by the U.S. Consumer Product Safety Commission:

Child-Resistant Packaging
Toy Guitar Strap Strangulations
Art Materials
Movable Soccer Goals Can Tip Over
Mesh Playpens
Child-Resistant Cigarette Lighters
Playground Cargo Net Strangulations
Baby Walkers
Caps for Toy Guns
Infant Cushion Ban
Infant Carrier Seats
Stroller Entrapment
Bucket Drownings
Baby Bath Rings—Drowning Hazard
Crib Toys
Strangulation on Wall Decorations
All-Terrain Vehicles
Burns on Hot Metal Playground Equipment
Poisonings with Iron-Containing Medicine
Automatic Garage Door Openers
Child Drownings in the Home
New Hair Dryers Prevent Electrocutions
Strings and Cords Can Strangle Children on Playground Equipment
Safety Devices
In-Line Roller Skates
Crib Corner Posts
Strings and Cords Can Strangle Infants
Bed Entrapment/Suffocation

Source: From the U.S. Consumer Product Safety Commission, Washington, DC. For updates call 1-800-638-2772.

The Canadian and American Cancer Societies and the Arthritis Foundations of the respective countries are examples of other agencies that alert the public to fraudulent health claims. Patients with cancer or arthritis are prime targets of quacks, and special vigilance is essential to protect these patients because of their greater desperation and vulnerability to deceptive claims. The Council of Better Business Bureaus also is alert to health frauds and provides public information on the reputability of companies, vendors, and service providers. Some companies have aligned themselves with voluntary and professional health organizations to lend credibility to their products. See, for example, the SmithKline Beecham Consumer Healthcare web site for information on the stop smoking product, Nicorette, endorsed by the American Cancer Society (www.nicorette.com). The American Dental Association has endorsed various toothpastes with fluoride for many years (see Issues and Controversies box).

The American Association of Retired Persons (AARP) is the largest membership organization lobbying and educating for consumer protection in health and related matters. It is an active member, for example, of the Postal Inspection campaign mentioned previously to curb mail fraud. As an advocacy organization for its growing segment of the population, it carries considerable influence in Washington, DC, where it is has its headquarters.

The Center for Science in the Public Interest and other consumer advocacy groups in Washington, DC and in Ottawa, lobby on behalf of consumers on specific issues such as nutrition, tobacco control, and pharmaceuticals. They serve as watchdogs for truth in labeling and truth in advertising. Most also have active publication programs with popular magazines such as *Consumer Reports* or newsletters subscribed through memberships (see http://www.consumerreports.org).

Most such official and voluntary agencies help protect against quackery and false advertising, but individuals remain vulnerable without self-protection. Education concerning recognition of symptoms requiring diagnosis is the first measure. The second need is education to select and to use wisely the available medical, dental, and hospital services when necessary, and safe forms of self-care.

ISSUES AND CONTROVERSIES

Professional, Voluntary, or Governmental Endorsement of Health Products?

Several professional and voluntary health organizations, and even some government agencies, have collaborated with private industry in developing or marketing some products. Everyone accepts that government has a role in stimulating and facilitating research in areas that may benefit the development of products and industries that will increase jobs and international competitiveness. It becomes more questionable when government and tax-exempt organizations such as voluntary health agencies and professional associations support or endorse specific health care products or services. A question arises whether tax-supported organizations create unfair competition in the marketplace, as when the U.S. Department of Health and Human Services joined Quaker Oats in promoting the nutritional value of high-fiber foods such as oatmeal. The same department also came under attack from some developers of Health Risk Appraisal instruments when the Centers for Disease Control developed its own Health Risk Appraisal. The government product could be made available at much lower cost and copied freely because it was in the public domain. The issue of unfair competition arises frequently in the health field.

Other issues arise with the endorsement by a voluntary or professional health association of a product such as toothpaste or a brand of food. The American Cancer Society's endorsement of Nicorette, the American Heart Association's offering of a "heart healthy" label to food products meeting their standards of lower fat and cholesterol, and the American Dental Association's endorsement of fluoride toothpastes, all came under attack. The questions raised included concerns about the possible conflict of interest if the companies were paying a fee to the health organizations or donating funds to the organizations. The Heart Association, for example, used its food-labeling plan for a short time as a fund-raising strategy that could provide a public service at the same time. They quickly abandoned this when questions were raised about the size of the fee and the difficulty of smaller companies paying such a fee to have their products endorsed.

One site on the world wide web is devoted to identifying and tracking health fraud: http://www.quackwatch.com. It contains a bibliography and a gallery of misleading ads with analyses. Students and instructors are invited to submit ads with analyses.

ALTERNATIVE AND COMPLEMENTARY HEALTH CARE

Struggling to distance itself from the stigma of quackery and to gain respectability in western countries is a range of practices identified as alternative and **complementary medicine** or health care. A survey reported in the *New England Journal of Medicine* in 1993 stated that one-third of Americans said they used at least one unconventional therapy in the past year. This was much higher than previously reported, forcing the mainstream medical and health professions to take notice of the apparently growing influence of this branch of services and therapies.

A 1994 to 1995 survey in Canada, where one might expect a lower use of alternative medicine given the universal access to conventional medical services, showed the proportion of the population using alternative and complementary health to be more than half, 5 percent within the past year. In Canada, 47 percent of people over 12 years of age had used a massage therapist, 27 percent had used a homeopath or naturopath, and 17 percent had used an acupuncturist. Other alternative or complementary providers such as herbalists, reflexologists, spiritual healers, and relaxation therapists were seen by less than 8 percent of the population. The two surveys cannot be compared directly because the Canadian survey did not count chiropractors as alternative therapists; the U.S. survey did.

One-third of the American sample saw providers for unconventional therapy. This group had an average of 19 visits to such providers during the previous year, with an average charge per visit of $27.60. These numbers indicate that alternative and complementary medical visits outnumber primary care physician visits. The costs, three-fourths of which were paid out of pocket, are comparable to the amount paid out of pocket annually by Americans for all hospitalizations. Chiropractors were the most frequently visited, used by 10 percent of the population in the past year, 70 percent of whom visited chiropractors with an average of 13 visits in 12 months. This fits with the most frequently reported medical condition, back problems, for which 36 percent used unconventional therapy in the past 12 months and 19 percent saw chiropractors or massage therapists.

One boost to the recognition of unconventional therapies was the establishment of an Office of Alternative Medicine by the U.S. National Institutes of Health (NIH). Another was the determination that almost 60 percent of American physicians refer patients to alternative practitioners and use such practices for their health care and that of their families. Then the FDA in 1996 took acupuncture needles off its list of "experimental" medical devices, recognizing that they were no longer experimental. In 1997 an NIH consensus panel endorsed acupuncture as clearly effective in relieving a variety of symptoms (postoperative pain and nausea and vomiting from chemotherapy and anesthesia). They found it possibly effective as well with migraines, arthritis, menstrual cramps, low-back pain, and tennis elbow. They also noted it has the advantage over many conventional Western medicines of having virtually no side effects.

Part of the shift in recognition given to alternative and complementary health care has been the growing emphasis on quality of life in treatment decisions as chronic and terminal illnesses. Side effects of western medicines and surgeries have exceeded the benefits some patients feel they have received from those treatments.

Herbal medicine spans the gap between conventional and unconventional treatments. Herbal medicine is integral to traditional medicine, but also to western medicine and pharmacy, which derive 25 percent of their modern drugs from higher plants. Indeed, the word "drug" derives from the Dutch word *droge,* which means to dry, as plants were dried for use as medicines. Scientists conduct thousands of studies each year on the chemistry, pharmacology, toxicology, and clinical use of hundreds of herbs. Most of these studies, conducted in Europe, seldom are reported in North American medical journals. Many industrialized countries have incorporated herbs and phytomedicines, or advanced herbal extracts, into the health care systems. Germany leads in this with a commission under the federal health agency that has reviewed the safety and efficacy of more than three-hundred herbs sold in German pharmacies.

Self-Care And Mutual Aid

Self-care and **mutual aid** are the largest segment of health care. What people do for themselves, their families and friends without personalized professional advice or intervention amounts to more than 95 percent of health care activity. People carry on much of it without symptoms as preventive self-care, including conscious lifestyle practices intended to avoid exposure to hazards, prevent diseases, or promote one's health. Some of it they do when symptoms or minor injuries occur, by way of self-medication with over-the-counter nonprescription drugs or first aid. Aging populations with chronic and degenerative conditions—incurable but controllable in their symptoms or their complications through self-management—account for a growing proportion of self-care and mutual aid. Some of this is through mutual aid in **self-help groups,** such as postcoronary groups, arthritis self-management groups, diabetes self-care groups, and others.

Potential Benefits to Society   Self-care and mutual aid have the potential to reduce costs of medical care and lost productivity and will contribute to an industry in which Canada and the United States have provided international leadership. The ten categories of cost-leading chronic diseases and conditions based on direct medical care expenditures, disability days, and lost productivity include:

1. cardiovascular diseases and events (hypertension, heart, and stroke);
2. musculoskeletal diseases (arthritis and rheumatism);
3. respiratory diseases (asthma, bronchitis, emphysema);
4. cancer;
5. sense-organ diseases (visual and hearing loss);
6. diabetes;
7. injury disability;
8. dental health; and
9. the wider range of emotional, mental, and addictive conditions.

The last group could move up the ranking to the extent that emotional, mental, and addictive conditions cause some of the other problems. All of these lend themselves to greater self-care and mutual aid, especially as the population ages and increases in education.

Demand and Growth for Self-Care   The North American health care systems have given insufficient place to educational and other patient decision-support technologies to keep pace with the appetite of the public for access to self-care and health information and for connection with others who have similar problems. These offer an enormous market for the private sector, a missed opportunity for government to save millions in direct costs of unnecessary medical services, and for industry to save additional billions in the indirect costs of absenteeism and lost productivity. The need to address these issues now and the potential to contribute more through self-care and mutual aid are multiplied by the aging of the baby-boom generation.

The needs and economic opportunities presented by self-care and mutual aid are to support more autonomous control of health by local populations, families, and individuals. These offer more effective ways of controlling the spiral of medical care costs and lost productivity than the financial patchwork of solutions being imposed on hospitals, health personnel, and taxpayers.

Home Testing   One example that falls in the gray area between consumer protection against commercial exploitation and the large opportunity for self-care to contribute to cost savings is home tests. Thermometers for mothers to test baby's temperature have been standard home-testing equipment for generations. Home-testing kits for blood sugar by diabetics have been well accepted by the medical profession for years. Home blood pressure monitoring devices for people with hypertension have become more professionally accepted after initial resistance from the medical profession and the American Heart Association. More controversial pregnancy testing kits have been on the market for several years. Home kits are also available on ovulation, cholesterol, rectal and colon cancer, bowel obstructions, urinary-tract infections, and the level of elements such as protein and ascorbic acid in urine.

The FDA and the Health Protection Branch of Health Canada have recently or expect soon to approve new self-test kits for HIV, hepatitis, some other cancers, strep throat, Lyme disease, blood-alcohol levels, substance abuse, and the bacteria that cause ulcers. The industry refers to these kits as **in-vitro diagnostic devices.** Laboratories and home self-test kits use these to expose a sample of bodily material such as blood or urine to a chemical to signal the presence or absence of a hormone or other element in the bodily material. These are part of a growing market for self-care products and at-home medical services including books, toll-free telephone hot lines, health-care CD-ROMs, and computer software.

Limitations in Self-Care and Mutual Aid   Self-care inevitably carries some risk of people delaying or denying themselves needed medical attention. Most agree, however, that the U.S. and

· · · · · · · · · · · · · · · · · · ·

Figure 21-3

"White-coat blood pressure" was long suspected of yielding higher than normal readings because patients felt a rush of anxiety in the presence of the health professional taking **sphygomanometer** readings. Home self-monitoring devices might relieve this problem, but might introduce others. On balance, home self-testing promises far greater advantages to the public than disadvantages. *Source:* Photo by Zafar, courtesy World Health Organization.

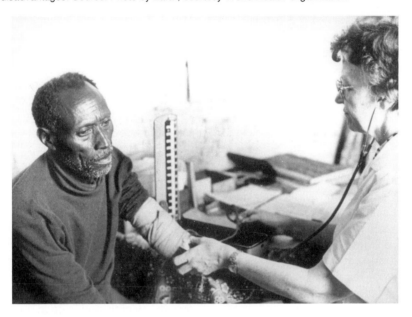

Canadian health care systems suffer from overuse more than underuse. Greater use of health services since the passage of Medicare and Medicaid has not accounted for much improvement in health status for the poor and previously underserved. Self-care lends itself to greater risks of health fraud because health professionals are not screening the decisions. Health professionals, however, for their quality assurance mechanisms and self-regulation have not provided universally sound decisions free of financial conflicts of interest.

Self-testing carries additional risks of misuse, unnecessary anxiety for misunderstood or incorrect results, and incorrect action in response to test results. The first home tests for pregnancy introduced in the mid-1970s took two hours, several steps, and the collection of the first urine the woman passed in the morning. They could be done only nine or

more days after a missed period. The latest generation of one-step pregnancy tests released in 1997 reveal the results in a minute, from urine at any time of the day, and as early as the first day after a missed period. The point is that the problems associated with the introduction of new self-care products should not be grounds to prohibit them or to discourage their use. Like all new technologies, the first users pave the way for improvements and simplifications for the average user.

The concern with some tests is less with the accuracy or simplicity of the technology than with the medical, emotional, and social counseling that the person might need in coping with the results (figure 21-3). When pregnancy home tests first appeared, the medical profession complained that women diagnosing themselves would put off seeing physicians, perhaps without the ability to cope with the test's results. Some public health officials and members of HIV/AIDS advocacy groups fear the same with the HIV tests on the market in the United States and under review by the Health Protection Branch in Canada. The kits allow people to collect blood samples and send them to labs, which they later call. This provides for privacy and convenience, but bypasses the counseling and referrals available to people tested through medical or public health channels. Home testing might preclude some of the other follow-up procedures built into medical and public health systems.

The Future of Self-Care   The public demand for self-care will only grow with the increase in chronic conditions of an aging population, the growing sophistication of the public about health matters, the self-care information increasingly available on the Internet, and new technologies. The FDA and Health Canada will expand their surveillance of products from presales only to include periodic testing or monitoring of some home-based devices. The range of self-test products will grow and will be easier and less invasive (requiring less penetration of the skin). Diabetic testing for glucose, for example, will not require a prick of the finger to draw blood. Instead, a device would scan and analyze the various elements in the skin, or draw blood into a pocket just beneath the skin, or use a laser to micropenetrate the skin painlessly. The rapid growth of the market will accelerate the development of these products because the potential profits will be great.

The connectivity of people with computers, cellular telephonic devices, and radio-linking devices will allow isolated or immobile people to have instant access to sophisticated diagnostic and monitoring capabilities. A widely remembered television commercial was for a signaling device that provided help for an older woman who cries out, "I've fallen and I can't get up!" This was the opening salvo in advertising of a wide range of devices to provide greater security for people living alone. Another product emerging in Britain consists of a computer and a set of urine-test sticks

that track the presence of two hormones present in a woman's menstrual cycle and determine when she is fertile. This simple, noninvasive home test could replace years of frustration and unnecessary visits to infertility clinics trying to help couples seeking a pregnancy.

PRIMARY CARE AND POPULATION HEALTH: THE COMMUNITY-INDIVIDUAL HEALTH LINK

Many Americans remain more susceptible than others to quackery and health fraud because they feel disconnected from a health and medical care system that they cannot afford or that denies them access or insurance. Measured against feelings of hopelessness, an annual insurance premium, or a day's hospital stay, a "quick cure" seems like a bargain to the vulnerable, especially the poor. This might also account in part for the avid use of self-care and mutual aid by the American public. The Canadian interest in alternative and complementary care could be attributed in part to some alienation from conventional medicine and in part to the coverage under some provincial health care systems of partial payment for services of some complementary practitioners. Chiropractors, for example, receive partial coverage of their services in most Canadian provincial health care plans. Many patients perceive chiropractors as more willing to take time to talk to their patients than they perceive physicians to be.

The gradual drift of the U.S. health care system to specialized medical care providers has limited the access of millions of Americans to basic and preventive health care services (figure 21-4). To include everyone in health and medical care requires reform of the U.S. system. Such reform was a top political priority for the 1990s.

A key to health care reform is primary health care. As conceived by the World Health Organization, it is a community-based concept of health care in which an individual's first contact with the system is with broadly trained, generalist physicians, nurses, and other professionals. These

· · · · · · · · · · · · · · · · · · · ·

Figure 21-4

Of countries with comparable standards of living, the United States has the lowest percentage of primary care physicians among all physicians. This means that more American physicians are specialists, which accounts in part for the higher cost of medical care in the United States. *Source:* Based on Asch, D. A., and J. Ende. 1992. The downsizing of internal medicine residency programs. *Ann Intern Med* 117:839; Jaen, C. R., K. C. Stange, and P. A. Nutting. 1994. Competing demands of primary care: a model for the delivery of clinical preventive services. *J Fam Prac* 38: 166; and Middelkoop, B. J. C., A. M. Bohnen, and A. Prins. 1995. Rotterdam general practitioners report (ROHAPRO): a computerized network of general practices in Rotterdam, The Netherlands. *J Epidem Community Health* 49:231.

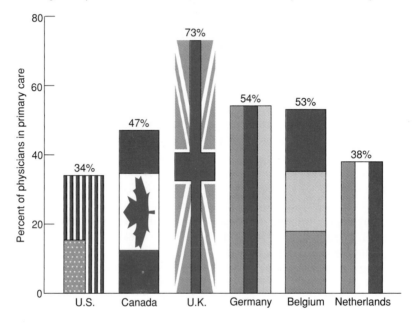

providers consider not only medical needs of individuals, but also their broader health needs and living situations. Primary care providers offer continuous, comprehensive care at lower costs than do health specialists. A system of health care based on a foundation of interdisciplinary, preventive, community-based, primary health care may be the most effective way to assure quality services at reasonable cost to the entire population.

To balance the seemingly incompatible goals of universal access to health care and control on costs, attention must focus on those who provide health care services. Health care depends so heavily on personnel and facilities, therefore any discussion about primary health care and health care reform needs to engage the various sectors and personnel who provide the services. The professional associations representing each of the provider disciplines, the insurers and the hospitals, have offices in Washington, DC and Ottawa to lobby for their place in health care reform. The recipients of services also have their consumer organizations there, as noted in the previous sections. The public health associations provide an interdisciplinary voice with concerns for balancing professional interests with population health interests. The voice for population health has argued for greater attention to the determinants of health rather than just the resources to provide services.

· · · · · · · · · · · · · · · · · · · ·
Figure 21-5

The resource-based planning model has prevailed in the development of financing and delivery of health care services since World War II. It produces a spiral of increased resources and increased demand for resources that drives the costs of health services upward even as a population's medical needs might be declining with improved health and living conditions. *Source:* Green, L. W. 1997. Building healthy, sustainable communities and social capital through participatory research. Houston: The 1997 John P. McGovern Award Lecture in Health Promotion, University of Texas Health Science Centre at Houston, School of Public Health, Center for Health Promotion Research and Development.

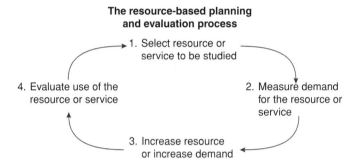

**The resource-based planning
and evaluation process**

1. Select resource or service to be studied

2. Measure demand for the resource or service

3. Increase resource or increase demand

4. Evaluate use of the resource or service

With agreement on the importance of primary health care and the determinants of population health, many systems, traditions, and attitudes will need to change to implement the necessary reforms. The education of health professions needs to be redirected toward health needs of the population, not only the medical needs. Health care financing policies need to favor primary care. Health personnel need to find reward in disease prevention. Television crews rush in for the medical miracles. They seldom show the successful outcome of prevention when something did not happen. Interdisciplinary efforts may mean allocation of responsibilities and power that individuals and regulatory agencies need to confirm. For health care reform to succeed, issues of health personnel availability, employment, and training must be considered within the context of the resource-based versus population-based planning and evaluation.

The Era of Resource-Based Planning and Evaluation

This drift of medical care to high technology and hospital-based resources to support that technology dragged health planning from a focus on outcomes to planning based on the cost of resources. Measurement and evaluation had to help justify, defend, and eventually contain the costs of the new technologies and resources. This refocused measurement and evaluation from the health outcomes in populations to the appropriate uses and applications of the resources. With that shift came the broader tendency in regional and community health planning toward a resource-based rather than population-based planning and development cycle. The hospitals, the personnel, and the technology became ends in themselves. As such they became the objects of measurement and evaluation in most health planning and development.

Increasing the Use of Health Services As shown in figure 21-5, increasing the use of health services had the effect of diverting attention away from the health needs of populations and toward their use or consumption of the resources and services offered. Government health agencies sponsored social and behavioral science research in the 1950s and 1960s focused mostly on increasing people's use of new technologies, services, and facilities. The Health Belief Model, for instance, emerged initially in the late 1950s to explain the results of studies on why people used or failed to use chest x-ray services to screen for tuberculosis. This influential model evolved in the 1960s to assess why people did not make greater use of immunization services and eventually to its more generic question of why people use health services.

Similarly, the PRECEDE-PROCEED model for health promotion planning and evaluation (see chapter 4) was first published as a cost-benefit evaluation model applied to decreasing the use of emergency room services by asthmatic adults.[1] It built initially on models of use of health services and family planning services. PRECEDE and other models in patient education were further developed and tested in the 1970s to understand patient "compliance" with prescribed medical regimens, another rapidly developing medical technology or resource. In each instance, the starting point for planning or research was a technology, facility, service, or other resource. The questions initially were how to increase the use of services. Later, the question became how to decrease the use of services.

Health Resources as Means or as Ends   The consequence of the resource-based planning and evaluation cycle for the health field is that it locked the development process into a spiral of justifying resources, services, and technologies as ends in themselves. These resources were becoming more numerous and more expensive. The cost of health care was escalating. After two decades of seeking to increase the use of services, health education's new order of business in the 1970s became the reduction of "overutilization" and unnecessary use of medical care services. In the United States, the President's Committee on Health Education in 1973, the Health Information and Health Promotion Act (PL 94-317) in 1974, and the

Health Maintenance Organization Act of 1973 sought to *reduce* the public's use of health services. They sought to do so, in part, by developing educational strategies and incentives to help the public to become more self-sufficient in health and to become better informed "consumers" of health care services. The HMO Act also sought to offer providers of services more incentives to reduce hospitalization by keeping their patients healthy rather than just treating their sicknesses and injuries.

This gave rise in the agencies and foundations funding health services research to an interest in the self-care movement. This movement grew out of the 1960s from a convergence of the women's movement, the do-it-yourself, self-help and self-improvement movements, and the emergence of mutual aid groups. Some of these fed on growing antiprofessionalism or at least some disenchantment with experts controlling people's lives or pocketbooks.

Search for the Magic Bullet   The resource-based planning and evaluation cycle had another effect on health and behavioral researchers. It caused them to reason by analogy from medical successes that their scientific quest should be to find the best intervention to achieve a specific type of health-related behavior change. Practitioners and the agencies funding health services and public health research eagerly embraced this search for magic bullet solutions to the behavioral change problems presented by medical care and public health. A generation of highly controlled randomized trials and fine-grained behavioral research ensued. These tested by trial and error specific ways to improve patient compliance. They included ways to reduce broken appointments, to educate mothers to restrain their tendency to bring a child to HMO or pediatric services for each earache or sore throat. They also emphasized ways to improve smoking cessation and to modify a range of specific consumer and self-care behaviors. The targets of the magic bullet "interventions" included "consumer" behaviors thought to account

---

[1]Green, L. W. 1974. Toward cost-benefit evaluations of health education: Some concepts, methods and examples. *Health Educ Monogr* 2 (Suppl. 1): 34.

for some of the "unnecessary" and "inappropriate" use of health services as much as those behaviors accounting for leading causes of death.

The magic bullet approach to behavioral research in health was nowhere more evident than in **smoking cessation** studies, which dominated the funded behavioral research in the 1970s and early 1980s. Social and behavioral researchers conducted hundreds of studies on each of several focused techniques for stopping smoking during this era. Smoking cessation research gained prominence with the growing recognition of tobacco as the leading cause of preventable deaths in western countries and from the concomitantly growing public demand for ways to quit smoking. The further possibility of pinpointing the relative cost-effectiveness of alternative smoking cessation methods made this work of interest to those trying to rationalize and finance preventive services within the evolving medical care system. These more precise measurement possibilities gave this line of research a status among the biomedical sciences that was difficult to match by other social, behavioral, and educational research initiatives in the health fields.

Reducing Use of Health Services   Health services funding agencies concerned with the cost-containment issues in health care use supported most of the applied social and behavioral research in health of that era. Researchers pursued these studies vigorously during the 1970s and early 1980s. The health resource imperative and the need to contain the cost centers of that resource drove the research priorities. Emergency room visits by poor people for routine care, for example, provided a focal point for American health services research because many of the costs in the ER could not be recovered from patients or fully from insurance or welfare systems. Cost savings or efficiencies from averting unnecessary visits to emergency rooms lent themselves to a precision of measurement of behavioral outcomes that seldom had to deal with the longer-term or messier issues of health outcomes and quality-of-life or social

outcomes. The motivation for funding such research, once again, had more to do with rationalizing the medical facilities or resources than with solving the health problem of a population.

The resource-based planning cycle also persisted in the education sector as new, sometimes expensive, educational technologies emerged in the 1970s. These refocused school health educators and researchers for a time away from comprehensive school health onto methods and techniques of classroom teaching. The disillusionment in health, education, and other sectors with the search for technological fixes, magic bullets, and one-size-fits-all packaged interventions has challenged the health and educational systems to find new methods and criteria to judge health care and schooling outcomes.

To these sources of disillusionment we can add those mentioned earlier in this chapter as the growing discontent of consumers and the public with commercial exploitation; fraud; and the institutional systems of health, social, and educational services. Add to this ferment the growing impatience and even hostility of the public with their passive role as subjects (objects) of research who feel exploited as individuals and sometimes compromised and maligned as groups. This is especially problematic for minority groups and disadvantaged communities, and practitioners working under adverse circumstances, when the results paint them in an unfavorable light.

Shifting from Resource-Based to Population-Based Planning and Evaluation

The alternative to the resource-based planning and evaluation cycle is the population-based planning and evaluation cycle, shown in figure 21-6. This process of planning and evaluation was implicit in early epidemiological approaches to public health planning that had prevailed in the communicable disease control eras of the nineteenth and early twentieth centuries in western countries. It continues in many developing countries, although they too have been caught up in the resource-based

• •

Figure 21-6

The population-based approach to planning and evaluation starts with the identification of a specific human population. This could be a population of patients using a clinical service or the population of a community served by a health service. *Source:* Green, L. W. 1997. Building healthy, sustainable communities and social capital through participatory research. Houston: The 1997 John P. McGovern Award Lecture in Health Promotion, University of Texas Health Science Centre at Houston, School of Public Health, Center for Health Promotion Research and Development.

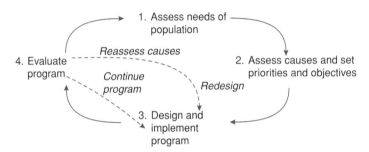

planning spiral as they seek to replicate the technological features of western medicine.

Phase 1 The population-based approach to planning and evaluation starts with the identification of a specific human population. This could be a population of patients using a clinical service or the population of students in a classroom. More to the point of its renaissance in health planning, the population-based approach prefers to conceive it as a population of people eligible to use (at risk of using) the clinical or educational service. The planners assess population needs beyond those of the individuals who appear for illness or injury treatment or beyond the people who turn out for educational events. The latter people may provide numerators against the denominator of the population.

   This initial focus on the denominator or population-at-risk is the critical distinction made implicitly in the emergence in the 1970s of health maintenance organizations (HMOs) and later community-oriented primary care (COPC) and managed care in the United States and population health elsewhere. It is also the distinction made implicitly in the 1974 Lalonde Report, *A New Perspective on the Health of Canadians*. It is made more explicitly in

the 1979 U.S. Surgeon General's Report on Health Promotion and Disease Prevention, *Healthy People,* and in the succession of countries adopting a planning-by-objectives approach to health promotion and disease prevention (United Kingdom, the Netherlands, Australia, New Zealand). Most of these built on the Canadian Lalonde Report and after 1979 on the American "Healthy People" experience and the World Health Organization's Primary Health Care and Health for All initiatives. Efforts to prevent disease or injury and to promote health become more compelling when an organization assumes responsibility for the population's health needs, regardless of the prevailing medical care resources.

Phase 2 The second phase of the population-based planning cycle is an assessment of causes of the health needs. Such assessments typically reveal a set of common causes that cut across multiple health problems among the leading causes of death, disability, illness, and injury. Most countries and communities understandably make these common risk factors such as alcohol, tobacco, poor nutrition or diet, and physical inactivity their priorities for the focus of limited health promotion and disease prevention resources. In 1986, the First

International Conference on Health Promotion produced the Ottawa Charter (figure 1.8), which helped reorient some of the exclusive focus of policy, programs, and practices away from these proximal risk factors. The shift that followed was to the more distal **risk conditions** that cause the risk factors, referred to as the "determinants of health." These included adequate housing; secure income; healthful and safe community and work environments; enforcement of policies and regulations controlling the manufacture, marketing, labeling, and sale of potentially harmful products; and the use of these products (e.g., alcohol and tobacco) where they can do harm to others. Some of these had been the dominant public health issues of earlier eras.

Assessing causes of the health needs may apply to a population of patients of clinical services, students in a school, employees in a workplace, or people in a community. It typically involves data collection from records or from observations or surveys, data reduction, and statistical analyses of the data. These steps are designed first to construct profiles or descriptions of the risk factors and risk conditions in the population. Assessing these statistical distributions in turn identifies the factors predisposing, enabling, or reinforcing the development or incidence of the most important risk factors or risk conditions in the population.

Phase 3 The third phase of the population-based planning model calls for the strategic application of data and knowledge about the causes identified in the second phase. These considerations lead to the selection or creation of programs that could influence change in the factors predisposing, enabling, or reinforcing the causes and thereby improve health outcomes. This and the second phase usually form the main subjects of textbooks and articles on program planning and implementation.

Phase 4 The fourth phase is the implementation and evaluation of the program or procedures implemented to meet the population needs. This phase leads logically to a reassessment of the needs of the population (phase 1). It can also lead through a short-loop feedback to the reassessment of assumptions or hypotheses formulated about causes in phase 2 or to the program itself to improve upon its construction or delivery or to continue it.

PROFESSIONAL PERSONNEL

How many and what kinds of health care workers does a population require? The terms supply and **requirements** are used in discussions about the health work force. In turn, the words demand and **need** are used in discussions of requirements.

Supply and Demand

Supply and demand are well-defined concepts in economics. *Supply* in the professional personnel context refers to the number of individuals in a specific occupational category who are seeking employment at the current pay level. *Demand* is the number of individuals in a specific occupational category that employers will employ at various wages. This is sometimes referred to as "economic demand" or "effective economic demand." Therefore supply and demand are different theoretical concepts. Economic theory describes what actually happens when demand draws on supply.

Need and *requirements* are less well and more variously defined terms. They are value judgments separate in concept from supply and demand. The "need for a specific health occupation" is defined as an adequate minimum quantity and quality of persons in that health occupation that widespread consensus holds ought to be available to the defined population for the purpose of restoring or maintaining their health. The additional requirements for health promotion or *improving* health may take the analysis beyond the health sector to workers in education and other sectors.

The requirement for a health occupation is implied in the match between the number of workers needed and the assumed level of their contribution to health goals. *Requirement* contains value judgments that reflect many considerations including economics, health priorities, traditional organization of health services, and political clout.

Seldom do planners have the data for a complete analysis of all four concepts of supply, demand, requirement, and need. In the next sections a summary of the supply and requirements for the health occupations in the United States will be given as an illustration of health resource analysis applicable to other countries and populations.

Health Care Services Personnel

The supply and requirements for the health care services work force change over time. Adjustments to shortages or oversupply of health care workers time sets off decades of chain responses in multiple sectors. The 1970s saw a time of rapid expansion in the number of physicians, nurses, pharmacists, and dentists. Between 1970 and 1980, the number of those graduating in medicine increased by 81 percent, nursing by 75 percent, pharmacy by 56 percent, and dentistry by 40 percent. The nation was in a resource-building era, as noted in the previous section, until the cost containment concerns of the late 1970s slowed this rapid expansion. As federal support was withdrawn, most of these professions peaked in the number of graduates by the mid-1980s.

By the end of the 1980s, the number of nursing and dental graduates dropped from the beginning of that decade by 18 percent and pharmacy graduates dropped by 12 percent. Only medical schools showed an increase of 3 percent in 1989 of the number of graduates over that in 1980. Whether these graduates represent an over- or undersupply is a matter of some debate, depending on assumptions about the organization of the health care system and understanding roles and responsibilities of health care providers. For example, projections by the Health Resources and Services Administration in 1988 were that supply would exceed requirements in selected health professions by the year 2000 (table 21-1).

Physicians The 90 percent increase in the number of physicians since 1970 represents a near doubling of the number of physicians per 100,000 population. Just as important as the ratio of physicians

Table 21-1

Projected Requirements and Supply for Selected Health Occupations for the Turn of the Century

	2000	
	Supply	**Requirements**
Medicine	708,600	637,000
Optometry	30,100	29,500
Pharmacy	198,600	193,000
Nursing*		
RN	1,799,000	1,743,000
LPN/LVN	630,200	585,400

Sources: Health Resources and Services Administration, 1988; Alliance for Health Reform, 1996; Council on Graduate Medical Education, *Fourth Report to Congress* and the Center for Health Professions, *Front and Center,* 2(1):1, 1997.

to total population is their distribution in practice and population. Approximately one-third of physicians practice primary care. This percent is in stark contrast to the 80 percent who were in primary care in 1931. In 1992 only 15 percent of medical school graduates chose primary health care. The financial incentives for specializing are tempting. General or family practice physicians have annual incomes that are 50 percent to 60 percent less than those of medical specialists (figure 21-7).

Physicians, like other North Americans, tend to congregate in metropolitan areas. Rural and inner city areas are not favored practice sites. The result is uneven distribution of health care services to the population. Medical schools have admitted a more ethnically diverse population and more women, although graduates do not reflect broader social diversity. In 1991 minorities constituted 22 percent of the U.S. population, but only 8 percent of practicing physicians. The application of women to U.S. medical schools nearly doubled in the six years from 1989 to 1995.

Making general practice attractive is the problem that must be resolved for the United States or the cry will continue that there is a shortage of

· · · · · · · · · · · · · · · · · · · ·
Figure 21-7

The prestige and glamour attached to medical and surgical specialties as a result of two decades of hospital dramas on television have made the family doctor and the primary care physician seem a throwback to a primitive era. The pitch in this ad is for strengthening of academic subjects in school to make today's children ready to handle tomorrow's technology. *Source:* The Advertising Council, the Business Roundtable, U.S. Department of Education, National Governors' Association, American Federation of Teachers, and the National Alliance of Business.

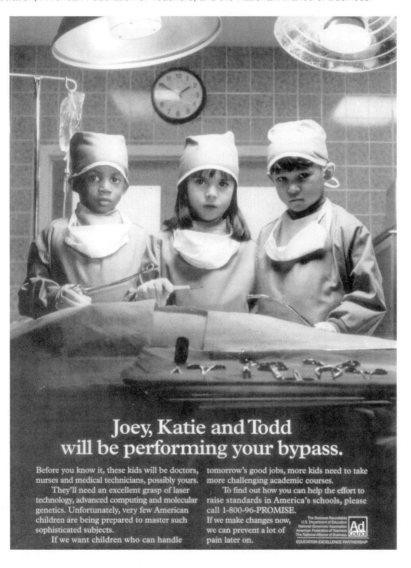

Joey, Katie and Todd will be performing your bypass.

Before you know it, these kids will be doctors, nurses and medical technicians, possibly yours.

They'll need an excellent grasp of laser technology, advanced computing and molecular genetics. Unfortunately, very few American children are being prepared to master such sophisticated subjects.

If we want children who can handle tomorrow's good jobs, more kids need to take more challenging academic courses.

To find out how you can help the effort to raise standards in America's schools, please call 1-800-96-PROMISE.

If we make changes now, we can prevent a lot of pain later on.

The Business Roundtable
U.S. Department of Education
National Governors' Association
American Federation of Teachers
The National Alliance of Business

Ad Council

EDUCATION EXCELLENCE PARTNERSHIP

physicians, when it is merely a shortage of general practitioners. To increase the availability of community-based primary care practitioners, a variety of strategies are considered that involve admission requirements to medical school; financial incentives for primary practice; curriculum changes that include community settings, retraining current specialists, and allowing more foreign medical graduates to practice in the United States. Some communities have been able to attract general practitioners by building a small but adequate hospital, providing office facilities, and guaranteeing a minimum salary.

For Canada, where patients must see general practitioners before they can be referred to specialists, the supply of family practice or general practice physicians has been less of a problem. The vast geographic dispersion of a small proportion of the Canadian population, where the farm population has declined like the U.S. farm population, makes the problem of recruiting physicians to rural and remote communities similar for both countries. Many other countries continue to support outreach through home visits by allied health personnel (figure 21-8). Nurse midwives provide for home deliveries covered by the Canadian health care plans, in lieu of hospital deliveries by obstetricians.

Another factor that drives up the cost of physician care is inefficient use of physician services. Too many physicians are taking too much valuable time doing tasks that others could do or should be trained to do. Others can be and are trained to take family and personal histories and to perform further duties. Examples are physicians' assistants, nurse practitioners, accredited record technicians, medical secretaries, medical transcriptionists, physical therapy aides, inhalation therapists, surgical technicians, darkroom technicians, dietitians, patient counselors, and diabetes educators.

Nurses   Chapter 20 on community health discussed the role nurses play in the health care system. As the largest health care profession, nurses

Figure 21-8

A primary health center in Pakthongchai district receives an emergency call from a neighboring village. The nurse midwife roars off on her motorbike. Access is achieved as a compromise between more clinical facilities and more outreach. *Source:* Photo by A. S. Kochar, courtesy World Health Organization.

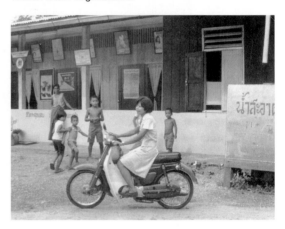

outnumber physicians by nearly three to one. Nurses and other allied personnel have assumed expanded roles in health services. Nurses have taken increased responsibility for patient education to help patients cope with emotional and learning aspects of self-care and rehabilitation. The potential for nurses and other allied health workers to bring a humanizing and preventive orientation back into a highly technological health care system gives them a most promising and central role in the future of community health and population health.

The number of nurses, as with physicians, has been subject to debates about shortages and oversupply. There was a 122 percent increase in the number of nurses from 1970 to 1.6 million in 1989. Such overall dramatic increases fail to show the rapid decrease in the number of nursing graduates in recent years, a 25 percent decrease from 1985 to 1989. Baccalaureate nursing levels are back to those of the early 1970s.

....
Figure 21-9

Oncology nurses provide emotional and highly technical support to cancer patients. *Source:* Johns Hopkins Oncology Center, the Johns Hopkins Medical Institutions.

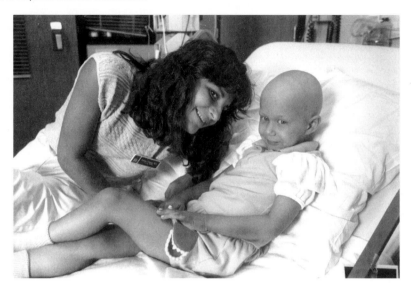

These decreases come at a time when health care providers report continuing and emerging shortages and maldistribution in key basic disciplines in nursing and allied health. Hospitals and nursing homes in particular report nursing shortages (figure 21-9). Increasing controls over rising health care costs are creating a demand for more community-based health care services provided by nonphysician practitioners.

Other Health Care Practitioners   Primary care engages health practitioners in education about health at some level. Certified health education specialists have primary training in health education and have passed a standardized examination. Their role in community and individual health education provides direction, support, and coordination to the health educational efforts of other health practitioners. The health education role is an important one in primary care.

The United States set as its goal for the year 2000 the development of an "appropriate" mix of personnel to support the expansion of access to primary and preventive care services. That mix includes primary care providers, for example, family physicians, general internists, pediatricians, nurse practitioners, physician assistants, and certified nurse midwives. Other health professionals have important primary care roles, including pharmacists, dentists, dental hygienists (figure 21-10), respiratory technicians and various other technicians and therapists, optometrists, dietitians, nutritionists, and social workers. These professionals need community ties that make primary health care community-based, not the medical care bureaucracy the current care system seems to many patients.

Accessibility   An adequate total supply of personnel, however, does not guarantee accessibility for all people. Other barriers—money, education,

· ·

Figure 21-10

Dental technicians, hygienists, and assistants provide a range of preventive and technical support services, freeing dentists to concentrate their more expensive time on surgical and restorative tasks. Such efficiencies throughout the health care system have their drawbacks, sometimes creating a more bureaucratic system, but no society has been able to sustain a system in which every individual sees the most specialized and highly trained practitioner for every symptom. *Source:* Photo by Marsha Burkes, courtesy The University of Texas Health Science Center at Houston.

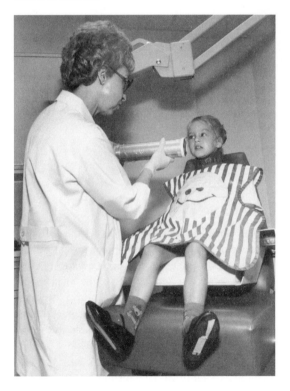

geography, or language—still keep too many people from needed health care. Many rural and inner city areas still experience shortages of health personnel despite the increases in supply. The designations of specific areas with shortages of health personnel encompass a broad range of areas. Although a majority of those areas are rural (nonmetropolitan) areas, urban areas contain about half

of the population who live in shortage areas. Efforts to identify these areas and a number of federal programs in the United States, including the National Health Service Corps, have attempted to correct the problems of access. The U.S. federal government has designated special population groups, such as American Indians, those who are Spanish-speaking, blacks, and the medically indigent, as having health personnel shortages. The estimated 30 million people who live in designated health personnel shortage areas in the United States approached the number who had no health insurance until 1996. Then President Clinton signed the Kennedy-Kassebaum Act that provided coverage for those who would lose health coverage if they changed jobs or a member of their family got sick. Many of the remaining uninsured are the same people as those in underserved areas, living in double medical jeopardy.

After passage of the Kennedy-Kassebaum bill, nearly 13 million of the roughly 110 million families in the United States—11.6 percent of families—still experienced difficulty or delays in obtaining medical care or did not get the care they needed during 1996. According to 1997 estimates from the Agency for Health Care Policy and Research (AHCPR), the most common barrier, experienced by 7.6 million families or roughly 60 percent of those reporting difficulty with access, was the inability to afford care. Other barriers included insurance-related problems, transportation problems, or difficulties securing childcare. Uninsured families were more likely to experience problems obtaining needed health care. More than 27 percent, or 3.3 million uninsured families, experienced barriers, including the inability to afford care. Hispanic families were more likely than white or black families to encounter problems—roughly 1.4 million Hispanic families (15 percent of Hispanic families) reported barriers. For nearly seven in ten of these Hispanic families, the problem was the cost of health care.

In developing countries, the problems of accessibility are compounded by poorer transportation and communications systems. People must bring

····················
Figure 21-11

A villager in Bangladesh brings his wife, with symptoms of tetanus, to a primary care center. Transportation and communication problems in developing countries compound their problems of access to health care. *Source:* Photo courtesy World Health Organization.

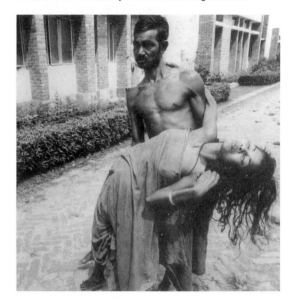

sick family members sometimes great distances by rudimentary and even primitive means of transport (figure 21-11) to receive basic or emergency health care. Greater use of ancillary health care personnel such as the "barefoot doctors" in China, the nurse-midwives in most countries, and multi-purpose workers in some, provide at least a liaison with more fully equipped primary care facilities and hospitals.

HOSPITAL FACILITIES

Supply and Distribution

Hospital facilities include short-term general and special hospitals. The issues of supply pertain to their bed capacity. The number of short-term general and special hospitals in many countries

was greater fifty years ago. Half a century ago, because of limited transportation, almost every little hamlet in the United States, for example, had its 15- or 20-bed hospital, poorly equipped, poorly serviced, and poorly administered, but accessible. With modern transportation it seemed logical to have fewer hospitals and to maintain only those hospitals with a large enough bed capacity to warrant extensive equipment and highly specialized personnel. The need for every town to have a hospital also seemed to diminish with the decline of communicable diseases. As a result, large, well-equipped, well-staffed, and well-administered hospitals erected in the large population centers have concentrated medical resources in the big cities and smaller cities with medical schools.

The old standard of four general hospital beds for every 1,000 inhabitants was attained in most western countries. Australia, Canada, England, Wales, Scotland, and the United States have close to four beds per 1,000 population as an average. Changing demographics and medical economics, however, have made it possible to meet a population's needs with half this number.

The uneven distribution of hospital beds in the United States was partially corrected by the Hill-Burton Hospital Survey and Construction Act of 1946. This law instituted a federal program that made more than $4.1 billion in grants to hospitals in all of the states during the twenty-nine years of its existence and added 496,000 beds to the nation's hospital system. These grants were made to local government hospitals, church hospitals, and nonprofit hospitals. A major U.S. shift occurred in the 1960s with the emphasis on neighborhood health centers and in the 1970s with the Health Maintenance Organizations Act. In Canada, the Universal Hospital Insurance and Diagnostic Services Act of 1957 provided federal cost sharing with all provinces for hospital care for all. By 1968, Canada passed the Federal Medical Care Act, expanding the provision of universal hospital care to universal medical outpatient care.

Hospices

In medieval Europe **hospice** referred to a place of shelter and rest for weary or sick travelers on long journeys. Dr. Cicely Saunders first used the term to describe specialized care for dying patients in 1967 when she established St. Christopher's Hospice in a residential suburb of London. The term today refers to a steadily expanding range of care in patients' homes, hospitals, and in freestanding facilities. The hallmark of hospice care is humane and compassionate **palliative** care for the whole person who has a terminal illness, rather than curative care for a disease.

Medical and nursing staffs of hospices cooperate closely with social workers to help patients and their families to adjust in a home-like atmosphere to terminal illness and to overcome their particular difficulties at a time that is potentially overwhelmingly stressful. For those facing death, bewildering and sometimes contradictory feelings emerge. A patient who is able to return home may need a variety of financial and visiting services to modify the home environment. The social worker can arrange such services and help the patients to feel more secure outside the protective care of the hospice or the

family to feel more secure with the patient in the hospice.

Hospice emphasizes quality rather than length of life; the entire family, not just the patient; and offers twenty-four-hour support to the patient and family. Using advanced methods of pain and symptom control, hospice care enables the patient to live as fully and comfortably as possible.

Sources: Wheatfields—A Sue Ryder Home for Cancer Patients. 1989. Leeds, England: The Sue Ryder Foundation; *The Basics of Hospice.* 1997. Arlington, VA: National Hospice Organization.

Characteristics

General Hospitals At the time the Hill-Burton program was becoming operational in 1948, the United States had 3.4 hospital beds per 1,000 population. As result of Hill-Burton, nearly 4,000 communities were aided in the construction of 6,549 public and nonprofit medical facilities.

Following the buildup of hospitals into the 1970s, there has been a steady decrease since 1975. At first the reduction in hospitals did not affect the continuing increase in admissions or discharges because the number of hospital beds continued to increase and Medicare made it possible for more people to be hospitalized. Since the early 1980s, a sharp decrease in hospital discharges (figure 21-12) has accompanied the cost-containment initiatives and new technologies for outpatient care. By 1990 there were 3.9 beds per 1,000 population, dropping back closer to the pre-Hill-Burton ratio. The average occupancy rate for general hospitals was about 67 percent in 1990 and the average stay 7.3 days. This compares with 10.5 days in Canada.

Continued reductions in the average stay in U.S. hospitals to 6.5 days in 1995 (while Canadian average stays have increased) have been most dramatic with maternity care and surgery. In 1970, the average duration of stay for an uncomplicated delivery in the United States was four days. By 1992, it was halved to two days. Today, a growing number of American insurers refuse to pay for more than twenty-four hours, and some even recommend release as early as eight hours after delivery. The risks in this trend are complications for new babies, including feeding problems, infections, dehydration, brain damage, and stroke.

Specialized Hospitals Hospitals have seen redistribution in their location and a change in types of hospitals. Between 1970 and 1990 tuberculosis hospitals decreased the most dramatically (94 percent) as this disease was being reduced in the overall population and drugs permitted outpatient treatment. As large state-run "warehouses" for the mentally ill were closed down, there was an

....

Figure 21-12

The U.S. rate of hospital discharges has dropped precipitously since 1983 at the same time the average duration of stay for most conditions has given way to outpatient treatment. *Source:* National Center for Health Statistics. 1997. *National health care survey: 1995 data highlights.* Atlanta, GA: Centers for Disease Control and Prevention, U.S. Department of Health and Human Services.

Rate of hospital discharges

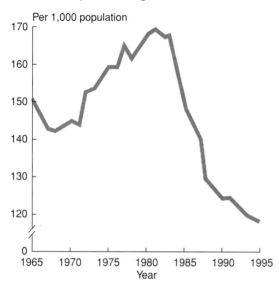

Table 21-2

Leading Medical Diagnoses Rendered in Emergency Departments

First-listed diagnosis	Number of visits in thousands
Open wound, excluding head	5,350
Contusion with intact skin surface	4,758
Acute upper respiratory infections, excluding pharyngitis	3,829
Otitis media and eustachian tube disorders	3,010
Open wound of head	3,001

Source: National Center for Health Statistics. *National health care survey: 1995 data highlights,* 1997. Atlanta, GA: Centers for Disease Control and Prevention, U.S. Department of Health and Human Services.

increase in small, private psychiatric hospitals (43 percent). It was not an even trade of populations; many from state institutions were left to the streets and were not the concern of privately run facilities.

Hospital Emergency Rooms Many hospital emergency rooms continue to be used as a primary source of care by those without insurance or other means of care. Emergency room visits have increased by over 50 percent in the last twenty years in Canada and the United States. The two leading causes of ER visits, as shown in table 21-2, are legitimate emergency care needs. The third and

fourth leading diagnoses in ERs, however, should not require emergency treatment. Common colds and earaches require no physician care in most instances, and create a strain on ER staff.

Hospital Costs The U.S. bill for hospital care passed $350 billion in 1995, up from $204 billion in 1990. American hospitals have an average of one staff for every two patients. The highly technological services offered by hospitals continue to increase. Such facilities as intensive care, open-heart surgery, radioisotope, and renal dialysis units have proliferated (figure 21-13). This addition of special facilities to a hospital's capacity has been one of the factors in rising hospital costs and the general inflation of the medical care dollar. By 1995 the average cost per day in a U.S. hospital was $968, up from $687 in 1990 and $245 in 1980. The average cost per stay in 1995 increased from $4,947 in 1990 to $6,229 in 1995.

Nursing Homes The number of beds in U.S. nursing homes nearly doubled between 1963 and 1983. The number of skilled nursing facilities has

Figure 21-13

New technologies have cost hospitals a large proportion of their increase in expenditures. Advanced diagnostic capabilities have led to some increase in the ordering of tests such as CAT scans that would not be justified by most standards of practice. Malpractice suits in a few instances when tests were not done have resulted in the ordering of tests as a form of defensive medical practice. *Source:* Photo courtesy Alberta Heritage Foundation for Medical Research.

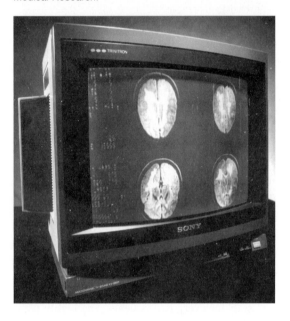

Figure 21-14

The proportion of patients served by home health care and nursing homes will increase as the population ages. The current distribution of people served by nursing homes shows the 65–84 years group as the largest, but proportionate to their population sizes, the 85 years and over group is more heavily represented in nursing homes. *Source:* National Center for Health Statistics. 1997. *National health care survey: 1995 data highlights.* Atlanta, GA: Centers for Disease Control and Prevention, U.S. Department of Health and Human Services.

Percent distribution of nursing home residents by age

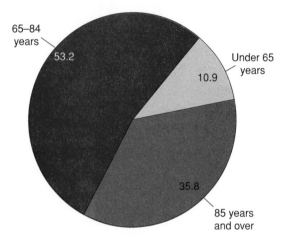

continued to increase, reaching 13,444 in the United States in 1996. This increase resulted in part from the coverage of the charges for certain types of nursing home care under the Medicare and Medicaid programs, which began in 1967. Some of the growth in nursing home use appears to be the result of placement in nursing homes of older patients who in earlier years would have been residents in state and county mental hospitals. With the aging of the population and an increasing life span, a greater need to care for the frail elderly (defined as those over 85) is expected (figure 21-14). Some of this need may be met through better home care service.

Home Health

The availability of home health services is often a factor in determining hospital staffing requirements and whether a patient must be hospitalized or can remain at home.

Staffing for a home health agency or a Visiting Nurse Association (VNA) usually includes the following personnel:

Nurses provide skilled nursing, specialized nursing, and liaison services.

- Skilled nursing includes general nursing services and technical procedures, such as intravenous (IV) therapy, catheterization, dressing wounds, and management of a physician-prescribed

· ·
Figure 21-15

Demographic trends alone will dominate many of the health care reforms seeking to control costs of medical and nursing home care in the years ahead. Today's well elderly and the aging baby boomers will require larger government outlays for medical, nursing, and home care even as the older population enjoys better health than in the past. *Source:* Photo by J. Chrétien, courtesy World Health Organization.

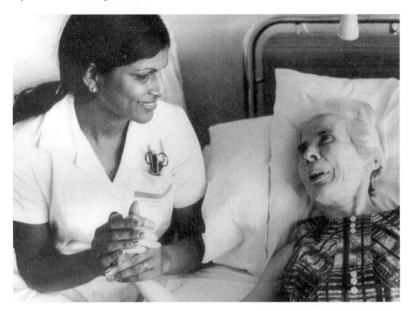

medical regime and instruction in patient care for the patient and family.
- Specialized nursing includes services of oncology clinical nurse specialists, a psychiatric mental health nurse, an enterostomal therapist, and pediatric nurse practitioners.
- A liaison nurse consults with local hospitals and nursing homes, provides information concerning VNA's services, and helps process the transition from the hospital to home (figure 21-15).

Therapists provide restorative physical therapy care for patients with stroke, fractures, and birth defects; occupational therapy for activities of daily living; and speech therapy for clients with communication problems related to speech, language, or hearing.

- *Home health aides,* certified paraprofessionals, provide personal care, such as bathing, grooming, bed changing, and grocery shopping.
- *Social workers* provide services that include evaluation, short-term counseling, and referral to community agencies.

The number of U.S. home health agencies approved for participation in the Medicare program increased appreciably between 1966 and 1970, the first four years of the Medicare program. After that the number of approved agencies remained stable at about 2,200 until 1985, when renewed growth occurred as a result of the new hospital discharge policies. Most of the earlier agencies were governmental health agencies or visiting nurse associations, but now proprietary home health agencies constitute 44 percent of the total, compared with 37 percent voluntary nonprofit and 19 percent government. The growth of the private share is a market response to the demand created by earlier discharges of patients from hospitals and the aging of the population.

HEALTH CARE SYSTEM COSTS

Growth in U.S. health care expenditure has been faster than growth of the total Gross National Product (GNP) for most of the last 35 years. The United States has exceeded other English-speaking and European countries in its increase in overall costs and in percentage of GNP. The United States spent 14.2 percent of its GNP on health in 1995, 40 percent more than Germany, the second highest spender. Canada was fifth among 14 OECD countries at 9.6 percent. The U.S. public share of all costs was 46 percent in 1995. That year, the United States spent $988.5 billion on health care, more than double what it was in 1985. The average amount spent per individual was $3,621. This is more than double $1800 (U.S.) spent per person by Canada in 1996. Despite paying the highest costs in the world, the United States lags behind other developed countries in vital health statistics such as infant mortality and immunization rates. The high-tech medical care system evolving in North America, Europe, and other countries is not a system that has extended health care as a right to all.

Changing Costs

Total U.S. health care costs surpassed the $1 trillion mark by 1997 and were projected to continue growing at a possibly accelerated rate (figure 21-16) based on demographic and technological trends. The government pays such a large amount of the total health care bill through Medicaid and Medicare, therefore it has an interest in controlling costs. The Clinton administration put top priority on health care reform to bring costs under control, at the same time trying to extend care to the 40 million Americans who were uninsured before 1997.

After failing to pass his comprehensive health care reform package in his first term, President Clinton proceeded to chip away at the problem with specific legislative packages for which Congress could share the credit or blame for passing or not passing.

Until 1997, hospital costs, physicians' fees, and other medical care services continued to rise faster than the inflation rate, despite the decline in duration of hospital stays resulting from incentives, regulations, and advances in medication, surgery, and other procedures. New incentives to minimize specialized care and hospitalization under managed care schemes in the United States and a tightening of referral from primary care in Canada, achieved a leveling off or slowing of the annual rate of increased costs in 1997. Nursing homes, rest homes, hospices, and home care as adjuncts to the general hospital have reduced the cost of hospitalization during the period of convalescence or dying. Patients who do not require the extensive care available in hospitals can recover as rapidly or die as peacefully in these homes at a lower cost and at even lower costs with good home health care services and self-care education for patients, families, and other caregivers.

Until the health insurance industry and large managed care organizations bought out many of the nonprofit community hospitals in the United States, the medical profession was the only industry in the United States that was free of market controls and governmental regulations. It had a virtual monopoly in the American economy, but physicians, always sensitive to the image of their profession, attempted to exercise supervision and discipline over members of the profession through professional associations and peer review within their local organizations in the United States and Canada. Instances of exorbitant medical charges have been substantiated. At the other extreme are the instances in which physicians have donated their professional services. It is not the extremes of overcharging or charity where the problem of the cost of medical care rests, but in the general inflation of prices in this relatively uncontrollable sector of the economy.

●●●●●●●●●●●●●●●●●●●●●●
Figure 21-16

National health expenditures topped $1 trillion in 1997. The rate of increase slowed briefly with managed care initiatives in the mid-1990s, then resumed its escalated rate as projected in 1992. *Source:* Health Care Financing Administration, Office of the Actuary; and U.S. General Accounting Office: *Access to health care: states respond.* 1992. Washington, DC: General Accounting Office; and U.S. Department of Health and Human Services 1998. *National health care expenditures.* Baltimore: Health Care Financing Administration, Office of National Health Statistics.

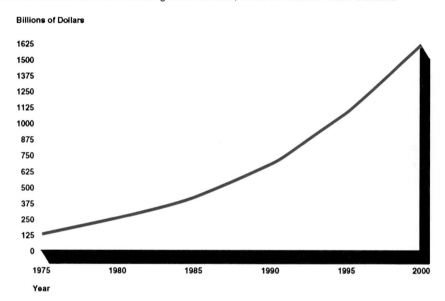

Note: Values after 1990 are estimates.

In the box titled "Controlling Costs of Personal Health Services," the economics of these trends, introduced in chapter 2, show ways in which costs could be controlled. Their further analysis would be beyond the scope of this text, but three major causes of cost increases (principally runaway hospital prices, more than one-third of the total costs) and the national policy initiatives to remedy or check these causes are shown.

A Community and Population Health Perspective on Health Costs

Education in Use of Health Services   The most effective use of health services and health insurance mechanisms requires an informed and concerned public. If the *ideal* health care system for some countries were installed tomorrow, it would be highly subject to disuse, misuse, and abuse by an unprepared public operating under the control of habits, attitudes, and expectations inculcated by a lifetime of coping with their traditional system. Many of the failures or temporary breakdowns in the implementation of new programs in various countries have been traced to problems of communication, knowledge, attitudes, and habits of consumers and practitioners. Health workers need to understand how their actions influence health outcomes and costs. Consumers need to understand how health care organization and escalating costs affect them. Without an understanding of the impact of health care decisions on taxes and insurance premiums, consumers are indifferent to costs

Controlling Costs of Personal Health Services

SOURCE OF COST INCREASES	**RECOMMENDED POLICIES**
Physician salaries or fees	Increasing use of paraprofessionals, advanced nurse practitioners, allied health, and other "physician-extender" personnel; also reductions in medical school enrollment, numbers allowed to go into specialties, incentives for practice in rural and remote areas, and reductions in foreign medical graduates admitted to practice in North America.
Unnecessary hospitalization, laboratory tests, length of stay, and elective surgery	Increased incentives for keeping patients out of hospitals by requiring outpatient surgery and allowing physicians to share in the profits of managed care organizations; also, peer review of medical practice, use review of hospital practice, and second opinions regarding suggested surgery (see table 21-3).
Increased use of medical services for conditions that might have been prevented and readmissions for chronic conditions not adequately controlled by patients	Increased emphasis on preventive medicine and health education, including occupational health, patient education, self-care education, mutual aid, support for family caregivers, health promotion, and environmental health (see examples in table 21-3).

when private insurance companies or the government pays the bill.

Participation in Planning   These problems would be more readily addressed in the planning of health care services if those who use the services are involved in planning them. Unless planning and implementation of services are closely tied at the community level, the best ideas of policy will not penetrate local practice and redistribution of expenditures.

Disease Prevention and Health Maintenance
Any new plan that makes health care more accessible and more acceptable to more people will place pressure on existing resources unless it is accompanied by a new orientation to prevention and health maintenance. A major criticism of the traditional fee-for-service structure of American medicine and scheduled reimbursement for office visits in the Canadian system is that they offer little in-

centive for the providers of services to give attention to prevention, health promotion, and health education. The rewards are tied almost entirely to treatment of the sick. When Americans and Canadians speak of health care, they usually mean medical treatment.

Continuing Education of Professionals   Health care professionals must become better trained to communicate effectively with patients and consumers and to place greater emphasis on disease prevention and health promotion with their patients (figure 21-17). This will call for expansion and reorientation of training programs for medical, nursing, and allied health professionals.

More Distal Determinants of Health   Shifting some of the attention from strictly medical and financing concerns to other determinants such as behavior or lifestyle and the environment puts a different spin on the health reform debate. The

Table 21-3

Costs of Treatment for Preventable Conditions in the United States

Condition	Overall magnitude in U.S.	Avoidable intervention*	Cost per patient†
Heart disease	7 million with coronary artery disease 500,000 deaths/yr 284,000 bypass procedures/yr	Coronary bypass surgery	$30,000
Cancer	1 million new cases/yr 510,000 deaths/yr	Lung cancer treatment Cervical cancer treatment	$29,000 $28,000
Stroke	600,000 strokes/yr 150,000 deaths/yr	Hemiplegia treatment and rehabilitation	$22,000
Injuries	2.3 million hospitalizations/yr 142,500 deaths/yr 177,000 persons with spinal cord injuries	Quadriplegia treatment and rehabilitation Hip fracture treatment and rehabilitation Severe head injury treatment and rehabilitation	$570,000 (lifetime) $40,000 $310,000
HIV/AIDS infection	1–1.5 million infected 118,000 AIDS cases (as of Jan. 1990)	AIDS treatment	$75,000 (lifetime)
Alcoholism	18.5 million abuse alcohol 105,000 alcohol-related deaths/yr	Liver transplant	$250,000

Drug abuse	Regular users:
	  1–3 million, cocaine
	  900,000, IV drugs
	  500,000, heroin
	Drug-exposed babies: 375,000
		Treatment of cocaine-exposed baby	$66,000 (5 years)

Low-birthweight baby	260,000 LBWB born/yr 23,000 deaths/yr	Neonatal intensive care for LBWB	$10,000
Inadequate immunization	Lacking basic immunization series: 20–30%, aged 2 and younger 3%, aged 6 and older	Congenital rubella syndrome treatment	$354,000 (lifetime)

Source: Office of Disease Prevention and Health Promotion. 1994. *For a healthy nation: returns on investment in public health.* Washington, DC: U.S. Department of Health and Human Services; and related analyses by Centers for Disease Control and Prevention, 1993–1997; and *Healthy People 2000: midcourse review and 1995 revisions.* 1996. Boston: Jones and Bartlett Publishers, pp. 4–5.

••••••••••••••••••••

Figure 21-17

Hospitals have taken more active community health education and health promotion roles in part to improve their image in the face of growing public cynicism about organized medicine. However they also do it because they see much of the preventable damage that arrives in their emergency rooms and beds with problems that could have been avoided with better understanding and more timely action. *Source:* St. Agnes Hospital, Baltimore.

That little chest pain you're ignoring could lose you a lot of heart muscle.

Cardiac care within the first hour could save your active life.

It can certainly increase your chances of saving heart muscle. And heart muscle sustains not only life...but the quality of life. It could mean the difference between living an active healthy life, or spending the majority of your life inactive.

Chance of saving heart muscle

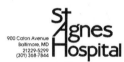

good treated within 1 hour | fair treated within 2-4 hours | poor treated after 4 hours

Act to survive with early cardiac intervention treatment.

Chest pain could mean a heart attack. Be prepared. At the first sign of heart pain, go to your

hospital immediately. Listen to what your heart is trying to tell you. It could save your life.

Check on the availability of early cardiac care at your community hospital.
For more information and a free brochure, write Raymond D. Bahr, M.D., CCU Medical Director.

The Paul Dudley White Coronary Care System ...20 years of promoting concepts in community cardiac care.
The Chest Pain Emergency Room...6 years experience in cardiac intervention.

St Agnes Hospital
900 Caton Avenue
Baltimore, MD
21229-5299
(301) 368-7844

A Daughters of Charity Hospital Serving the Community Since 1862. A Tradition of Caring for 125 years

This information made possible by a grant from the National Emergency Medicine Association through its National Heart Research Project. 11 West Pennsylvania Avenue, Towson, MD 21204.

community and population health perspective on health services emphasizes consumer participation in planning, issues of distribution and education for appropriate use of health care resources, preventive health maintenance, communication with patients, reorientation of health professional training, and reorientation of health systems in concert with other sectors. Each of these will have the ef-

fect, in part, of shifting some concern, if not resources, to the broader societal determinants of health. The remainder of this chapter comments specifically on national health plans from the community health perspective.

SOCIALIZED MEDICAL SERVICES

Medical services are socialized when the government administers them. More than fifty nations have national medical service programs, and nearly all of these are socialized programs. For generations the federal, state, and local governments in the United States have socialized various services—mail service, education, and police and fire protection—but only parts of their medical systems. A city that sells water or electricity to its residents is engaged in the socialization of an economic enterprise.

Personal health care services vary from one nation to the next. The first national medical program was the German Sickness Insurance Plan, but the Swedish and Canadian programs have been of special interest to Americans. These programs have similarities and dissimilarities and represent basic types of national medical programs. Sweden's is truly national; Canada's "national" health insurance system is really an interlocking set of ten provincial and two territorial health insurance plans.

Sweden

Economists generally agree that Sweden has the best-structured and administered national health program. Sweden's experience in pension programs, maternal and infant care programs, geriatrics programs, and welfare programs was excellent preparation for establishing in 1955 the System of Medical Care and Sickness Benefit insurance.

Access   The national health insurance program covers all Swedish citizens and alien residents. The national health insurance system is a principal means of creating socioeconomic equality while also functioning as a financing instrument and one

· ·

Figure 21-18

The organization of health care in Sweden features an integrated distribution of facilities such that areas of small population concentration have adequate primary care resources, but can access more specialized hospital services at more centralized levels. The system provides universal care at less cost per person than the United States. Sweden also enjoys better health statistics by most indicators. *Source:* The Swedish Institute. 1991. *Fact sheet prepared for Swedish information service abroad.* Stockholm: The Institute.

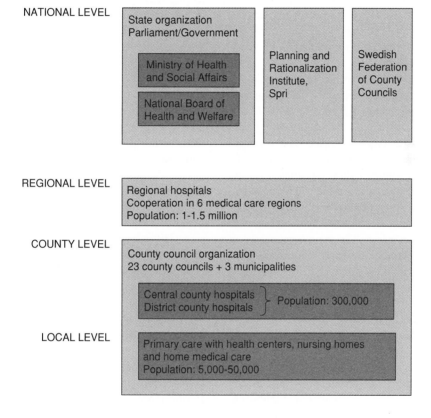

of state control and supervision. The system is based on the fundamental principle that all citizens are entitled to good health and equal access to health and medical care, regardless of their economic circumstances or where they live.

Organization The Ministry of Health and the National Board of Health and Welfare (figure 21-18) administer Sweden's program. It is nevertheless highly decentralized. On the local level each county has a county council elected by the local people responsible for local problems. A managing committee composed of a delegate from the county council, a physician, and a supervisory official conducts necessary business between meetings of the county council. Physicians who are government employees receive a straight salary dependent on rank but irrespective of specialty. The government operates hospitals.

Financing The social insurance office makes payments under the national health insurance system when a person seeks medical and dental care and hospital treatment. The patient pays a standard charge set by the county council for public outpatient services. Costs covered by the national system include consultation with a physician, birth control counseling, x-rays, lab tests, and referrals. Costs not covered include physical, occupational, and speech therapy. A ceiling caps costs for those with catastrophic illness. Dental coverage up to 60 percent is included in the system.

Medical care costs have increased, but at 7.2 percent still remain well below the American 14.2 percent and the Canadian 9.5 percent of GNP. The percent of Sweden's GNP devoted to medical care expenditures has actually decreased. The system is financed primarily by income taxes levied by the county councils. General state subsidies level out differences in income between the county councils.

The Swedish system enjoys a high level of public confidence, and its universality contrasts with the current U.S. system. The main weaknesses of the Swedish system are the lack of integration between services, high proportion of direct referrals to hospitals, long waiting lists for some types of treatment, some limited choice, and insufficient incentives for health personnel to improve the productivity and efficiency of the health sector.

Canada

Known to Canadians as "Medicare," their health care system insures access to universal, comprehensive coverage for medically necessary hospital care, and in-patient and out-patient physician services. While Americans have been concerned about having the technologically best health care system in the world, Canadians have been concerned about building an equitable and universally accessible system, with portability of rights to care from one province to another. Surface similarities between the two systems mask the underlying value differences between Canada and the United States.

Organization The Canadian system, as with any system of health care, reflects the national political structure and philosophy (see "Milestones" box). Canadians are traditionally more accepting than their American neighbors of the role of government in social and human services. Canada considers health a right and a national responsibility. Canadian patients have freedom of choice in selecting their *primary* health care providers in the first instance. They are obliged to see a primary care provider before they can expect to use the services of specialists, which must be by referral but still with freedom of choice. The medical profession is independent and self-regulating. Physicians are not salaried, but instead are reimbursed on a fee-for-service basis, with fee schedules established independently by each province. Hospitals are not government owned, but are locally controlled, nonprofit organizations.

Financing The federal government provided approximately half the funding in the past through transfer of tax revenue to the provinces and territories. The ten provinces and two territories are covering an increased share and find privately-funded expenditures rising from 24 percent in 1985 to 28 percent in 1994 (figure 21-19). They also administer their own programs and have the final say about how much is spent and how resources are allocated. Many of the key features of the Canadian system such as access, affordability, and comprehensiveness have long been policy goals in the United States with bipartisan appeal. Furthermore, in most respects the program does not violate the traditional practice of medicine. The system is decentralized, with increasing autonomy given to local governments regarding the scope and provision of health care services. Providers of care are reimbursed in a manner similar to that of the United States. The main difference is that the provincial government in Canada is a single payer, whereas most American physicians and hospitals must deal with multiple insurance carriers. While some incentives to affect distribution of physicians have been adopted, there are few real restraints on specialization or location of practice. The provinces agreed in 1993 to a 10

Canadian Milestones in Health Insurance and Health Services

1919 National Health Plan first proposed.

1947 First universal Hospital Insurance Plan introduced in Saskatchewan.

1957 Federal Hospital Insurance and Diagnostic Services Act (50/50 cost sharing between federal and provincial governments).

1961 Universal Hospital Plans in all provinces.

1962 First Universal Medical (physician) Care Plan in Saskatchewan.

1968 Federal Medical Care Act (50/50 cost sharing with provinces).

1972 Medical Plans in all provinces and the two territories.

1974 Minister of Health, Marc Lalonde, issued report, *A New Perspective on the Health of Canadians,* in which the three determinants of health other than medical care (lifestyle, genetics, and environment) were given greater importance.

1977 Established Programs Financing (EPF) replaced 50/50 cost sharing to put the federal transfers to provinces and territories on a per capita basis.

1979 Hall Commission reported that extra-billing by doctors, requiring their patients to supplement what the provincial plan paid the doctor for specific services, threatened to create a two-tiered system.

1984 Canada Health Act passed, establishing the five principles for universality, accessibility, comprehensiveness, public administration, and portability of health care coverage across provinces.

1986 Minister of Health, Jake Epp, issued report on *Achieving Health for All,* simultaneously with the international Ottawa Charter for Health Promotion, giving renewed attention to determinants and strategies for health other than medical care.

1996 Federal government contributions to provincial health and social programs consolidated into a new single block transfer payment, the Canada Health and Social Transfer.

1997 National Health Care Forum issued report concluding that "The answer to the genuine need and desirability of health care reform will not be found in increased spending on health care. At the same time, emerging knowledge about non-medical interventions demands action at all levels of society."

••••••••••••••••••••••

Figure 21-19

Health care expenditures in Canada show the dominance of provincial governments over private sector and other sources (workers' compensation payments, municipal and federal direct payments for specific groups including First Nations and Armed Forces). *Source:* Health Canada data for 1996, analyzed by Manitoba Centre for Health Policy and Evaluation. 1997. *What drives health care expenditures?* Winnipeg: The Manitoba Centre for Health Policy and Evaluation.

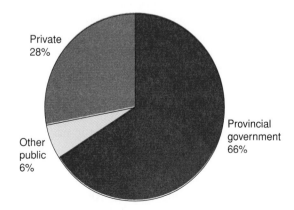

. . . .
Figure 21-20

Canada's system removes the out-of-pocket cost barrier to primary care, which results in more equitable distribution of basic health care services for the population. *Source:* Photo by James H. Peacock, Calgary, courtesy Alberta Heritage Foundation for Medical Research, Edmonton.

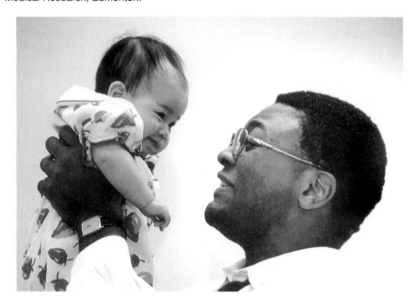

percent reduction in medical school enrollments to control the escalation of costs that are now understood to be driven by oversupply of physicians.

Access Public access to personal health services improves with the removal of economic barriers to care (figure 21-20). Canada has seen some shift in resource **allocation** from rich to poor. Poor people have increased their use of physicians, as have the middle- and upper-income groups. Not all problems related to access can be solved merely through changes in financing, however, and certain inequities persist. For example, the poor still use hospital emergency rooms more for primary health care problems than other income groups, indicating that physician maldistribution may be a persistent problem in primary care.

Use of Services Use of services has not increased at the alarming rate originally projected in some quarters. If Canada's experience is any

guide, a national health insurance scheme does not necessarily create a "flood" of people seeking unnecessary medical care.

Cost Containment In 1996 Canadians spent $75.2 billion on health care, which was $2,510 per person, less than in 1992. Health care costs were 9.5 percent of the GNP, down from the 1992 peak figure of 10.2 percent. This compares with U.S. figures at $3,621 per person (in U.S. dollars, about 1.3 times higher than Canadian dollars), 14.2 percent of the GNP. Costs present problems for Canada as for the United States. Hospital cost inflation in Canada has less to do with higher use than with increases in earnings of hospital workers and intensity of care. The structure of reimbursement and the organization of medical practice are further contributing to the cost crisis. Hospital insurance was passed ten years before the physician reimbursement portion (see "Milestones" box), therefore incentives were put in place to hospitalize patients rather than to treat them in more cost-effective **ambulatory health care services** or settings. Global budgets are negotiated in advance for each hospital. There is a substantial degree of freedom of expenditures within the budget. If at the end of a fiscal year an institution has an operating surplus, the government does not necessarily reclaim the surplus. This provides the hospitals with an incentive to economize.

Health Care as a Right Canadians discovered that granting health care as a "right" has been costly, but Canada spends a lower percentage of its gross national product on health care than does the United States, less per capita, and its rate of increase has been lower than that of the United States. Canada's vital statistics are generally better than those of the United States. Consumers have virtually no out-of-pocket expenses for regular hospital and medical care. Some provincial plans have imposed cost-sharing provisions for hospital stays, but the amounts are nominal. At the same time, Canada has an active supplementary insurance market, primarily for drugs, dental care, private rooms in hospitals, and other services not covered by the program.

Health Education and Promotion Canada has educated the health care consumer about overuse of services and how to use the system more effectively. Some emphasis has been given to health promotion to support better health habits and conditions of living. Community health promotion has greater support in some Canadian provinces than in most states of the United States. The National Health Care Forum reported to the Prime Minister in 1997 the findings and recommendations from its two-year study of the Canadian system. The Forum said that, taken alone, spending more money on health care was not the key to sustaining the system, but that health could be improved and maintained more effectively through strategic investments in more distal determinants of health, including positive childhood development, employment, and social support. The 1997 budget of

the Government of Canada responded with a pledge of over $300 million over three years for a health care transition fund, an integrated Canadian Health Information System, and restored funding levels for community action programs for children and prenatal nutrition.

U.S. PROGRAMS

Throughout U.S. history, Americans have attempted in various ways to make medical care available. Industrial firms and other employers have provided medical and hospital services for employees and their dependents. For generations the medical profession has used a sliding scale of fees based on the ability of the patient to pay. Socialized medicine was selectively in existence in the United States before the turn of the century. The federal government has provided medical and hospital care for members of the armed services and their dependents, war veterans, federal prison inmates, American Indians on reservations, foreign service personnel, and various categories of government employees. The federal government, with the state and local governments, has provided medical and hospital services for families on welfare. A universal program to ensure access and equity in health services, however, has never materialized. Although there are many different names for health insurance plans used currently, three main types include private insurance, Health Maintenance Organizations (HMOs), and Preferred Provider Organizations (PPOs). These have come increasingly under managed care arrangements.

Private Insurance

Private or fee-for-service health insurance is the traditional health care policy in the United States. Commercial insurance companies were once reluctant to initiate health insurance but began with hospital insurance where **actuarial data** were available and costs were reasonably stable and predictable. Success with hospital insurance encouraged the companies to expand to medical insurance and, finally, insurance for physician visits. Voluntary, noncommercial organizations have developed insurance programs for groups and individuals.

Insurance is a financial contract that exchanges average costs as prepaid premiums for variable costs as guaranteed payments in the event of loss or specific expenses. It is not possible to predict the medical and hospital expenses for one person for the next year, but it is possible to predict total medical and hospital expenses for a million people. From such population data, insurance premiums are determined and medical and hospital costs are spread among many rather than falling heavily on a few.

Extent of Coverage In 1995, approximately 85 percent of Americans had some form of health insurance. Approximately 75 percent of those covered had private health insurance and Medicaid covered 8 percent. Losses of jobs during the recession and cutbacks on benefits to employees meant an increase in the number of those without health coverage. In 1995 it was estimated that 41 million Americans had no health insurance. Among those uninsured, 60 percent were working but at low-paying service or retail industries that did not offer insurance benefits. With the passage in 1996 of the Kennedy-Kassebaum Act, insurance coverage was assured by the government for those who were losing health insurance when they changed jobs or a family member became ill.

Health insurance coverage varies among sectors of the population. The people least likely to have coverage are those between 18 and 24 years of age. Twenty-eight percent of this age group lacked insurance in 1995, compared to the nearly complete coverage by Medicare or private supplemental insurance of the over-65 age group. People in the Northeast and Midwest are more likely to have health insurance than those in the South and West. Nearly one-third of those of Hispanic origin lack insurance coverage (figure 21-21), 21 percent of African Americans, and 14 percent of White Americans.

················

Figure 21-21

Health insurance and Medicaid provisions for children vary widely across the states. Children, therefore, are at great risk of having no coverage or at best uneven coverage with no continuity of care. Hispanic children, especially if foreign born and without American citizenship, are the most likely to be without health insurance. *Source:* Photo by Marsha Burke, courtesy University of Texas Health Science Center at Houston.

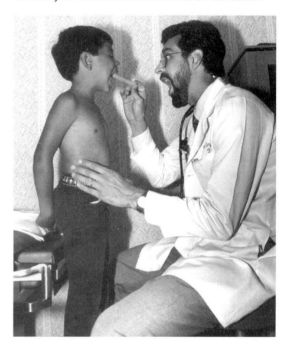

Types of Coverage Fee-for-service insurance provides the most choice of doctors and hospitals. While such plans usually pay some doctor and most hospital expenses, most do not cover preventive services such as physical checkups or immunizations and limit well-child care. Of the 734 million visits made to doctors' offices in 1996, 21 percent were paid for by private fee-for-service insurance (figure 21-22), down from 36 percent in 1991. In addition to medical care, many insured people have plans that include dental insurance of varying generosity.

· · · · · · · · · · · · · · · · · · · ·

Figure 21-22

Although private insurance still paid for the largest proportion of physician office visits in the United States in 1996, decreasing portions of that were fee-for-service private insurance and increasing portions were HMO or other managed care insurance arrangements. *Source:* Woodwell, D. A. 1997. National ambulatory medical care survey: 1996 summary. *Advance data from vital and health statistics,* no. 295. Hyattsville, MD: National Center for Health Statistics.

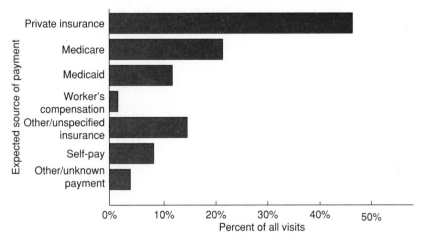

NOTE: Sum of percents may exceed 100 because more than one source of insurance may be reported per visit.

There are two basic kinds of fee-for-service coverage: basic and major medical. Basic protection pays toward the costs of a hospital room and care received in the hospital. It covers some hospital services and supplies, such as x-rays and prescribed medicine. Basic coverage also pays toward the cost of surgery and/or some doctor visits. Major medical insurance takes over where basic coverage leaves off. It covers the cost of long, high-cost illness or injuries. Some policies combine both types of insurance into a "comprehensive plan."

The insured person pays three kinds of costs: a monthly premium, an annual deductible, and coinsurance toward costs. The deductible, which might be $250 in a typical plan, must be paid each year before the insurance payments begin. After the deductible amount for the year is paid, the policyholder shares the remaining bill with the insurance company. In a typical arrangement the policyholder's **coinsurance** portion of the shared bill may be 20 percent and the insurer pays 80 percent. Most fee-for-service plans have a "cap"—the highest amount an individual will have to pay for medical bills in a given year. A cap is reached when deductible and coinsurance payments exceed a certain amount, which may be as low as $1,000 or as high as $5,000. The insurance company pays the full amount in excess of the cap for items it covers.

Health Maintenance Organizations (HMOs) and Other Managed Care Arrangements

HMOs, prepaid health plans, experienced substantial growth in the United States, from 175 in 1976 to 650 in 1997. HMOs served over 67 million people in 1997, more than three times as many as in 1985. The number of people projected for enrollment in HMOs is expected to continue to increase

Milestones in Managed Care

1789   The Reverend Edward Wigglesworth assessed the health of Americans and produced the first American mortality tables.

1851   An early voluntary mutual protection association organized in San Francisco and established a hospital to provide care for its members.

1910   First example of an HMO, known then as a "prepaid group practice," at the Western Clinic in Tacoma, Washington, for lumber mill owners and employees.

1929   First rural farmers' cooperative health plan created by a doctor in Elk City, Oklahoma. Baylor Hospital in Houston, Texas, also provided prepaid care to 1,500 teachers. Ross-Loos Clinic established in Los Angeles as a forerunner of HMOs.

1932   The AMA adopted a strong opposition to prepaid group practices, endorsing instead indemnity-type insurance.

1937   In southern California, Kaiser Foundation Health Plan began financing medical care for workers building an aqueduct in the desert. By 1990s, this plan covered sixteen states and 7.3 million members.

1944   New York City employees received the Health Insurance Plan (HIP) of Greater New York as an early HMO for government workers. It now covers 1.1 million members.

1960   Kerr-Mills Act passed as forerunner of Medicare and Medicaid.

1965   Lyndon Johnson signed Medicare-Medicaid amendments to the Social Security Act (PL 88-97).

1967   Initial enrollment in Medicare for people aged 65 and over was 19.5 million. In 1996 it was 38.1 million.

1973   Congress passed HMO Act to ensure access to employer-based insurance markets and authorized start-up funding.

1977   Carter administration reduced barriers to HMO creation; enrollment jumps from 6.3 million in 1977 to 67 million in 1997.

1978   First preferred provider organization (PPO) created when a benefits consulting firm in Denver negotiated discounts with physicians not in the contracted network of an HMO.

1994   HMO and PPO enrollment reach 51 million, each accounting for 25 percent of the health plan market.

1997   Acquisitions, alliances, and mergers produced conglomerates of hospitals, insurance payers, and practitioners as managed care systems designed to provide comprehensive care.

Sources: Managing managed care. *Washington Post* 1997. Editorial. 25 Dec; Fisher, I. 1998. HMO premiums rising sharply, stoking debate on managed care. *NY Times,* 11 Jan. Meyers, E. 1997. The evolution of managed care. *Academic Nurse* 14(2):13.

to 90 million in 2000, 148 million in 2010. These projections, however, preceded the growing disenchantment of consumers with their HMOs, first noted in 1997. Eroding confidence in HMOs was reflected in the declining stock prices on Wall Street during a year when the stock market was booming in most sectors.

Between the passage of the Social Security Act in 1934 and the amendments in 1965 that created Medicare and Medicaid, most of the significant advances in ensuring greater access to medical care were made by private insurance companies and states. Then came the 1960s, discussed in the previous chapter (p. 695) as a period of ferment in the health care system. Some of the more significant events during the twentieth century in the development of managed care are shown in the "Milestones" box. Of particular note during this period was the evolution of the health maintenance organization concept.

Health maintenance organizations (HMOs), sometimes identified merely as prepaid group practice, have faced criticism of becoming bureaucratized and cold-hearted in their management of illness. The programs often have been subsidized, at least at the outset, but in the main, these have been self-sustaining enterprises. Four principles characterize an HMO. It is

1. an *organized system* of health care that accepts the responsibility to provide or otherwise ensure the delivery of
2. an agreed-upon set of *comprehensive health maintenance and treatment services* for
3. a voluntarily *enrolled group* of people in a geographical area and
4. is reimbursed through a *prenegotiated and fixed periodic payment* made by or on behalf of each person or family enrolled in the plan.

These four principles of HMO development are further defined and described by Congress in the Health Maintenance Organization Assistance Act of 1973.

An Organized System   An HMO must be capable of bringing together directly, or arranging for, the services of physicians and other health professionals with the services of inpatient and outpatient facilities for preventive, acute, and other care, and any other health services that a defined population might reasonably require. The system is organized in such a way as to ensure for the enrollee the most efficient and effective entry into the health care system. It also promises continuity of care for the enrolled population through linkages between the components of organization.

In nearly all HMOs, members are assigned or choose one doctor to serve as a primary care doctor. This doctor monitors the member's health and provides most of the medical care, as in the Canadian and Swedish systems, referring to specialists and other health care professionals as needed. In some HMOs doctors are salaried and have offices in the same location. In other arrangements, independent doctors contract with the HMO to take care of patients. These are called individual practice associations (IPAs), with doctors located in scattered locations in their own private offices.

Comprehensive Health Maintenance and Treatment Services   The HMO must be capable of providing or arranging for the provision of the health services that a population might require, including primary care, emergency care, acute inpatient hospital care, and inpatient and outpatient care and rehabilitation for chronic and disabling conditions. Primary care, one of the keystones of the HMO, emphasizes those services aimed at preventing the onset of illness or disability, at the maintenance of good health, and at the continuing evaluation and management of early complaints, symptoms, problems, and the chronic aspects of disease. Typical services include doctor visits, hospital stays, emergency care, surgery, lab tests, x-rays, and therapy. HMOs typically provide preventive care such as office visits, immunizations, well-baby checkups, mammograms, and physicals.

An Agreed-Upon Set of Services   The consumers and the HMO agree on which services will be purchased from the HMO in return for the prepayment figure. The benefit schedule for population groups may differ because some HMOs may have groups or enrollees paid for by Medicare, Medicaid, or employer-employee arrangements.

An Enrolled Group   Members of an HMO are those people who voluntarily join the HMO through a contract arrangement in which the enrollee (or head of household) agrees to pay the fixed monthly or other periodic payment (or have it paid on his or her behalf) to the HMO. Enrollees agree to use the HMO as their principal source of health care if they become ill or need care.

Type of Coverage   Those enrolled in an HMO pay a monthly premium. This is a fixed fee that covers the agreed-on set of services. There may be a small **copayment** for each office visit, such as a $5 fee for a doctor visit or $25 fee for hospital emergency room treatment. Rather than completing multiple forms usually required by fee-for-service insurance, members present a card, like a credit card, at the doctor's office or hospital.

Preferred Provider Organizations (PPOs)

This type of organization is a combination of the traditional fee-for-service plan and an HMO. Like the HMO, the consumer-member has a limited number of doctors and hospitals to choose from. When members use one of the "preferred" providers, most of the medical bills are covered. Usually there is a small copayment for each visit. Some services require a deductible and coinsurance. PPOs also use a primary care doctor to monitor members' health. Most cover preventive care such as doctor visits, well-baby care, immunizations, and mammograms. PPOs also allow members to use doctors who are not part of the plan and still receive some coverage. Usually the member will pay a larger portion of the bill when using someone other than a preferred provider.

Medicare

The United States launched its first widespread program of socialized medicine in 1965, when the Medicare Act was passed. Medicare was established as a federal health insurance program for Americans age 65 and older, for certain disabled Americans under age 65, and people of any age who have permanent kidney failure. It is not necessary to have Social Security or government work credits to be eligible for Medicare. In 1991 Medicare covered approximately 35 million people, of whom about 3 million were disabled and some 150,000 were kidney disease patients.

Medicare is administered by the Health Care Financing Administration of the U.S. Department of Health and Human Services. Commercial insurance companies and managed care organizations serve as agents or intermediaries for the program. Claimants under the program fill out a form and mail it to the designated insurance company serving as agent for the government.

Medicare has two basic forms of coverage—Part A provides hospital insurance and Part B provides supplemental medical insurance for costs such as payments for doctors and related services and supplies ordered by a doctor. All who meet the eligibility requirements can partici-

pate in Part A of Medicare free. Part B requires payment of a premium.

Medicare hospital insurance, Part A, is financed mainly from a portion of the Social Security payroll tax (the FICA) deduction. The Medicare part of the payroll tax is 1.65 percent from the employee and 1.45 percent from the employer; 15.3 percent for self-employed people. The optional Medicare medical insurance, Part B, is financed by the monthly premiums paid by enrollees and from general federal revenues. The monthly premium in 1997 was $43.80. The premiums pay about 25 percent of the cost of the Part B program, and general tax revenues pay about 25 percent. For coverage of health care costs, patients pay a $100 **deductible** and monthly premiums, then Medicare pays for 80 percent of covered services.

Part A: Hospital Insurance   Medicare hospital insurance pays for up to 90 days of inpatient care (including hospital care and related posthospital home care and physical therapy) per benefit period. For the first 60 days, Medicare pays for all covered services, except for a deductible. In 1997 the deductible was $760 per benefit period. Those services include a semiprivate room, regular nursing service, operating room, drugs, lab tests, x-rays, medical supplies, and rehabilitation services. From days 61 to 90, Medicare continues to pay for these services, but the beneficiary must pay a daily coinsurance amount.

Medicare also pays for skilled nursing or rehabilitation services up to 100 days. Hospital insurance pays for all covered services for the first 20 days. For the next 100 it pays for all covered services except for a daily coinsurance amount, which was $95 per day in 1997. Medicare makes a careful distinction between skilled nursing care and "custodial care." Those who are medically trained provide the former, and Medicare pays for such services. The latter type of care includes help with dressing, walking, or eating, which does not required skilled care; therefore, Medicare does not pay for such services.

Medicare and Managed Care

The section titled "Part B: Medical Insurance" explains how Medicare Part B works if you receive your benefits through the traditional fee-for-service (pay-as-you-go) delivery system. As a Medicare beneficiary, you also have the option of receiving physician and other health care services through coordinated care plans that have contracts with Medicare, such as health maintenance organizations (HMOs), and competitive medical plans (CMPs).

In a coordinated care plan, a network of health care providers (physicians, hospitals, skilled nursing facilities, etc.) usually offers medical services to plan members on a prepaid basis. Services usually must be obtained from the professionals and facilities that are part of the plan. If you enroll in a plan that has a contract with Medicare, a Medicare claim will seldom need to be submitted on your behalf. Medicare pays the plan a set amount and the plan provides your medical care. Additionally, instead of paying Medicare's deductible and coinsurance as you would under fee-for-service care, most coordinated care plans charge enrollees a monthly premium and nominal copayments.

Most plans serving Medicare beneficiaries are required to provide all Medicare hospital and medical benefits available in the plan's service area. Some plans also provide benefits beyond what Medicare pays for, such as preventive care, prescription drugs, dental care, hearing aids, and eyeglasses.

Source: HCFA, 1992 and 1997.

Medicare pays the full cost of home health visits by an approved agency. There is no limit to the number of covered visits for intermittent skilled nursing care and physical or speech therapy. A 20 percent copayment does apply to medical equipment such as wheelchairs or hospital beds. Medicare can help pay for hospice care for terminally ill beneficiaries up to a maximum of two 90-day periods and one 30-day period and one extension.

Part B: Medical Insurance This supplemental insurance pays for doctor services and many other medical services and supplies that are not covered by the hospital insurance part of Medicare. Each year before Medicare medical insurance begins paying for covered services, beneficiaries must meet the annual medical insurance deductible, which was $100 in 1997. After the deductible is met, Medicare will usually pay 80 percent of the approved charges for covered services during the rest of the year.

The Medicare law specifically prohibits federal interference in the physician-patient relationship, but this also precludes monitoring of quality. Free-dom of choice is guaranteed—there is no "preferred" group of physician providers (see box titled "Medicare and Managed Care").

Services Not Covered Medicare does not pay for custodial care, most nursing home care, most care outside the United States, dental care, routine checkups, prescription drugs, routine foot care, hearing aids, and eyeglasses. Many private insurance companies sell insurance to pay for costs not covered by Medicare. Such "Medigap" coverage varies among states and was standardized in 1992 to a core package of benefits.

Medicaid

Title XIX of the Social Security Act, also called the Kerr-Mills medical assistance plan (Medicaid), provides medical care not only for indigents 65 years of age and older but for those of any age who are defined as medically indigent (figure 21-23). This program is a joint enterprise of the federal and state governments, which subsidize all of the costs.

Like Medicare, the Medicaid "Grants to States for Medical Assistance Programs" was addressed exclusively to the problem of purchasing power and made little or no effort to deviate from "usual and customary fees" to hospitals and physicians or from the prevailing organization of delivery systems. Both programs under PL 89-97 were established on the assumption that the existing delivery systems would respond to the needs and demands of the population if sufficient fees for services were provided. The increased demand contributed to increased prices. The two programs rose from $5 billion in their initial year to over $124 billion in 1996 for Medicare and over $120 billion for Medicaid.

Federal Requirements

The purpose of Medicaid was to provide medical assistance for the "medically indigent" families with dependent children, the aged, the blind, and the disabled. The law extended coverage to rehabilitation and other services to help such families attain independence and self-care. The distinguishing mechanism of this plan is that it authorizes appropriations on a fiscal-year basis for payments to states that submit approved plans. The act required that state plans must

1. cover the entire state
2. contribute at least 40 percent of the nonfederal share,
3. provide for a fair hearing to any individual whose claim is denied or delayed,
4. provide for administration of the state program or supervision of locally administered plans,
5. designate a single state agency for administration or supervision of the plan,
6. provide reports to the Secretary of Health and Human Services,
7. provide safeguards for confidentiality of records,
8. provide that all individuals wishing to make application for medical assistance under the plan have an opportunity to do so, and
9. designate an authority for establishing and maintaining standards for participating institutions.

· ·

Figure 21-23

Medically indigent families with dependent children (particularly prevalent in single-parent families) are eligible for Social Security payments to the dependents of disabled or deceased beneficiaries and for Medicaid for their medical care requirements. *Source:* U.S. Social Security Administration and Advertising Council.

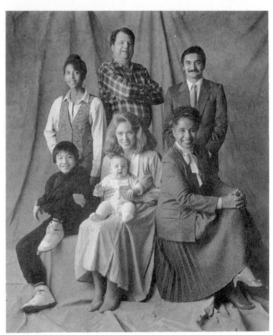

Can you guess who's eligible for Social Security?

They all are.

Because Social Security isn't just for retirement; it's for people of all ages.

If your life is somehow cut short, it will pay survivors benefits to your family, even if you're years from retirement.

If a serious illness or injury prevents you from working, it can provide disability payments.

Now you can find out what your benefits might be with a free Personal Earnings and Benefit Estimate Statement from Social Security. Using our records of your Social Security earnings and the future income information you provide us, we'll give you an estimate of what you can expect—not only for retirement, but in disability and survivors benefits as well.

Write to Dept. 74, Pueblo, Colorado 81009, and we'll send you a simple form you can complete to get your own Personal Earnings and Benefit Estimate Statement.

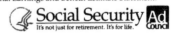

Social Security Ad Council
It's not just for retirement. It's for life.

Assessment   Consider some of the implications of these nine requirements. Numbers 1 and 2 clearly distinguish Medicaid from Medicare as a *state* plan. Number 3 places emphasis on repairing damage that should be prevented by requirements 8 and 9. From an educational perspective, number 8 should require states to include coordinated programs to ensure that all eligible beneficiaries know of their eligibility and that all applicants know of and have access to sources of assistance in maneuvering the application process. According to a survey in California, 95 percent of the potential beneficiaries and many of the community workers interviewed confused Medi-Cal (the California name for Medicaid) with *welfare* and with Medicare. (Some thought it was a soft drink!) Even among those using the program, 90 percent thought Medi-Cal was the same as welfare. The welfare stigma is found to be highly unsettling for most users, a cause of misuse, and a clear deterrent to use by potential beneficiaries.

The coverage of preventive services by Medicaid varies widely from state to state. New federal requirements for states to cover prenatal and infant care services have been implemented by states at considerable cost but still without the systematic coverage provided in other countries.

Cost Containment   Of high concern to state and federal governments are uncontrolled growth of health care costs and the lack of physicians and other providers willing to treat Medicaid patients. Under traditional fee-for-service arrangements neither the state nor any other entity monitors the physician's provision of services. These arrangements are inadequate in terms of controlling costs and ensuring quality care.

Medicaid costs were increasing an average of 10 percent a year in the 1980s. In 1989, they began to rise even more rapidly, nearly doubling between 1990 and 1995. As the federal contribution to Medicaid has declined, states have picked up a larger share of the costs. In 1995 federal and state spending on Medicaid totaled $120 billion,

with benefits paid for 36.3 million aged, blind, disabled, or poor persons with families. The number of beneficiaries increased by 44 percent between 1990 and 1995 to over 36 million. Extended health insurance coverage for children under new legislation in 1998 should increase it more.

The distribution of costs with the Medicaid system varies by population group. For example, while 27 percent of Medicaid recipients are on Supplemental Security Income, these mostly elderly recipients account for nearly 70 percent of Medicaid expenditures. Aid to Families with Dependent Children (AFDC) became Temporary Aid to Needy Families (TANF) in July 1997. TANF gives state broad authority to determine eligibility and benefit levels. To qualify for matching federal Medicaid funds a state must provide medical coverage for all persons who receive assistance under TANF.

Managed Care   To deal with the costs, access problems, and aging of the overall population, states have increasingly turned to managed care delivery systems. These systems are a continuum of models that share a common approach. At one end of the continuum are prepaid models that pay organizations a per capita amount each month to provide or arrange for all covered services. At the other end of the spectrum are primary care case management models similar to traditional fee-for-service arrangements. The difference with managed care is that providers receive a per capita management fee to coordinate a patient's care in addition to reimbursement for the services they provide. Common to all managed care models in the Medicaid program is the use of a primary care physician to control and coordinate the delivery of health services in a cost-conscious manner.

By 1995 all states had at least one managed care program in place. Four key issues to resolve in managed care systems include planning for implementation, making enrollment mandatory, setting capitation rates, and educating beneficiaries about the program.

● ●

Figure 21-24

Health care reform has benefited from new information systems and technologies giving health care workers access to records and the latest scientific information. This has improved evidence-based practice, but has also raised new and complicating ethical issues. How these issues will affect community health services, especially disease prevention and health promotion, was widely debated and discussed in professional meetings during the 1990s. *Source:* PhotoDisc/Business and Occupation.

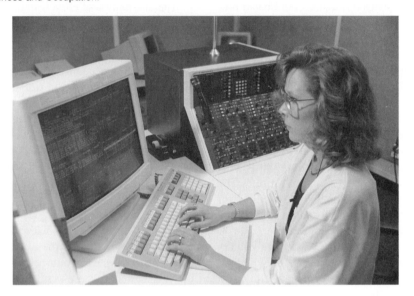

HEALTH CARE REFORM

Faced in the 1990s with escalating costs, a huge deficit, an aging population, new technologies and managed care plans, the role of lifestyle and community in health, a new administration in the White House, and bipartisan support, the United States was poised for major health care reform. After President Clinton's proposal and some thirty other health care proposals ran the gauntlet of economic, political, social, and philosophical considerations, none were passed. Canadians elected a new government and sent their members of Parliament to Ottawa with a clear message that preserving and renewing (if not reforming) their health care system was their highest priority. A survey conducted by Harvard School of Public Health in 1995 in both countries revealed that Americans and Canadians remain wedded to their respective approaches to health care (figure 21-24).

Health care reform proposals continue to fall into three main groups: (1) market-based proposals to assist some people now without insurance to purchase it, (2) "pay-or-play" plans in which employers either provide insurance to employees or pay taxes to finance an alternate public system, and (3) proposals for a single-payer health care system like Canada's. Most plans aim to hold down the soaring costs of health care and to enable those without health insurance to have access to the health care system. A smaller number of proposals would insure the costs of long-term care. Almost all proposals require new financing to meet start-up expenses or shifting of costs from the private to the public sector.

While Washington moves cautiously toward health care reform, various states have taken creative steps toward reform at home. Through community participation, Oregon has established

National Objectives to Ensure Clinical Preventive Services

Objectives target
- increasing receipt of recommended services,
- increasing access to primary care,
- removing financial barriers to receipt of services,
- ensuring clinical preventive services for publicly funded programs,
- ensuring provision of recommended preventive services by clinicians,
- ensuring access to clinical preventive services by local public health departments, and
- increasing the representation of racial and ethnic minority groups among health professionals.

priorities for health care services for which it will pay. Preventive services lead the list. While the proposed rationing of services stirs strong emotional debate, it acknowledges limits to services the state can afford to pay. Under the Hawaii health plan called QUEST, Medicaid, State General Assistance, and the State Health Insurance Program are joined to form a large purchasing pool that will buy health care coverage for 150,000 individuals. Through a process of competitive bidding among managed care plans Hawaii hopes to hold costs down. Minnesota has several proposals for reform to extend coverage to the uninsured.

Health care reform will be difficult. Most fundamentally, health care reform will not only mean looking at our wallets, it will mean looking at our values. Do we really concur with the principles of Alma-Ata that health is a fundamental human right? If we believe health is a right, how do we express and pay for that value in a system that provides liberty, justice—and health care—for all?

SUMMARY

Community and population health are concerned with the health outcomes for whole populations and the context within which people live. The cur-

rent health care systems are mostly concerned with treating sickness, not preventing disease or injury, nor with enhancing health. While Americans and Canadians are rightfully proud of advances in medical care, the United States lags behind other developed countries in some health care indicators and matches some less developed countries in infant mortality. Canadians worry increasingly about their access to specialized care as the baby-boom generation approaches retirement. Americans spend billions on "miracle" cures and quick weight loss, while over 30 million Americans have no health insurance. The increased specialization of medical services, the aging of the population, and uncontrolled health care costs have forced health care reform in the United States, a "health care renewal" in Canada, to the top of the national agenda of both countries. How the system is reformed will depend as much on fundamental values as on current circumstances.

The countries that rank higher than the United States in life expectancy and infant mortality statistics have a national health program (either financing or providing services). They also have lower per capita costs for health care than does the United States. Comparison with Canada has been most instructive for policy development in the United States, and vice versa.

Most health insurance in the United States is not prevention-oriented. It is *sickness* rather than *health* insurance. It gives partial rather than comprehensive benefits and fails to control either costs or quality.

Various proposals for restructuring the health care system have been introduced by public and private groups. Recognizing the inadequacy of the Social Security amendments on Medicare and Medicaid to provide health insurance for the elderly and the medically indigent, health care reform debates continue. Cost containment remains a compelling consideration in all proposals, and this led to an emphasis on competitive and free-market mechanisms in the political climate of the 1980s. The outcome of the health care reform initiatives of the Clinton Administration were beaten back by the health insurance industry and Congress. Reforms in Canada and the United States proceed piecemeal, but with substantial impact on costs, access, prevention, and quality of care.

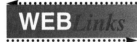

WEB *Links*

http://www.fda.gov/fdahomepage.html
U.S. Food and Drug Administration

http://www.hwc.ca/links/english.html
Canadian Consumer Health Information

http://www.cpsc.gov
U.S. Consumer Product Safety Commission

http://www.consumerreports.org
Consumer Reports magazine

http://www.meps.ahcpr.gov/publicat.htm
Agency for Health Care Policy and Research

QUESTIONS FOR REVIEW

1. Explain the paradox that of the developed countries, the United States and Canada have neither the highest level of health nor the greatest life expectancy?
2. Why is health education of the poor an urgent need?
3. Why does health fraud tend to flourish?
4. Why might an adult wear a charm around his or her neck to keep sickness away?
5. How can the communications media protect the public from health fraud?
6. Is the U.S. hospital admissions rate too high or too low? Why?
7. What is the ratio of physicians to population in your community or country, and what is your appraisal of the situation?
8. How does your country measure up to the standard of four hospital beds per 1,000 people?
9. Why are the average number days of stay in hospitals decreasing?
10. To what extent should the number of nursing homes and personal care homes in your community be increased in the next ten years?
11. Why are medical and hospital costs increasing at a greater rate than the cost-of-living index?
12. What would be your proposal for paying hospital and medical care for low-income families not on welfare?
13. Why are Americans often slow in paying their medical and hospital bills?
14. What are some arguments for and against the federal government totally subsidizing education in the medical, dental, and other health professions?
15. Why should the consumer of medical services have a voice in how the costs of these services are to be paid?

READINGS

Fisher, E. B., V. Strunk, L. K. Sussman, V. Arfken, R. K. Sykes, J. M. Munor, S. Haywood, D. Harrison, and S. Bascom. 1996. Acceptability and feasibility of a community approach to asthma management: the Neighborhood Asthma Coalition (NAC). *J Asthma* 33(6):367.

This is one of the most thorough applications of the PRECEDE-PROCEED model (see chapter 4) in recent projects demonstrating the effectiveness of careful planning of a community approach to self-care and personal health management of a chronic condition.

Lorig K, and Associates. 1996. *Patient Education: A Practical Approach.* 2d ed. Thousand Oaks, London, New Delhi: Sage Publications.

This book presents state-of-the-art methods of carrying out the patient education function of personal health services. See especially pp. 216–223 for an application of the PRECEDE-PROCEED model to arthritis.

McGowan, P., and L. W. Green. 1995. Arthritis self-management in Native populations of British Columbia: An application of health promotion and participatory research principles in chronic disease control. *Can J Aging* 14 (suppl. 1):201.

This case study shows the steps by which Native Canadians were engaged in an active process of planning and adapting an arthritis self-management program, based on Lorig's work (see previous reference), to their needs. Illustrates how the PRECEDE-PROCEED model and participatory research apply in a multicultural setting for self-care and mutual aid.

National Forum on Health. 1997. *Canada health action: building on the legacy.* Ottawa: National Forum on Health and Minister of Public Works and Government Services.

This is the final report of the National Forum on Health, appointed by Prime Minister Jean Chrétien in 1994. It renews the call of reports by previous Ministers of Health, Marc Lalonde and Jake Epp, for a refocusing of attention from health care alone in the health care reform debates to a wider concern for determinants of health beyond medical care. See the report also on the Internet at http://www.nfh.hwc.ca.

BIBLIOGRAPHY

Barer, M. L., T. R. Marmor, and E. M. Morrison. 1995. Editorial. Health care reform in the United States: on the road to nowhere (again)? *Soc Sci Med* 41:453.

Bloom, J. R., J. A. Alexander, and B. A. Nuchols. 1997. Nurse staffing patterns and hospital efficiency in the United States. *Soc Sci Med* 44:147.

Carson, A. J., and M. K. Pichora-Fuller. 1997. Health promotion and audiology: the community-clinic link. *J Acad of Rehabilitative Audiol* 30:29.

Davis, D. A., M. A. Thomson, A. D. Oxman, and R. B. Haynes. 1995. Changing physician performance: A systematic review of the effect of continuing medical education strategies. *J Am Med Assoc* 274:700.

Dignan, M., R. Michielutte, K. Blinson, H. B. Wells, L. D. Case, P. Sharp, S. Davis, J. Konen, and R. P. McQuellon. 1996. Effectiveness of health education to increase screening for cervical cancer among eastern-band Cherokee Indian women in North Carolina. *J National Cancer Inst* 88:1670.

Earp, J. L., M. Alpeter, L. Mayne, C. Viadro, and M. S. Omalley. 1995. The North Carolina breast cancer screening program—Foundations and design of a model for reaching older, minority, rural women. *Breast Can Res & Treatment* 35:7.

Eisenberg, D. M., R. C. Kessler, C. Foster, F. E. Norlock, D. R. Calkins, and T. L. Delbanco. 1993. Unconventional medicine in the United States: prevalence, costs, and patterns of use. *N Engl J Med* 328:246.

Federal, Provincial and Territorial Advisory Committee on Population Health. 1996. *Report on the health of Canadians.* Ottawa: Health Canada.

Fraser, W. 1997. Randomized controlled trial of a prenatal vaginal birth after cesarean section education and support program. *Am J Obstet Gynecol* 176:419.

Hagdrup, N. A., E. J. Simoes, and R. C. Brownson. 1997. Health care coverage: traditional and preventive measures and associations with chronic disease risk factors. *J Community Health* 22:387.

Han, Y., L. C. Baumann, and B. Cimprich. 1996. Factors influencing registered nurses teaching breast self-examination to female clients. *Cancer Nursing* 19:197.

Heywood, A., D. Firman, R. Sanson-Fisher, and P. Mudge. 1996. Correlates of physician counseling associated with obesity and smoking. *Prev Med* 25:268.

Hiddink, G. J., J. G. A. J. Hautvast, C. M. J. van Woerkum, C. J. Fieren, M. A. van't Hof. 1995. Nutrition guidance by primary-care physicians: perceived barriers and low involvement. *Eur J Clin Nut* 49:842.

Lairson, D. R., P. Hindson, and A. Hauquitz. 1994. Equity of health care in Australia. *Soc Sci Med* 41:475.

Laitakari, J., S. Miilunpaolo, and I. Vuori. 1997. The process and methods of health counseling by primary health care personnel in Finland: A national survey. *Patient Educ Couns* 30: 61.

Lomas, J. 1993. Diffusion, dissemination, and implementation: Who should do what? In *Doing More Good than Harm: The Evaluation of Health Care Interventions,* edited by K, S. Warren and F. Mosteller. New York: Annals of the New York Academy of Sciences, Vol. 703, pp. 226–37.

Macarthur, A., C. Macarthur, and S. Weeks. 1995. Epidural anaesthesia and low back pain after delivery: a prospective cohort study. *Brit Med J* 311:1336.

McKell, C. J., C. Chase, and C. Balram. 1996. Establishing partnerships to enhance the preventive practices of dietitians. *J Can Dietetic Assoc* 57:12.

Morrison, C. 1996. Using PRECEDE to predict breast self-examination in older, lower-income women. *Am J Health Behav* 20(2):3.

Olson, C. M. 1994. Promoting positive nutritional practices during pregnancy and lactation. *Am J Clin Nutr* 59 (suppl.):525S.

Pedersen, A., M. O'Neill, and I. Rootman, eds. 1994. *Health promotion in Canada: provincial, national and international perspectives.* Toronto: W. B. Saunders Canada.

Rivo, M. L., H. L. Mays, and D. A. Kindig. 1995. Managed health care: implications for the physician workforce and medical education. *J Am Med Assoc* 274:712.

Roemer, M. I. 1993. National health systems throughout the world. *Annu Rev Public Health* 14:335.

Selby-Harrington, M., J. R. Sorenson, D. Quade, S. C. Stearns, A. S. Tesh, P. L. N. Donat. 1995. Increasing Medicaid child health screenings: The effectiveness of mailed pamphlets, phone calls, and home visits. *Am J Public Health* 85:1412.

Shappert, S. M. 1997. Ambulatory care visits to physician offices, hospital outpatient departments, and emergency departments: United States, 1995. National Center for Health Statistics. *Vital Health Stat* 13(129).

Van Veenendaal, H., D. R. Grinspun, and H. P. Adriaanse. 1996. Educational needs of stroke survivors and their family members, as perceived by themselves and by health professionals. *Patient Educ Couns* 28:265.

Wiggers, J. H., and R. Sanson-Fisher. 1997. Practitioner provision of preventive care in general practice consultations: association with patient educational and occupational status. *Soc Sci Med* 44:137.

Wong, M. L., R. Chan, J. Lee, D. Koh, and C. Wong. 1996. Controlled evaluation of a behavioural intervention programme on condom use and gonorrhoea incidence among sex workers in Singapore. *Health Educ Res* 11:423.

Zuckerman, M., L. G. Guerra, D. A. Drossman, J. A. Foland, and G. G. Gregory. 1996. Health-care-seeking behaviors related to bowel complaints—Hispanics versus non-Hispanic whites. *Digestive Dis & Sci* 41:77.

Appendix A

Areas of Community Health Specialization

Area of specialization	Differentiating characteristics (pertaining to the area of specialization and illustrative ways it contributes to improved health)	Illustrative jobs and job settings (for graduates of the area of specialization)
Biostatistics The application of statistical procedures, techniques, and methodology to characterize or investigate health problems and programs	Biostatistics is concerned with such activities as the collection, organization, retrieval, and analysis of data; design of experiments; and application of techniques of inference and probability to the examination of biological, social, and environmental data. Biostatistics closely interacts with the field of epidemiology, while also extending into the congruent areas of vital statistics and demography, computer systems programming and analysis, and program planning and evaluation. The specialty helps to anticipate needs and improve decision making with regard to health problems, programs, and technologies through (1) the development and operation of ongoing statistical information systems concerned with vital events, health status, and program operations and (2) the proper design and carrying out of studies, and the analysis and interpretation of data obtained from such studies.	In local and state agencies employment includes the collection, tabulation, and analysis of statistics bearing on all aspects of health problems and programs. In state, provincial, federal, and academic settings employment includes providing assistance to investigators in the design, performance, and data analysis of research on health problems, and programs. In academic institutions employment includes training health workers in the use and interpretation of statistics and carrying out research to discover improved ways of using statistical measures and procedures.
Epidemiology The science devoted to the systematic study of the distribution and determinants of disease or disability	Epidemiology determines disease frequencies and trends in populations, and those factors that increase or reduce disease and disability. Epidemiology has both a descriptive and an analytical role. In the former, and in conjunction with the field of biostatistics, it makes use of statistical methods to determine morbidity, mortality, prevalence, incidence and	In health agencies at all levels epidemiologists are employed in the design and execution of studies or information systems concerned with ascertaining the distribution and determinants of disease or disability. In academic settings epidemiologists teach, do research, and assist clinical investigators in the study of disease and in the evaluation of new or

Based on Hall, T. L., R. S. Jackson, and W. B. Parsons. 1980. *Schools of public health, trends in graduate education.* DHHS Pub No (HRA) 80–45, Washington, DC: Division of Associated Health Professions, Public Health Service; American College of Preventive Medicine. 1993. *What is preventive medicine?* Washington, DC: The College; A brighter future for you and the world begins with a career in environmental health. 1997. Washington, DC.

715

Area of specialization	Differentiating characteristics (pertaining to the area of specialization and illustrative ways it contributes to improved health)	Illustrative jobs and job settings (for graduates of the area of specialization)
Epidemiology—cont'd	case fatality rates, and estimates of risk of developing specific diseases in a given population. In its analytical role, epidemiology uses a variety of techniques to examine and evaluate data that seek to identify predisposing, precipitating, and prolonging factors bearing on disease and disability. By developing new or improved information on the distribution and determinants of disease, epidemiology helps the health care system design better ways to prevent, detect, and treat disease and disability.	improved measures for disease prevention, therapy, and rehabilitation.
Health services administration The application of skills in resource management to accomplish the effective and efficient delivery of health services	Areas of expertise relevant to this specialization include those of planning, organizing, directing, controlling, policy formulation and analysis, financial management, economics, accounting, and operations research. While persons with prior professional degrees are not uncommon, students in specialized programs of health services administration tend to have recent bachelor's degrees or to have been practicing administrators without other advanced training. Health services administrators seek to ensure that the resources available for the promotion, protection, and restoration of health are applied as effectively and efficiently as possible, consistent with the scientific knowledge base that exists about health and disease.	Health services administrators are employed at all levels of government and in the private sector to plan, implement, manage, coordinate, and evaluate programs for the delivery of health care and to design administrative systems appropriate to the needs of the population being serviced.
Public health practice and program management The application of specialized knowledge and skills to the planning, implementation, management, and evaluation of activities carried out relevant to selected types of health professional disciplines and health problems or target populations	This area of specialization encompasses many of the identifiable public health programs and activities, some of which are organized according to the demographic characteristics of the target population (maternal and child health, gerontology), others according to a health problem or organ system (mental health, dental public health), and still others according to professional discipline (nursing, social work). Specialists in each of these	Employed at all levels of government and in the private and educational sectors, these specialists assume leadership roles in community-based health care, health promotion and disease prevention programs and systems; apply technical expertise to planning, implementation, and evaluation of technical programs within a defined organizational framework; and carry out training and research activities.

Area of specialization	Differentiating characteristics (pertaining to the area of specialization and illustrative ways it contributes to improved health)	Illustrative jobs and job settings (for graduates of the area of specialization)
Public health practice and program management—cont'd	programmatic areas usually have a prior professional degree in one or more health disciplines in addition to specialty training relevant to their field of choice. They seek to integrate the body of knowledge of the basic discipline (medicine, nursing, etc.) with skills relevant to public health practice (planning, program, development, etc.) to design and implement programs appropriate to specific health needs.	
Health education The process of influencing health-related social and behavioral change in human populations by predisposing, enabling, and reinforcing voluntary decisions and actions conducive to health	Health education specialists use specific methods, skills, and program strategies to help people change to healthful lifestyles, make more efficient use of health services, adopt self-care practices wherever possible, and participate actively in the design and implementation of programs that affect their health. Skills in the social and behavioral sciences, communication dynamics, educational theory, and community organization are relevant to this specialty, which has given leadership to health promotion.	Employment is available in many different types of agencies in the public and private sectors to identify social and health needs of population groups, adapt the health care delivery system to the needs of individuals and communities, develop and implement patient education in health care and community settings, and use the media effectively as a means of achieving the above. Health education and health promotion programs in schools, companies, and clinical and other community settings employ health educators.
Environmental sciences Those specialties concerned with the identification and control of factors in the natural environment that affect health	Environmental sciences specialists are concerned with the relationships between the characteristics of the natural environment (air, water, soil, chemicals, etc.) and mental and physical health. This information is used to establish limits on pollutants that the environment can absorb without detrimental effects, to develop control technology, and to implement controls as necessary for the benefit of human and animal populations. The educational background of most environmental scientists usually includes disciplinary training in one or more of the natural sciences plus advanced courses in those aspects of environmental health relevant to their primary discipline.	Employment is available at all levels of government, public and private organizations, and industry to provide technical knowledge and methods in the investigation, planning, controlling, and regulation of matters pertaining to environmental health hazards. In addition, employees carry out basic and operational environmental research procedures and provide training to community workers and interest groups in methods and techniques of environmental protection.

Area of specialization	Differentiating characteristics (pertaining to the area of specialization and illustrative ways it contributes to improved health)	Illustrative jobs and job settings (for graduates of the area of specialization)
Occupational safety and health The identification of health and safety hazards related to work and the work environment, and prevention and control of these hazards	In collaboration with many disciplines such as medicine, nursing, statistics, engineering, and psychology, this area of specialization seeks to minimize ill health, injury, and maladjustments to work that may occur as a result of a person's association with work and the work environment.	In industry, occupational safety and health specialists are concerned with establishing the causes and effects of industrial health problems and the implementation of acceptable control methods. In government they are involved with monitoring morbidity and mortality associated with the work environment, formulating and enforcing safety standards, investigating specific health and safety problems, and planning and implementing appropriate health programs. Those employed by academic institutions are involved with the training of specialists in this field and with research.
Nutrition The study of the interaction between nutrients, nutrition, and health; and the application of sound nutritional principles to improve or maintain health	One specialty in nutrition is concerned primarily with the scientific study in laboratory and clinical settings of the effects of nutrients on growth, developments, and health; the other specialty is concerned with the application of specialized nutrition knowledge and skills to improve or maintain the health of target population groups. In the former category are found persons with basic preparation in biochemistry, medicine, and related sciences; in the latter are persons with training in dietetics, clinical nutrition, and related fields.	Employment opportunities for specialists in nutrition exist at all levels of government and in private agencies, institutions, and industry. Examples of typical job activities include the assessment of nutritional problems in individuals and population groups, development and implementation of programs to change patterns of food consumption, and fundamental research into human and animal nutrition.
Biomedical and laboratory practice Various specialty disciplines that use laboratory techniques for the diagnosis and treatment of disease, and for the investigation of conditions affecting health status	The two main defining characteristics of this broad area of specialization are (1) the type of facilities and equipment used and (2) the fact that it is concerned with the scientific investigation in individuals of biological and biochemical processes that affect or reflect health status. Specialists working in this area may be primarily concerned with the development of new knowledge or with the application of existing laboratory-based techniques for the maintenance of health and for the prevention, early detection, and treatment of disease, on an individual-case basis and in mass screening and prevention programs.	Those trained in this specialty are employed at all levels of government, in medical and academic institutions, and in public and private laboratories. Illustrative job opportunities include laboratory research for the detection and treatment of disease, and the planning and operation of training programs concerned with the basic training of laboratory personnel and with their needs for continuing education.

Area of specialization	Differentiating characteristics (pertaining to the area of specialization and illustrative ways it contributes to improved health)	Illustrative jobs and job settings (for graduates of the area of specialization)
Preventive medicine and community medicine The application of clinical medicine and public health skills to understand and reduce risks of disease, disability, and death in individuals and populations	Preventive medicine (in the United States) and community medicine (in Canada) specialists manage programs in public or community health and conduct research to prevent and control disease; provide direct patient care; use scientific methods to identify health and safety hazards in the workplace and work to prevent occupational illness and injury; work to improve preventive and primary care services to underserved and high-risk populations; assess and eliminate environmental health hazards.	Preventive medicine and community medicine specialists work in varied community settings. Examples of activities include revival of an inactive tuberculosis control program, management of an inner-city clinic for sexually transmitted diseases, development of a statewide breast cancer screening initiative, development of a community health center in an underserved urban area, identification of drinking water safety problems, and development of a program to evaluate the health of a population living near a hazardous waste site.
Public health nursing The application of nursing and public health principles to promote the physical, mental, and social well-being of people and communities	Public health (PH) nurses provide health counseling and education to individuals, families, and communities. They are concerned with individual health in the broader community context, which may include: being the liaison with multiple community agencies to meet health needs; staff public health clinics; demonstrate patient care to family caregivers, but not generally provide direct patient care; serve on community boards and committees to affect health policy and services; organize and implement educational programs.	PH nurses play a key role in many community programs. For example, they promote maternal and infant health through such activities as counseling parents on health matters; assisting parents in developing skills to deal with health needs of their children; urge regular health exams and immunization; help parents secure screening services; teach home nursing and parenting skills; assist in improving social conditions that affect health; recognize and report child abuse.
Other Although they do not fit within any of the preceding categories, various other specialties make important contributions to community health. These specialties are defined in different ways, such as by disciplinary background (e.g., behavioral and social sciences) or by the kinds of phenomena under consideration (e.g., the study and treatment of health problems in an international setting).		Employment opportunities exist primarily at the federal state levels, in academic institutions, and in some private agencies and foundations. Skills of particular relevance to this broad area of specialization include the collection and analysis of data pertinent to the health status of defined populations, and the planning, development, and operation or evaluation of programs designed to deal with particular health needs.

Common Job Titles— Public and Community Health

Administrator

Director (of a specific service or program)

Health administrator

Health care administrator

Health officer

Health science manager

Health services administrator

Health services manager

Hospital administrator

Nursing home administrator

Analyst

Computer specialist

Demographer

Epidemiologist

Systems analyst

Dentist

Public health dentist

Engineer

Air pollution engineer

Environmental engineer

Product safety engineer

Waterworks engineer

Enviornmental Health Specialists

Environmental technician

Sanitarian

Health Educator

Community health educator

Health promotion specialist

Patient educator

Public health educator

School health educator

Worksite health promotion manager

Hygienist

Dental hygienist

Industrial hygienist

Inspector

Food and drug inspector

Hospital inspector

Milk and food inspector

Nursing home inspector

Laboratory Technician/Technologist

Biochemical technologist

Food technologist

Laboratory technician

Microbiology technologist

Radiological technologist

Veterinary lab technician

Nurse

Industrial health nurse

Mental health nurse

Nurse practitioner

Occupational health nurse

Public health nurse
School nurse
Visiting nurse

Nutritionist
Community nutritionist
Public health nutritionist
School nutritionist

Physician
Aerospace physician
District health officer
Health officer
Industrial health physician
Medical officer of health
Occupational health physician
Public health physician
School health physician

Planner
Facilities planner
Health planner
Manpower planner
Program planner
Services planner

Scientist
Anthropologist
Bacteriologist
Behavioral scientist
Biologist
Chemist
Dairy scientist
Ecologist

Entomologist
Microbiologist
Parasitologist
Psychologist
Social scientist
Sociologist
Soil scientist
Zoologist

Social Worker
Medical social worker
Mental health counselor
Public health social worker
Psychiatric social worker

Statistician
Analyst
Biometrician
Biostatistician
Survey statistician
Vital statistician

Therapist
Occupational therapist
Physical rehabilitation therapist
Physical therapist
Recreation therapist
Speech therapist
Vocational rehabilitation therapist

Veterinarian
Public health veterinarian
Vector control technician

U.S. Schools of Public Health and Graduate Public Health Programs*

GRADUATE SCHOOLS OF PUBLIC HEALTH

University of Alabama at Birmingham School of Public Health, 210 Ryals Building, 1665 University Blvd., Birmingham, AL 35294-0022, (205) 934-7730, Dean: Eli I. Capilouto, DMD, MPH, ScD, (1978) 12/31/00

Boston University School of Public Health, School of Medicine, 80 East Concord St., A-407, Boston, MA 02118-2394, (617) 638-4640, Dean: Robert F. Meenan, MD, MPH, MBA, (1981) 12/31/01

University of California at Berkeley School of Public Health, 19 Earl Warren Hall, Berkeley, CA 94720 (510) 642-2082, Dean: Patricia A. Buffler, PhD, (1946) 7/1/00

University of California at Los Angeles School of Public Health, Center for the Health Sciences, Box #951772, Los Angeles, CA 90095, (310) 825-6381, Dean: A. A. Afifi, PhD, (1960) 12/31/98

Columbia University School of Public Health, 600 West 168th St., New York, NY 10032, (212) 305-3929, Dean: Allan Rosenfield, MD, (1946) 12/31/01

Emory University, Rollins School of Public Health, 1518 Clifton Road NE, Atlanta, GA 30322, (404) 727-8720, Dean: James W. Curran, MD, MPH, (1978) 12/31/97

Harvard School of Public Health, 677 Huntington Ave., Boston, MA 02115, (617) 432-1025, Dean: Harvey V. Fineberg, MD, PhD, (1946) 7/1/00

University of Hawaii School of Public Health, 1960 East-West Road, Honolulu, HI 96822, (808) 956-8066, Interim Dean: D. William Wood, PhD, (1965) 10/22/98

University of Illinois at Chicago School of Public Health, 2121 West Taylor Street, Chicago, IL 60612, (312) 996-6620, Dean: Susan C. Scrimshaw, PhD, (1972) 7/1/99

The Johns Hopkins University School of Hygiene and Public Health, 615 North Wolfe St., Baltimore, MD 21205-2179, (410) 955-3540, Dean: Alfred Sommer, MD, MHS, (1946) 7/1/99

Loma Linda University School of Public Health, Loma Linda, CA 92350 (909) 824-4578, Dean: Richard H. Hart, MD, DrPH, (1967) 12/31/96

University of Massachusetts School of Public Health and Health Sciences, 108 Arnold House, Amherst, MA 01003-0037, (413) 545-1303, Dean: Stephen H. Gehlbach, MD, MPH, (1970) 12/31/00

University of Michigan School of Public Health, 109 South Observatory St., Ann Arbor, MI 48109-2029, (313) 763-5454, Dean: Noreen M. Clark, PhD (1946) 12/31/99

University of Minnesota School of Public Health, Box 197, Mayo Memorial Building, 420 Delaware St., SE, Minneapolis, MN 55455-0381, (612) 624-6669, Dean: Edith D. Leyasmeyer, PhD, MPH, (1946) 7/1/00

---

*Accredited by the Council on Education for Public Health as of Mar 1997. The date in parentheses noted for each school or program represents the year first accredited or preaccredited.

State University of New York (SUNY) University at Albany, School of Public Health, One University Place, Rensselaer, NY 12144-3456 (518) 402-0283, Dean: David Carpenter, MD, (1993) 12/31/01

University of North Carolina School of Public Health, CB 7400 Rosenau Hall, Chapel Hill, NC 27599-7400, (919) 966-3215, Dean: Michel A. Ibrahim, MD, MPH, PhD, (1946) 7/1/01

The Ohio State University School of Public Health, College of Medicine, M-116 Starling Loving Hall, 320 W. 10th Avenue, Columbus, OH 43210-1240, (614) 293-3907, Interim Director: Randall E. Harris, MD, PhD, (1985) 10/22/98

University of Oklahoma College of Public Health, Health Sciences Center, P.O. Box 26901, 801 NE 13th St., Oklahoma City, OK 73104-5072, (405) 271-2232, Dean: Elisa T. Lee, PhD, (1967) 7/1/99

University of Pittsburgh Graduate School of Public Health, 111 Parran Hall, 130 De Soto Street, Pittsburgh, PA 15261, (412) 624-3001, Dean: Donald R. Mattison, MD, (1950) 7/1/99

University of Puerto Rico School of Public Health, Medical Sciences Campus, PO Box 365067, San Juan, Puerto Rico 00936, (787) 764-5975, Acting Dean: Alida Galletti, EdD, (1956) 12/31/01

Saint Louis University School of Public Health, O'Donnell Hall, 4th Floor, 3663 Lindell Blvd., St. Louis, MO 63108, (314) 977-8100, Dean: Richard S. Kurz, PhD, (1983) 7/1/00

San Diego State University Graduate School of Public Health, San Diego, CA 92182-4162, (619) 594-5922, Acting Director: John Elder, PhD, MPH, (1982) 7/1/98

University of South Carolina School of Public Health, Columbia, SC 29208, (803) 777-5032, Interim Dean: Dianne S. Ward, EdD, (1977) 7/1/01

University of South Florida College of Public Health, 13201 Bruce B. Downs Blvd. (MDC-56), Tampa, FL 33612-3805, (813) 974-6603, Dean: Charles Mahan, MD, (1987) 7/1/98

University of Texas-Houston School of Public Health, PO Box 20186, Houston, TX 77225, (713) 500-9050, Dean: R. Palmer Beasley, MD, MS, (1969) 12/31/97

Tulane University School of Public Health and Tropical Medicine, 1430 Tulane Avenue, New Orleans, LA 70112, (504) 588-5397, Dean: Paul K. Whelton, MD, MSc, (1947) 12/31/02

University of Washington School of Public Health and Community Medicine, Box 357230, Seattle, WA 98195, (206) 543-1144, Dean: Gilbert S. Omenn, MD, PhD, (1970) 12/31/98

Yale University Department of Epidemiology and Public Health, School of Medicine, PO Box 208034, 60 College St., New Haven, CT 06520-8034, (203) 785-2867, Dean of Public Health and Chair: Michael Merson, MD (1946) 7/1/99

GRADUATE PROGRAMS IN COMMUNITY HEALTH EDUCATION

California State University-Long Beach MPH and MS Programs in Community Health Education, Health Science Department, College of Health & Human Services, 1250 Bellflower Blvd., Long Beach, CA 90840, (310) 985-4057, Chair: Mohammed Forouzesh, PhD (1990) 7/1/97

California State University-Northridge MPH Program in Community Health Education, Dept. of Health Science, School of Communication, Health & Human Services, 18111 Nordhoff St., Northridge, CA 91330, (818) 677-2997, Director: Ronald Fischbach, PhD, (1971) 10/22/98

East Stroudsburg University MPH Program in Community Health Education, Health Department, East Stroudsburg, PA 18301, (717) 422-3702, Chair: William C. Livingood, PhD, (1990) 12/31/99

Hunter College MPH Program in Community Health Education, School of Health Sciences, CUNY, 425 E. 25th St., New York, NY 10010, (212) 481-5111, Director: Marilyn Iris Auerbach, DrPH, MPH, (1972) 12/31/99

University of Illinois at Urbana-Champaign MSPH Program in Community Health Education, Department of Community Health, 1206 S. Fourth St., Champaign, IL 61820, (217) 333-2307, Head: Lee Crandall, PhD, (1983) 7/1/98

New York University MPH Program in Community Health Education, Department of Health Studies, School of Education, 35 W. 4th St., Suite 1200, New York, NY 10012, (212) 998-5780, Chair: Vivian P.J. Clarke, EdD, (1971) 7/1/01

University of Northern Colorado MPH Program in Community Health Education, Department of Community Health & Nutrition, College of Health & Human Sciences, Greeley, CO 80639, (970) 351-2755, Coordinator: William G. Parkos PhD, (1989) 12/31/98

San Jose State University MPH Program in Community Health Education, Department of Health Science, School of Applied Sciences and Arts, San Jose, CA 95192, (408) 924-2970, MPH Director: Kathleen Roe, DrPH, (1974) 12/31/99

Temple University MPH Program in Community Health Education, Department of Health Education, College of Health, Physical Education, Recreation & Dance, 304 Seltzer Hall, Philadelphia, PA 19122, (215) 204-8726, Coordinator: Alice J. Hausman, PhD, MPH, (1985) 7/1/01

University of Wisconsin at La Crosse MPH Program in Community Health Education, Department of Health Education and Health Promotion, 203 Mitchell Hall, La Crosse, WI 54601, (608) 785-8163, Director: Gary D. Gilmore, MPH, PhD, (1992) 7/1/97

GRADUATE PROGRAMS IN COMMUNITY HEALTH/PREVENTIVE MEDICINE

Arizona Graduate Program in Public Health, Arizona State University and University of Arizona, Arizona Health Sciences Center, Tucson, AZ 85724, (520) 626-9112, Interim Director: Carlos C. Campbell, MD, MPH, (1994) 9/23/96

California State University-Fresno MPH Program, Department of Health Science, School of Health and Human Services, 2345 E. San Ramon Ave., Fresno, CA 93740-0030, (209) 278-4014, Coordinator: Sanford M. Brown, MPH, PhD, (1996) 10/22/98

University of Colorado MSPH Program, Department of Preventive Medicine & Biometrics, School of Medicine, Health Sciences Center, 4200 E. Ninth Ave., Box C-245, Denver, CO 80262, (303) 315-8357, Director: Phoebe Lindsey Barton, PhD, (1985) 12/31/98

University of Connecticut MPH Program, Department of Community Medicine and Health Care, School of Medicine, Farmington, CT 06030-1910, (860) 679-3351, Director: Holger Hansen, MD, DrPH, FACE, (1984) 7/1/00

Florida International University Graduate Program in Public Health, Department of Public Health, North Miami Campus, 3000 N.E. 145th St., North Miami, FL 33181-3600, (305) 919-5877, Director: H. Virginia McCoy, PhD, (1993) 7/1/99

The George Washington University MPH Program, School of Medicine & Health Sciences, 23001 St., NW, Box 32, Washington, DC 20037, (202) 994-2807, Associate Dean for Public Health Programs: Richard K. Riegelman, MD, MPH, PhD, (1990) 12/31/00

University of Miami MPH Program, Department of Epidemiology and Public Health, School of Medicine, PO Box 016069, Miami, FL 33101, (305) 243-6759, Director: Peggy O'Hara, PhD, (1982) 7/1/99

University of Southern Mississippi MPH Program, Center for Community Health, College of Health & Human Sciences, Southern Station, Box 5122, Hattiesburg, MS 39406-5122, (601) 266-5437, Interim Director: Agnes Hinton, DrPH, (1993) 7/1/97

University of Medicine & Dentistry of New Jersey-Robert Wood Johnson Medical School and Rutgers, The State University of New Jersey Graduate Program in Public Health, Environmental & Occupational Health Sciences Institute (EOHSI), 681 Frelinghuysen Rd., Piscataway, NJ 08855-1179, (908) 445-0199, Director: George G. Rhoads, MD, MPH, (1986) 12/31/02

University of New Mexico MPH Program, School of Medicine, 2400 Tucker NE, Albuquerque, NM 87131, (505) 272-4173, Director: Nina B. Wallerstein, DrPH, (1996) 7/1/01

Oregon MPH Program, Oregon Health Sciences University, Oregon State University and Portland State University, Department of Public Health, OSU, 256 Waldo Hall, Corvallis, OR 97331-6406, (541) 737-3825, Director: Rebecca J. Donatelle, PhD, (1996) 10/22/98

University of Rochester MPH Program, School of Medicine and Dentistry, 601 Elmwood Avenue, Rochester, NY 14642, (716) 275-2194, Director: Sarah Trafton, JD, (1978) 7/1/99

University of Tennessee at Knoxville MPH Program, Department of Health, Leisure & Safety Sciences, College of Human Ecology, 1914 Andy Holt Ave., Knoxville, TN 37996-2710 (423) 974-6674, Head: Charles B. Hamilton, MPH, DrPH, (1969) 7/1/00

Tufts University School of Medicine Combined MD/MPH Program, Department of Community Health, 136 Harrison Avenue, Boston, MA 02111, (617) 956-6807, Director: Lydia Mayer, MD, MPH, (1992) 7/1/97

Uniformed Services University of the Health Sciences Graduate Programs, Department of Preventive Medicine and Biometrics, School of Medicine, 4301 Jones Bridge Rd., Bethesda, MD 20814-4799, (301) 295-3050, Director: Kenneth E. Dixon, MD, MPH, (1985) 7/1/98

University of Utah MPH and MSPH Programs, Department of Family and Preventive Medicine, School of Medicine, 50 N. Medical Drive, Salt Lake City, UT 84132, (801) 581-7234, Director: Charles C. Hughes, PhD, (1978) 12/31/97

Virginia Commonwealth University MPH Program, Department of Preventive Medicine and Community Health, Medical College of Virginia, P.O. Box 980212, Richmond, VA 23298-0212, (804) 828-9785, Chair: Jack O. Lanier, DrPH, FACHE, (1996) 7/1/99

Medical College of Wisconsin MPH Programs, Department of Preventive Medicine, 8701 Watertown Plank Rd., Milwaukee, WI 53226, (414) 456-4510, Director: William W. Greaves, MD, MSPH, (1991) 7/1/98

COUNCIL ON EDUCATION FOR PUBLIC HEALTH

1015 Fifteenth Street, NW, Suite 402
Washington, DC 20005
phone: (202) 789-1050
fax: (202) 789-1895

The date in parentheses noted for each school or program represents the year first accredited or preaccredited. The second date indicates the conclusion of the current accreditation term; the next scheduled review must take place prior to that date.

Glossary

abatement   Removal or discontinuance of a nuisance.

abortion   Termination of a pregnancy before it is carried to full term, either by induced means (legal and illegal abortions) or by involuntary means (spontaneous abortion).

accessibility   The distribution of health resources (for example, personnel and facilities) such that people in need are able to avail themselves of the resources with reasonable convenience and at reasonable cost.

accident   The official designation of an occurrence in a sequence of events that produces unintentional injury, death, or property damage.

acid rain   Sulfur oxide pollutants carried in rain clouds.

acquired immunity   Resistance to disease resulting from previous exposures that produced the disease and the antibodies against subsequent exposures.

active immunity   Resistance to disease resulting from the host's body producing its own antibodies, either from exposure to the disease or from artificial introduction of the antigenic substance by vaccination or immunization.

active life expectancy   Years before death in which individuals are able to perform activities of daily living and to function relatively independently.

actuarial data   Information used to predict the average risks of deaths or other vital events, based on population experience in a recent period.

adaptation   The process by which an organism, person or population makes a successful change to accommodate new circumstances. Some scholars argue that adaptation is the most generalizable measure of health.

addiction   A derangement in cellular metabolism causing physiological and psychological dependence on a substance.

adolescence   The years between childhood and adulthood, defined biologically by the advent of reproductive sex characteristics.

adulthood   The years following adolescence, beginning with any age defined by the community, by custom, or by legal responsibilities and rights.

Aedes aegypti   The mosquito found to be the transmitter of yellow fever by Walter Reed and colleagues in 1900.

age-adjusted rate   The total rate for a population, adjusted to ignore the age distribution of the specific population by multiplying each of its age-specific rates by the proportion of a standard (for example, national) population in that age group, then adding up the products.

ageism   The stereotyped perceptions of aging that result in prejudice or discrimination against elderly people.

agent   An epidemiological term referring to the organism or object that transmits a disease or injury from the environment to the host.

age-specific rate   The incidence (number of events during a specified period of time) for a specific age group, divided by the total number of people in that age group.

aging   The process of growing older, especially referring to the period in which body functioning declines.

air exchange rate   The frequency with which inside air is replaced with outside air.

ALARA   As low as is reasonably achievable, a principle applied to control some pollutants where an absolute standard (MPC) or a cost-benefit analysis cannot be applied to set a permissible limit on emissions or concentrations.

allocation   A distribution of resources to specific categories of expenditure.

Alzheimer's disease   A syndrome characterized by symptoms associated with loss of mental capacities and functioning; often equated with senility.

ambient   Surrounding condition of environment, usually referring to air quality or noise.

ambulatory care services Those health services provided to patients who are not placed in beds, usually performed in outpatient clinics.

amniocentesis A procedure for extracting fluid from the uterus of a pregnant women to use for screening and diagnosis, especially in relation to birth defect possibilities.

anaerobic Without oxygen, referring in this book to pathogenic organisms, such as *Clostridium botulinum,* that do not produce toxin in free air.

Anopheles The mosquito found, by Ronald Ross in India and Battista Grassi in Italy in 1898, to be responsible for transmitting malaria.

anorexia nervosa A compulsive nutritional disorder in which the obsession to lose weight leads to self-starvation.

antenatal care Medical, nursing, and educational services to the expectant mother, ideally begin during the first trimester of pregnancy; more commonly called prenatal care.

antibiosis Antagonism to specific organisms.

antibodies Protein molecules formed in the blood stream by exposure to a foreign substance such as an invading organism, later they are available to bind to the same substance and prevent its growth and reproduction.

antigen A substance that causes the production of antibodies when introduced into the body.

antiseptic Any substance used to kill or retard the growth of potentially harmful microorganisms, first discovered by Lister.

appropriation The placement of funds in a budget category previously authorized; the final step in the legislative process of initiating action in the administrative branch.

aquifers Large underground rock formations containing water that has percolated down from the earth's surface via cracks and faults.

arthritis A range of diseases afflicting the joints, including rheumatoid arthritis—an inflammatory disease with onset usually between the ages of 20 and 45—and osteoarthritis, which affects only older persons and weight-bearing joints, notably hips and knees.

asbestos A flameproof product used widely in the past as insulation material in buildings, now known to produce a toxic dust that causes lung diseases.

asepsis Sterilization methods for killing pathogenic organisms in wounds or on surfaces that might infect patients during clinical procedures.

atherosclerosis A thickening and hardening of arteries from fatty deposits of plaque making the blood vessels less elastic and narrower so that blood flow is impeded or clots may block the flow of blood. A form of arteriosclerosis.

atmosphere The air surrounding the earth or any community or environment.

atrophy The withering or weakening of an organ, muscle or faculty due to lack of activity or use.

attributable risk The proportion of a specific disease or cause of death that can be blamed on a particular risk factor.

authority The power to take action legally or constitutionally.

authorization The step in legislative action in which resource allocations are made possible.

automatic-protective strategies Those preventive methods that bypass the motivation and decisions of people by structuring the environment in such a way that choices of action are minimized.

bacteriology The branch of science concerned with the study of microorganisms, the contributions of which were critical to the control of communicable diseases at the turn of the twentieth century.

bacteriostasis An arrest in the multiplication of bacteria, enabling the host's natural defenses to destroy the invading organism.

barriers The obstacles to performing a prescribed action or to carrying out a program.

behavioral diagnosis Delineation of the specific health actions most likely to effect a health outcome.

behavioral objective A statement of a desired outcome that specifies who is to demonstrate how much of what actions by when.

bereavement The loss of loved ones—one of the transitions most commonly experienced by elderly people, requiring adaptation and coping by the individual and the community.

bioassay Assessment of chemical substances in animal or plant tissue.

biotic potential The highest possible birthrate for a population, thought to be around 50 per 1000 in human population.

Black Death The common name for bubonic plague, a disease transmitted by fleas that became pandemic in past centuries.

block grants Funds transferred from one level of government to another with minimal earmarking of how they must be spent.

BOD Biochemical oxygen demand, an indicator of the amount of organic waste in water based on the amount of oxygen required to decompose it.

botulism A disease caused by a toxin produced by a spore-forming organism that is found in soils and that contaminates vegetables and other foods.

building codes Ordinances restricting the materials and standards of construction to assure safe habitation of indoor spaces.

bulimia A compulsive eating disorder in which the dual obsessions to eat and to lose weight lead to bingeing on large quantities of food, then purging or vomiting.

Byzantine Referring to the Eastern Roman Empire; connoting bureaucracy, luxury, and decadence.

carcinogen A cancer-causing substance.

cardiorespiratory fitness The combination of health benefits associated with aerobic exercise, including a more efficient heart, a stronger diaphragm, a slower resting heart rate, and lower levels of cholesterol and fibrin in the blood and arteries.

cardiovascular disease A group of conditions including heart disease, hypertension, atherosclerosis, stroke, rheumatic heart disease, and other disorders of the heart or blood vessels.

cardiovascular fitness The combination of heart rate (resting pulse), circulation, and other physiological signs resulting from adequate functioning and conditioning of the heart and circulatory system.

carriers Those hosts that continue to harbor the infectious agents even after their own recovery, making them a risk to the health of others.

cause-specific rate A death rate for a given disease or cause of death, such as the heart disease death rate, based on the number of deaths attributed to a specific cause divided by the total population at the midpoint of the period of measurement.

CDC Centers for Disease Control, a part of the Public Health Service in the U.S. Department of Health and Human Services. Renamed Centers for Disease Control and Prevention in 1996.

cerebrovascular disease Atherosclerosis specifically in the arteries of the brain, often resulting in stroke.

chemotherapy The treatment of an illness or condition with chemical substances. In the case of mental illness, the use of alkaloids has reduced the need to keep patients in hospitals.

chlorination Treatment of water with chlorine, which kills all bacteria pathogenic to man at concentrations above 0.2 PPM.

Clean Air Act The legislation passed by the U.S. Congress in 1965, renewable every 5 years, providing for federal assistance and standards for air pollution control.

coalition A group of individuals, usually representing organizations or agencies in a community, working together on an issue of mutual concern.

coercive strategies Preventive methods that bypass the motivation and decisions of people by dictating or precluding choices.

coinsurance The portion of medical care costs required by an insurance plan to be paid by the insured.

coliform test A standard bacteriological examination of drinking water safety, using *E. coli* organisms as an indicator of fecal contamination.

common law The unwritten rules of society honored by courts because they have been established by custom or by previous court decisions.

communicable disease A potentially harmful organism or its toxic products that can be transmitted from one human host, reservoir, or lower animals to susceptible human hosts.

community For most purposes in this book, the term is applied to a group of inhabitants living in a somewhat localized area under the same general regulations and having common norms, values, and organizations.

community health The health status of a defined population, and a field of practice encompassing and coordinating at the local level the overlapping aspects of school health, public health, employee health, maternal and child health services, environmental health protection, and the personal health practices of individuals and families.

community health education Any combination of learning experiences designed to facilitate voluntary actions in individuals or groups that will be conducive to the health of people in a locality.

community health events High-visibility activities such as marathon races or health fairs that provide some combination of publicity, recreation and health information and involve a broad spectrum of the community.

community health promotion Any combination of educational and social supports for people taking greater control of, and improving their own or the health of population of a geographically defined area.

community health protection Actions taken through enforcement of regulations or through environmental modification to prevent the exposure of a community to health risks.

community health services   Actions taken by a community to ensure access of residents to health care and to assure the quality of the care.

complementary medicine   Health care interventions not widely taught at medical schools or generally available at hospitals.

conservation   The wise use of resources; the most effective use of the environmental resources necessary for survival and quality of life.

contamination   The presence of toxins or pathogenic organisms on inanimate objects such as food, soil, water, or fomites.

convalescence   The period following the acute phases of an illness during which some symptoms and potential infectiousness continue to exist, so continuing rest or isolation is needed.

copayment   The provision in health insurance plans requiring the insured to pay a percentage of the cost of care after paying the deductible.

coping   The process of adjusting to stress in a constructive manner.

coronary artery disease   Narrowing of the heart vessels due to deposits of cholesterol and fat, thus weakening the function of the heart and increasing the risk of myocardial infarction.

coronary heart disease   Atherosclerosis specifically in the arteries of the heart muscle.

corrosivity   The potential of a substance to oxidize or rust metals and other surfaces with which it comes in contact.

cost-benefit analysis   A procedure for policy decisions, based on a comparison of the expense of a program with its expected monetary yield or savings.

crude death rate   The total number of deaths divided by the total population, usually multiplied by 1000 so that the result can be expressed as annual number of deaths per 1000 population.

decibel   A measure of noise intensity, based on just noticeable differences in sound.

decontamination   The killing or removing of pathogens or toxins in or on inanimate objects.

deductible   That part of the cost of care that health insurance policies require the insured to pay before the policy pays.

defection   The period during or following convalescence from an infectious disease during which organisms are still being cast off by the body, so isolation may continue to be necessary.

defervescence   The period following the most acute phase of an infectious illness during which symptoms subside but relapse remains probable without continuing treatment or rest.

deinstitutionalization   The policy or practice of placing mentally ill patients back in the community, made possible by drugs that control the symptoms of illness.

demand   The economic concept of consumer desire for a product or service resulting in greater tendency to purchase or acquire it by other means and thereby to affect its supply or price.

demography   The study of human population growth, decline, and movement, using measures of fertility, mortality, and migration.

deregulation   An administrative strategy to reduce governmental responsibility for surveillance and enforcement.

desertification   The transformation of arable or habitable land to desert, usually as a result of change in climate or destructive land use.

diabetes   A metabolic disease that affects the arteries as a result of failure to metabolize carbohydrates.

diffusion   The spread in a population, over time, of a new idea or innovation.

disabling injury   An injury that results in death, permanent disability, or any duration of temporary total disability.

disability-free life expectancy   Years of life lived without disabling illness or injury.

disaster plans   The detailed procedures to be followed in the event of a catastrophe such as a tornado, flood, or nuclear accident.

disease   A harmful departure from the normal state of a person or other organism.

disinfection   The killing or removing of organisms capable of causing infection.

disintegration of personality   The process of failing to cope with stress constructively; the opposite of coping.

DPT   The trivalent vaccine, given in a single inoculation, that inoculates against diphtheria, pertussis, and tetanus.

diffusion   The process by which an idea, innovation, behavior, disease, or other transmissible thing spreads in a population, described over time by an S-shaped growth curve showing the cumulative number of people reached or changed.

disability-free longevity   A new epidemiological measure of longevity in which years of dependency are subtracted from total longevity to give greater weight to quality of life years, not just quantity.

dysgenic   Conditions or changes that produce poor genetic or evolutionary outcomes.

early adopters   The segment of the population accepting a new idea or practice soon after the innovators but before the middle majority, and who tend to be opinion leaders for the middle majority.

E-codes   Classification of injuries according to the International Classification of Disease (ICD) coding for emergency medical care.

ecology   The study of the interaction of life-forms with their environment.

economy of scale   The point in the growth of a program or service at which each additional element of service costs less to produce.

educational diagnosis   The delineation of factors that predispose, enable, and reinforce a specific health behavior.

educational strategies   Preventive methods that seek to assure that people are able to take voluntary action based on informed decisions.

efficiency   The ability to function as needed with a minimum of energy expenditure, and to meet emergencies or special demands.

emergency medical services system   The coordinated resources responsible for urgent medical care, including ambulance service, communications, and medical facilities and personnel.

Employee Assistance Program   A somewhat standardized offering of counseling and referral to troubled employees with the intent of improving their performance by reducing or eliminating their dependence on or misuse of alcohol or drugs.

enabling factor   Any characteristic of the environment that facilitates health behavior, and any skill or resource required to attain the behavior.

endemic   Epidemiological term referring to a disease or condition that persists within a geographical area.

enforcement   Action taken to assure compliance with the law or legislative intent.

environment   All factors external to the organism that may impinge on its behavior or well-being.

EPA   Environmental Protection Agency, a federal agency of the U.S. Department of Health and Human Services responsible for air and water quality standards.

epidemic   Widely and rapidly spreading disease, more than an outbreak but less than a pandemic.

epidemiological diagnosis   The delineation of the extent, distribution, and causes of a health problem in a defined population.

epidemiology   The study of disease transmission, development, and consequences in populations to identify causes and distributions of diseases.

etiologies   The origins or causes of a disease or condition under study; the first steps in the natural history of a disease.

evaluation   The comparison of an object of interest against a standard of acceptability.

excise tax   A tax on the manufacture, sale, or use of certain products such as alcohol or tobacco to generate revenue for a government or to control consumption, or both.

exercise   Physical activity consciously undertaken in a structured and repetitive way for the purpose of improving or maintaining physical fitness.

ex officio   Serving as a member of a committee or board because of one's official position rather than by election.

extramural   Activities such as research conducted outside the agency.

facilitators   Those enabling factors helping to overcome barriers.

family   A group of two or more people related by birth, marriage, or adoption and residing together in a household.

family planning   The process of establishing the preferred number and spacing of children in one's family and selecting the means by which this objective is achieved.

family violence   Spouse abuse, child abuse by parents, child-to-parent abuse, sexual abuse of family members, and most common of all, child-to-child abuse.

farm safety survey   A procedure for the assessment of hazardous conditions on a farm.

fastigium   The period during which a disease is at its most acute or intense expression of symptoms.

fatal accidents   Official classification of events producing injuries resulting in one or more deaths within 1 year.

fecundity   The state and degree of being capable of conceiving and giving birth to offspring.

federal   The level of government representing the collective interests of states.

federalism   That system of governance emphasizing the powers retained by states making up a federation.

fetal death rate   The number of deaths of fetuses with gestations of 20 weeks or more per 1000 total births (i.e., live births plus fetal deaths).

filtration   Removal of particulate matter in water by percolation through a layer of sand or other porous material.

fitness   The condition of being physically, mentally, and socially at a high level of efficiency.

flash mix   The first step in rapid sand filtration method of water treatment, in which aluminum sulfate is added to the water to congeal suspended matter as a floc that can be trapped or filtered.

flocculation   Trapping particles suspended in water by adsorption and settling.

fluorocarbon propellants   Inert gases used in some pressurized containers to propel other gases because they do not react with other gases, but they do release chlorine in the upper atmosphere when exposed to ultraviolet rays.

fomites   Inanimate objects other than water, milk, food, air, and soil that might be contaminated and provide vehicles of disease transfer; examples include plates, glasses, clothing, bed linen, and handrails.

food poisoning   The common term for either of two reactions: (1) a toxic reaction to a food that is itself poisonous, or (2) a reaction to food that has transmitted a pathogen or toxin.

formative evaluation   Steps taken to assess the appropriateness and performance of a program before it is fully launched, with the specific purpose of improving its form and delivery.

frank cases   Those individuals whose disease becomes known through symptoms.

full-time equivalent   A measure of staffing or personnel requirements based on counting each full-time employee as 1 and each part-time employee as a fraction of 1.

functional health   That state of health enabling one to carry out social responsibilities and to be a productive member of the community.

genocide   The systematic killing (elimination) of a race or nation of people.

geriatrics   The field of professional practice addressed to the health needs of the elderly.

gerontology   The field of research devoted to the processes and problems of old age.

global warming   The gradual increase of the temperature of earth's lower atmosphere as a result of greenhouse gases allowing radiation from the sun to reach the earth unimpeded and to trap heat at earth's surface.

greenhouse effect   The accumulation of gases, especially carbon dioxide, in the atmosphere, causing heat to be held next to the earth.

groundwater   Naturally occurring underground reservoirs used by many small communities and a few large cities as their source of water.

habituation   The incorporation of a pattern of behavior into one's life-style to the degree that it is performed virtually without thought, but does not necessarily entail physical or psychological dependence.

HACCP   Hazard Analysis Critical Control Points, a standard for assessment by food industry of food production processes at critical points where contamination or its prevention could occur.

harm reduction   An approach to public health that acknowledges the inevitability of some incidence and prevalence of a problem, but seeks to minimize the damgage done by it.

health   A state of complete physical, mental, and social well-being, not merely the absence of disease (WHO), or the ability of an organism to adapt to its environment and circumstances.

health care organization   The pattern of arrangements for access to medical, dental, nursing, and related facilities, resources, and services in a community.

health education   Any combination of learning experiences designed to elicit, facilitate or maintain voluntary actions conducive to the health of individuals, groups, or communities.

health field concept   The classification of factors influencing health under four categories: environment, human biology, behavior, and health care organization.

health fraud   Promotion of a health or medical product or service with an intent to deceive.

health promotion   Any combination of educational, organizational, economic, and social supports for conditions of living and behavior of individuals, groups, or communities conducive to health.

Health Systems Agency   A U.S. federally mandated, state-approved organization to carry out systematic assessments of a region's health needs and to develop health service goals and implementation plans for that geographical area.

heart attack   Insufficient supply of blood to the heart muscle, causing the failure of the muscle to function.

high-pressure food processing A method of preserving certain foods by using water pressure instead of heat, thereby preserving vitamins and minerals while killing bacteria.

HMO Health Maintenance Organization, a group offering comprehensive, prepaid health coverage for both physician and hospital services.

homeless Any person who routinely sleeps in bus, railway, airport, or subway terminals, in abandoned buildings, or outside.

home rule A grant of authority from the state to counties through statutes or constitutions allowing local self-determination and ability to levy local taxes for specific purposes.

home safety survey A procedure for the assessment of hazardous conditions in a home.

hospice Care provided to terminally ill patients in their last months, with emphasis on pain and symptom control, and on support for the whole family.

host A concept in epidemiology referring to an individual who harbors or is at risk of harboring a disease or condition.

host resistance The capacity of a person or population to ward off disease through natural or acquired defenses.

hypercholesterolemia Elevated cholesterol levels in the blood, resulting from high percentages of saturated animal fats in the diet and leading to increased risk of heart and vascular diseases.

hypertension A vascular disease associated with increased risk of stroke, the cause of which is unknown but which is easily diagnosed, treated, and controlled. Also called high blood pressure.

hypothermia A drop in deep body temperature under 95° F (35° C), which typically develops in isolated elderly people over a period of days.

immunity Resistance to a specific disease.

immunization The process of producing antibodies that protect the individual from a disease by introducing an antigenic substance into the body.

incidence A measure of frequency of occurrence based on the number of new cases appearing over a given period of time (usually one year).

incubation The period and process during which organisms are growing within their host, within an egg, womb, or artificial incubator.

industrial safety Injury control in a branch of trade or production on a broad geographic scale.

infant mortality The number of deaths of live-born children under 1 year of age per 1000 live births.

infection The successful invasion of a host by pathogens under such conditions as will permit them to multiply and harm the host.

infectious disease A communicable disease that results in a reaction of the host to the invading organism, producing abnormalities in the host and usually killing the invading pathogen.

informed consent A medical-legal doctrine that holds providers responsible for ensuring that consumers or patients understand the risks and benefits of a procedure or medicine before it is administered.

injunction An official order restraining a person or organization from continuing an action or maintaining a condition that is deemed a nuisance.

injuries Bodily damage caused by trauma.

injury control The prevention or limitation of harm to health either through prevention of, or through the protection of, victims of accidents, natural disasters, or intentional violence.

innovators The segment of the population first to adopt a new idea or practice, usually based on information from sources outside the community.

insurance A financial contract by which a company collects average costs (premiums) from the insured in exchange for guaranteed payment of variable costs in the event of certain types of loss.

intentional injury Homicide, suicide, assault, battery, rape, and most instances of family violence.

in-vitro diagnostic devices Products used in laboratories and in home self-test kits to expose a sample of bodily material such as blood or urine to a chemical which signals the presence or absence of a hormone or other element in the bodily material.

irradiation A method for decontaminating food by damaging the genetic material of bacteria so they cannot survive or multiply, without making the food radioactive or increasing human exposure to radiation.

isolation Segregation of an infected person or lower animal until the danger of conveying infection has passed.

jurisdiction The boundaries within which an agency or official has authority.

laboratory services Analytical bioassays for clinical, environmental, toxicological, forensic, and related assessments.

latchkey syndrome Pattern of problems associated with children who come home from school and have no guardian to supervise them.

late adopters That portion of a population who are among the last to accept an innovation.

late majority The segment of the population most difficult to reach through mass communication channels or to convince of the need to adopt a new idea or practice, sometimes because they cannot afford it or cannot get to the source, or because of cultural or language differences or other difficulty.

lead paint Any paint containing more than 0.06% lead.

leisure The use of time not devoted to work.

life expectancy The average number of years that an individual of a given age can expect to live, based on the longevity experience of the person's population.

life span A biological estimate of the maximum number of years a species is expected to live, based on the longest living cases observed and inherited characteristics.

lifestyle A complex pattern of habituated behavior that is socially and culturally conditioned and may be health-related but not necessarily health-directed.

local public health agency The officially designated authority for the planning and execution of facilities, programs, and services to protect and promote a community's health.

longevity The expected duration of life, based on life-table analyses of age-specific death rates.

malaria An infectious tropical disease involving cycles of fever, sweating, and chills, transmitted by the infected female *Anopheles* mosquito's bite carrying the parasite *Plasmodium* from the red blood cells of another victim.

managed care The organization of hospitals, doctors, and other providers into groups to enhance the cost-effectiveness and quality of health care.

mandatory programs Programs required by law, usually for one level of government regulated by the next higher level.

market testing The placement of a message or product in a commercial context to determine how it influences consumer behavior.

maturation The psychosocial process of developing mental, emotional, moral and social skills, and the biological process of gaining physical growth and sexual characteristics that mark the life span.

maternal mortality The number of women dying from complications of pregnancy or childbirth per 100,000 live births.

Medicaid A state-operated program of medical reimbursement for the medically indigent in the United States.

Medicare A federal program of health insurance for the elderly in the U.S.; the general term for the universal health care system in Canada.

mental health The emotional and social well-being and psychological resources of the individual.

metastasis The spread of cancerous cells from the site of the original development of the cancer.

miasma Noxious air or vapors. A belief that "bad air" causes disease.

miasma phase A period of the nineteenth century in which disease transmission efforts were directed at controlling "bad air."

middle majority The segment of the population who adopt a new idea or practice after the innovators and early adopters but before the late adopters, usually influenced by a combination of mass media, interpersonal communication, and endorsements by famous personalities or organizations of which they are members.

MPC Maximum permissible concentration, a standard applied to radiation.

mutation The adaptation of a species or strain of organism from one generation to another as a result of the survivors of the previous generation reproducing themselves, the effect being that an organism originally susceptible to a germicide or antibiotic can become resistant to it.

mutagenic A substance or process that results in abnormalities produced by damage to the genes.

mutual aid Support and reciprocal help provided by people who share a common condition or illness or other problem.

natural history of health The theoretical cycle describing what would maintain health in the absence of any social organization.

natural immunity Resistance to disease conferred by genetic inheritance.

natural increase The growth (or decline) of population attributable to births minus deaths in a given year.

need The assessed problem or aspiration requiring intervention or fulfillment.

neonatal mortality   The number of deaths of infants under 28 days of age per 1000 live births.

NIH   National Institutes of Health, a part of the U.S. Public Health Service.

NIOSH   National Institute for Occupational Safety and Health, a component of the U.S. Centers for Disease Control and Prevention.

nitrogen cycle   The continuous natural process of organic waste decomposition.

nitrogen oxides   Air pollutants arising from all combustion.

normal   That which is expected and tolerated by the community. What is considered normal in one community may be considered abnormal in other communities.

norms   A sociological concept describing the expected patterns of behavior in a population, based on the prevalence of the behavior.

nosocomial infection   Disease incurred in a hospital environment, especially threatening because the extensive use of antibiotics and antiseptics in hospitals has produced resistant strains of pathogens there.

nostrum   A secret or patented substance or device for which false therapeutic claims are made.

nuclear winter   The series of expected consequences of the massive cloud of dust and smoke that would be produced by extensive nuclear explosions.

nuisance   A condition that adversely affects or injures one or more persons. A **public nuisance** is one that affects many people.

obesity   The condition of being significantly overweight, as determined by skinfold measurements, body mass, or ratio of weight to height. Obesity is usually defined as 120 percent or more of ideal weight for height and age, based on statistical tables.

occupational injury   Injury arising out of and in the course of gainful employment, regardless of where the accident occurs.

occupational safety   Injury control in specific worksite.

official agency   A tax-supported or governmental authority.

official health agency   A governmental organization designated as having authority in some sphere of health.

oncogenic   Substances or processes that produce cancer.

OSHA   Abbreviation referring either to the Occupational Safety and Health Act of 1970 or to the Occupational Safety and Health Administration, a federal agency of the United States.

outbreak   Two or more illnesses linked to a common source.

outcome evaluation   The comparison of the results of a program or intervention against ultimate objectives of the program or against some other standard of acceptability.

ozone   One of the gases contributing to pollution in the lower atmosphere and to protection against ultraviolet radiation in the upper atmosphere.

PAHO   Pan American Health Organization, which also serves as the WHO Regional Office for the Americas.

palliative   care focused on the control of symptoms rather than on treatment of the disease.

pandemic   A widespread epidemic, usually affecting several countries and sometimes the entire globe.

passive immunity   Protection against disease conferred at least temporarily by the mother's antibodies in the infant or by serum from another person.

pasteurization   Heating a medium to a certain temperature for a given time period required to kill pathogenic organisms.

pathogenic   Disease-producing.

patient package insert   A statement listing appropriate uses of a medication and its possible side effects, required to be inserted in the packaging of medical products to be used by consumers.

perinatal   Stillborn and early neonatal deaths covering the period from 28 weeks of pregnancy to 1 week following birth.

permanent disability   Any degree of permanent impairment of the body, such as amputation, loss of vision, and other crippling nonfatal injuries.

physical activity   Body movement of any type that may contribute to physical fitness, depending on type, intensity, frequency, and duration.

physical fitness   One or more effects of physical activity on the health of the circulatory, respiratory, muscular, skeletal, or digestive system.

physiological efficiency   The ability of an organ or system to carry out its biological function with a minimum of stress.

planning   The process of establishing priorities, diagnosing causes of problems, and allocating resources to achieve objectives.

poison control center   An emergency information source for the diagnosis and management of injuries caused by poisonous substances.

poisoning   Damage caused by the chemical effect of a toxic substance ingested, injected, or on the skin.

police power   The authority of the people, vested in their government, to promote and protect their general welfare.

population   An aggregate of people or other elements.

population health   The status of a category of people with respect to their well-being and the determinants of that status.

population health promotion   Any combination of educational, organizational, policy or regulatory interventions to support actions or conditions of living conducive to the health of a population.

postneonatal mortality   The number of deaths of infants from 28 days to 365 days of age per 1000 live births.

predisposing factor   Any characteristic of a patient, consumer, student, or community that motivates behavior related to health.

prematurity rate   The percentage of babies born who weigh 2500 grams (5;n1;fs;d2 pounds) or less.

prenatal care   Medical services and counseling, combined with the personal protective and health promotion actions of the pregnant woman and her family, on behalf of the unborn fetus.

preretirement counseling   Preparation of older employees for the transition from working to nonworking status.

prevalence   A measure of frequency of occurrence based on the number of cases (old and new) existing at a given time.

price   The market value placed on a consumer good by the effects of supply and demand.

primary health care   As used in North America, refers to medical diagnosis and treatment of most symptoms not requiring specialist or hospital care; as used by WHO, refers to an approach to community health encompassing principles of the Alma Ata Declaration.

process evaluation   Assessment of the ongoing delivery or conduct of the program or method to determine its appropriate implementation and acceptability, short of assessing its outcomes.

prodrome   That stage of the disease process in the individual that precedes the acute manifestation of symptoms.

Professional Standards Review Organizations   Peer review groups created by federal legislation in 1972 to assure the maintenance of standards in medical and hospital practices and to restrain cost increases.

psychiatry   Discipline or medical specialty that concerns itself with the diagnosis, treatment, and cure of mental disorders.

puberty   The period of development during which the child develops adult sexual characteristics.

public nuisance   A condition sufficiently objectionable to invoke police power of the health department or other local authority.

public pool   A swimming facility used by people other than the owners or their families.

puerperium   Following birth.

pumice   Small bits of light, expanded lava found in volcanic ash.

quackery   False medical or health claim for a worthless product or procedure.

quality assurance   An approach to evaluation based on measure of the proficiency or quality of services rendered rather than on health outcomes achieved.

quarantine   The segregation or detention of susceptible individuals who have been exposed to a communicable disease.

radon   Naturally occurring radiation from soil or rocks, permeating buildings to produce indoor pollution.

rate   Any ratio that contains an element of time. Most common method of comparison used in epidemiology.

recreation   The act or process of refreshing or recovering after work or stress.

rehabilitation   The restoration to the fullest degree of physical, mental, social, vocational, and economic usefulness of which an individual is capable.

reinforcing factor   Rewards or punishments following or anticipated as a consequence of a health behavior.

relative risk   The ratio of deaths or cases of a disease in those who have a particular characteristic (e.g., age, sex, or a risk factor) to those deaths or cases not having that characteristic.

relative-risk ratio   The rate of the disease or condition in the exposed population divided by the rate in the unexposed population.

Renaissance   Literally, rebirth; referring to a period following the Dark Ages in Europe when the arts and sciences, including health, flowered again after having been denigrated as unworthy and ungodly pursuits.

requirements   The assessed resources needed to implement a program, to overcome barriers, and to accomplish its objectives.

reservoir   The natural habitat of an infectious agent, where it lives and multiplies until it can be transmitted to a susceptible host.

rhinitis   A respiratory condition characterized by nasal congestion and inflammation, associated with allergic reactions to food and other substances.

risk conditions   The factors in the environment underlying or determining risk factors.

risk factors   Those characteristics of the individual that predispose him or her to greater probability of developing a disease.

roentgen   A unit of radiation dosage equal to the amount of ionizing radiation required to produce one electrostatic unit of charge per cubic centimeter of air. Abbreviated R.

Salmonella   A pathogenic organism sometimes present in uncooked meat or unpasteurized milk and producing acute gastrointestinal distress after being ingested.

scholasticism   Philosophical systems of thought based on assumptions about God, truth, and ideology rather than on observable realities. This approach ruled human affairs during the Dark Ages and was displaced by realism and science during the Renaissance.

school health education   Any combination of learning experiences conducted in the school setting to predispose students to and enable them to carry out future decision making and behavior conducive to health.

school health program   The main channel of health promotion, health services, and health protection for children, consisting of health education, school health services, and a healthful school environment.

sedentary living   A pattern of physical activity insufficient in vigor, duration, or frequency of movement to maintain fitness.

sediment   Material that settles on the bottom of a body of water.

sedimentation   The removal of floc in the treatment of water by collecting it at the bottom of settling tanks.

self-care   Any combination of actions taken with or without professional consultation to protect one's health, to self-manage symptoms or prevent complications of existing illness, or to cope with the emotional and social consequences of one's medical condition.

self-help groups   People joining in loosely organized association to meet periodically with the purpose of learning from each other and supporting each other in coping with a common problem or condition.

skinfold measures   Measurement of subcutaneous fat by means of calipers on areas such as biceps, triceps, trunk, thighs, or calves.

slum   An area in which any four of the criteria of substandard housing are met.

smog   The atmospheric result of the photochemical reaction of hydrocarbons and sulfur oxides produced by sunlight.

smoking cessation   Process or methods used to help individuals give up cigarettes, cigars or pipes.

social diagnosis   Assessment of the factors influencing the quality of life.

social health   The capacity of individuals to work productively and to participate actively in the life of their community.

social history of health   A theoretical cycle describing what happens to the natural history of health when social organization is imposed on it.

social pathology   Failures of adjustment leading to antisocial acts that are destructive to other individuals or to community property.

socialization   A process of developing behavioral patterns or life-style through modeling or imitating socially important persons.

sovereignty   Independent power or authority residing in a state.

society   The larger community of people who share a common government, cultural heritage, territory, or some combination of these; a community of communities; sometimes synonymous with nation or population.

sphygomanometer   A device using an inflatable cuff, a stethoscope, and a mercury meter to measure blood pressure.

spontaneous generation   An early theory of how maggots and other larvae ("worms") appeared on rotted food and infested flesh, disproved when scientists observed the laying of eggs by flies and lice.

statutory law   Those rules of society established by legislation.

stroke   Cerebrovascular disease caused by a thrombus (blood clot) in an artery of the brain.

subclinical infection   The existence of disease that does not manifest itself as a frank case.

subcutaneous fat   Nonmuscular tissues beneath the skin.

substandard housing   Houses or apartments failing to meet criteria established by city ordinances or building codes, based usually on national standards.

sulfur oxide   A pollutant of air, arising primarily from burning of sulfur-containing coal and fuel oil.

summative evaluation   The assessment of outcomes or impact of a program, service, intervention, or method.

Superfund   A special-purpose budget set aside for a large task that is limited in time, such as cleaning toxic waste sites.

supply   The available resource, service, or product in response to need or demand.

supply and demand   The economic factors determining the price of a consumable product or service.

surface water   Water above ground in runoff sources such as streams. Surface water used to supply a community is usually stored in a reservoir, treated, and piped to homes and other use sites.

synergistic   When two or more factors combine to produce an effect that is greater than the sum of their individual effects.

temperature inversion   A layer of warm air above a layer of cooler air that prevents surface air from carrying pollutants from the lower atmosphere and dispersing them.

teratogenic   Health problems or abnormalities produced in the fetus by chemical or infectious agents introduced during pregnancy.

thoracic   Of or pertaining to the chest and lungs.

triage   A method of sorting casualties or patients into degrees of severity to set priorities on the order or methods of treatment.

turbidity   A cloudy state of otherwise clear liquid, caused by particulate matter suspended in the liquid.

unintentional injury   Term currently preferred by public health experts in place of the term *accident* to emphasize health consequences and to avoid the implication that the injury-causing event was necessarily uncontrollable.

vector   Any animal that harbors and transfers disease from one human host to another, or from intermediate animal hosts to human hosts.

vehicle   An inanimate object or a living thing that can act like a vector or an intermediate host or reservoir for transmission of disease.

ventilation   The transfer of outside air and inside air and the control of temperature, humidity, and movement of air.

vital index   The difference between births per 1000 population and deaths per 1000 population, reflecting the rate of natural increase.

victim blaming   Excessive dependence on policies or methods of intervention that assume people have potential for change or control when the social or other determinants of their health are beyond their control.

voluntary health agency   A nongovernmental organization devoted usually to a particular set of health problems, operating on funds donated by the public.

well-being   A good or satisfactory condition of existence.

WHO   World Health Organization.

YPLL Years of potential life lost,   a measure of the longevity of a population giving greater weight to premature deaths proportionate to the years before age 65 or age 75 that the deaths occurred.

zoning   The restriction on types of buildings or facilities that can be constructed or operated in specific areas of a community.

zoonoses   Diseases transmitted to human populations by vertebrate animals rather than by arthropods (insects, spiders, ticks, etc.) or other invertebrates.

Index